MANAGEMENT OF THE PERIMENOPAUSE

MANAGEMENT OF THE PERIMENOPAUSE

PRACTICAL PATHWAYS IN OBSTETRICS AND GYNECOLOGY

James H. Liu, MD
Arthur H. Bill Professor
Chair, Department of Reproductive Biology
Case School of Medicine
Chair, Department of Obstetrics and Gynecology
University MacDonald Women's Hospital
Cleveland, Ohio

Margery L. S. Gass, MD
Professor, Clinical Obstetrics and Gynecology
Department of Obstetrics and Gynecology
University of Cincinnati College of Medicine
Cincinnati, Ohio

McGRAW-HILL
Medical Publishing Division

New York Chicago San Francisco Lisbon London Madrid Mexico City Milan
New Delhi San Juan Seoul Singapore Sydney Toronto

The McGraw-Hill Companies

Management of the Perimenopause

1 2 3 4 5 6 7 8 9 0 DOC/DOC 0 9 8 7 6

ISBN 0-0-142281-1

This book was set in Melior by International Typesetting and Composition.
The editors were Karen G. Edmondson and Penny Linskey.
The production supervisor was Sherri Souffrance.
The cover designer was Cathleen Elliott.
The indexer was Susan Hunter.
RR Donnelley was printer and binder.

This book is printed on acid-free paper.

NOTICE

Medicine is an ever-changing science. As new research and clinical experience broaden our knowledge, changes in treatment and drug therapy are required. The authors and the publisher of this work have checked with sources believed to be reliable in their efforts to provide information that is complete and generally in accord with the standards accepted at the time of publication. However, in view of the possibility of human error changes in medical science, neither the editors nor the publisher nor any other party who has been involved in the preparation or publication of this work warrants that the information contained herein is in every respect accurate or complete, and they disclaim all responsibility for any errors or omissions or for the results obtained from use of the information contained in this work. Readers are encouraged to confirm the information contained herein with other sources. For example and in particular, readers are advised to check the product information sheet included in the package of each drug they plan to administer to be certain that the information contained in this work is accurate and that changes have not been made in the recommended dose or in the contraindications for administration. This recommendation is of particular importance in connection with new or infrequently used drugs.

Cataloging-in-Publication data for this title is on file with the Library of Congress.

Perimenopause : practical pathways in obstetrics and gynecology / edited by James H. Liu, Margery L.S. Gass.
p. ; cm.
Includes index.
ISBN 0-07-142281-1 (alk. paper)
1. Perimenopause. I. Liu, James H. II. Gass, Margery L.S.
[DNLM: 1. Perimenopause. 2. Dyslipidemias—complications. 3. Genital Diseases, Female—complications. 4. Genital Diseases, Female—therapy. 5. Hormone Replacement Therapy. WP 580 P4446 2006]
RG188.P47 2006
618.1'75—dc22 2006041969

Contents

SECTION 3 PATHOPHYSIOLOGY

SECTION 4 HORMONE THERAPIES

SECTION 5 PREVENTIVE HEALTH STRATEGIES

Contributors

Lesley M. Arnold, MD *(Chapter 15)*
Associate Professor of Psychiatry
Director of Women's Health Research Program
Department of Psychiatry
University of Cincinnati College of Medicine
Cincinnati, Ohio

Karen L. Ashby, MD *(Chapter 10)*
Assistant Professor Reproductive Biology
Case School of Medicine
University Hospitals of Cleveland
Cleveland, Ohio

Michael S. Baggish, MD *(Chapter 17)*
Professor, Obstetrics and Gynecology
University of Cincinnati

Chairman
Obstetrics and Gynecology
Good Samaritan Hospital

Director, Obstetrics and Gynecology Residency
Training Program
TriHealth Hospitals
Cincinnati, Ohio

Shari S. Bassuk, ScD *(Chapter 19)*
Epidemiologist
Division of Preventive Medicine
Brigham and Women's Hospital
Boston, Massachusetts

E.O. Bixler, PhD *(Chapter 5)*
Professor
Sleep Research and Treatment Centre
Department of Psychiatry
Pennsylvania State University College of Medicine
Hershey, Pennsylvania

Elizabeth V. Brandewie, MD *(Chapter 22)*
Department of Obstetrics and Gynecology
Wilson Memorial Hospital
Sidney, Ohio

Paul D. DePriest, MD *(Chapter 12)*
Associate Chief of Staff
Department of Obstetrics and Gynecology

Associate Professor
Division of Gynecologic Oncology
Department of Obstetrics and Gynecology
University of Kentucky Medical Center
Lexington, Kentocky

Robert R. Freedman, PhD *(Chapter 3)*
Professor
Psychiatry and Obstetrics and Gynecology
Wayne State University School of Medicine
Detroit, Michigan

Margery L. S. Gass, MD *(Chapters 1 and 20)*
Professor, Clinical Obstetrics and Gynecology
University of Cincinnati College of Medicine
Cincinnati, Ohio

Rebecca D. Jackson, MD *(Chapter 23)*
Professor of Medicine
Department of Internal Medicine
Division of Endocrinology, Diabetes and Metabolism
The Ohio State University
Columbus, Ohio

Thomas Janicki, MD *(Chapter 11)*
Associate Clinical Professor
Reproductive Biology
Case School of Medicine
Director, Pelvic Pain Center
Department of Obstetrics and Gynecology
MacDonald Women's Hospital
University Hospitals of Cleveland
Cleveland, Ohio

Sona Kashyap, MD *(Chapter 16)*
Practicing Endocrinologist
Lancaster Endocrinology
Lancaster, SC

Sheryl A. Kingsberg, PhD *(Chapter 6)*
Associate Professor
Departments of Reproductive Biology and Psychiatry
Case Western Reserve University School of Medicine
Chief, Division of Behavioral Medicine
Department of Obstetric and Gynecology
University MacDonald Women's Hospital
Cleveland, Ohio

Robert Krikorian, MD *(Chapter 4)*
Associate Professor
Department of Psychiatry
University of Cincinnati
Cincinnati, Ohio

James H. Liu, MD *(Chapters 8 and 9)*
Arthur H. Bill Professor
Chair, Department of Reproductive Biology
Case School of Medicine
Chair, Department of Obstetrics and Gynecology
University MacDonald Women's Hospital
Cleveland, Ohio

Carol J. Mack, MPH, MSHS, PAC *(Chapter 18)*
Physician Assistant
Women's Health Research Center

JoAnn E. Manson, MD *(Chapter 19)*
Chief, Division of Preventive Medicine
Brigham and Women's Hospital
Professor of Medicine and the Elizabeth F. Brigham Professor of Women's Health
Harvard Medical School
Boston, Massachusetts

Ken N. Muse, MD *(Chapter 7)*
Associate Professor
Department of Obstetrics and Gynecology
University of Kentucky
Lexington, Kentucky

W. Jerry Mysiw, MD *(Chapter 23)*
Bert C. Wiley Chair and Associate Professor of Physical Medicine and Rehabilitation
Department of Physical Medicine and Rehabilitation
The Ohio State University
Columbus, Ohio

Shahla Nader, MD *(Chapter 16)*
Professor, Department of Internal Medicine and Obstetrics and Gynecology
University of Texas-Houston
Houston, Texas

Robert W. Rebar, MD *(Chapter 2)*
Clinical Professor
Department of Obstetrics and Gynecology
University of Alabama
Birmingham, Alabama

Paul A. Robb, MD *(Chapter 21)*
Assistant Professor
Obstetrics and Gynecology, REI Division
Medical College of Wisconsin
Milwaukee, Wisconsin

Elizabeth A. Shaughnessy, MD, PhD *(Chapter 13)*
Assistant Professor
Surgical Director of the Breast Consultation Center
Division of Surgical Oncology
Department of Surgery
University of Cincinnati Medicine Center
Cincinnati, Ohio

Shubhangi Shidham *(Chapter 23)*
Clinical Fellow
Division of Endocrinology, Diabetes, and Metabolism
Department of Endocrinology, Diabetes, and Metabolism
Ohio State University
Columbus, Ohio

James A. Simon, MD *(Chapter 18)*
Clinical Professor
Department of Obstetrics and Gynecology
George Washington University
Washington, DC

Cynthia A. Stuenkel, MD *(Chapter 14)*
Clinical Professor of Medicine
Division of Endocrinology and Metabolism
University of California, San Diego
La Jolla, California

Maida Taylor, MD, MPH *(Chapter 24)*
Clinical Professor
Department of Obstetrics, Gynecology and Reproductive Sciences
University of California, San Francisco
San Francisco, California

Fred R. Ueland, MD *(Chapter 12)*
Assistant Professor
Division of Gynecologic Oncology
Department of Obstetrics, and Gynecology
University of Kentucky Medical Center
Lexington, Kentucky

J. R. van Nagell, Jr. *(Chapter 12)*
Professor and Director
Division of Gynecologic Oncology
Department of Obstetrics, and Gynecology
University of Kentucky Medical Center
Lexington, Kentucky

A.N. Vgontzas, MD *(Chapter 5)*
Director, Center for Sleep Disorder Medicine
Endowed Chair in Sleep Disorders Medicine
Professor of Psychiatry
Department of Psychiatry
Pennsylvania State University College of Medicine
Hershey, Pennsylvania

Daniel B. Williams, MD *(Chapter 21)*
Professor and Director
Center for Reproductive Health
Cincinnati, Ohio

Elizabeth A. Wise, MD *(Chapter 18)*
Research Assistant
James A. Simon, MD, PC
Washington, DC

Foreword

Interest in the phenomenon of menopause has surged over the past decade, as burgeoning numbers of postwar baby boomer women began entering the menopausal transition. Thus began a campaign for more information on menopause-related symptoms and strategies for their amelioration and a better understanding of the role of menopause in healthy aging. Targeted efforts, such as conferences and initiatives and enhanced research funding by the National Institutes of Health of the Department of Health and Human Services, have helped stimulate new scientific exploration of the menopause and its sequelae. As a result, we have dramatically expanded our basic and clinical knowledge base on the biology of the menopause transition and the effects of estrogen and other therapies on symptoms and various conditions and diseases associated with the menopause and estrogen deficiency.

This book focuses on the "Perimenopause," which encompasses the menopausal transition (from the reproductive period through the final menstrual period) and 1 year of the postmenopause. It is a time of dynamic fluctuations in sex hormone levels and profound changes in many nonreproductive as well as reproductive tissues. Because it is associated with increased reporting of various symptoms ranging from hot flashes and night sweats, uterine bleeding problems, vulvovaginal atrophy and musculoskeletal and sleep problems to depression and loss of sexual desire, the perimenopause may have a highly negative impact on quality of life for many women. This innovative, multidimensional book offers clinicians a better understanding of the processes at work and practical treatment strategies to address many of these symptoms.

Recent findings show significant variation in the symptom experience of women transitioning the menopause, and indicate that there is no "universal menopause syndrome." Importantly, race/ethnicity (as well as other host characteristics such as body mass index, diet, physical activity, and smoking) may have a significant role in the presentation and severity of many symptoms and outcomes associated with the menopause as well as responses to various therapeutic interventions. It is vital, therefore, that attention is paid to the social and cultural context in which the menopause is experienced in order to develop and/or customize efficacious new strategies for more diverse populations.*

A present challenge in reducing the burden of menopause- and age-related disorders and diseases and in promoting healthy aging lies in enhancing the availability of, and access to reliable, updated information and health-care options for women. This book is an excellent step forward in this direction.

Sherry Sherman, PhD
Program Director
Clinical Aging and Reproductive Hormone Research
National Institute on Aging
National Institute of Health

* NIH State-of-the-Science Panel, National Institutes of Health State-of-the-Science Conference Statement: Management of Menopause-Related Symptoms. *Ann Intern Med.* 2005;142:1003–1013.

Preface

Management of the Perimenopause is intended to be a practical guide for the clinician who is assisting women as they transition from the reproductive years to the postreproductive years. The book deals primarily with the problems and health concerns that can be encountered in the transition. We would like to emphasize that a healthy lifestyle is central to this transition, and that it is very important to encourage all women to include good nutrition, physical activity, and appropriate attention to mental, emotional, spiritual, and relationship health. However, these important topics are beyond the scope of this book.

Most chapters follow a format that includes basic information about the topic with key points highlighted, an algorithm outlining the author's recommended approach to the condition, guiding questions for the clinician, and case studies that illustrate how the information might be applied. Select references are included within each chapter to amplify the basic information provided, since the book is not intended to serve as a reference text on menopause.

We hope the reader will enjoy the format of this book and that it will assist the reader in enabling women to manage their menopause transition more smoothly.

James Liu, MD
Margery L. S. Gass, MD

Acknowledgments

We would like to thank our many colleagues for their participation in this book. We greatly appreciate their generous contribution of time and expertise in preparing these chapters. We also thank our respective partners, Lynn Liu, PhD, and Frederick Gass, PhD, for their support and understanding.

James Liu, MD
Margery Gass, MD

MANAGEMENT OF THE PERIMENOPAUSE

PHYSIOLOGY OF THE PERIMENOPAUSE

1 Perimenopause Perspective

Margery L. S. Gass

Introduction

KEY POINT

The perspective of a woman and her clinician can affect recommendations and actions.

Perimenopause refers to the years of transition from the reproductive to the nonreproductive segment of a woman's life. For some women it is a barely noticeable milestone. Their menstrual cycles cease uneventfully and the transition carries little to no impact. For others, it is a phase of life significant for the physical, psychological, or emotional effects. This chapter addresses how the perspective of the woman and her clinician can affect recommendations and actions.

The literal meaning of perimenopause derives from the Greek *peri* (around, near), *men* (month), and *pausis* (a break, stop, or rest).[1] As will be seen in greater detail in Chap. 2, perimenopause is usually a brief 3–4-year time frame encompassing the last menstrual period. Menopause is the permanent cessation of menses secondary to decreased ovarian function.[2] In the case of natural menopause, the diagnosis is retrospective, requiring 12 months of amenorrhea.

Significant strides have been made toward understanding perimenopause, both through basic research and data gathered from several longitudinal studies. Cohort studies in the United States, Australia, and Sweden have followed women with hormone levels and questionnaires that span the perimenopausal transition (Table 1-1). Details of the interplay among the inhibins, follicle-stimulating hormone, luteinizing hormone, estrogen, progesterone, and androgens can be found in Chap. 2.

Table 1-1. **LONGITUDINAL PERIMENOPAUSE COHORT STUDIES**

Study Name	Location	Number in Study	Ages at Baseline	Date Begun
Malmo Perimenopausal Project	Malmo, Sweden	160	48	1977
Massachusetts Women's Health Study	Massachusetts	2570	45–55	1981
Seattle Midlife Women's Health Study	Seattle, WA	508	35–55	1990
Melbourne Women's Health Study	Melbourne, Australia	438	45–55	1991
Study of Women's Health Across the Nation	Seven sites across United States	Cross sectional 16,065 Longitudinal 3,306	40–55 42–52	1995

A Perimenopausal Syndrome?

Attempts to distill a universal menopausal syndrome from the many symptoms reported at midlife have had a variety of results. The Study of Women's Health Across the Nation (SWAN study) reported the occurrence of symptoms in a cross-sectional survey of 14,906 women in the United States aged 40–55 years including Caucasian (7448), African American (4163), Hispanic (1859), Japanese (811), and Chinese (625) subgroups.[3]

KEY POINT

The hot flush is the most universal symptom of perimenopause, but the percent of women affected varies in different settings.

Of all of the symptoms analyzed in SWAN, two clusters occurred frequently enough in all groups to be used in the final analysis. The first cluster was labeled psychosomatic symptoms and included such terms as irritable, tense, blue or depressed, forgetful, and headaches. The second cluster was labeled vasomotor symptoms and included hot flushes and night sweats. However, symptom reports varied across the different racial/ethnic groups. The perimenopausal women reported more psychosomatic symptoms than the pre- or postmenopausal women. The postmenopausal women (defined as 12 months of amenorrhea) had more vasomotor symptoms.

In a prospective study, 172 Australian women completed a checklist of 33 symptoms annually as they transitioned to and through perimenopause. Although women in this age group reported numerous symptoms, the only symptoms that appeared to be related to perimenopause were vasomotor episodes, vaginal dryness, and breast tenderness. Breast tenderness decreased through the transition while vasomotor symptoms and vaginal dryness increased.[4]

A cross-sectional study of 1329 Chinese women, aged 46–54, on the agrarian island of Kinmen found that sleep disturbance, backaches, and joint pain were the most frequently reported symptoms.[5] However, only vasomotor and urogenital symptoms were significantly associated with menopause. The prevalence of vasomotor symptoms was low, with hot flushes noted by 15% and night sweats by 8% of the cohort.

One particularly interesting cross-sectional study from China surveyed 402 urban professional women and 404 rural farming women, ages 41–60. Hormone levels were performed in a subset of 209 women.[6] Hormone levels were comparable between groups, but the professional women were more symptomatic than the farming women ($P < 0.01$). Of all of the symptoms reported, only hot flushes correlated with hormone levels. Greater prevalence of symptoms was also associated with feelings of becoming older, sad, or lost. The authors concluded that symptom reporting is related to more than just biological factors.

Hot flush reporting varies in different cultures around the world. Japanese, Indonesian, and Mayan women have been noted to report substantially fewer hot flushes than other women who have been studied.[7] The reasons for these differences are not fully understood.

The variability of findings in these reports illustrates the need to conduct studies in a more organized and systematic manner. To date, the basic elements of a menopausal syndrome are hot flushes and symptoms of vaginal atrophy, both of which vary greatly from woman to woman. Other symptoms are even less consistent across cultures and geographic sites.

Changing Perspectives

Attitudes toward menopause in the medical profession have shifted over the years. John Friend of the eighteenth century was reportedly of the opinion that menopause was a benefit to women's health as they aged.[8] Toward the end of the nineteenth century, the Landau clinic in Berlin purportedly treated menopause as an estrogen deficiency state analogous to thyroid deficiency.[9] Positive views of menopause were promulgated in the past by such prominent physicians as Novak, whose textbook of gynecology has been well respected for over half a century. The very first edition in 1941 stated "...there are many women to whom the menopause comes as a boon, with striking improvement in general health and well-being..." He later writes, "...two facts may be considered as clearly established: (1) that in only a small minority of women are the characteristic menopausal symptoms sufficiently severe to interfere materially with health and happiness, as measured roughly by the necessity for medical attention, and (2) that many of the symptoms often complained of by women in the fifth decade of life are wrongly attributed to the menopause."[9] This last phrase has been verified by the results of the symptom studies cited previously.

KEY POINT

Attitudes of the medical profession toward menopause have ranged between viewing menopause as a beneficial occurrence and viewing it as a deficiency disease.

During the last few decades of the twentieth century, menopause was largely viewed as an estrogen deficiency disease. In 1999, the American Association of Clinical Endocrinologists reported in their guidelines for the management of menopause that the association "believes that menopause is a state of hormone deficiency that should be treated."[10]

Scholars of medical history have suggested that a confluence of events in the 1930s and 1940s including the better understanding of physiology and the greater availability of potential therapies, such as diethylstilbestrol (DES) and later conjugated equine estrogens (Premarin), promoted a medicalization of menopause.[11] Similar scenarios involving widespread application of newly discovered therapies are not uncommon in medicine whether related to drugs or devices (e.g., thyroid medication being used for overweight adolescents, radiation therapy for thymus and acne problems, and laser treatments for a variety of ailments).

Women and their clinicians who share the perspective that menopause is a hormone deficiency state will be far more inclined to turn to hormone therapy (HT) as the logical course for both symptomatic and asymptomatic situations. Women who view menopause as a marker of aging may also be more inclined to take HT. It is not uncommon to hear a woman state that her skin seems "better" on HT. Issues of quality of life may subtly influence a woman's perspective on menopause even when those issues are not clearly related to hormone levels.

KEY POINT

The majority of women have a neutral to positive attitude toward menopause.

Although women themselves express a wide range of negative to positive attitudes toward menopause, the majority of them view menopause in a neutral to positive light. A telephone survey of 750 women found that 42% expressed a neutral attitude and 36% conveyed a positive attitude toward menopause.[12] Data from large cohort studies support these findings.[13]

Menopause Perspective and Hormone Therapy

HT has been highly effective in the treatment of vasomotor symptoms and has eclipsed earlier remedies such as Lydia Pinkham's Vegetable Compound and lesser-known products. The use of therapies that predated HT appears to confirm that there has long been a number of women who seek therapy of some sort for their perimenopausal symptoms.

For many years in recent history, the most widely used prescription intervention for menopause has been HT. Not only was HT used liberally for menopausal symptoms, it was being increasingly used as preventive therapy for many purposes on the basis of observational findings (see Chaps. 19 and 20). However, even in times of great popularity, HT was used far more extensively by Caucasians than by other ethnic groups.

In the Third National Health and Nutrition Examination Survey 1988–1994 (NHANES 3), ever use of HT by 3479 women over age 60 was reported to be 40% (confidence interval [CI], 37–41%) for non-Hispanic White women, 24% (CI, 20–29%) for Mexican American women, and 20% (CI, 14–25%) for non-Hispanic Black women.[14] There are many possible explanations for the differential use of HT among various ethnic groups. Factors to be considered include access to medical care, quality of medical care, patient skepticism, reluctance to take medications, lack of financial resources for nonessential medication, and more pressing medical/social concerns, to name a few. Attitude, or perspective, toward menopause could also influence the likelihood of using HT. The SWAN study found that African American women had a significantly more positive attitude toward menopause than other ethnic groups.[15,16] A much smaller study found that 197 low-income African American women had a similar occurrence of symptoms compared to Caucasian groups but reported them as not very bothersome.[17] Such a finding could result from milder hot flushes or simply a different cultural attitude toward them.

KEY POINT

Women who have undergone hysterectomy are far more likely to initiate and continue HT than those who have not had a hysterectomy.

One striking difference in HT use occurs between the group of women who experienced a natural menopause and those who had a surgical menopause or even a hysterectomy without oophorectomy. NHANES 3 revealed that 51% of women who had a hysterectomy reported use of HT while only 20% of women with a natural menopause reported using HT.[14] One reason for this discrepancy in usage could relate to the fact that some surgically menopausal women are younger than the average age of natural menopause. Some clinicians and patients may believe that hormone supplementation is appropriate until the average age of menopause as a means of simulating the normal duration of the female reproductive stage of life. Furthermore, there is a widely held belief, confirmed by the SWAN study, that women with a surgical menopause were more likely to have symptoms than women with a natural menopause.[3] In addition, women undergoing hysterectomy are engaged with the medical establishment, where discussions of the risks and benefits of HT are more likely to occur. Postoperative complaints of hot flushes can be easily addressed with HT.

There are other factors that may contribute to greater use of HT among women who have had a hysterectomy, not the least of which is that these women will not experience uterine bleeding, the major nuisance side effect of HT. Bleeding is a reason why many women who start HT discontinue it. Awareness of this fact may make the therapy more attractive to the clinician as well as the patient who has had a hysterectomy.

Large, randomized, controlled trials have challenged the view that the majority of postmenopausal women will benefit from HT (see Chaps. 19 and 20).[18–20] Time will tell if the pendulum will swing back from the perspective of menopause as a pathologic deficiency state to a more neutral position. It is slowly becoming apparent that conditions such as coronary disease and osteoporosis, once thought to be closely related to a negative impact of menopause may not be so negatively linked: (1) the rate of increase in death from coronary heart disease does not accelerate at menopause (Fig. 1-1), and (2) short-term rapid loss of bone mineral density at menopause may simply be an unloading of extra mineralization that occurred at puberty for reproductive purposes.[21]

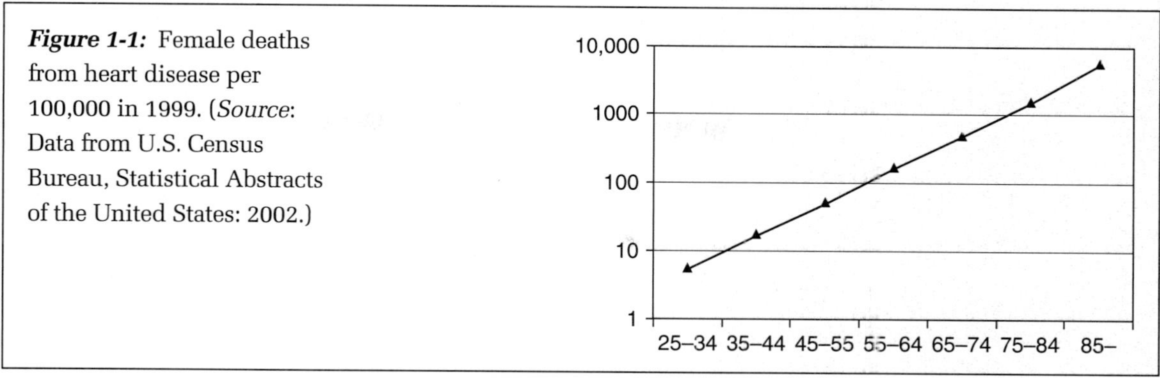

Figure 1-1: Female deaths from heart disease per 100,000 in 1999. (*Source*: Data from U.S. Census Bureau, Statistical Abstracts of the United States: 2002.)

Approach to the Perimenopausal Patient

KEY POINT

Be aware of both clinician and patient perspectives toward menopause.

In approaching the perimenopausal patient, it is important to know how she is experiencing this phase in her life. Two women may have the same number of hot flushes per day. One finds them very distracting and disruptive; the other views them as a nuisance, but manageable. The patient's perspective, chief complaint or concern, remains the starting point for the patient-clinician encounter. It will guide the clinician in how best to meet the needs of the patient. During this process, clinicians should be conscious of their own attitudes and beliefs regarding menopause.

The schema in Fig. 1-2 provides a conceptual overview of an annual office visit for a perimenopausal woman, starting with the woman's health agenda. If her primary reason for the visit is health preservation, an update of personal health and family history can be undertaken. The update will allow an enumeration of health strengths and vulnerabilities. Health-promoting behavior should be reinforced and encouraged; preventive measures can be discussed for areas of vulnerability. Input from the patient about her health goals and values will assist both parties in arriving at a course of action that is most likely to meet with success.

For the woman who presents primarily because of a complaint or a concern, time needs to be devoted to understanding the nature and context of the problem. Some problems could be manageable for the patient, were it not for the context. For example, hot flushes that would be manageable under ideal circumstances are not manageable because the individual is concurrently under high stress at work or at home. She feels she just cannot tolerate any additional

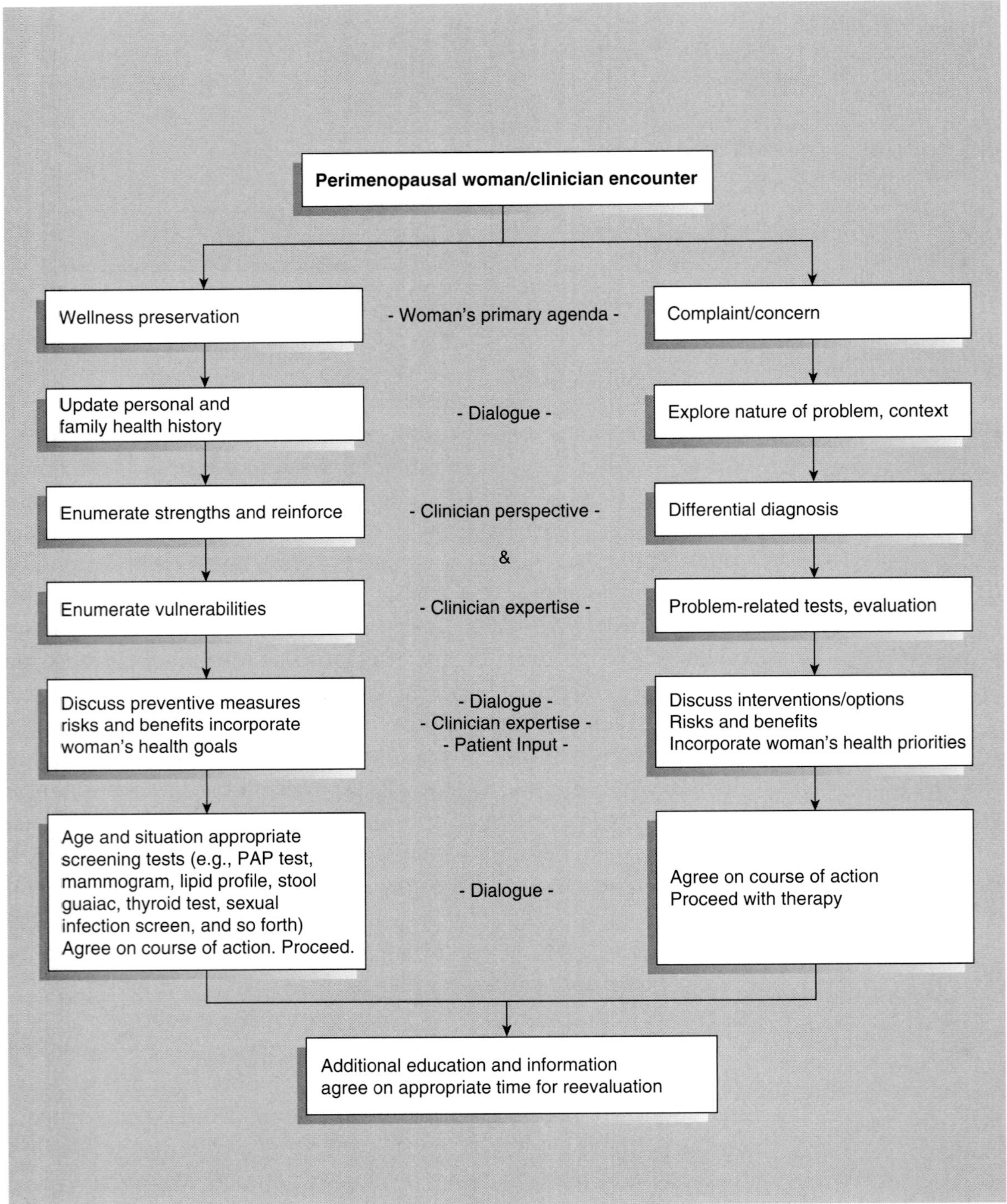
Perimenopausal woman/clinician encounter
Wellness preservation
- Woman's primary agenda -
Complaint/concern
Update personal and
family health history
- Dialogue -
Explore nature of problem, context
Enumerate strengths and reinforce
- Clinician perspective -
Differential diagnosis
&
Enumerate vulnerabilities
- Clinician expertise -
Problem-related tests, evaluation
Discuss preventive measures
risks and benefits incorporate
woman's health goals
- Dialogue -
- Clinician expertise -
- Patient Input -
Discuss interventions/options
Risks and benefits
Incorporate woman's health priorities
Age and situation appropriate
screening tests (e.g., PAP test,
mammogram, lipid profile, stool
guaiac, thyroid test, sexual
infection screen, and so forth)
Agree on course of action. Proceed.
- Dialogue -
Agree on course of action
Proceed with therapy
Additional education and information
agree on appropriate time for reevaluation

Figure 1-2

stress. Another example of contextual importance might be the woman who complains of low libido. She subconsciously minimizes the potential libido-lowering effect of recent marital difficulties and wonders if menopause is to blame for her low desire (see Chap. 6).

After a thorough exploration of the specific concern and the context, a differential diagnosis can be established and problem-related tests can be arranged. Test results and the pros and cons of various treatment options are reviewed with the patient in consideration of her goals and value system. The approach should lead to a course of action that will be acceptable to the patient and beneficial as well. The patient who presents with a problem will also need the components of the health maintenance visit at the same time or at a follow-up visit.

Both the health maintenance visit and the problem-oriented visit should include education on issues where the patient has misconceptions or incomplete understanding. Screening tests appropriate for the patient's age and situation should be recommended (e.g., Pap test, mammogram, lipid profile, stool guaiac, thyroid test, sexually transmitted infection tests, and so forth). The next step can be discussed and agreement can be reached on the time for reevaluation. Women should be informed that their healthy lifestyle is the most important thing they can do for themselves in order to remain healthy through perimenopause and beyond.

With the rapid arrival of new medical information, it is important to emphasize to patients that guidelines may change from one year to the next. The goal for clinicians is to stay abreast of new information and to convey that information to patients at each visit. Should patients see or hear something in the media that troubles them or contradicts what they heard in the office, they should feel free to call or make an appointment to discuss it.

It is the view of the editors that perimenopause is a natural, healthy phase of a woman's life. Just as menarche and puberty herald the beginning of the reproductive phase, menopause and the climacteric represent the conclusion of that phase. Both are normal and natural. Both, however, can result in troubling symptoms and medical conditions for some women. This book will address health maintenance as well as the management of symptoms and medical problems common to this stage of life.

Subsequent chapters will describe perimenopause in greater detail, focus on specific symptoms and common health problems of this stage in life, and discuss various treatments and preventive care options.

Guiding Questions

- What is your personal attitude toward menopause?
- What is the attitude of the patient toward menopause?
- Is the visit for health maintenance or for a problem?
- What are the patient's health priorities?
- Is the treatment plan consistent with good medical practice and the patient's health priorities and preferences?

What's the Evidence?

Evidence exists to support the view that menopause is a natural and normal transition in a woman's life that is inherently neither healthy nor unhealthy. It brings with it different risks and benefits for each individual in much the same way that puberty and pregnancy have different health consequences for individual women.

Discussion of Cases

CASE 1

A 41-year-old gravida 2, para 2, 5 ft 6 in., 125-lb Caucasian presents with a complaint of skipping menses the last 6 months. Her menses had been regular until then. The bleeding after skipping a month or two is much heavier. The patient is otherwise in good health and has no other symptoms. Her weight has been stable. A complete history and physical examination revealed no health problems. The patient had undergone tubal sterilization at age 34.

What is the patient's main concern?

Irregular, heavier menses.

What is the most likely diagnosis?

In the absence of hot flushes and in the presence of heavier bleeding over the last few months, the most likely diagnosis is anovulatory bleeding with estrogen dominance and a relative progesterone deficiency.

Are laboratory tests necessary?

A thyroid-stimulating hormone level and a prolactin level can be ordered for completeness to exclude thyroid disorders and hyperprolactinemia. A urine pregnancy test can be obtained if there is uncertainty regarding pregnancy in a patient. Hormone levels are

generally not necessary in this setting as her cycle pattern could indicate an ovulatory dysfunction seen in the perimenopause. Furthermore, follicle-stimulating hormone and estradiol levels vary markedly from day to day in the perimenopause and thus offer no additional useful information in most cases. Depending on the degree and duration of menorrhagia, a complete blood count might be appropriate.

Is an endometrial biopsy or sonogram indicated?

If the pelvic examination is unsatisfactory or abnormal, a sonogram might be useful. If the bleeding pattern is highly abnormal, very heavy, has persisted a long time or if the patient is obese and thus at higher risk for hyperplasia, an endometrial biopsy would be indicated. In other cases with short-term irregular bleeding, treatment could be initiated first. If the bleeding did not improve with treatment in the next couple cycles, an endometrial biopsy would be necessary (see Chaps. 9 and 21).

What are the treatment options?

Since the patient has no need for contraception, a simple therapy would be to replace progesterone in her cycle (see Chap. 20). She is obviously still producing estrogen. With her pattern of skipping cycles, the progestogen can be conveniently administered the first 10–14 days of the month. For the menorrhagic patient with a normal or shortened cycle interval, the progestogen may be more effective if given in what should be the luteal phase, days 19–28 in a normal length cycle or on days 16–25 in a shorter cycle. In many cases, the progestogen given early in the short cycle can gradually be moved back to days 19–28 of the cycle, thereby spacing out the cycle to the usual 4-week interval. Any patient whose bleeding pattern is not regulated by progestogen therapy should have further evaluation with endometrial biopsy, hysteroscopy, sonohysterogram, or dilation and curettage of the uterus to look for polyps, intracavitary fibroids, hyperplasia, or cancer (see Chaps. 9 and 21).

What about other treatment options?

Combined estrogen plus progestin hormonal contraceptives would be especially beneficial for the healthy, nonsmoking woman who also desires contraception or who is having intermittent, troubling hot flushes. Disadvantage: Natural menopause will be camouflaged (see Chap. 21).

What about expectant management?

If the patient is not disturbed by the menstrual pattern and she is not at risk of significant anemia, expectant management is an appropriate option. Depending on the degree of irregularity and menorrhagia, an endometrial biopsy and iron supplements should be considered.

References

1 *The American Heritage Dictionary of the English Language.* 4th ed. Boston, MA: Houghton Mifflin Company; 2000.

2 World Health Organization Scientific Group. *Research on the Menopause in the 1990s.* Geneva, Switzerland: World Health Organization; 1996. Technical Report Series 866.

3 Avis NE, Stellato R, Crawford S, et al. Is there a menopausal syndrome? Menopausal status and symptoms across racial/ethnic groups. *Soc Sci Med.* 2001;52:345–356.

4 Dennerstein L, Dudley EC, Hopper JL, et al. A prospective population-based study of menopausal symptoms. *Obstet Gynecol.* 2000;96: 351–358.

5 Fuh J, Wang S, Lu S, et al. The Kinmen women-health investigation (KIWI): a menopausal study of population aged 40–54. *Maturitas.* 2002;21:S51–S58.

6 Zhao G, Wang L, Yan R, et al. Menopausal symptoms: experience of Chinese women. *Climacteric.* 2003;3:135–144.

7 Kronenberg F. Hot flashes: epidemiology and physiology. *Ann NY Acad Sci.* 1990;592:52–86.

8 Andrist LC, MacPherson KI. Conceptual models for women's health research: reclaiming menopause as an exemplar of nursing's contribution to feminist scholarship. *Ann Rev Nurs Res.* 2001;19:29–60.

9 Novak E. *Gynecology and Female Endocrinology.* Boston, MA: Little, Brown and Company; 1941.

10 AACE Medical guidelines for clinical practice for management of menopause. *Endocr Pract.* 1999;5(6):355–366.

11 Bell S. The medicalization of menopause. In: Formanek R, ed. *The Meanings of Menopause: Historical, Medical, and Clinical Perspectives.* London: The Analytic Press; 1990.

12 Kaufert P, Boggs PP, Ettinger B, et al. Women and menopause: beliefs, attitudes, and behaviors. The North American Menopause Society 1997 Menopause Survey. *Menopause.* 1998;5:197–202.

13 Avis ND, McKinlay SM. A longitudinal analysis of women's attitudes toward the menopause: results from the Massachusetts Women's Health Study. *Maturitas.* 1991;13:65–79.

14 Friedman-Koss D, Crespo CJ, Bellantoni MF, et al. The relationship of race/ethnicity and social class to hormone replacement therapy: results from the Third National Health and Nutrition Examination Survey 1988–1994. *Menopause.* 2002;9:264–272.

15 Sommer B, Avis N, Meyer P, et al. Attitudes toward menopause and aging across ethnic/racial groups. *Psychosom Med.* 1999;61:868–875.

16 Pham KT, Grisso JA, Freeman EW. Ovarian aging and hormone replacement therapy. Hormonal levels, symptoms, and attitudes of African American and White women. *J Gen Intern Med.* 1997;12: 230–236.

17 Holmes-Rovner M, Padonu G, Kroll J, et al. African American women's attitudes and expectations of menopause. *Am J Prev Med.* 1996;12:420–423.

18 Hulley S, Grady D, Bush T, et al. Randomized trial of estrogen plus progestin for secondary prevention of coronary heart disease in postmenopausal women. *JAMA*. 1998;280:605–613.

19 Writing Group for the Women's Health Initiative Investigators. Risks and benefits of estrogen plus progestin in healthy postmenopausal women. *JAMA*. 2002;288:321–333.

20 The Women's Health Initiative Steering Committee. Effects of conjugated equine estrogen in postmenopausal women with hysterectomy. The Women's Health Initiative Randomized Controlled Trial. *JAMA*. 2004;291:1701–1712.

21 Järvinen T, Kannus P, Sievanen H. Estrogen and bone: a reproductive and locomotive perspective. *J Bone Miner Res*. 2003;18: 1921–1931.

2 Endocrine Changes and Stages of the Menopausal Transition

Robert W. Rebar

Introduction

The menopausal transition, as the name implies, is a period of dynamic change in a woman's life. The primary changes that occur are hormonal and are reflective of the process of ovarian aging. The hormonal changes are commonly associated with the development of certain signs and symptoms. Simultaneously, physiological and social changes are occurring that make it difficult to distinguish the effect of ovarian aging from the effects of aging in general.

As is true for the initiation of reproductive life at puberty, the end of reproductive life at menopause, defined as the last menstrual period, does not occur at a defined chronological age. Moreover, the physiological changes associated with the menopausal transition do not occur over a definite interval of time.

KEY POINT

Change is the hallmark of the menopausal transition.

Although all women who survive beyond the average age of menopause, a little over 51 years of age, pass through the menopausal transition, relatively little was known about the changes that do occur until recently. Because the menopausal transition is now the focus of intense investigation, it is likely that this period in a woman's life will be better characterized in just a few years than it is at the present time.

The Stages of Reproductive Aging Workshop (STRAW), held in July 2001, attempted to articulate stages for the menopausal transition and to address the confusing nomenclature for this period in life so that investigators and clinicians might communicate more clearly and precisely. The staging system proposed is easier to understand in the context of what is known about the physiological changes that occur. In this chapter, these changes will be described and the staging system will be discussed in detail.

Endocrine Changes Before and During the Menopausal Transition

OVARIAN CHANGES

The number of oocytes increases to a peak of 7–20 million at 20–24 weeks of fetal age.[1] From that time onward, the number decreases. Most actually degenerate by the process of atresia, such that only 1–2 million are present at birth and only 200,000–400,000 oocytes remain by the time of the first ovulation.[2] No more than 300–400 oocytes are released at ovulation over the reproductive lifespan of the woman. It appears that the loss of oocytes accelerates after the age of 38 years, and very few oocytes remain by the last menstrual period.[3]

In addition to the continuing decrease in the number of oocytes and the associated decrease in the thickness of the ovarian cortex in which the oocytes are found within their follicles, there is a progressive decrease in the total volume of the ovary over time. Ovarian size begins to decrease after the age of 30 with significant reductions in ovarian volume each decade until the age of 70.[4] Consistent with the decrease in volume, ultrasound visualization of the ovaries of women in their forties reveals fewer small, early antral follicles than are present in younger women.[5]

HORMONAL CHANGES

GONADOTROPINS, ESTRADIOL, AND PROGESTERONE It has been clear for several years that hormonal variability is the hallmark of the years during the menopausal transition. Typical characteristics of menstrual cycles associated with the menopausal transition are summarized in Table 2-1.

The first detailed information was provided by Sherman and Korenman in the mid-1970s.[6,7] Data from six menstrual cycles from women 46–51 years of age were compared to those from cycles in younger women. The older women had shorter follicular phases and lower levels of estradiol throughout the menstrual cycle than women younger than 35 years of age. Moreover, levels

Table 2-1. **MENSTRUAL CYCLES DURING THE MENOPAUSAL TRANSITION**

Regular cycles may continue up to the very last menstrual period
Variable cycles may occur, with some being ovulatory and others anovulatory
Cycles may become shorter, due to a shortened follicular phase, or may become longer as a result of anovulation
FSH levels may be increased at times, particularly early in the follicular phase
Estradiol levels may be increased, decreased, or normal
Progesterone levels may be normal or decreased in apparently ovulatory cycles

Abbreviation: FSH, follicle-stimulating hormone.

of follicle-stimulating hormone (FSH) were increased throughout the menstrual cycle despite estradiol concentrations that might have been expected to suppress FSH. Other studies have noted normal estradiol levels in cycles of some women over age 40.[8,9] Progesterone levels in these short ovulatory cycles may well be normal.

More recent studies have documented a monotropic rise in serum FSH throughout the menstrual cycle with reproductive aging.[10] FSH first increases early in the follicular phase of the menstrual cycle. The fact that this increase is functionally important is documented by the observation that elevated levels of FSH early in the follicular phase reduce the likelihood of pregnancy for infertile women undergoing in vitro fertilization and embryo transfer.[11–13]

KEY POINT

Menstrual cycles are of variable length during the menopausal transition.

Clinicians have recognized for many years that menstrual cycles during the menopausal transition may sometimes be short, long, or of normal length. Ovulatory and anovulatory cycles may occur in random sequence. Gonadotropin and steroid excretion during menstrual cycles and menopausal transition have been characterized recently.

We measured estrone-3-glucuronide (E1G) and pregnanediol glucuronide (PdG) excretion, major urinary metabolites of estradiol and progesterone, and monitored follicular growth and endometrial development by transvaginal ultrasound in a single cycle in 35 women aged 40–50 years and compared the data to those from 50 cycles in women under age 35.[15] Only three of the cycles in the older women were frankly anovulatory. Abnormal E1G and PdG patterns were identified frequently and included earlier increases in E1G and decreased PdG excretion as well as increased, reduced, or erratic excretion of E1G compared to the cycles in the younger women. At least one other group has documented that estrogen production early in the menopausal transition may be normal or even higher than in young, reproductive-aged women in the face of increased pituitary FSH secretion (Fig. 2-1).[14]

More recently, we collected first-morning urine samples for 4 years from one woman who was 48.5 years of age and having regular menstrual cycles at the time the collections were initiated.[16] During the first year, she had 11 episodes of vaginal

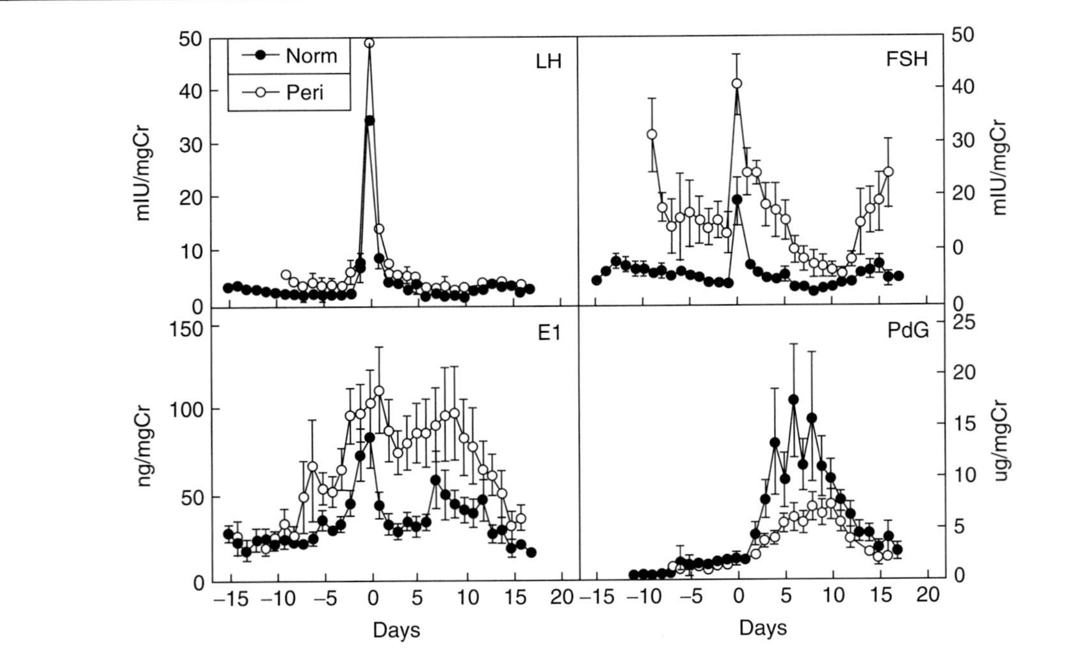

Figure 2-1: Mean (± standard error of the mean) first-morning urinary concentrations of luteinizing hormone (LH), follicle-stimulating hormone (FSH), estrone conjugates (E1), and pregnanediol glucuronide (PdG) excretion corrected for creatinine and standardized to the day of the midcycle LH surge (day 0) in 11 regularly menstruating perimenopausal women (open circles) compared with 11 younger women (closed circles). E1 was higher in the perimenopausal women ($P = 0.015$) and PdG was lower ($P = 0.015$). (*Source*: Santoro N, Brown JR, Adel T, et al. Characterization or reproductive hormonal dynamics in the perimenopause. *J Clin Endocrinol Metab.* 1996;81:1495.)

bleeding (Fig. 2-2A). While being monitored over the first 2 months, she had persistently elevated and menopausal levels of urinary β-FSH. Levels were intermittently elevated thereafter, at times two- to fourfold greater than concentrations seen in midreproductive-aged women, with periodic increases in

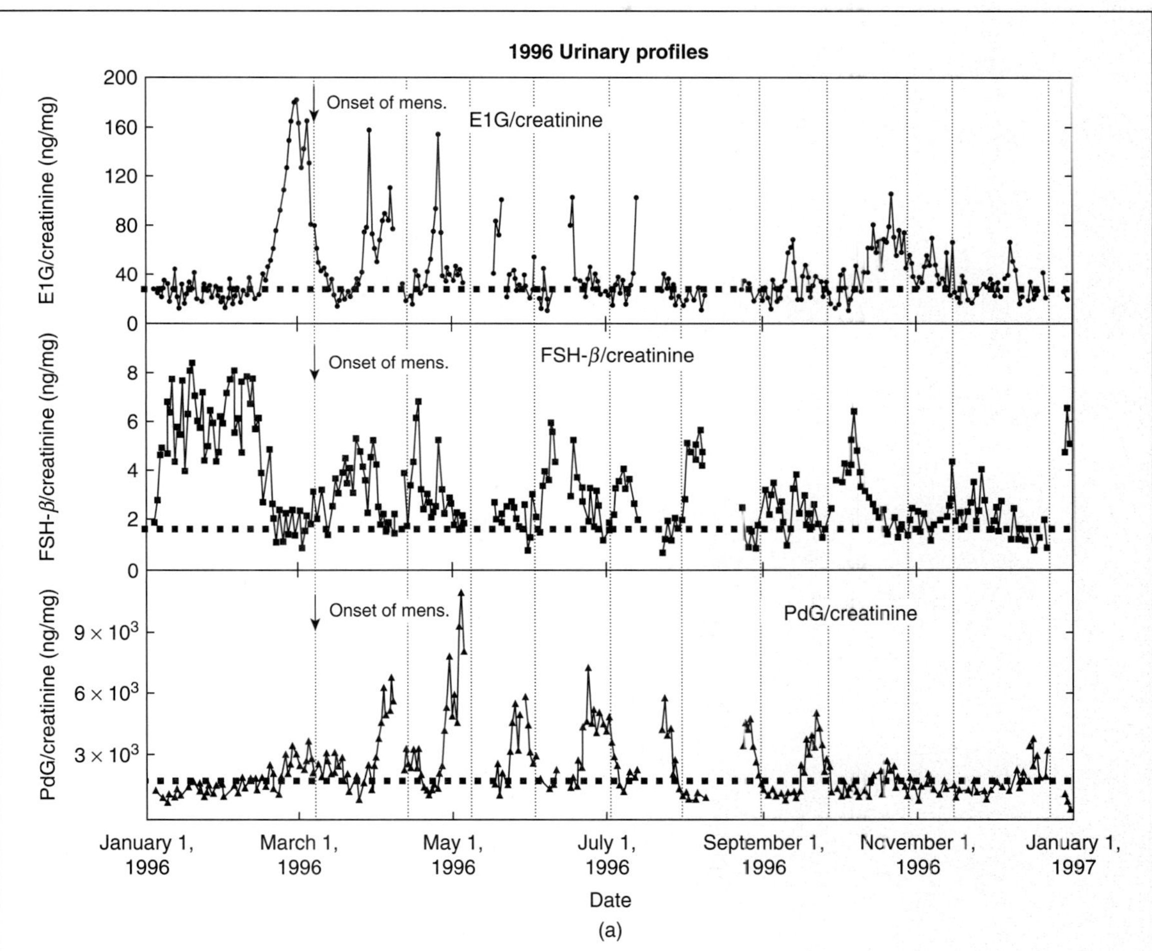

Figure 2-2: First-morning urinary concentrations of estrone-3-glucuronide (E1G), β-follicle-stimulating hormone (β-FSH), and pregnanediol glucuronide (PdG) excretion normalized to creatinine in one perimenopausal woman over a 4-year period beginning at age 48.5 years. The vertical, dashed lines represent the onset of vaginal spotting or bleeding, as recorded by a diary. The bold, horizontal dashed lines represent the mean values for perimenopausal women during the follicular phase of the menstrual cycle, as established for the laboratory. Panels A–D each depict a year from 1996 through 1999. (*Source*: Liu JH, Kao L, Rebar RW, et al. Urinary β-FSH subunit concentrations in perimenopausal and postmenopausal women: a biomarker for ovarian reserve. *Menopause.* 2003;10:526.)

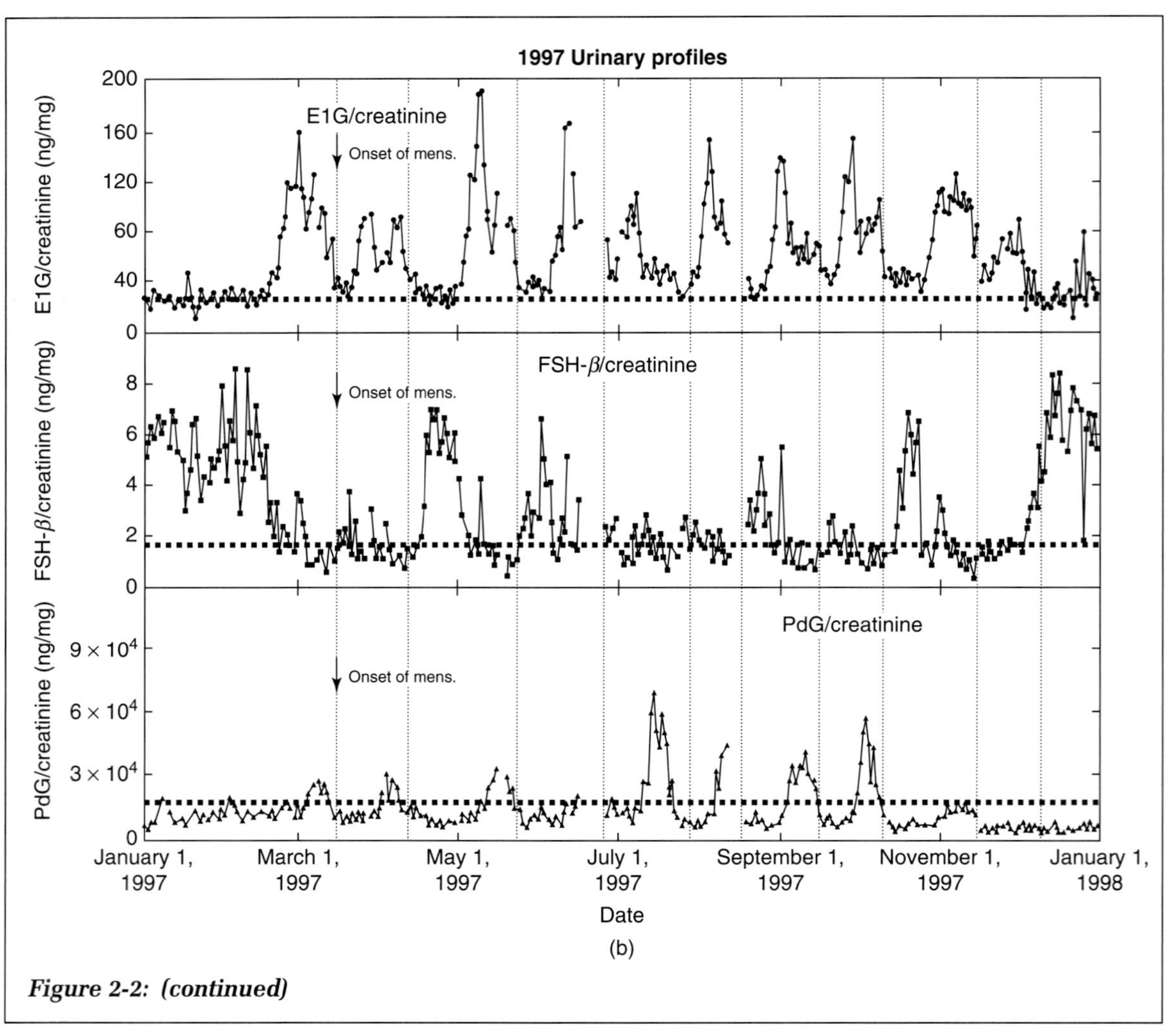

Figure 2-2: (continued)

KEY POINT

Circulating FSH levels are elevated during the menopausal transition and after menopause, but the increase in FSH may begin several years earlier.

E1G. Increases in PdG prior to menses suggest that 8 of the 11 cycles were ovulatory.

During the second year, urinary β-FSH concentrations were often elevated above levels seen in younger women (Fig. 2-2B). Excretion of E1G remained similar to that in the younger women. There were 10 episodes of vaginal bleeding, and 7 were preceded by increases in PdG indicative of ovulation. During the third year, urinary β-FSH concentrations were elevated even more often but did fall to levels typical of the midreproductive years on many occasions (Fig. 2-2C). Excretion of E1G was largely in the normal reproductive range, whereas PdG

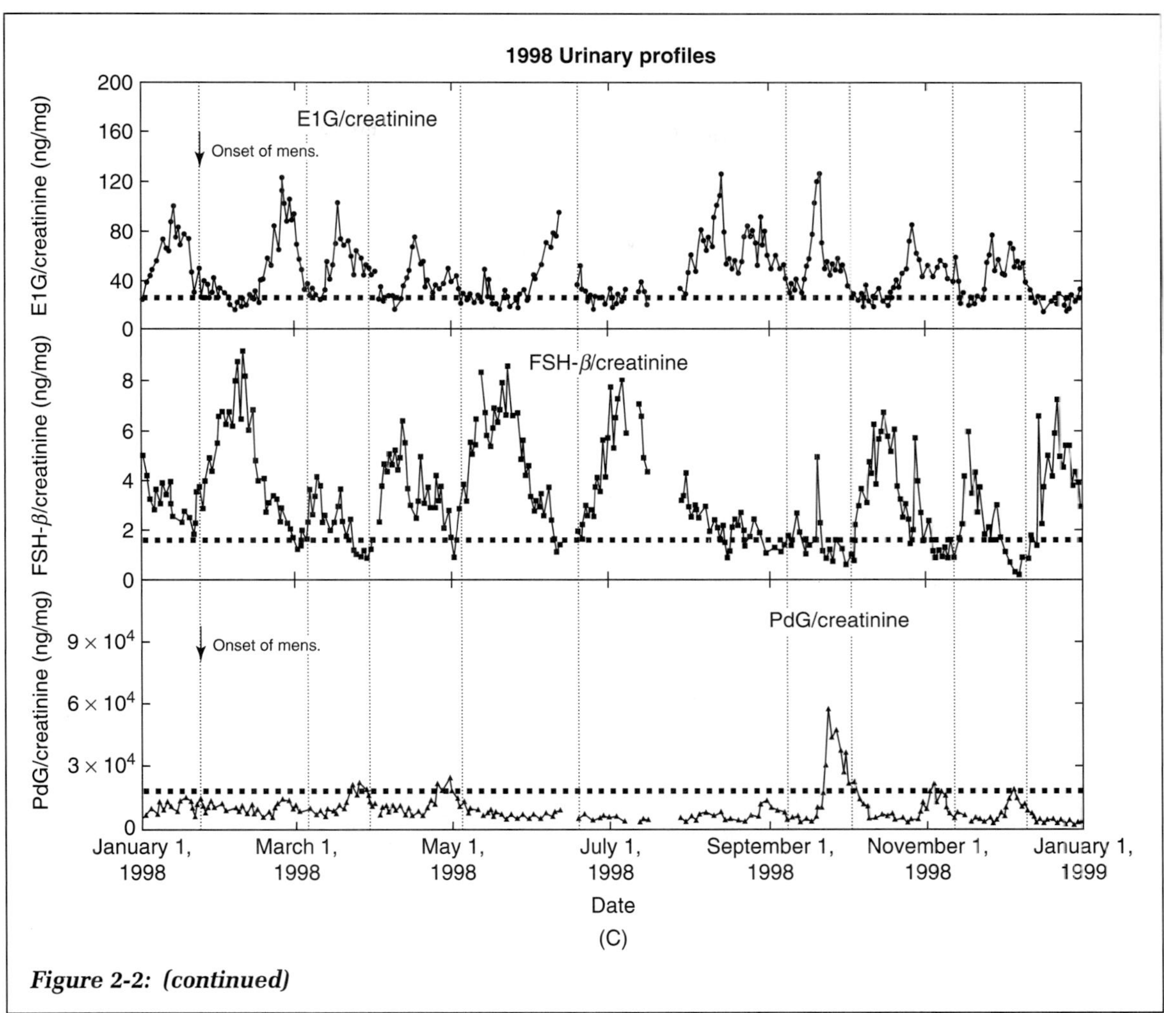

Figure 2-2: (continued)

excretion was generally less than seen during ovulatory menstrual cycles in younger women. However, six of the nine reported episodes of vaginal bleeding were preceded by elevations in PdG that, although low, appeared indicative of ovulation. During the fourth year, the number of bleeding episodes decreased to seven (Fig. 2-2D). There were fewer consistent increases in E1G during the follicular phase, and urinary β-FSH excretion increased for many days. The subject reported severe vasomotor symptoms for most of the year. Only three of the bleeding episodes were preceded by small, but discernible, increases in PdG.

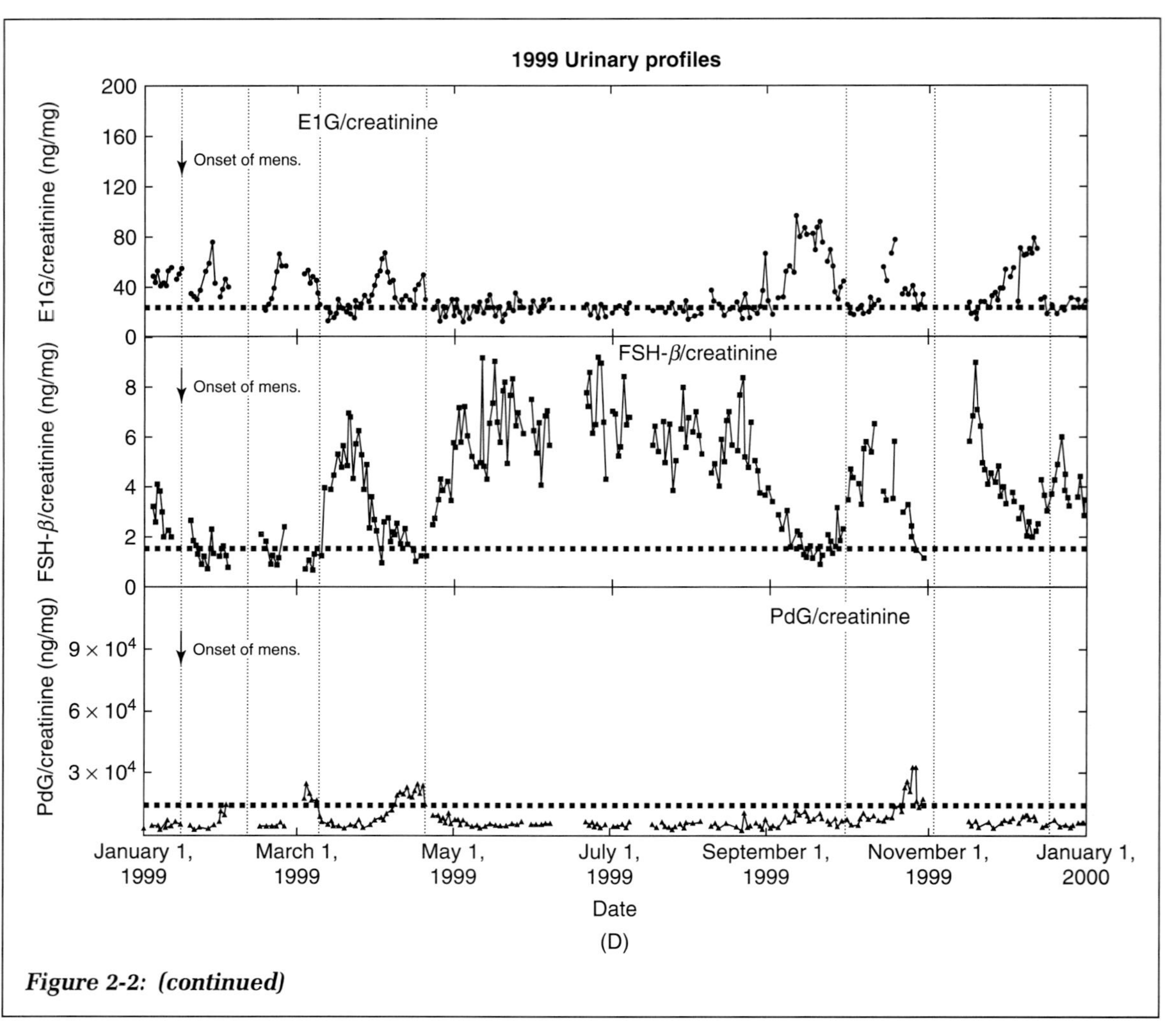

Figure 2-2: (continued)

INHIBINS Although the patterns of other reproductive hormones during the normal menstrual cycle have been known for many years, it is only in the last decade that the changes in circulating inhibins have been documented.[17] Inhibins are peptides synthesized by granulosa cells in response to FSH and secreted into the follicular fluid and ovarian venous effluent. Inhibins, as the name implies, inhibit FSH secretion. Thus, FSH stimulates the secretion of inhibins from granulosa cells and in turn is suppressed by inhibins.

Inhibins consist of two dissimilar peptides, known as the alpha and beta subunits, linked by disulfide bonds. Two forms of inhibin, inhibins A and B, have been identified. Each is composed of an identical alpha subunit and distinct but related beta subunits. Thus, there are three subunits for inhibins: alpha, beta-A, and beta-B. Inhibin A contains the beta-A subunit and inhibin B contains the beta-B subunit.

There is considerable evidence to indicate that the circulating concentrations of inhibins A and B are under differential control. Inhibin A, together with estradiol, appears to be synthesized and secreted by the dominant ovarian follicle and the ensuing corpus luteum.[17,18] Inhibin B, on the other hand, is synthesized and secreted by small antral follicles.[17,18]

The patterns of inhibins A and B differ through the menstrual cycle.[17] Concentrations of inhibin A tend to mirror those of estradiol. In contrast, concentrations of inhibin B closely parallel those of FSH during the luteal-follicular transition and the early follicular phase. There is a midcycle peak, but during the luteal phase, inhibin B concentrations decrease to their lowest values during the cycle.

The fact that the increase in concentrations of FSH in the follicular phase that is observed as women age is specifically related to a fall in circulating concentrations of inhibin B was documented by observing that inhibin B levels decrease as FSH levels increase.[19–21] Inhibin A levels were unchanged and estradiol levels were actually higher in the older than in the younger women in this study. Data from the cross-sectional Melbourne Women's Midlife Health Project indicate that inhibin B levels fall prior to the decrease in estradiol, consistent with the hypothesis that declining concentrations of inhibin B provide a mechanism for allowing FSH levels to rise in an effort to maintain estradiol levels at the same levels as observed in younger women (Fig. 2-3).[20,21] In this study, levels of inhibin A did not fall until late in the menopausal transition, close to the final menstrual period (FMP). Thus, it has been postulated that inhibin B levels reflect the number of follicles recruited from the pool of primordial follicles, and the size of this pool decreases with age, as noted previously.[3] Burger and colleagues have concluded that the earliest endocrine change marking entry into the menopausal transition is a major fall in inhibin B, presumably reflecting that the number of ovarian follicles has fallen to a critically low number.[21,22]

Androgens It appears that circulating androgen levels decrease with age but do not decrease abruptly during the menopausal

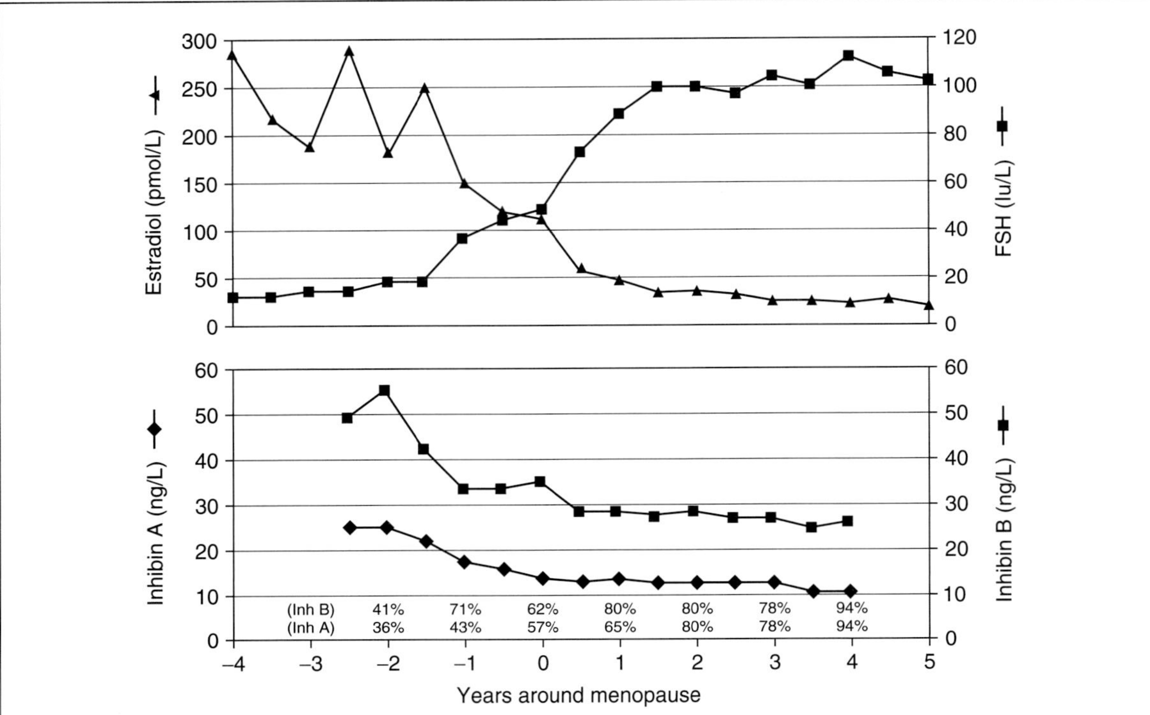

Figure 2-3: Geometric means of (A) follicle-stimulating hormone (FSH) and estradiol, and (B) inhibins A and B normalized to the final menstrual period (FMP) (0). The horizontal axis represents time in years relative to the FMP, with negative years indicating before, and positive years after, the FMP. The percentages above the timescale in panel B indicate the percentages of measured inhibins A and B at or below the assay sensitivity. (*Source*: Burger HG, et al. Prospectively measured levels of serum follicle-stimulating hormone, estradiol, and the dimeric inhibins during the menopausal transition in a population-based cohort of women. *J Clin Endocrinol Metab.* 1999;84: 4025.)

KEY POINT

Androgen levels decline slowly with age but do not fall abruptly at menopause; in fact, free androgen levels actually increase during the menopausal transition.

transition or at menopause. Longcope and colleagues (1986) did not observe any significant change in testosterone (T) and androstenedione (A) levels in the 80 months preceding the FMP.[23] However, they noted that mean concentrations of T in all their subjects, including those still having cyclic menses, were significantly less than those of a group of normal young women sampled on days 5–7 of the menstrual cycle. Another group reported a sharp fall in total serum T with age, noting that levels in a 40-year-old woman were approximately 50% of those in a woman aged 21.[24] Free T concentrations decreased in a similar fashion.

In the Melbourne Women's Midlife Health Project, there were no significant decreases in either total T concentrations or the T-sex hormone-binding globulin (SHBG) ratio (also known as the free androgen index [FAI]) as a function of changing menopausal status.[25,26] In fact, the FAI increased by 80% from 4 years before the FMP to 2 years after because of a concomitant decrease in SHBG levels during this same time interval (due no doubt to the decrease in circulating estradiol levels). Levels of the major adrenal androgen, dehydroepiandrosterone sulfate, decreased slowly with age, as has been reported by others, but the levels were not related to the FMP.

Symptoms Associated with Reproductive Aging

KEY POINT

The menopausal transition, heralded by menstrual irregularity, has been estimated to last about 4 years and ends with the FMP.

As detailed in subsequent chapters in this book, numerous symptoms are associated temporally with the menopausal transition. The Massachusetts Women's Health Study, a prospective cohort study involving over 2500 women aged 45–55, noted that the median age at the FMP was 51.3 years.[27] The median age at what was termed perimenopause, based on appearance of menstrual irregularity, was 47.5 years, with the length of the typical menopausal transition estimated at nearly 4 years. Smokers, and possibly nulliparous women, were found to have earlier menopausal transitions.

Most of the symptoms appear due to declining levels of estrogen in the circulation. In fact, clinicians have known for many years that removal of the ovaries in premenopausal women reproduces the symptoms commonly associated with the menopausal transition and menopause. Several prospective studies have now documented that symptoms can even precede the onset of menstrual irregularity associated with the menopausal transition.[28,29] Indeed, we noted that 50% of women consider the onset of symptoms in this period of life, rather than the FMP, to signal the onset of menopause.[30] Data from the Melbourne Women's Midlife Health Project suggest that symptoms associated with the late premenopause and early menopausal transition can be combined.[28] Symptoms that appear to specifically relate to the hormonal changes of the menopausal transition include vasomotor symptoms (i.e., hot flushes and night sweats), vaginal dryness, and breast tenderness. Hot flushes, night sweats, and vaginal dryness increase and breast tenderness decreases as estrogen levels fall in the late menopausal transition.

KEY POINT

Symptoms may be absent, mild, or severe and may precede or follow onset of the menopausal transition.

Definitions and Stages of the Menopausal Transition

The World Health Organization has defined menopause as the permanent cessation of menstruation resulting from loss of

KEY POINT

Menopause is the permanent cessation of menstruation as a result of loss of ovarian activity.

ovarian follicular activity.[31] As defined by STRAW, the menopausal transition begins with variations in menstrual cycle length in a woman who has levels of FSH in the early follicular phase that are increased above levels found in regularly menstruating women under the age of 35 and ends with the FMP (Fig. 2-4).[32] Perimenopause, which literally means "about or around the menopause," begins at the same time as the menopausal transition and ends one year after the FMP. The STRAW report suggested that because the terms *perimenopause* and *climacteric* are not used consistently, they should be used only with patients and in the lay press and not in scientific papers.

The STRAW report further divides reproductive and postreproductive life into several stages. The anchor for the entire staging system is the FMP, and the age range and duration for each of the stages varies. Five stages, numbered negatively from the FMP (considered 0) precede, and two stages, numbered positively, follow the FMP. Stage –5 refers to the early, stage –4 to the peak,

Final menstrual period (FMP)

Stages:	–5	–4	–3	–2	–1	0	+1	+2
Terminology:	Reproductive			Menopausal transition		Postmenopause		
	Early	Peak	Late	Early	Late*	Early*		Late
				Perimenopause				
Duration of stage:	Variable			Variable		ⓐ 1 yr	ⓑ 4 years	Until demise
Menstrual cycles:	Variable to regular	Regular		Variable cycle length (*>7 days different from normal*)	≥2 Skipped cycles and an interval of amenorrhea (*≥60 days*)	*Amen x 12 mos*	None	
Endocrine:	Normal FSH		↑FSH	↑FSH		↑FSH		

**Stages most likely to be characterized by vasomotor symptoms.* ↑ *= elevated*

Figure 2-4: The STRAW staging system for normal reproductive aging in women (see text for explanations). (*Source*: Soules MR, Sherman S, Parrot E, et al. Executive summary: Stages of Reproductive Aging Workshop (STRAW). *Fertil Steril.* 2001;76:874 with permission from American Society for Reproductive Medicine.)

and stage –3 to the late reproductive period. A woman's peak fertility occurs in her mid- to late-twenties (stage –4), after which it progressively decreases until menopause. The decrease in fertility is likely an early sign of reproductive aging preceding the monotropic increase in FSH levels and changes in menstrual cyclicity. However, fertility was not included in the staging system because relative fertility in an individual is nearly impossible to measure and is codependent on the fertility of the male partner. Stage –2 refers to the early and stage –1 refers to the late menopausal transition.

Stage +1a refers to the first year after the FMP, stage +1b refers to years 2–5 postmenopausal, and stage +2 refers to the later postmenopausal years after 5. The participants agreed that the first 5 years after menopause should be included in stage +1 (early) postmenopause because this time interval encompasses a further dampening of ovarian hormone function to a permanent low level as well as accelerated bone loss. Stage +2 (late postmenopause) has a definite beginning but its duration varies because it ends with death. Further divisions may be warranted as women live longer and more information is accumulated.

KEY POINT

The proposed staging system for the menopausal transition will be modified as additional information is acquired.

By the late reproductive years (stage –3), FSH levels are significantly elevated in the early follicular phase compared to those observed in regularly menstruating women but menses remain regular. Although it is more difficult for women in this stage to conceive and spontaneous abortions are more common, pregnancy is still possible. In the early menopausal transition (stage –2), a woman's menstrual cycles remain regular, but the duration changes by 7 days or more. Pregnancy is even more unlikely but still possible. The late menopausal transition (stage –1) is characterized by two or more skipped menstrual periods and at least one intermenstrual interval of 60 days or more. Pregnancy is extremely unlikely, but still possible. Menopause is determined in retrospect, after a woman has had a year of amenorrhea.

These definitions are not perfect but represent definitions that the participants in the STRAW conference could accept. They will no doubt be modified in the future. Data indicate that women with 3–11 months of amenorrhea will likely become menopausal within 4 years.[33] Women over the age of 45 who have a year of amenorrhea have a 9 in 10 chance of not having another spontaneous menstrual period.[34] Symptoms were not included because it has been observed that symptomatology varies markedly among ethnic groups, cultures, socioeconomic groups, and climates. Furthermore, the symptoms do not correlate closely with the menstrual cycle or with the endocrine changes occurring during the menopausal transition. Although the participants considered it premature to consider pelvic sonography in attempting to stage individuals, they recognized the potential use of antral follicle counts (e.g., those measuring 2–10 mm in diameter) as a future adjunct.

The participants did not believe that this staging system should be applied to women who smoke cigarettes (which is known to advance the age of menopause), those at the extremes of body weight (body mass index <18 kg/m^2 or >30 kg/m^2), those who do heavy aerobic exercise (>10 h/week), those with chronic menstrual cycle irregularity, those who have had a hysterectomy, or those who have abnormal uterine (e.g., fibroids) or ovarian anatomy (e.g., endometriomas). In addition, there are recent data, most notably from the Study of Women's health Across the Nation (SWAN), that suggest that patterns of change may differ among racial groups.[35,36] Further studies are needed to determine if such differences affect the proposed staging system.

Identifying the Menopausal Transition and Menopause

Women who present with irregular menses or amenorrhea (for 3 or more months) prior to the age of 45 may be entering the menopausal transition but should be evaluated for the major causes of amenorrhea. A careful history and physical examination should be conducted. Basal levels of LH, FSH, and prolactin should be measured in such individuals, with further evaluation predicated on the results of these tests.

Women who are 45 years or older and present with irregular menses or amenorrhea are much more likely to be in the menopausal transition (Fig. 2-5). Thus, it makes much more sense to merely measure basal FSH. If changes typical of menopause accompany the change in menses, it may not be necessary to measure FSH levels unless the patient is particularly anxious. It is rarely necessary to measure FSH in women aged 50 or older. FSH levels >15 mIU/mL are typical of the menopausal transition as measured in most laboratories. Values <15 mIU/mL are present intermittently in women

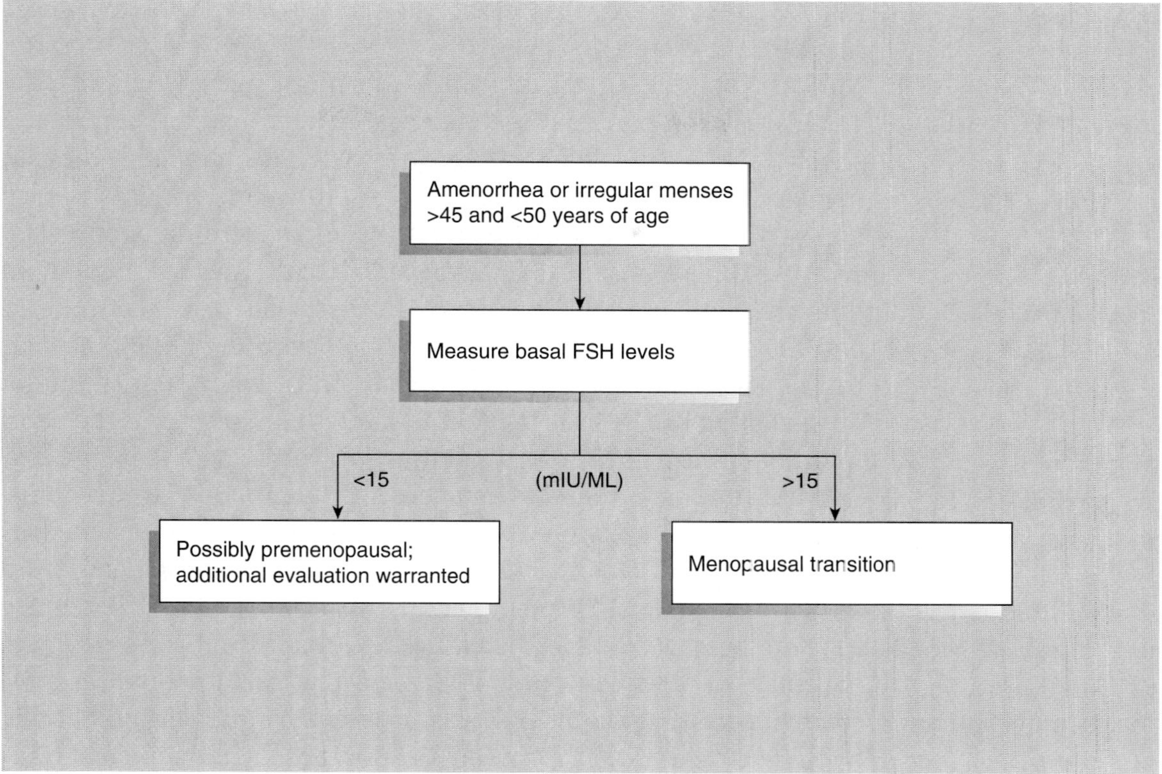

Figure 2-5: Approach to the woman with amenorrhea or irregular menses who is between 45 and 50 years of age.

during the menopausal transition, but such normal levels indicate the need for further evaluation.

It is also important to remember that irregular menses in women in this age group may well indicate anovulation and be associated with an increased risk of endometrial hyperplasia. Thus, endometrial sampling may be warranted for women with a history of irregular menses of more than 6 months.

Because, as noted previously, symptoms of estrogen deficiency may precede or follow any objective changes associated with the menopausal transition, the presence of symptoms should not lead the clinician to conclude that menopause is approaching. Symptoms that seem typical of menopause and estrogen deficiency may be indicative of a less common disorder, including undiagnosed hyperthyroidism or even a pheochromocytoma or gastrointestinal tract tumor secreting serotonin.

What's the Evidence?

Menopausal transition is a dynamic phase in a woman's life. Distinguishing changes associated with aging from those associated specifically with the end of reproductive life is a challenge indeed. However, the greatest difficulty at present is determining exactly where in the menopausal transition an individual woman is. Because this phase of life is of variable length, it is not possible to tell any woman for how many more years she will continue to ovulate and to have menses at any time before the FMP. It is clear that fertility has decreased, and the end of reproductive life is approaching by the time that FSH levels are increased in the early follicular phase of the cycle, but this does not appear to be the first sign of the approaching menopause. A distinguished group of clinical investigators from Australia, led by Henry Burger, has suggested that a fall in inhibin B levels may be the first easily detected hormonal change of the menopausal transition, but this will require further observations and discussion. A change in the frequency of menses is probably the first obvious sign of the menopausal transition in most women and was selected by individuals at the STRAW conference as signaling the onset of the menopausal transition. Ongoing prospective studies will no doubt lead to changes in our understanding of this stage of life and to the ability to explain more about this period of life to individual women.

Discussion of Cases

CASE 1

A 46 year-old woman presents complaining of hot flushes, night sweats, and difficulty sleeping. Her lack of sleep is interfering with her job. On questioning, she notes that her menses have become somewhat irregular, occurring at 22–40-day intervals over the past 6 months, whereas they previously had occurred at 29–32-day intervals.

What testing will confirm that this woman is in the menopausal transition?

Measurement of a basal FSH level is indicated, reveals a concentration of 16 mIU/mL, and is consistent with the menopausal transition.

What therapy, if any, would you offer this patient?

If she has no contraindication, menopausal hormone therapy (HT) is likely to aid this patient. The lowest dose of estrogen that is effective in alleviating her symptoms should be provided and may well be as little as 0.3 mg

of conjugated estrogens daily. Either oral or transdermal estrogen may be used. Because she is still menstruating, it is important to tell her that irregular menses are likely to continue. It makes sense to add a progestogen (such as micronized progesterone 100 mg or medroxyprogesterone acetate 5 mg/day) for 14 days at 1–2-month intervals to minimize any risk of endometrial hyperplasia.

If the patient does have a contraindication to the use of HT, data indicate that a selective serotonergic reuptake inhibitor (SSRI) may be effective in helping alleviate her symptoms. However, no therapy yet identified is as effective as estrogen in treating vasomotor symptoms.

CASE 2

A 49-year-old woman presents with irregular menses at 20–60-day intervals, hot flushes, night sweats, insomnia, and weight gain of 20 lb over the preceding year. She tells you that she owns a bakery together with her husband.

On physical examination, her blood pressure is 130/85, and her pulse rate is 104 beats/min. She has a fine tremor of her hands and fasciculations of her tongue. Remainder of the physical examination is normal. Her vaginal mucosa is well estrogenized.

What testing is warranted in this patient?

Although this woman is near the age of menopause, her symptoms are not entirely consistent with her entering the menopausal transition. In fact, her pulse rate, hot flushes, tremor, and fasciculations may suggest hyperthyroidism. Confusing in this regard is her weight gain, but this may be explained by the fact that she has access to food and hyperthyroidism increases appetite. Thus, basal levels of FSH, TSH, and thyroxine (T4) are warranted. In this patient, the findings reveal an FSH of 21 mIU/mL, a TSH of 0.2 μU/mL, and a T4 of 20.2 μg/dL.

What therapy is indicated for this patient?

It would appear that this patient has hyperthyroidism and is also in the menopausal transition. Appropriate therapy for the hyperthyroidism should be provided first. If she continues to have symptoms associated with estrogen deficiency after she is euthyroid, then this problem can be addressed.

REFERENCES

1 Baker TG. A quantitative and cytological study of germ cells in human ovaries. *Proc R Soc Lond B Biol Sci.* 1963;158:417.

2 Block E. A quantitative morphological investigation of the follicular system in newborn female infants. *Acta Anat.* 1953;17:201.

3 Richardson SJ, Senikas V, Nelson JF. Follicular depletion during the menopausal transition: evidence for accelerated loss and ultimate exhaustion. *J Clin Endocrinol Metab.* 1987;65:1231.

4 Pavlik EJ, DePriest PD, Gallion HH, et al. Ovarian volume related to age. *Gynecol Oncol.* 2000;77:410.

5 Flaws JA, Langenberg P, Babus JK, et al. Ovarian volume and antral follicle counts as indicators of menopausal status. *Menopause.* 2001; 8:175.

6 Sherman BM, Korenman SG. Hormonal characteristics of the human menstrual cycle throughout reproductive life. *J Clin Invest.* 1975;55: 699.

7 Sherman BM, West JH, Korenman SG. The menopausal transition: analysis of LH, FSH, estradiol, and progesterone concentrations during menstrual cycles of older women. *J Clin Endocrinol Metab.* 1976;42:629.

8 Reyes FI, Winter JS, Faiman C. Pituitary ovarian relationships preceding the menopause. I. A cross-sectional study of serum follicle-stimulating hormone, luteinizing hormone, prolactin, estradiol, and progesterone levels. *Am J Obstet Gynecol.* 1977;129:557.

9 Lee SJ, Lenton EA, Sexton L, et al. The effect of age on the cyclical patterns of plasma LH, FSH, estradiol and progesterone in women with regular menstrual cycles. *Hum Reprod.* 1988;3:851.

10 Klein NA, Battaglia DE, Fujimoto VY, et al. Reproductive aging: accelerated ovarian follicular development associated with a monotropic follicle-stimulating hormone rise in normal older women. *J Clin Endocrinol Metab.* 1996;81:1038.

11 Scott RT, Toner JP, Muasher SJ, et al. Follicle-stimulating hormone levels on cycle day 3 are predictive of in vitro fertilization outcome. *Fertil Steril.* 1989;51:651.

12 Cahill DJ, Prosser CJ, Wardle PG, et al. Relative influence of follicle stimulating hormone, age, and other factors on ovarian response to gonadotrophin stimulation. *Br J Obstet Gynaecol.* 1994;101:999.

13 Toner JP, Philput CB, Jones GS, et al. Basal follicle-stimulating hormone level is a better predictor of in vitro fertilization performance than age. *Fertil Steril.* 1991;55:784.

14 Santoro N, Brown JR, Adel T, et al. Characterization or reproductive hormonal dynamics in the perimenopause. *J Clin Endocrinol Metab.* 1996;81:1495.

15 Rebar RW, Cedars MI, Liu JH. Premature ovarian failure: a model for the perimenopause? In: Lobo RA (ed). *Perimenopause.* New York: Springer-Verlag; 1997:7.

16 Liu JH, Kao L, Rebar RW, et al. Urinary β-FSH subunit concentrations in perimenopausal and postmenopausal women: a biomarker for ovarian reserve. *Menopause.* 2003;10:526.

17 Groome NP, Illingworth PJ, O'Brien M, et al. Measurement of dimeric inhibin B throughout the menstrual cycle. *J Clin Endocrinol Metab.* 1996;81:1401.

18 Roberts VJ, Barth S, El-Roeiy A, et al. Expression of inhibin/activin subunits and follistatin messenger ribonucleic acids and proteins in ovarian follicles and the corpus luteum during the menstrual cycle. *J Clin Endocrinol Metab.* 1993;77:1402.

19 Klein NA, Illingworth PJ, Groome NP, et al. Decreased inhibin B secretion is associated with the monotropic rise of FSH in older, ovulatory women: a study of serum and follicular fluid levels of dimeric inhibin A and B in spontaneous menstrual cycles. *J Clin Endocrinol Metab.* 1996;81:2742.

20 Burger HG, Dudley EC, Cui J, et al. Early follicular phase serum FSH as a function of age: the roles of inhibin B, inhibin A, and estradiol. *Climacteric.* 2000;3:17.

21 Burger HG, Dudley EC, Robertson DM, et al. Hormonal changes in the menopause transition. *Recent Prog Horm Res.* 2002;57:257.

22 Burger HG, Cahir N, Robertson DM, et al. Serum inhibins A and B fall differentially as FSH rises in perimenopausal women. *Clin Endocrinol.* 1998;48:809.

23 Longcope C, Franz C, Morello C, et al. Steroid and gonadotropin levels in women during the perimenopausal years. *Maturitas.* 1986;8:189.

24 Zumoff B, Strain GW, Miller LK, et al. Twenty-four hour mean plasma testosterone concentration declines with age in normal premenopausal women. *J Clin Endocrinol Metab.* 1995;80:1429.

25 Burger HG, Dudley EC, Hopper JL, et al. The endocrinology of the menopausal transition: a cross-sectional study of a population-based sample. *J Clin Endocrinol Metab.* 1995;80:3537.

26 Burger HG, Dudley EC, Cui J, et al. A prospective longitudinal study of serum testosterone, dehydroepiandrosterone sulphate and sex hormone binding globulin levels through the menopause transition. *J Clin Endocrinol Metab.* 2000;85:2832.

27 McKinlay SM. The normal menopause transition: an overview. *Maturitas.* 1996;23:137.

28 Mitchell ES, Woods NF. Symptom experiences of midlife women: observations from the Seattle midlife women's health study. *Maturitas.* 1996;25:1.

29 Dennerstein L, Dudley EC, Hopper JL, et al. A prospective population-based study of menopausal symptoms. *Obstet Gynecol.* 2000;96:351.

30 Anderson E, Hamburger S, Liu JH, et al. Characteristics of menopausal women seeking assistance. *Am J Obstet Gynecol.* 1987;156:428.

31 World Health Organization Scientific Group. *Research on the Menopause in the 1990s.* Geneva, Switzerland: World Health Organization; 1996. Technical Report Series 866.

32 Soules MR, Sherman S, Parrot E, et al. Executive summary: Stages of Reproductive Aging Workshop (STRAW). *Fertil Steril.* 2001;76:874.

33 Garamszegi C, Dennerstein L, Dudley E, et al. Menopausal status: subjectively and objectively defined. *J Psychosom Obstet Gynaecol.* 1998;19:165.

34 Wallace RB, Sherman BM, et al. Probability of menopause with increasing duration of amenorrhea in middle-aged women. *Am J Obstet Gynecol.* 1979;135:1021.

35 Manson JM, Sammel MD, Freeman EW, et al. Racial differences in sex hormone levels in women approaching the transition to menopause. *Fertil Steril.* 2001;75:297.

36 Lasley BL, Santoro N, Randolf JF, et al. The relationship of circulating dehydroepiandrosterone, testosterone, and estradiol to stages of the menopausal transition and ethnicity. *J Clin Endocrinol Metab.* 2002;87:3760.

AGING AND NEUROCOGNITIVE CHANGES

Hot Flash Management

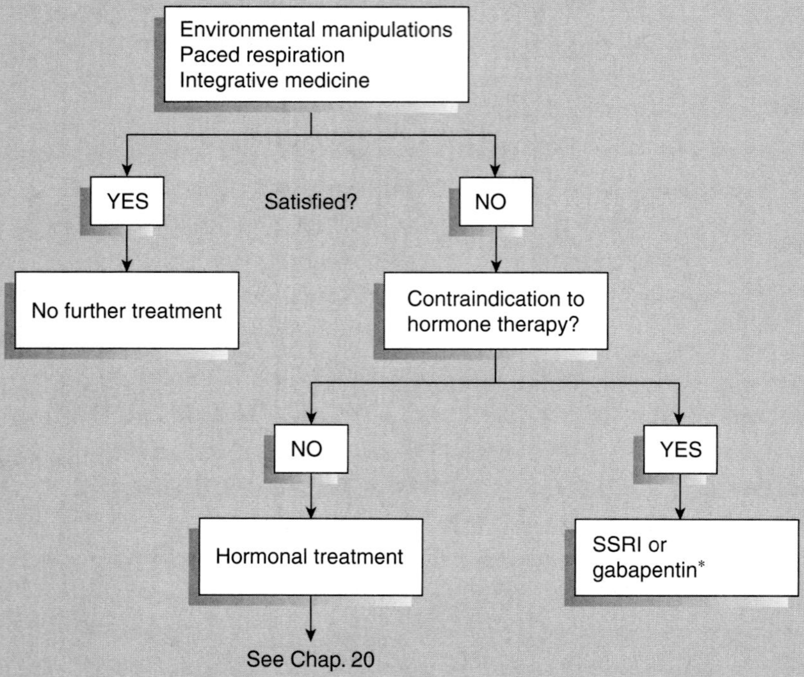

*Neither drug is FDA approved for this indication.

3 Management of Hot Flashes

Robert R. Freedman

Introduction

Hot flashes are the most common symptom of the climacteric and occur in the majority of women by the time of postmenopause. The Study of Women's Health Across the Nation (SWAN study) found that the percentage of women reporting hot flashes ranged from 25.2% at age 40–43 to 46.4% at age 52–55.[1] Other studies have found the prevalence among naturally menopausal women to be 68%[2] and 82%[3] in the United States. In premenopausal women undergoing oophorectomy, the prevalence of hot flashes is about 90%.[4]

Although there are no major risk factors for menopausal hot flashes, cultural factors do affect their reports. Women from China report hot flashes at rates of 10–25%[5] and Indonesian women report them at rates of 10–20%.[6] Reasons for these differences are not known. It is possible that women from Eastern cultures demonstrate physiological hot flash events in the same manner as Western women but are acculturated not to report them. It is also possible that they do have fewer physiological hot flashes, possibly due to dietary and other environmental factors.

Physiology

Descriptive

KEY POINT

Hot flashes are a heat dissipation response.

Hot flashes are generally described as sensations of intense internal heat, superior to the sternum, accompanied by sweating, flashing, and chills. Sweating is reported most frequently in the face, neck, head, and chest. Hot flashes generally last about 2–4 minutes, but may persist for much longer. Feldman[3] found that 64% of women surveyed reported hot flashes from 1 to 5 years, with a median of 4 years. About 40% of women reported a premonition that a hot flash was about to occur.

Objective

Peripheral vasodilation, as evidenced by increased skin temperature and blood flow, occurs over virtually the entire body surface (Fig. 3-1).[7–9] The whole-body sweat rate during hot flashes has been measured to be about 1.3 g/min, with more sweat occurring in the upper half of the body.[10] Skin conductance, an electrical measure of sweating, also increases during hot flashes, and can be used objectively to indicate them.[11,12] It has been shown that an increase in skin conductance of 2 μmho/30s, measured over the sternum, corresponds with patient self-reports in 95% of hot flashes recorded in the laboratory and 77–86% of those recorded during ambulatory monitoring.[11,12]

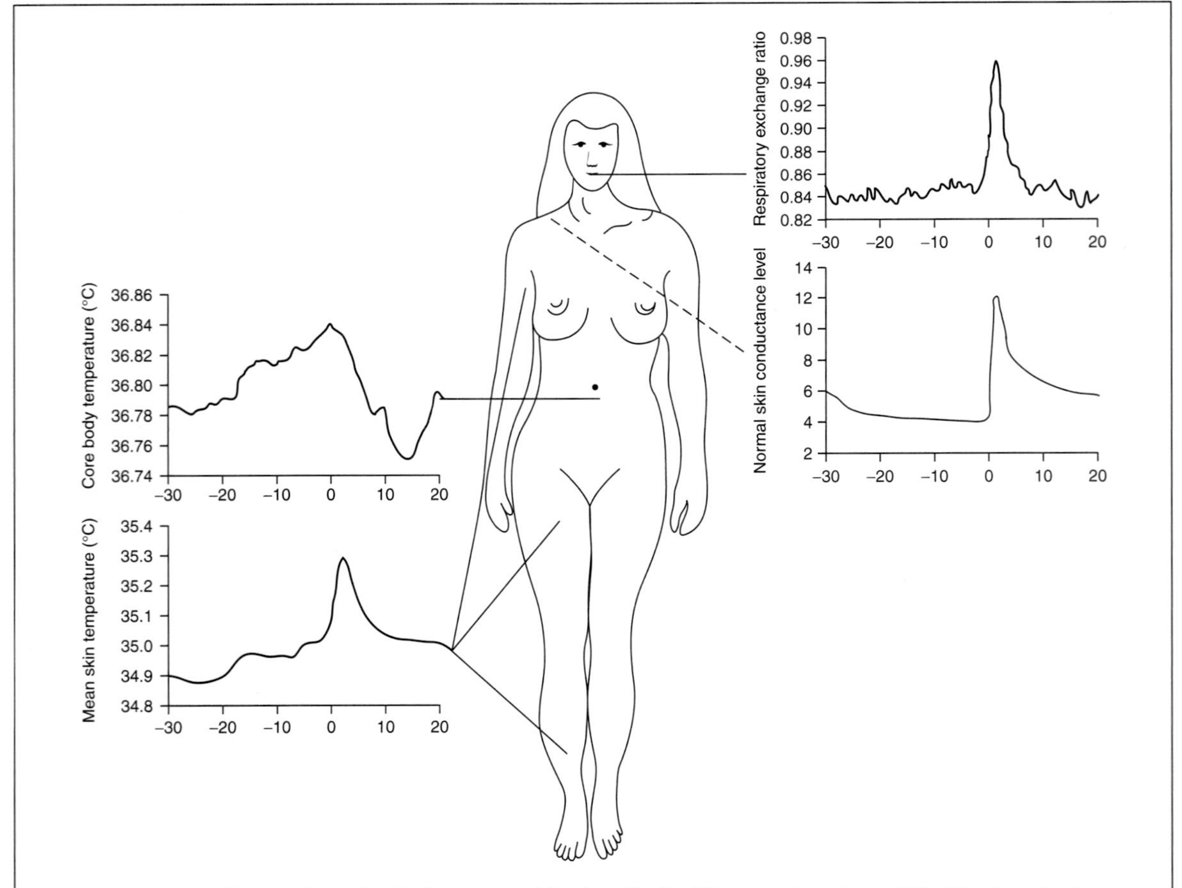

Figure 3-1: Peripheral physiological events of the hot flash. (*Source*: Freedman RR. Biochemical, metabolic, and vascular mechanisms in menopausal hot flashes. *Fertil Steril.* 1998;70:332–7.)

Humans regulate core body temperature (T_c) between an upper threshold, where sweating and peripheral vasodilation occur, and a lower threshold, where shivering occurs. The temperature range between the two thresholds is considered the thermoneutral zone. If T_c were elevated in women with hot flashes, their symptoms of sweating and peripheral vasodilation could be explained. However, measurements of esophageal,[13] rectal,[14] and tympanic[15] temperatures were not found to be elevated prior to hot flashes. These studies all found declines of about 0.3 EC following hot flashes, probably due to increased heat loss (peripheral vasodilation) and evaporative cooling (sweating). However, esophageal and rectal temperatures have long thermal lag times, and respond too slowly to appear along with the rapid peripheral events of the hot flash.[16] Additionally, it has been shown that tympanic temperature does not reliably measure T_c because it is affected by peripheral vasodilation and sweating.[17]

KEY POINT

Hot flashes are triggered by small elevations in core body temperature acting within a reduced thermoneutral zone.

Several studies were conducted in which T_c was recorded with an ingested radiotelemetry pill, which responds more rapidly than esophageal and rectal temperatures. We found that small but significant increases in core body temperature preceded 65–76% of hot flashes recorded in the laboratory, whereas rectal temperature did not change.[7,14] Small elevations in T_c may, therefore, be the triggering event for the majority of hot flashes.

Elevations in T_c can be caused by increased metabolic rate (heat production) and by peripheral vasoconstriction (decreased heat loss). We sought to determine whether either of these factors accounted for the core body temperature elevations preceding hot flashes. Significant elevations in metabolic rate (about 15%) occurred, but were simultaneous with sweating and peripheral vasodilation and did not precede the T_c elevations (Fig. 3-1). Peripheral vasoconstriction did not occur. Thus, increased metabolic rate and peripheral vasoconstriction did not account for the core body temperature elevations in these women.

Small increases in heart rate, about 7–15 beats/min occur at the same time as the peripheral vasodilation and sweating.[13]

Endocrinology

ESTROGEN

Because hot flashes accompany the decline of estrogen in the vast majority of naturally and surgically menopausal women, there is little doubt that estrogens play a role in the genesis of hot flashes.

KEY POINT

Estrogen levels do not differ between symptomatic and asymptomatic women.

However, estrogens alone do not appear to be responsible for hot flashes because there is no correlation between the presence of this symptom and plasma,[18] urinary,[19] and vaginal concentrations.[20] No differences in unconjugated plasma estrogen concentrations were found in symptomatic versus asymptomatic women.[21] Additionally, clonidine significantly reduces hot flash frequency in some but not all studies without altering circulating estrogen values.[22]

GONADOTROPINS

Because gonadotropins become elevated at menopause, their possible role in the initiation of hot flashes has been investigated. Although no differences in luteinizing hormone (LH) concentrations were found between women with and without hot flashes,[23] a temporal association was found between LH pulses and hot flash occurrence.[24,25] However, subsequent investigation revealed that women with a defect of gonadotropin-releasing hormone (GnRH) secretion (isolated gonadotropin deficiency) had hot flashes but no LH pulses, and women with abnormal input to GnRH neurons (hypothalamic amenorrhea) had some LH pulses but no hot flashes.[25] Additionally, hot flashes occur in hypophysectomized women, who have no LH release,[26] in women with pituitary insufficiency and hypoestrogenism,[27] and in women with LH release suppressed by GnRH analog treatment.[28,29] Thus, LH cannot be the basis for hot flashes.

OPIATES

It was observed that alcohol-induced flashing in subjects taking chlorpropamide, a drug that stimulates insulin release and lowers blood glucose, was related to opiate receptor activation.[30] Lightman and colleagues[31] subsequently found that naloxone infusion significantly reduced hot flash and LH pulse frequencies in six postmenopausal women. However, DeFazio and associates[32] attempted to replicate this study and found no effects. Tepper and co-workers[33] found that plasma β-endorphin concentration decreased significantly before the occurrence of menopausal hot flashes, whereas Genazzani and colleagues[34] found significantly increased values preceding hot flashes. Thus, there is no consistent evidence of the involvement of an opioidergic system in menopausal hot flashes.

CATECHOLAMINES

There is considerable evidence that norepinephrine plays an important role in thermoregulation, mediated in part through α_2-adrenergic receptors.[35] Injection of norepinephrine into the preoptic hypothalamus causes peripheral vasodilation, heat loss, and a subsequent decline in T_c.[35] Additionally, there is considerable evidence that gonadal steroids modulate central noradrenergic activity.[36]

KEY POINT

Central noradrenergic activity is elevated before and during hot flashes and narrows the thermoneutral zone.

3-Methoxy-4-hydroxyphenylglycol (MHPG) is the main metabolite of norepinephrine and reflects whole-body sympathetic activation.[37] Basal levels of plasma MHPG are significantly higher in symptomatic than in asymptomatic postmenopausal women, and increase significantly further with the occurrence of each hot flash.[38] It was subsequently shown that plasma vanillylmandelic acid (VMA), the peripheral metabolite of norepinephrine, does not change with hot flashes,[7] lending support to the hypothesis that central norepinephrine levels are elevated in symptomatic women.

Clonidine, an α_2-adrenergic agonist, reduces central noradrenergic activation and hot flash frequency.[39–41] Conversely, yohimbine, an α_2-adrenergic antagonist, increases central noradrenergic activation and triggers hot flashes.[42] These data support the hypothesis that α_2-adrenergic receptors within the central noradrenergic system are involved in the initiation of hot flashes and that brain norepinephrine is elevated in this process.

Thermoregulation and Hot Flashes

Circadian Rhythms The circadian rhythm of T_c is well-known, and similar variations in other thermoregulatory parameters, such as heat conductance and sweating, have also been demonstrated. These patterns suggest that the thermoregulatory effector responses of hot flashes might also demonstrate temporal variations. A previous study showed circadian rhythmicity of self-reported hot flashes in some menopausal women, but no physiological data were collected.[43] We therefore recorded sternal skin conductance level and T_c (with the telemetry pill) in symptomatic and asymptomatic postmenopausal women using 24-hour ambulatory monitoring.[21] Cosinor analysis demonstrated a circadian rhythm ($P < 0.02$) of hot flashes with a peak around 18.25 (Fig. 3-2). This rhythm lagged the circadian rhythm of T_c in symptomatic women by about 3 hours. T_c values of the symptomatic women were lower than those of the asymptomatic women ($P < 0.05$) from 00.00 to 04.00, and at 15.00 and 22.00. The majority of hot flashes were preceded by elevations in T_c, a statistically significant effect ($P < 0.05$). The

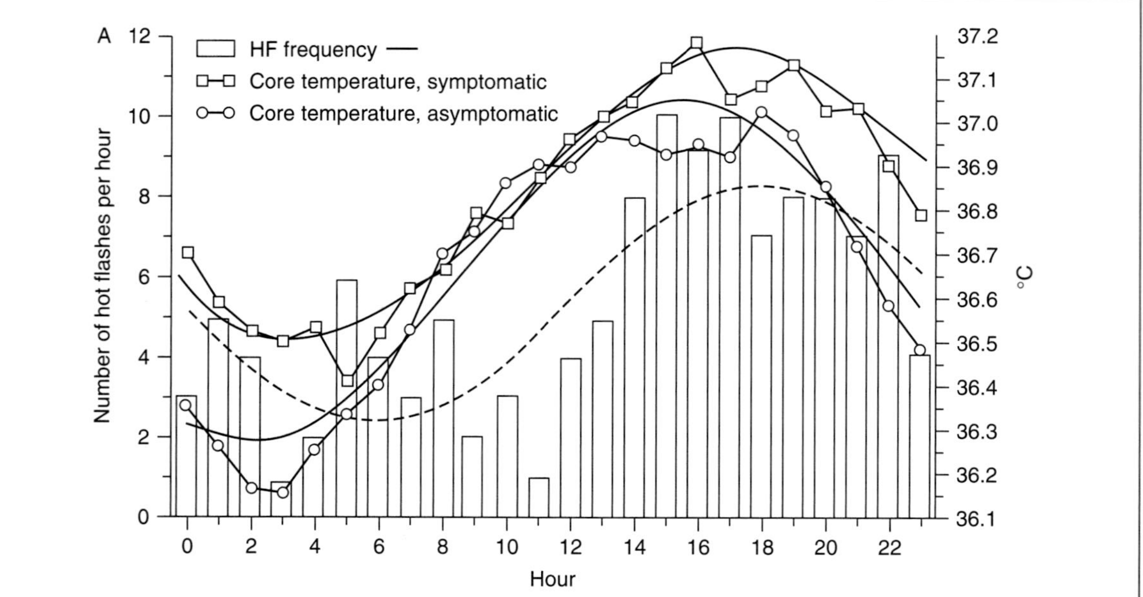

Figure 3-2: Hot flash (HF) frequency and core body temperature over 24 hours. Hot flash frequency in 10 symptomatic women shown as bars. Curves: Best-fit cosine curve for hot flash frequency (-----): 24-hour core temperature data for 10 symptomatic women (–) with best-fit cosine curve (—): 24-hour core temperature data in six asymptomatic women (□—□) with best-fit cosine curve (·····). (*Source*: Freedman RR, Norton D, Woodward S, et al. Core body temperature and circadian rhythm of hot flashes in menopausal Women. *J Clin Endocrinol Metab.* 1995;80(8):2354–2358. The Endocrine Society.)

mean core temperature associated with hot flashes (36.82 ± 0.04°C) was significantly higher ($P < 0.05$) than the mean core temperature during periods when there were no hot flashes (36.70 ± 0.005°C). These data are consistent with the hypothesis that elevated T_c serves as part of the hot flash triggering mechanism.

Increased thermosensitivity at menopause has been noted in the literature for many years, and is reflected in reports of increased hot flash frequency and duration during warm weather.[44,45] Peripheral heating has been demonstrated to provoke hot flashes in most symptomatic women.[11,46] As noted above, T_c in humans is regulated by hypothalamic centers between the T_c thresholds for sweating and peripheral vasodilation and for shivering. According to this mechanism, the heat dissipation responses of hot flashes (sweating, peripheral vasodilation) would be triggered if body temperature were elevated above the sweating threshold lowered.

Three separate investigations have found that small elevations in T_c precede the majority of menopausal hot flashes.[7,11,14] Since these elevations also occur in asymptomatic women, they do not explain the entire triggering mechanism.[47] However, if the thermoneutral zone were sufficiently narrowed in asymptomatic women, the T_c elevations would be a likely trigger. This appears to be the case.

A study was conducted in which the thermoneutral zone was measured to be 0.0 EC in symptomatic postmenopausal women and 0.4 EC in asymptomatic postmenopausal women.[48] Sweating rates were significantly higher in the symptomatic women, and hot flashes were triggered by T_c elevations produced by body heating and exercise.

Animal studies have shown that increased brain norepinephrine narrows the width of the thermoneutral zone.[35] Conversely, clonidine reduces norepinephrine release, raises the sweating threshold, and reduces hot flashes in symptomatic women.[49] Estrogen ameliorates hot flashes by raising the sweating threshold in symptomatic women.[50]

Thus, it is proposed that elevated brain norepinephrine narrows the thermoregulatory interthreshold zone (thermoneutral zone) in symptomatic postmenopausal women, and that small elevations in core body temperature trigger hot flashes when the sweating threshold is crossed (Fig. 3-3).

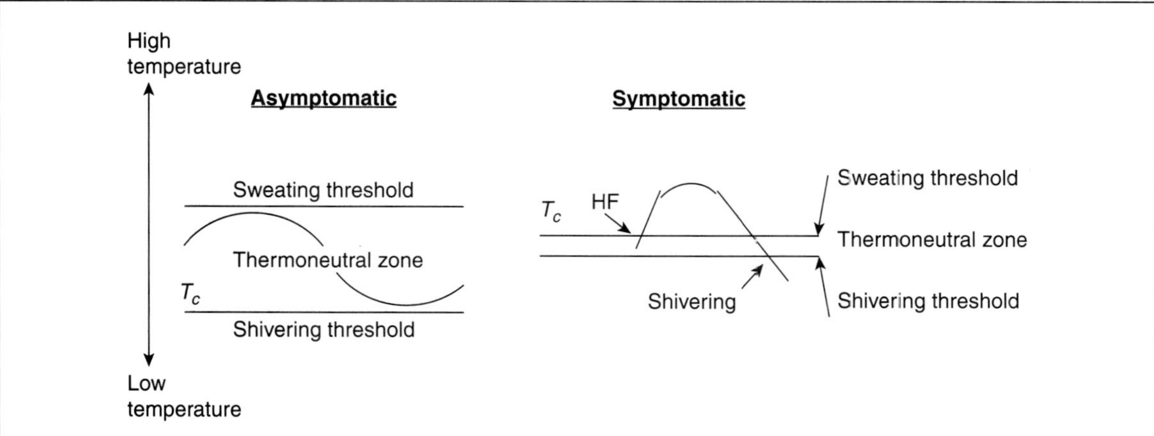

Figure 3-3: Small core body temperature (T_c) elevations acting within a reduced thermoneutral zone trigger HFs in symptomatic postmenopausal women.

Treatment

Introduction

KEY POINT

HT should no longer be regarded as the first line of treatment for hot flashes.

Until recently, hormone therapy (HT) was considered the treatment of choice for menopausal hot flashes. However, recent data from the Women's Health Initiative demonstrate increased risks for breast cancer, coronary heart disease, stroke, thromboembolism, and dementia with HT use, although women in that trial were, on average, older than those usually experiencing hot flashes.[56] Nonetheless, HT need not be regarded as the first line of treatment for this symptom.

Estrogen levels fluctuate substantially during the perimenopause as does the occurrence of hot flashes. Accordingly, the need for treatment may not remain constant during this period.

Environmental Manipulations

Research reviewed above suggests that hot flashes are triggered by small elevations in T_c acting within a reduced thermoneutral zone. Additionally, it has been shown that hot flashes occur more frequently in warm than in cold rooms and that they can be triggered by peripheral heating. Accordingly, measures to reduce ambient heat and T_c will reduce the occurrence of hot flashes. Lowering the room temperature, dressing in layers, and drinking cold liquids instead of hot ones are all thought to be helpful. Small fans and personal air conditioners may be useful in the workplace.

Behavioral Treatments

KEY POINT

Methods of cooling the body will reduce hot flashes.

We have presented evidence that central sympathetic activation is increased in women with hot flashes. Behavioral relaxation methods have been shown to reduce sympathetic activity in normal subjects and in some clinical populations.[51] Therefore, we treated seven menopausal women with hot flashes using a combination of progressive muscle relaxation exercises and slow deep breathing.[52] Seven additional women were assigned to receive a control procedure, alpha wave EEG biofeedback. The relaxation procedure significantly reduced objective symptoms recorded in the laboratory and diary-reported hot flash frequency (by about 50%) compared to the control procedure. This investigation demonstrated that a combination of muscle relaxation exercises and slow deep breathing significantly reduce hot flash frequency in a small group of subjects. However, because two treatment procedures were combined, it was not possible to determine which component was responsible for the therapeutic effect. The physiological data showed that respiration rate was the only recorded variable that was significantly altered during training.

KEY POINT

Paced respiration reduces hot flash frequency by about 50%.

Therefore, a second study was performed in which one group of subjects received slow, deep breathing alone, another group received muscle relaxation exercises alone, and a third group received alpha EEG biofeedback.[53] Treatment outcome was assessed by ambulatory monitoring of sternal skin conductance responses, described previously. Only the paced respiration group showed a significant decline in hot flash frequency (about 50%), decreased respiration rate, and increased tidal volume. There were no significant changes shown by the other two groups.

We then sought to determine if reduced sympathetic activation was the mechanism by which paced respiration ameliorates hot flashes.[54] We therefore measured plasma MHPG, epinephrine, norepinephrine, and platelet α_2-receptors during paced respiration or alpha EEG biofeedback in 24 symptomatic women. Treatment outcome was again assessed by ambulatory monitoring of sternal skin conductance. The paced respiration group showed a significant decline in hot flash frequency (again about 50%) compared to no change in the control group. However, there were no significant changes in any biochemical measure for either group. Thus, the mechanism through which paced respiration reduces hot flash frequency remains to be determined.

Two other small studies[55,56] have also found significant amelioration of hot flashes through behavioral relaxation procedures. Thus, behavioral treatments should be recommended to women for whom environmental measures do not provide sufficient symptom control.

Acupuncture has been investigated as a treatment for hot flashes. One randomized trial compared acupuncture to a control acupuncture intervention (shallow needle placement) and to oral estrogen. The estrogen treatment experienced a 90% decrease in hot flashes and the two acupuncture groups both experienced a 50% decrease.[57]

Prescription Therapies

Several Selective Serotonin Reuptake Inhibitors Estrogen is the only Food and Drug Administration (FDA)-approved therapy for hot flashes and is 90% effective. The therapies described below are currently not FDA-approved but studies have shown them to reduce hot flashes.

Several selective serotonin reuptake inhibitors (SSRIs), including venlafaxine, paroxetine, and fluoxetine, have been shown to be reasonably effective in the treatment of hot flashes. A randomized clinical trial of venlafaxine in 229 women reporting at least 14 hot flashes/week found reductions in hot flash scores of about 60% for 75 and 150 mg/day.[58] Reported side effects included nausea and vomiting (5–10%) as well as dry mouth, decreased appetite, constipation, and occasionally orgasmic dysfunction.

A randomized clinical trial of paroxetine[59] found significant declines in hot flash scores of 62% (12.5 mg/day) and 65% (25 mg/day), compared to 38% for the placebo group. Reported side effects include nausea, somnolence, decreased appetite and orgasmic dysfunction.

Increased sweating is listed as a potential side effect for many SSRIs and can add confusion to the treatment setting. It is important that SSRIs be discontinued in a dose-tapered manner.

Gabapentine This anticonvulsant has been used to treat hot flashes, although the mechanism of action is completely unknown. A randomized clinical trial of 59 women found a reduction in hot flash frequency of 45% at a dose of 900 mg/day.[60] Dizziness, lightheadedness, and peripheral edema were the most commonly reported side effects.

Clonidine Several small clinical trials have found that clonidine, given orally or transdermally, reduces hot flash frequency by about 50%.[39, 40] However, since clonidine reduces blood pressure, hypotension is a significant problem. Additionally, clonidine can cause sedation, constipation, and dry mouth.

For a discussion of the management of hot flashes with hormones, phytoestrogens, and herbs, see Chaps. 20 and 24.

PACED RESPIRATION: A BEHAVIORAL INTERVENTION FOR HOT FLASH MANAGEMENT

When a staff member approached us for advice about a nonpharmacologic treatment for a family member who had been treated for breast cancer, we set about developing a behavioral intervention for hot flashes. The treatment we developed centers around a slow, controlled diaphragmatic breathing technique (paced respiration). The patient is instructed to find a quiet area in which she can sit and employ the technique with as few distractions as possible. For 15 minutes in the morning and evening, the woman practices the technique by inhaling slowly (5-second count) and exhaling slowly (5-second count), using diaphragmatic breathing. Once the woman becomes accustomed to this technique, she can use the paced respiration as an intervention when she feels a hot flash beginning. Because this is a conscious intervention, it cannot, of course, be used for hot flashes that occur during sleep.

Discussion of Cases

CASE 1

A 49-year-old woman with intermittent menstrual cycles began experiencing frequent hot flashes, which were disturbing at work and home. She tried dressing in layers, reducing the room temperature, and paced respiration for several months, but was still experiencing substantial discomfort. She was placed on Paxil 10 mg/day. She initially experienced daytime sedation for several weeks, which resolved. She reported that the frequency and severity of her symptoms decreased "by over 50%" and that she was considerably more comfortable. No further treatment was required.

CASE 2

A 50-year-old woman with recent breast cancer treated with chemotherapy experienced frequent, severe hot flashes. She refused all pharmacological treatments and stated she did not expect complete resolution of her hot flashes. She began practicing paced respiration using the regimen described here, paying particular attention to the onset of symptoms. Her symptom frequency was reduced by about half, and she was satisfied with this result. No further treatment was recommended.

Guiding Questions

- How frequent and severe are the vasomotor symptoms?
- Are they manageable or does the woman desire assistance in managing them?
- Is she willing to try environmental measures and/or paced respirations first?
- Does she understand and accept that these measures provide improvement but rarely completely eliminate hot flashes?
- Does the woman understand the natural course of hot flashes to be gradual improvement over time?
- Is it obvious that the woman needs prescription medication and is willing to accept any associated side effects?

What's the Evidence?

Data continue to be acquired regarding the mechanisms associated with vasomotor symptoms. The α_2-adrenergic receptors, norepinephrine, and core body temperature all appear to play an important role. The narrowed thermoneutral zone plays a key role. Numerous alternative therapies have been promoted for the

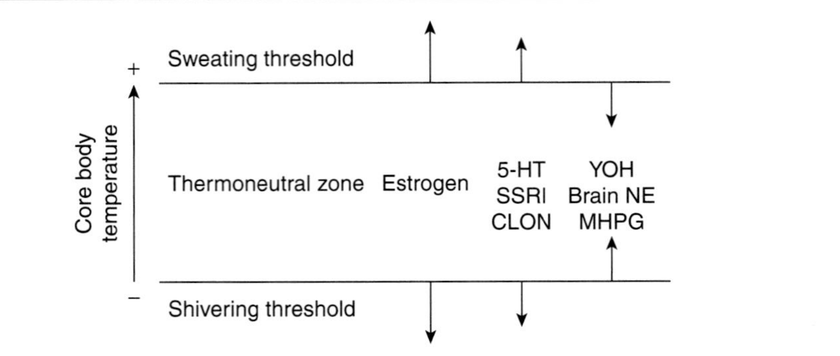

We have shown that the thermoneutral zone is narrowed in symptomatic women. Elevated brain norepinephrine (NE) in animals reduces this zone. Yohimbine (YOH) elevates brain norepinephrine and should reduce this zone. Conversely, clonidine (CLON) should widen it.

MHPG, 3-methoxy-4-hydroxyphenylglycol (the primary NE metabolite); 5-HT, serotonin; SSRI, selective serotonin reuptake inhibitor.

Figure 3-4: Compounds that may expand or reduce the thermoneutral zone.

alleviation of vasomotor symptoms, but for most of them the studies have yielded mixed results. Environmental management and paced respirations have supportive studies and provide the patient with measures that she can utilize with minimal cost and minimal risk. The use of nonestrogen prescription therapies such as SSRIs may modify the thermoneutral zone (see Fig. 3-4).

References

1 Gold EB, Sternfeld B, Kelsey JL, et al. Relation of demographic and lifestyle factors to symptoms in a multi-racial/ethnic population of women 40–55 years of age. *Am J Epidemiol.* 2000;152:463–473.

2 Neugarten BL, Kraines RJ. “Menopausal symptoms” in women of various ages. *Psychosom Med.* 1965;27:266–273.

3 Feldman BM, Voda A, Gronseth E. The prevalence of hot flash and associated variables among perimenopausal women. *Res Nurs Health.* 1985;8:261–268.

4 Chakravarti S, Collins WP, Newton JR, et al. Endocrine changes and symptomatology after oophorectomy in premenopausal women. *Br J Obstet Gynaecol.* 1977;84:769–775.

5 Tang G. Menopause: the situation in Hong Kong Chinese women. In: Berg G, Hammar M, eds. *The Modern Management of the Menopause.* Vol. 8. New York: Parthenon; 1994:47–55.

6 Flint M, Samil RS. Cultural and subcultural meanings of the menopause. *Ann NY Acad Sci.* 1990;592:134–148.

7 Freedman RR. Biochemical, metabolic, and vascular mechanisms in menopausal hot flashes. *Fertil Steril.* 1998;70:332–337.

8 Ginsburg J, Swinhoe J, O'Reilly B. Cardiovascular responses during the menopausal hot flash. *Br J Obstet Gynaecol.* 1981;88:925–930.

9 Sturdee DW, Reece BL. Thermography of menopausal hot flashes. *Maturitas.* 1979;1:201–205.

10 Molnar GW. Body temperature during menopausal hot flashes. *J Appl Physiol Respir Environ Exercise Physiol.* 1975;38:499–503.

11 Freedman RR. Laboratory and ambulatory monitoring of menopausal hot flashes. *Psychophysiology.* 1989;26:573–579.

12 Freedman RR, Woodward S, Norton D. Laboratory and ambulatory monitoring of Menopausal hot flashes: comparison of symptomatic and asymptomatic women. *J Psychophysiology.* 1992;6:162166.

13 Kronenberg F, Cote LJ, Linkie DM, et al. Menopausal hot flashes: thermoregulatory, cardiovascular, and circulating catecholamine and LH changes. *Maturitas.* 1984;6:31–43.

14 Freedman RR, Woodward S. Core body temperature during menopausal hot flashes. *Fertil Steril.* 1996;65:1141–1144.

15 Tataryn IV, Lomax P, Bajorek JG, et al. Postmenopausal hot flashes: a disorder of thermoregulation. *Maturitas.* 1980;2:101–107.

16 Molnar GW, Read RC. Studies during open heart surgery on the special characteristics of rectal temperature. *J Appl Physiol.* 1974;36:333–336.

17 Skiraki K, Nobuhide K, Sagawa S. Esophageal and tympanic temperature responses to core blood temperature changes during hyperthermia. *J Appl Physiol.* 1986;61:98–102.

18 Askel S, Schomberg DW, Tyrey L, et al. Vasomotor symptoms, serum estrogens, and gonadotropin levels in surgical menopause. *Am J Obstet Gynecol.* 1976;126:165–169.

19 Stone SC, Mickal A, Rye F, et al. Postmenopausal symptomatology, maturation index, and plasma estrogen levels. *Obstet Gynecol.* 1975; 45:625–627.

20 Hutton JD, Jacobs HS, Murray MAF, et al. Relation between plasma esterone and estradiol and climacteric symptoms. *Lancet.* 1978;1: 671–681.

21 Freedman RR, Norton D, Woodward S, e al. Core body temperature and circadian rhythm of hot flashes in menopausal women. *J Clin Endocrinol Metab.* 1995;80:2354–2358.

22 Schindler AE, Muller D, Keller E, et al. Studies with clonidine (Dixarit) in menopausal women. *Arch Gynecol.* 1979;227:341–347.

23 Campbell S. Intensive steroid and protein hormonal profiles on postmenopausal women experiencing hot flashes and a group of controls. In: Campbell S, ed. *Management of the Menopause and Post-Menopause Years*. London: MTP Press; 1976.

24 Casper RF, Yen SSC, Wilkes MM. Menopausal flashes: a neuroendocrine link with pulsatile luteinizing hormone secretion. *Science*. 1979;205:823–825.

25 Gambone J, Meldrum DR, Laufer L, et al. Further delineation of hypothalamic dysfunction responsible for menopausal hot flashes. *J Clin Endocrinol*. 1984;59:1097–1102.

26 Mully G, Mitchell RA, Tattersall RB. Hot flashes after hypophysectomy. *Br Med J*. 1977;2:1062.

27 Meldrum DR, Erlik Y, Lu JKH, et al. Objectively recorded hot flashes in patients with pituitary insufficiency. *J Clin Endocrinol Metab*. 1981;52:684–687.

28 Casper RF, Yen SSC. Menopausal flashes: effect of pituitary gonadotropin desensitization by a potent luteinizing hormone releasing factor agonist. *J Clin Endocrinol Metab*. 1981;53:1056–1058.

29 DeFazio J, Meldrum DR, Laufer L, et al. Induction of hot flashes in premenopausal women treated with a long-acting GnRH agonist. *J Clin Endocrinol Metab*. 1983;56:445–448.

30 Leslie RDG, Pyke DA, Stubbs WA. Sensitivity to enkephalin as a cause of non-insulin dependent diabetes. *Lancet*. 1979;1:341–344.

31 Lightman SL, Jacobs HS, Maquire AK, et al. Climacteric Flashing: clinical and endocrine response to infusion of naloxone. *Br J Obstet Gynaecol*. 1981;88:919–924.

32 DeFazio J, Vorheugen C, Chetkowski R, et al. The effects of naloxone on hot flashes and gonadotropin secretion in postmenopausal women. *J Clin Endocrinol Metab*. 1984;58:578–581. Tepper R, Neri A, Kaufman H, Schoenfield A, Ovadia J. Menopausal hot flashes and plasma β-endorphins. *Obstet Gynecol*. 1987;70:150–152.

33 Genazzani AR, Petraglia F, Facchinetti F, et al. Increase of proopiomelanocortin-related peptides during subjective menopausal flashes. *Am J Obstet Gynecol*. 1984;149:775–779.

34 Brück K, Zeisberger E. Adaptive changes in thermoregulation and their neuro-pharmacological basis. In: Schönbaum E, Lomax P, eds. *Thermoregulation: Physiology and Biochemistry*. New York: Pergamon; 1990:255–307.

35 Insel PA, Motulskey HJ. Physiologic and pharmacologic regulation of adrenergic receptors. In: Insel PA, ed. *Adrenergic Receptors in Man*. New York: Dekker;1987:201–336.

36 Lambert GW, Kaye DM, Vas M, et al. Regional origins of 3-methoxy-4-hydroxyphenylglycol in plasma: effects of chronic sympathetic

nervous activation and denervation, and acute reflex sympathetic stimulation. *J Autom Nerv Syst.* 1995;55:169–178.

37 Freedman RR, Woodward S. Elevated α_2-adrenergic responsiveness in menopausal hot flashes: pharmacologic and biochemical studies. In: Schönbaum E, Lomax P, eds. *Thermoregulation: The Pathophysiological Basis of Clinical Disorders.* Basel: Karger; 1992:6–9.

38 Clayden JR, Bell JW, Pollard P. Menopausal flashing: double blind trial of a non-hormonal medication. *Br Med J.* 1974;1:409–412.

39 Laufer LR, Erlik Y, Meldrum DR, et al. Effect of clonidine on hot flashes in postmenopausal women. *Obstet Gynecol.* 1982;60:583–589.

40 Schmitt H. The pharmacology of clonidine and related products. *Handb Exp Pharmacol.* 1977;39:299–396.

41 Freedman RR, Woodward S, Sabharwal SC. α_2-adrenergic mechanism in menopausal hot flashes. *Obstet Gynecol.* 1990; 76: 573–578.

42 Albright DL, Voda AM, Smolensky MH, et al. Circadian rhythms in hot flashes in natural and surgically-induced menopause. *Chronobiol Int.* 1989;6:279–284.

43 Molnar GW. Menopausal hot flashes: their cycles and relation to air temperature. *Obstet Gynecol.* 1981;57(Suppl. 6):52–55.

44 Kronenberg F, Barnard RM. Modulation of menopausal hot flashes by ambient temperature. *J Therm Biol.* 1992;17:43–49.

45 Sturdee DW, Wilson KA, Pipili E, et al. Physiological aspects of menopausal hot flash. *Br Med J.* 1978;2:79–80.

46 Freedman RR. Core body temperature variation in symptomatic and asymptomatic postmenopausal women: brief report. *Menopause.* 2002;9:399–401.

47 Freedman RR, Krell W. Reduced thermoregulatory null zone in postmenopausal women with hot flashes. *Am J Obstet Gynecol.* 1999;181: 66–70.

48 Freedman RR, Dinsay MD. Clonidine raises the sweating threshold in symptomatic but not in asymptomatic postmenopausal women. *Fertil Steril.* 2000;74:20–23.

49 Freedman RR, Blacker CM. Estrogen raises the sweating threshold in postmenopausal women with hot flashes. *Fertil Steril.* 2002;77: 487–490.

50 Hoffman JW, Benson H, Arns PA, et al. Reduced sympathetic nervous system responsivity associated with the relaxation response. *Science.* 1982;215:190–192.

51 Germaine LM, Freedman RR. Behavioral treatment of menopausal hot flashes: evaluation by objective methods. *J Consult Clin Psychol.* 1984;52(6):1072–1079.

52 Freedman RR, Woodward S. Behavioral treatment of menopausal hot flashes: evaluation by ambulatory monitoring. *Am J Obstet Gynecol.* 1992;167(2):436–439.

53 Freedman RR, Woodward S, Brown B, et al. Biochemical and thermoregulatory effects of behavioral treatment for menopausal hot flashes. *Menopause.* 1995;2(4):211–218.

54 Irvin JH, Domar AD, Clark C, et al. The effects of relaxation response training on menopausal symptoms. *J Psychosom Obstet Gynecol.* 1996;17:202–207.

55 Wijima K, Melin A, Nedstrand E, et al. Treatment of menopausal symptoms with applied relaxation: a pilot study. *J Behav Ther Exp Psychiatry.* 1997;28(4):251–261.

56 Wyon Y, Wijma K, Nedstrand E, et al. A comparison of acupuncture and oral estradiol treatment of vasomotor symptoms iin postmenopausal women. *Climacteric.* 2004;7:153–64.

57 Loprinzi CL, Kugler JW, Sloan JA, et al. Venlafaxine in management of hot flashes in survivors of breast cancer: a randomized controlled trial. *Lancet.* 2000;356:2059–2063.

58 Stearns V, Beebe KL, Iyengar M, et al. Paroxetine controlled release in the treatment of menopausal hot flashes: a randomized controlled trial. *JAMA.* 2003;289:2827–2834.

59 Guttuso T Jr, Kurlan R, McDermott MP, et al. Gabapentin's effects on hot flashes in postmenopausal women: a randomized controlled trial. *Obstet Gynecol.* 2003;101:337–345.

60 MacLennan JE, Lester S, Moore V. Oral oestrogen replacement therapy versus placebo for hot flashes (Cochrane Review). *Cochrane Database Syst Rev.* 2001;1: CD002978.

61 Notelovitz M, Lenihan JP, McDermott M, et al. Initial 17beta-estradiol dose for treating vasomotor symptoms. *Obstet Gynecol.* 2000;95: 726–731.

62 North American Menopause Society. Role of progestogen in hormone therapy for postmenopausal women: position statement of The North American Menopause Society. *Menopause.* 2003;10:113–132.

63 North American Menopause Society. Estrogen and progestogen use in peri- and postmenopausal women: September 2003 position statement of The North American Menopause Society. *Menopause.* 2003;10:497–507.

64 Writing Group for the Women's Health Initiative Investigators. Risks and benefits of estrogen plus progestins in healthy postmenopausal women. *JAMA.* 2002;288:321–333.

65 Bullock JL, Massey FM, Gambrell RD Jr. Use of medroxyprogesterone acetate to prevent menopausal symptoms. *Obstet Gynecol.* 1975;46: 165–168.

66 Schiff I, Tulchinsky D, Cramer D, et al. Oral medroxyprogesterone in the treatment of postmenopausal symptoms. *JAMA.* 1980;244: 1443–1445.

67 Loprinzi CL, Michalak JC, Quella SK, et al. Megestrol acet`ate for the prevention of hot flashes. *N Engl J Med.* 1994;331:347–352.

68 Casper RF, Dodin S, Reid RD. The effect of 20 μg ethinyl estradiol/ 1 mg norethindrone acetate (Minestrin™), a low-dose oral contraceptive, on vaginal bleeding patterns, hot flashes, and quality of life in symptomatic perimenopausal women. *Menopause.* 1997;4:139–147.

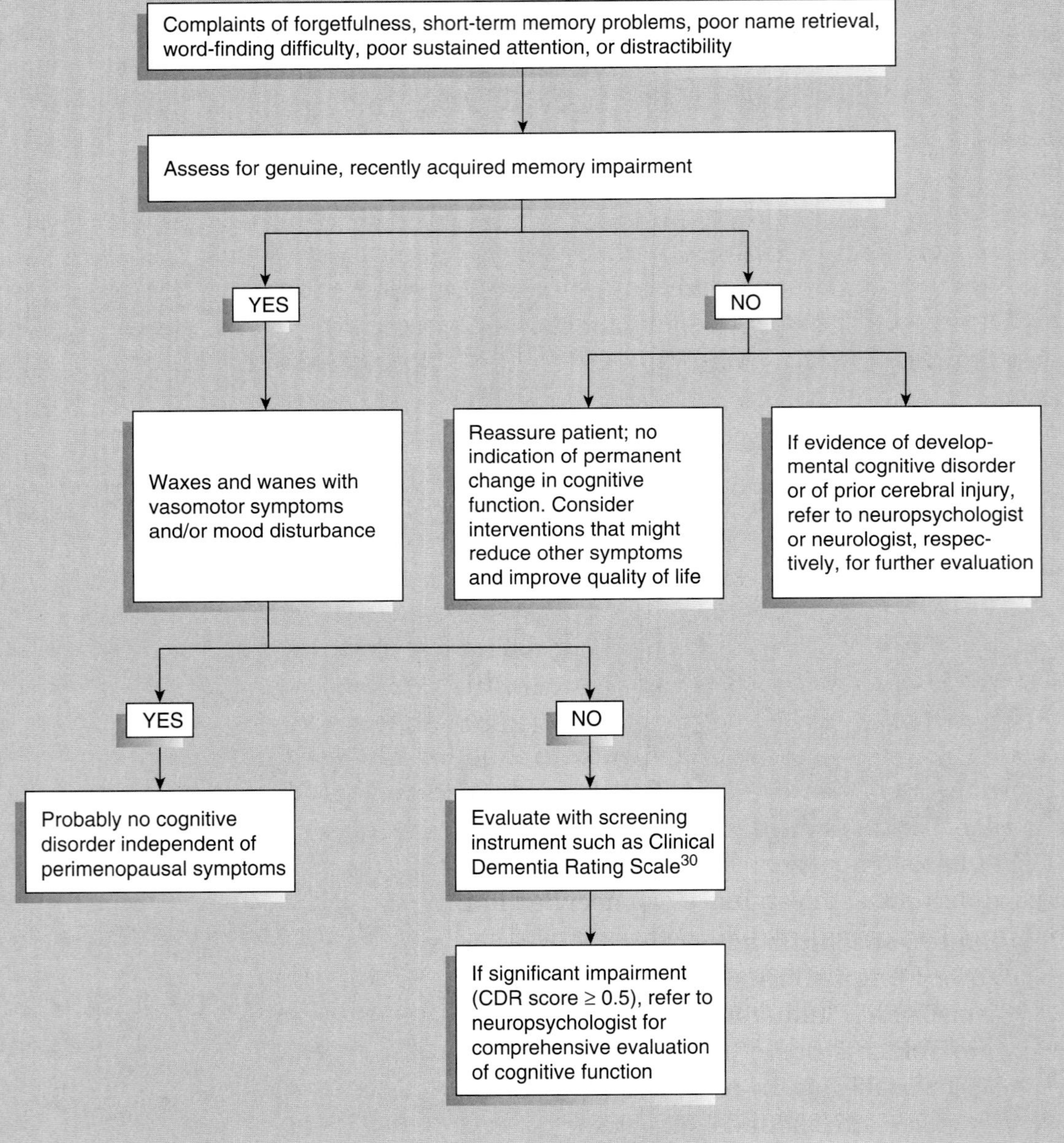
Pathway for Assessment of Memory Complaints During Perimenopause
Complaints of forgetfulness, short-term memory problems, poor name retrieval, word-finding difficulty, poor sustained attention, or distractibility
Assess for genuine, recently acquired memory impairment
YES
NO
Waxes and wanes with vasomotor symptoms and/or mood disturbance
Reassure patient; no indication of permanent change in cognitive function. Consider interventions that might reduce other symptoms and improve quality of life
If evidence of developmental cognitive disorder or of prior cerebral injury, refer to neuropsychologist or neurologist, respectively, for further evaluation
YES
NO
Probably no cognitive disorder independent of perimenopausal symptoms
Evaluate with screening instrument such as Clinical Dementia Rating Scale30
If significant impairment (CDR score ≥ 0.5), refer to neuropsychologist for comprehensive evaluation of cognitive function

4 Cognitive Changes in Perimenopause

Robert Krikorian

Introduction

Neurocognitive function in the perimenopause has not been well characterized. Unlike childhood and old age, periods for which there are extensive studies of cognitive function, there is a dearth of research concerning changes in cognition during middle age. There is a need for more empirical study of this important and complex phase of maturation. This chapter will review existing data in this regard.

Understanding cognitive changes in women during perimenopause is complicated by the fact that two processes, aging and the menopause transition, occur concurrently. Several factors can affect cognitive function and confound its evaluation, including alterations of reproductive hormone levels, concomitant vasomotor and mental symptoms, and the fact that the perimenopausal period extends for several years during which time age-related neurological decline also may occur. In addition, the course of perimenopause can be quite variable across individuals, making it difficult to identify characteristic neurocognitive manifestations.

While the termination of reproductive capability certainly is a sign of aging, it is not clear how the timing or course of reproductive aging is related to organism aging more generally or to brain aging specifically. Despite the fact that survival after menopause has increased twofold over the last 100 years, maximum reproductive age has not changed.[1] The stability of maximum reproductive age suggests that changes in the levels of reproductive hormones are independent of overall organism aging. On the other hand, the endocrinological changes associated with perimenopause are controlled by age-related brain changes and are not always benign with respect to other tissues and organ systems; for example, there is ample demonstration of negative effects on bone mineral density. While life span may not affect the onset of perimenopause, some of the processes intrinsic to perimenopause may influence organism aging. In addition, there are indications that the endocrinological changes inherent in reproductive aging may affect cognitive-cerebral function. There would appear to be both primary and secondary interactions of brain function with reproductive aging. There are data supporting the notion that the onset of reproductive senescence is influenced by the hypothalamic- pituitary system[2] and age-related aberrations of central circadian control.[3] An ancillary and provocative observation is that better intellectual function in childhood is strongly associated with onset of menopause at later age and this relationship is not attributable to the typically predictive factors including social status, education, physical development, smoking, and alcohol consumption.[4]

KEY POINT

Understanding cognitive function during perimenopause is complicated by the vasomotor and mental symptoms often experienced during the menopause transition and potentially by age-associated neurocognitive decline.

The issues under consideration in this chapter concern whether cognitive change is, indeed, manifested during perimenopause and whether the many endocrine-driven perturbations that result in reproductive senescence or other age-associated processes contribute to such effects. Animal and human research has established that reproductive hormones, especially estrogen, are involved in neural processes in brain regions that mediate cognitive function.[5] Such studies range from observational research assessing changes in cognition after menopause, to hormone replacement studies, and to investigations of normally cycling women in whom measurable differences on specific cognitive function tasks have been demonstrated at different phases in the cycle. All of this research has implicated a role for reproductive hormones in cognition.

Estrogen has been studied most extensively, and there has been considerable work demonstrating the neurobiological basis for estrogen effects on cognition, indicating that estrogen may be one of the most important hormones with respect to cognitive function. The empirical basis for positing that estrogen is important for cognitive function, especially memory, has led to the expectation that the alterations in the levels of reproductive hormones during the menopause transition would be associated with deterioration of brain function and cognitive aging. This inference is

KEY POINT

The importance of estrogen actions in the neural mediation of memory function has been established; however, it is not clear that ET improves memory or is neuroprotective.

based on the assumption that the brain depends on estrogen for normal function, even in the postmenopausal milieu; that is, if the reduction of endogenous estrogen is associated with decline in cognition, exogenous replacement would be expected to restore normal function. While this is a reasonable expectation and positive neural actions of estrogen have been established, the efficacy of estrogen therapy (ET) for enhancement of memory function or prophylaxis against memory impairment has not been clearly demonstrated. There are numerous methodological issues that make the study of ET a daunting task. Some of these issues include the healthy user bias that confounds observational studies, issues of dosage, regimen, and route of administration of estrogen, and cohort differences, in particular the age at which ET is initiated.

Cognitive Aging

Data from the United Nations Population Division, compiled in 2003, indicate that the median age in industrialized countries will rise from 37 years in 2000 to 50 years in 2050. Accordingly, industrialized cultures, including the United States, are moving toward a time when a near majority of the female population will be postmenopausal and risk of age-associated cognitive decline will affect a very substantial portion of the population as a whole. It is expected that the prevalence of dementia in the United States will increase from 4 to 14 million cases by the year 2050, and advancing age represents the greatest single risk factor for the development of neurodegenerative disorders.[6]

Measurable cognitive impairment and neuropathological changes predate clinical manifestations and diagnosis of dementia by several years and are suggestive of a disease process with latent and malignant phases.[6] The development of Alzheimer's disease (AD) has been characterized as an extended process marked by a preliminary period of *initiation* involving a number of mechanisms, most prominently inflammation, apoptosis, and oxidative stress, followed by *propagation*, in which self-reinforcing molecular cascades accelerate pathogenesis.[7] Brain regions most vulnerable to the damaging effects of inflammation, apoptosis, and free radical generation are those involved in memory and higher-order cognition. These phases (initiation and propagation) have been linked to early clinical manifestations (such as mild cognitive impairment [MCI]) and dementia (AD), respectively. Thus, age-related changes in cognitive function are a significant concern, even during middle age—a period during which processes affecting neurodegeneration already may have begun.

KEY POINT

Neurodegenerative processes develop over many years and diseases such as AD tend to affect new learning, memory, and adaptational functions.

MCI has been recognized as a condition representing the initial clinical manifestation of the neurodegenerative processes associated with AD and other potentially dementing conditions.[8] MCI is defined as significant memory impairment in the relative absence of generalized intellectual and functional deficiency. The notion of early, isolated memory impairment corresponds with neuropathological evidence indicating early cell loss in entorhinal cortex and within the hippocampus (regions mediating new learning and memory consolidation), and subsequent progression to more widespread degeneration of medial temporal lobe and neocortical structures.[9] Longitudinal studies have documented rates of progression from MCI to AD ranging from 10 to 15% per year. In samples of individuals with MCI, the prevalence rates of AD are 50–60% after 5 years.[8,10]

In general, so-called normal age-related cognitive decline is similar in nature, albeit not in extent, to the manifestations of dementia. These manifestations include, most prominently, decline of executive function and memory abilities as well as diminished speed of information processing. Individuals with incipient dementia demonstrate diminished metabolic activity in the frontal, temporal, and parietal lobes.[11] Executive and working memory processes associated with prefrontal and other neocortical regions are crucial to initial information storage and encoding, while medial temporal lobe structures, including the hippocampus, mediate integration of episodic information and consolidation of new learning. Accordingly, the cerebral structures that mediate problem-solving, learning, and adaptational functions appear to be the most vulnerable to the deleterious effects of age and neurodegenerative disease.

Cognitive-Cerebral Function in Perimenopause

Estrogen Effects on Cognitive-Cerebral Function

Epidemiological evidence has been cited in the past to suggest that women may have greater risk than men for AD. This view has been challenged by more recent data,[12] although there may be differentially higher risk for women among the very old. Nonetheless, there are gender differences in brain structure and physiology produced by differences in gonadal hormones during early development, and decline in cerebral function following menopause may be related to diminished estrogen levels at gender-specific sites in the brain.

KEY POINT

Estrogen actions in brain mediate a number of nonreproductive functions, most prominently memory.

Estrogens have multiple effects in many brain regions mediated through a variety of mechanisms.[13] These actions involve sustaining and regulating neural function as well as prophylaxis against neural damage. Among the many mechanisms of action, the more important with respect to cognitive function are regulation of serotonergic, cholinergic, and catecholamine neurotransmitter systems, inhibition of β-amyloid protein production, regulation of glucocorticoid levels, and modulation of dendritic connections in the hippocampus.[13] In addition, estrogen has potent neurotrophic effects in the hippocampus during development and in other brain regions in adulthood, in particular neocortex and hippocampus.[14] Neocortex and hippocampus are the regions that mediate selective attention, working memory, and episodic memory functions. Direct neural effects have been detected in animal studies in which estrogen has been shown to induce production of new dendritic spines and to have synaptogenic effects in the hippocampus. In humans, estrogen actions occur in the brain regions that mediate cognition, in particular medial temporal lobe structures involved in episodic memory function. Enhancing effects on brain structures and on cognitive function can be observed in a relatively brief time frame. Functional brain imaging using single photon emission computerized tomography (SPECT) has shown increased cerebral blood flow, especially in the medial temporal lobe (hippocampal region) following short-term ET, and these changes have been associated with improved verbal memory performance.[13] More recently, it has been shown that elderly menopausal women involved in ET had generally greater regional cerebral blood flow that increased with duration of ET. The most prominent increases involved hippocampal structures, and significant improvement in memory ability was observed in comparison with subjects who did not receive ET.[15]

To the extent that there is increased vulnerability for dementia resulting from the decline of endogenous estrogen after menopause, there would appear to be gender-specific opportunity for treatment with estrogenic agents. However, such therapeutic effects have yet to be demonstrated definitively. Earlier studies seemed to indicate that ET might act as a protective factor against age-associated decline and dementia. In addition, ET was thought to improve cognition in nondemented older women as well as serve as an ameliorative agent for women with dementia. However, more recent data have raised the possibility that ET may worsen rather than improve cognition in the elderly.

A number of intervention studies indicated improved memory, and especially improved verbal memory, in postmenopausal women receiving ET.[16,17] These earlier studies involved relatively younger women who had undergone surgical menopause and, therefore, a rapid decline of endogenous estrogen levels. In these studies, a positive correlation of memory performance with measured serum estrogen levels was observed. Memory enhancement was shown with treatment protocols of 2–12 weeks' duration. This time course is consistent with observations in normally cycling young women who show changes in verbal and spatial task performance associated with different menstrual cycle phases, a period of several days.

Observational studies have also produced positive findings.[18] These studies, of course, are not interventional, and tend to be clinical- or community-based and often do not involve a prospective design. However, one recent community-based observational study that included a prospective design also indicated protective effects against the development of AD .[19] Observational studies are also susceptible to the healthy user bias, a sampling issue that results in a greater proportion of healthy and/or higher socioeconomic status (SES) subjects among the estrogen users than among nonusers. Since both health and SES are inversely related to cognitive impairment and risk for dementia, a component of the beneficial effect observed for estrogen users might be associated with those subjects' general health and demographic characteristics. On balance, the data suggest that estrogen improves or maintains cognition in younger women and, when initiated in middle age, may lower risk for development of age-related cognitive decline in late life.

KEY POINT

There is some empirical support for the notion that ET may maintain memory function in younger, menopausal women. However, there are recent indications of a negative effect on cognition when initiated in late life.

However, recent studies indicate that when ET is initiated later in life, and particularly at the stage of MCI or after the onset of dementia, it has no effect or may increase impairment.[20] This important result from a randomized, controlled trial of women with mild and moderate AD emphasizes the significance of the timing of the introduction of ET. This effect contrasts sharply with findings of observational studies indicating markedly beneficial effects on cognition, and especially for verbal memory of ET when introduced in healthy postmenopausal women.[18,19] Most recently, data from the Women's Health Initiative Memory Study, utilizing a double-blind, randomized, placebo-controlled design, found no benefit of estrogen plus progestin treatment with respect to mild cognitive decline in a very large cohort of women who were enrolled at age 65 and older.[21] Findings from the same trial also indicated that this therapy increased risk for dementia twofold, compared with women in the placebo arm.[22]

Discussion of Cases

CASE 1

A 42-year-old woman scheduled an appointment with her gynecologist specifically because of subjective memory problems that had persisted for about a year. She described forgetfulness, more difficulty recall names of familiar people, and diminished ability to focus and sustain attention on tasks. She had experienced night sweats, hot flushes, sleep disturbance, and occasional irritability over the last several months. The event that precipitated this visit was forgetting an appointment for lunch with a close friend. She is the primary homemaker, although her husband and children help her at home most of the time. There has been no change in her ability to complete tasks at home, although she has felt more overwhelmed, especially when entertaining guests. She is an interior designer and has her own business and works about 35 h/week, and felt that she was able to perform at work effectively and meet the expectations of her clients. However, she experiences more anxiety and feels less competent than formerly. Within the past year, her teenage daughter began menses, has become less cooperative and helpful at home, and has been spending more time with friends. The patient suspects that she may have a boyfriend but her daughter denies it. This has been a concern for the patient and has increased her stress. However, during an extended family vacation when the patient felt that family relationships were harmonious, she felt relaxed and was able to sleep undisturbed for longer periods. In this context of reduced stress, she did not notice the memory and attention problems. There is no prior depression or other psychiatric disturbance. She takes no medication but has increased consumption of soy foods during the last year.

This assessment suggests that the cognitive symptoms are concomitants of the perimenopausal symptoms and of the increased environmental stress that this patient has experienced. The context specificity and temporal relationship of the memory problems with the vasomotor symptoms and the stressful environment supports this impression. She would likely benefit from reassurance regarding the basis for her cognitive symptoms and from counseling regarding ways to reduce stress, especially with respect to the symptomatic period of the menopause transition. One would expect that this sort of intervention might lead to enhancement of cognitive resources and a reduction of related symptoms.

Perimenopausal Symptoms

The course and severity of perimenopausal symptoms vary across individuals. Symptoms may begin in the earliest stages of the menopause transition, although they generally tend to be most prominent in the later phases.[23] Many women in Western cultures experience relatively dramatic symptomatic changes during perimenopause, especially during the last year during which menstrual cycles occur and the first year following the final cycle. While women in some non-Western cultures characteristically experience fewer and less severe symptoms (the Japanese culture) or no symptom at all (the Mayan culture), it is noteworthy that the time course of the female climacteric is not changed in these cultures. Cross-cultural differences in symptom manifestation suggest the possibility that environmental factors such as diet and level of physical activity may have a significant moderating impact on physiology and the psychological experience of the menopause transition, and there are data suggesting that level of physical activity is associated with mood regulation.[24]

The most prominent symptoms are the vasomotor symptoms, hot flushes, and night sweats. But central nervous system (CNS) and psychological symptoms, such as sleep disturbance, migraine, and mood changes are common as well. Concentration and memory problems also are reported, often in association with these symptoms. There is also evidence that dysthymia and irritability may be associated with vasomotor symptoms. Rates of mood disturbance vary during the course of reproductive senescence and are highest in women during perimenopause, lowest in older postmenopausal women, and at moderate levels in early postmenopausal women.[25] Furthermore, vasomotor symptoms appear to contribute to depressive symptoms even in the absence of perceived sleep disturbance and regardless of levels of estradiol, findings supporting the notion that mood changes in perimenopause are a concomitant of vasomotor symptoms.[26]

An important question concerning cognitive function during perimenopause is whether the cognitive symptoms that many women report represent functional changes related to perturbations of reproductive hormones, secondary concomitants of the other symptoms, or age-associated changes. While there are some observational studies that document complaints of memory impairment in perimenopausal women, there are very few that utilize formal evaluation to assess the neuropsychological status of these women, and the existing empirical data would seem to indicate that when memory complaints occur in perimenopause, they are related to other symptoms.

The assessment of perceived memory function and associated symptoms in the Seattle Midlife Women's Health Study represents one of the better observational studies of memory and perimenopausal symptoms.[27] It incorporated a longitudinal design with annual evaluations for up to 8 years. The memory assessment was based on a questionnaire inquiring about several categories of everyday memory ability such as forgetfulness. Subjects rated their memory ability but were not evaluated with objective procedures. The results indicated that while nearly 50% of the sample endorsed memory problems, relatively few rated the problems as serious. Negative health status and depressive symptoms were correlated with all categories of perceived memory difficulty at each phase of perimenopause. While these associations cannot be viewed as indicating that poor health, increased symptomology, and mood disturbance caused the memory difficulties, they are suggestive. Furthermore, younger women in earlier phases of perimenopause reported more memory difficulty, and those women, regardless of age or stage, who had relatively less symptomology reported less memory disturbance. As noted in another investigation, although 62% of midlife women reported subjective decline in memory, it is not clear whether these results represent measurable changes in memory or other aspects of cognition.[28]

One of the few studies that objectively evaluated symptoms and memory function in perimenopause with neuropsychological tests failed to find significant decline in neuropsychological measures of memory function.[29] In this study, vasomotor symptoms, memory complaints, and neuropsychological tests of memory ability were administered to premenopausal and perimenopausal women. Perimenopausal women endorsed significantly more symptoms and memory complaints than premenopausal women. However, there was no significant difference in memory performance on neuropsychological measures between perimenopausal and premenopausal women. In addition, a significant association between memory complaints and psychological distress was found. The findings suggested that memory complaints in perimenopausal women were related to symptoms rather than to objectively measured cognitive difficulty. This study did not analyze differences with respect to the stage of perimenopausal, control for possible age differences between the groups, or address the endocrinological differences between the premenopausal and perimenopausal women. Such demographic and endocrinological factors are particularly salient. If there were little or no difference in demographic and endocrinological factors, this fact would enhance the meaningfulness of the finding that there was no difference in memory ability between the groups. Nonetheless, this research provides additional corroboration for the notion that memory complaints are closely linked to symptoms during perimenopausal and that women with forgetfulness and other symptoms may not demonstrate measurable memory disorder.

CASE 2

A 48-year-old woman was seen in the clinic for a regular examination. She had not had a menstrual cycle for 15 months and felt that the moderate vasomotor symptoms associated with the menopause transition had largely resolved. On further questioning, she described an increase in word-finding difficulty and problems with short-term memory that had persisted and possibly worsened over a 2-year period. The memory problems were more troubling as they sometimes interfered with performance in her part-time job as well as increased inefficiency at home. She felt that she was not able to get as much done at work or at home, often because she lost track of her intentions or goals when performing tasks. She also tended to begin tasks but leave them undone for extended periods, something that formerly had been uncharacteristic. She reported that her husband seemed to notice the memory changes and that her daughter had confronted her about her forgetfulness on several occasions. She was not using hormone therapy. The patient was generally healthy with some arthritis, moderate weight gain during the last several years, and slightly elevated blood pressure. There was no psychiatric or neurological history and no major change in medication or alteration in environmental factors that might affect cognitive function. Her sleep habits were not changed, and she denied that she was experiencing mood disturbance.

In order to evaluate the apparent memory decline more objectively, the Clinical Dementia Rating (CDR) scale[30] was administered during the office visit. Her CDR score was 0.5, which is consistent with questionable dementia or MCI. This suggested a modest but meaningful decline in memory ability that was affecting functioning to a significant extent. In view of this, she was referred for more comprehensive evaluation by a neuropsychologist to determine the nature and extent of the cognitive impairment and to obtain baseline data against which the results of future studies might be compared.

Verbal Memory Ability in Young and Middle-Aged Women

Because declining memory function is the cardinal sign of cognitive aging and the chief complaint of aging women, memory ability is the most salient function to evaluate during adult development. We have accumulated memory performance data for 361 young adult and middle-aged women ranging in age from 18 to 59 years. Cross-sectional samples were recruited from among university students and community-dwelling women. All of the women were healthy, and none were referred from clinical programs or were receiving hormone replacement. The age range of this sample represents a substantial portion of the reproductive life span, specifically, from prime childbearing years through menopause. The memory measure used in this study was the Verbal Paired Associate Test (V-PAL).[31] This type of memory task requires subjects to form novel associations between common words (e.g., garden–note). It is a widely used memory measure that makes demands on executive function resources as well as memory consolidation ability. It is among the most sensitive tasks for evaluating age-associated memory decline. A verbal intelligence estimate[32] and a measure of mood disturbance[33] were also administered.

Six age cohorts were generated, each comprising a 6-year age range. Table 4-1 shows that there were statistical differences between the cohorts on the IQ measure. However, intelligence estimates for all the cohorts were in the average range (101–110), and the statistical differences do not reflect meaningful variation on this factor. Also shown in Table 4-1 are large group differences

Table 4-1. **DEMOGRAPHIC INFORMATION AND MOOD IN YOUNG AND MIDDLE-AGED WOMEN**

Age Cohort	*Education (Years)*	*PPVT**	*POMS-TMD†*
18–24	13.2	103.1	31.8
25–31	14.2	102.8	28.9
32–38	13.9	101.8	52.2
39–45	14.5	108.4	42.4
46–52	14.4	106.5	21.3
53–59	14.1	110.3	10.8

Abbreviations: PPVT, Peabody Picture Vocabulary Test (Ref. 32) standard score equivalent (IQ estimate); POMS-TMD, Profile of Mood States-Total Mood Disturbance score (Ref. 33).

Note: All data represent group means, except cohort age ranges.

*Overall cohort difference at $P < 0.05$.

†Overall cohort difference at $P < 0.001$.

in levels of mood disturbance, which were confirmed statistically. It is notable that the women in cohort 6, all of whom were postmenopausal, endorsed the lowest levels of mood disturbance, suggesting that after menopause there is less emotional upheaval, a common observation. In addition, higher levels of mood disturbance were observed during the perimenopausal years, especially in cohorts 3 and 4. Most importantly, mood disturbance scores were not correlated with memory performance ($P > 0.14$), suggesting that emotional factors were not related to memory ability in this sample. Ancillary correlational analyses also showed that there was no significant association of memory performance with mood within any individual group.

Figure 4-1 shows that memory performance declined with age. Post hoc analyses indicated a significant difference between the groups attributable to lower memory scores for cohorts 5 and 6 as compared with both cohort 1 and cohort 2. Given that this is a cross-sectional investigation, it is possible that these age differences do not reflect age-related decline in memory performance but

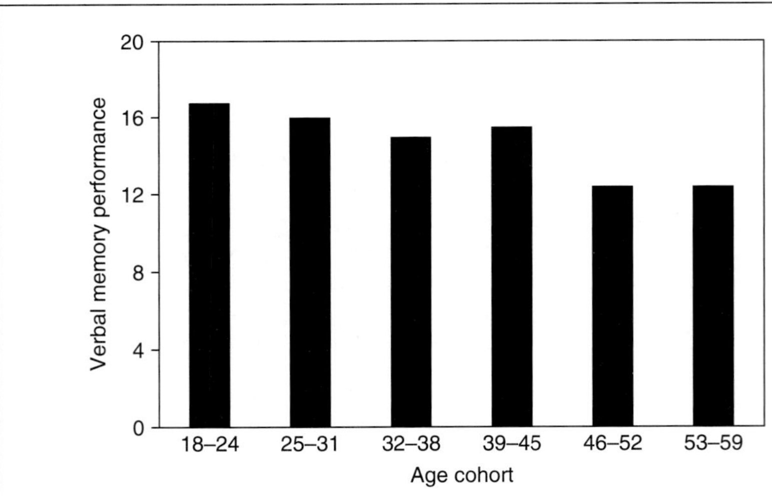

Figure 4-1: Age differences in verbal memory performance. Statistical differences in verbal paired associate learning performance (Ref. 31) were demonstrated in this cross-sectional study. Women in the two oldest cohorts exhibited significantly worse performance than women in the two youngest cohorts suggesting an age-related effect on memory function in healthy, untreated peri- and postmenopausal women.

rather inherent differences in memory ability between the cohorts. However, this concern is mitigated substantially because the age categories are relatively narrow and are continuous across the entire age range. Overall, the data demonstrated a relatively constant decline in performance. Accordingly, it is likely that the obtained age differences represent genuine change in memory performance, which would suggest that the perimenopausal and postmenopausal women in this sample experienced a decline in memory ability. This decline corresponds to the phase of perimenopause in which there is the greatest reduction in estrogen levels,[34] suggesting the possibility that this hormonal change mediated the difference in memory performance. However, the fact that the memory decline was observed in the oldest cohorts allows for the possibility that other, age-related factors contributed to this effect.

Guiding Questions

- Are the memory problems truly recently acquired rather than lifelong difficulties?
- What is the nature of the memory difficulty?
- To what extent do the memory problems impair everyday functioning?
- Are the memory problems associated with environmental changes that have increased cognitive demands in general, caused increased stress, or produced a persistent distraction?
- Do the memory problems vary in accordance with the presence or absence of vasomotor symptoms and/or mood disturbance?
- Has there been a past depressive episode, in particular associated with the premenstrual or postpartum periods?

What's the Evidence?

Much of the available data would seem to indicate that concentration and memory problems experienced during perimenopause are related to vasomotor symptoms and possibly mediated by the same mechanisms that produce such symptoms—the perturbations of reproductive hormones. Under this view, memory complaints should be temporary and might be expected to be resolved with the termination of the menopause transition. This view is supported by the observational studies and questionnaire data and at least in part by an investigation using an objective measure of memory ability.

However, there may also be a genuine decline in memory ability during perimenopause that has not been adequately investigated to this point and which, ironically, may be masked by the reports of vasomotor symptoms and other subjective changes. The preliminary data presented in Fig. 4-1 suggest that age-related changes in memory function might occur during perimenopause. The cohort data indicated that healthy, untreated women show objective decline in memory performance during age periods that correspond to late perimenopause and early postmenopause. It may be that this sort of effect has not been observed previously because it has not been studied objectively with longitudinal or closely spaced cross-sectional samples. Clearly, these findings require replication.

For some women, such changes in memory represent benign age-related effects but for others they may indicate initiation of a pathological process that will accelerate over time and ultimately produce dementia. Both scenarios exist and it may ultimately be possible to differentiate these conditions and, thereby, predict outcome on the basis of changes in memory function during perimenopause. This would allow intervention during the initiation stage of the neurodegenerative course.[35] However, at this time, the instrumentation that would allow such prediction does not exist.

Conclusion

Certainly, there is a need for more comprehensive and objective empirical study of cognitive function during the perimenopausal period. Given the prospects for an increasing number of older adults with cognitive deterioration, prevention, early detection, and amelioration of the neurodegenerative process represent the optimal means of coping with this problem. However, preventive and early intervention approaches remain underdeveloped options to date. The development and application of accurate detection of pathological, age-associated cognitive impairment is a highly significant public health issue because we are on the threshold of a virtual epidemic of dementia, given the demographics and health status of our aging population. Understanding memory decline in middle age and during the perimenopause is an important first step in this endeavor. Such knowledge could be utilized along with an understanding of how hormone therapy might be used to preserve and ameliorate cognitive-cerebral function as a means of greatly reducing the risk for dementia.

If decline in memory initiated by menopause is confirmed, this might be taken as an indication for instituting a course of ET in the late phase of the perimenopause, especially in light of the evidence of prophylaxis for those receiving such treatment in midlife. This may enhance memory function and help to lower risk for future decline. Data from an animal model support a hypothetical basis for such a prophylactic effect with respect to midlife ET in the context of coronary artery disease as well as for worsening of the disease with institution of replacement therapy later in life.[36] Similarly, recent data from the Women's Health Initiative Memory Study has indicated a negative effect on memory of combined estrogen and progestin therapy in women who began treatment late in life.[21] It is quite possible that these cardiovascular and cerebral effects have common etiological mechanisms, possibly involving estrogen-induced inflammatory processes that would increase risk for both cardiovascular illness and neurodegenerative conditions such as AD.[37] The complexity of the mechanisms of estrogen's effects and possible interactions of ET with life-stage-specific processes require that we perform careful studies of both reproductive and nonreproductive effects at different phases of development in order to understand if and how estrogen may be used as a beneficial agent. While ET is a theoretically attractive concept, it is not clear that it is a beneficial intervention, even if administered for a limited period at the time of menopause.

References

1 Brody JA, Grand MD, Frateschi LJ, et al. Epidemiology and aging: maximum reproductive age unaffected by increase life expectancy in the twentieth century. *Aging.* 1998;10:170.

2 Reame NE. Neuroendocrine regulation of the perimenopause transition. In: Lobo RA, Kelsey J, Marcus R, eds. *Menopause: Biology and Pathobiology.* San Diego, CA: Academic Press; 2000:95.

3 Wise PM. Estrogens: protective or risk factors in brain function? *Prog Neurobiol.* 2003;69:181.

4 Richards M, Kuh D, Hardy R, et al. Lifetime cognitive function and timing of natural menopause. *Neurology.* 1999;53:308.

5 McEwen BS. Estrogen actions throughout the brain. *Recent Prog Horm Res.* 2002;57:357.

6 Katzman R, Kawas C. The epidemiology of dementia and Alzheimer disease. In: Terry RD, Katzman R, Bick KL, eds. *Alzheimer Disease.* New York: Raven Press; 1994.

7 Cotman CW. Homeostatic process in brain aging: the role of apoptosis, inflammation, and oxidative stress in regulating healthy neural circuitry in the aging brain. In: Stern PC, Carstensen LL, eds. *The Aging Mind.* Washington, DC: National Academy Press; 2000:114.

8 Petersen RC, Doody R, Kruz A, et al. Current concepts in Mild Cognitive Impairment. *Arch Neurol.* 2001;58:1985.

9 Morrison JH. Age-related shifts in neural circuit characteristics and their impact on age-related cognitive impairment. In: Stern PC, Carstensen LL, eds. *The Aging Mind.* Washington, DC: National Academy Press; 2000:83.

10 Morris JC, McKeel DW, Storandt M. Very mild Alzheimer's disease: informant-based clinical, psychometric, and pathologic distinction from normal aging. *Neurology.* 1991;41:469.

11 Small GW, Ercoli LM, Silverman DH, et al. Cerebral metabolic and cognitive decline in persons at genetic risk for Alzheimer's disease. *Proc Natl Acad Sci U S A.* 2000;97:6037.

12 Ruitenberg A. Incidence of dementia: does gender make a difference? *Neurobiol Aging.* 2001;22:575.

13 McEwen BS, Alves SE. Estrogen actions in the central nervous system. *Endocr Rev.* 1999;20:279.

14 Greene JD, Miles K, Hodges JR. Neuropsychology of memory and SPECT in the diagnosis of dementia of Alzheimer type. *J Neurol.* 1996;243:175.

15 Maki PM, Resnick SM. Longitudinal effects of estrogen replacement therapy on PET cerebral blood flow and cognition. *Neurobiol Aging.* 2000;21:373.

16 Sherwin B. Estrogenic effects on memory in women. *Ann N Y Acad Sci.* 1994;743:213.

17 Wolf OT, Kudielka BM, Hellhammer DH, et al. Two weeks of transdermal estradiol treatment in postmenopausal elderly women and its effect on memory and mood: verbal memory changes are associated with the treatment induced estradiol level. *Psychoneuroendocrinology.* 1999; 24:727.

18 Jacobs DM, Tang MX, Stern Y, et al. Cognitive function in nondemented older women who took estrogen after menopause. *Neurology.* 1998;50:368.

19 Zandi PP, Carlson MC, Plassman BL, et al. Hormone replacement therapy and incidence of Alzheimer disease in older women: the Cache County Study. *JAMA.* 2002;288:2123.

20 Mulnard RA, Cotman CW, Kawas C, et al. Estrogen replacement therapy for treatment of mild to moderate Alzheimer's disease. *JAMA.* 2000;283:1007.

21 Rapp SR, Espeland MA, et al. Effect of estrogen plus progestin on global cognitive function in postmenopausal women. *JAMA.* 2003; 289:2663.

22 Schumaker SA, Legault C, Rapp SR, et al. Estrogen plus progestin and the incidence of dementia and mild cognitive impairment in postmenopausal women. *JAMA.* 2003;289:2651.

23 Soules MR, Sherman S, Parrott E, et al. Executive summary: stages of reproductive aging workshop (STRAW) Park City, Utah, July 2001. *Menopause.* 2001;8:402.

24 Joffe H, Hall JE, Soares CN, et al. Vasomotor symptoms are associated with depression in perimenopausal women seeking primary care. *Menopause.* 2002;9:389.

25 Avis NE, Crawford S, Stellato R, et al. Longitudinal study of hormone levels and depression among women transitioning through menopause. *Climacteric.* 2001;4:243.

26 Slaven L, Lee C. Mood and symptom reporting among middle-aged women: the relationship between menopausal status, hormone replacement therapy, and exercise participation. *Health Psychol.* 1997;16:203.

27 Woods NF, Mitchell ES, Adams C. Memory functioning among midlife women: observations from the Seattle Midlife Women's Health Study. *Menopause.* 2000;7:257.

28 Maki P, Hogervorst E. HRT and cognitive decline. *Baillieres Best Pract Res Clin Endocrinol Metab.* 2003;17:105.

29 Pickholtz JL. Self-assessment of memory function and memory test performance in perimenopausal women. *Diss Abstr Int: Sci Eng.* 2001;16:4423.

30 Hughes CP, Berg L, Danziger WL, et al. A new clinical scale for the staging of dementia. *Br J Psychiatry.* 1982;140:566.

31 Krikorian R. Independence of verbal and spatial paired associate learning. *Brain Cogn.* 1996;32:219.

32 Williams K, Wang JJ. *Technical References to the Peabody Picture Vocabulary Test-third edition.* Circle Pines, MN, American Guidance Service, 1997.

33 McNair D, Lorr M, Droppleman L. *Manual for the Profile of Mood States.* San Diego, CA: Educational and Industrial Testing Service; 1992.

34 Burger HG, Dudley EL, Robertson DM, et al. Hormonal changes in the menopause transition. *Recent Prog Horm Res.* 2002;57:257.

35 Russo-Neustadt AA, Beard RC, Huan YM, et al. Physical activity and antidepressant treatment potentiate the expression of specific brain-derived neurotrophic factor transcripts in the rat hippocampus. *Neuroscience.* 2000;101:305.

36 Koras RH, Clarkson TB. Considerations in interpreting the cardiovascular effects of hormone replacement therapy observed in the WHI: timing is everything. *Menopausal Med*[s8]. 2003;10:8.

37 Marriott LK, Hauss-Wegrzyniak B, Benton RS, et al. Long-term ET worsens the behavioral and neuropathological consequences of chronic brain inflammation. *Behav Neurosci.* 2002;116:902.

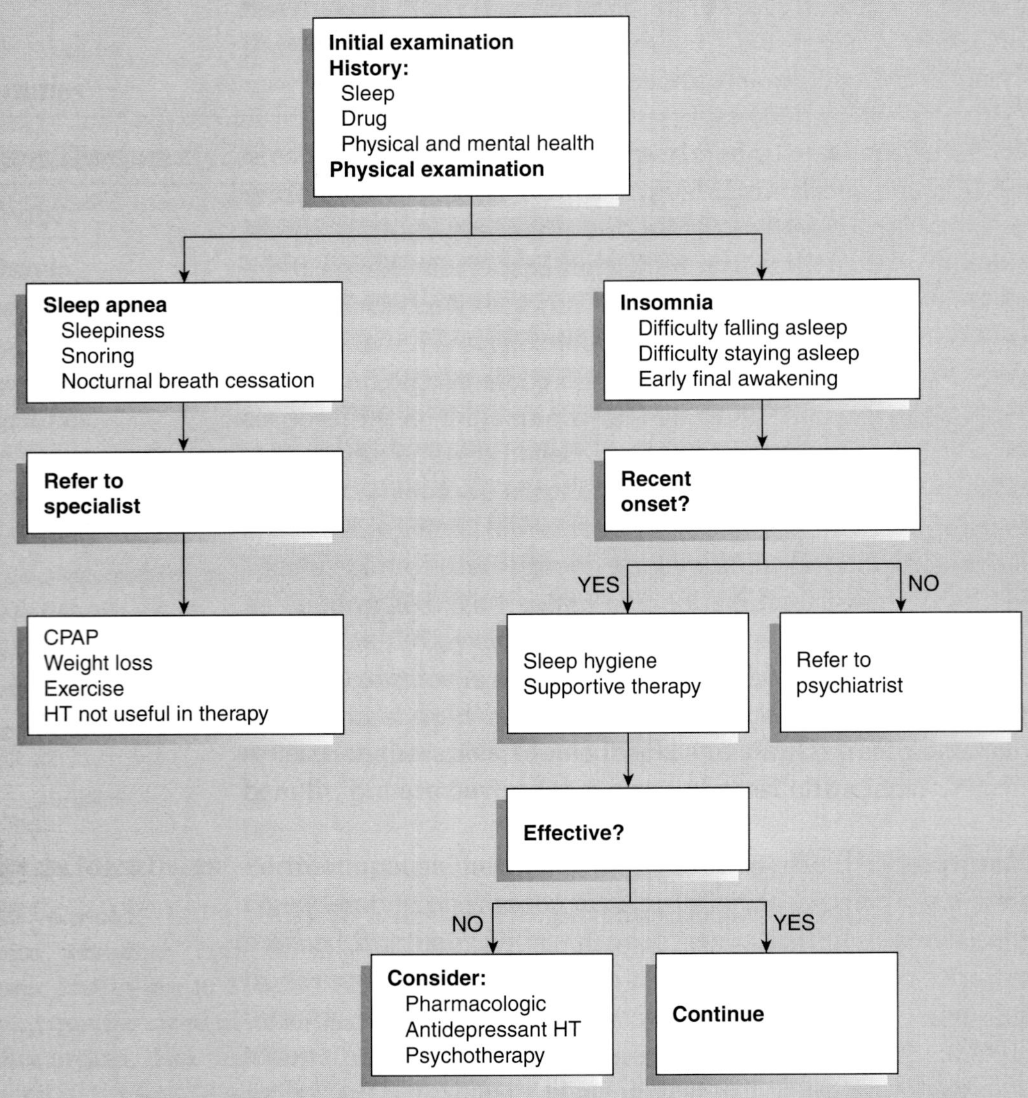

Diagnosis and Management of Sleep Disturbance
Initial examination
History:
Sleep
Drug
Physical and mental health
Physical examination
Sleep apnea
Sleepiness
Snoring
Nocturnal breath cessation
Insomnia
Difficulty falling asleep
Difficulty staying asleep
Early final awakening
Refer to specialist
Recent onset?
YES
NO
CPAP
Weight loss
Exercise
HT not useful in therapy
Sleep hygiene
Supportive therapy
Refer to psychiatrist
Effective?
NO
YES
Consider:
Pharmacologic
Antidepressant HT
Psychotherapy
Continue

5 Sleep Disorders in Perimenopausal and Menopausal Women, Diagnosis and Clinical Management

E.O. Bixler
A.N. Vgontzas

Introduction

KEY POINT

Incidence of insomnia and sleep apnea increase during the perimenopause.

The most common sleep disturbances observed in midlife women are complaints of inadequate sleep (insomnia) or disordered breathing during sleep (sleep apnea). Increases in both types of sleep disturbance are associated with midlife women as they approach menopause.

However, whether increased complaints of insomnia are directly linked to changes in hormonal levels is somewhat controversial. On the other hand, the association between sleep apnea and changes in hormonal levels is more clearly established. We will review the available evidence to support the association between both types of sleep disturbance and changing hormone levels and summarize guidelines for their diagnosis and management.

Insomnia

Subjective Complaint

Insomnia has been traditionally defined as a problem with difficulty falling asleep and staying asleep, or with an early final awakening.[1] More recently, the complaint of awakening feeling unrefreshed was added.[2] Insomnia is considered to be the most common sleep disorder.[1] Prevalence estimates, however, vary considerably depending upon the definition used.[3] Earlier studies employing the definition of a problem with falling asleep, staying asleep, or early final awakening reported estimates in the order of 33%. If the question employed was phrased as occasional insomnia or insomnia with no duration restriction, the estimates reported were lower (e.g., about 25%). When prevalence estimates required chronicity, then the prevalence reported was even lower (e.g., about 10%).

Insomnia has been found to be associated with a wide range of variables.[3] The class of variables most consistently reported is the association with psychopathology. For example, insomnia is commonly employed as a diagnostic criterion for psychiatric disorders and conversely, psychopathology is commonly present in patients with insomnia. The strong association between insomnia and psychopathology has been repeatedly demonstrated in terms of improvement in one dimension by treatment in another. Finally, there are longitudinal epidemiologic data that demonstrate that the presence of insomnia at baseline is associated with increased risk for new-onset major depression at follow-up.

KEY POINT

Women are at greater risk for insomnia than men.

There is a strong consensus that women are at a greater risk for insomnia than are men.[1,3] This may be at least partially explained by the finding that women are also more at risk for depression. This increased risk for depression includes the milder dsythymic depression, which is the most common depressive disorder associated with insomnia.

There is consensus that the prevalence of insomnia increases with age.[1] In a large general sample, aged 3–94 years, Lugaresi observed that the prevalence of the complaint of insomnia increased in both men and women at a similar rate until age 40.[4] After age 40, the prevalence of insomnia in women showed a dramatic increase compared to men. Based on this observation, he speculated that this increase in prevalence at age 40 for women was associated with the onset of menopause. This speculation was confirmed in another study based on a subsample of a very large cohort established by the American Cancer Society.[5]

There have been several studies specifically designed to assess the association between menopause and insomnia.[6,7] The consensus is that menopause is associated with an increase in complaints of insomnia with only a few studies not finding any association when evaluated using cross-sectional analysis. There is also consensus that the presence of hot flushes increases the risk for a complaint of insomnia.

KEY POINT

Vasomotor symptoms increase the risk for insomnia.

Vasomotor symptoms increase the risk for insomnia. Insomnia does, however, also occur in perimenopausal women who are not experiencing hot flushes.

Many of the studies assessing the association between insomnia and menopause did not control for age leaving open the question of whether changes due to age could account for the association between insomnia and menopause. A recent study from the Wisconsin Sleep Cohort evaluated sleep patterns in 589 women followed up for 4 years. This study controlled for both age and body mass index (BMI) and observed that a complaint of difficulty initiating sleep was associated with perimenopause but not with postmenopause.[8]

KEY POINT

Difficulty initiating sleep is associated with perimenopause.

Difficulty initiating sleep is associated with perimenopause. In addition, the complaint of dissatisfied sleep was associated with both perimenopause and postmenopause. However, no other sleep complaints were associated with either perimenopause or postmenopause, including waking up during the night, awakening too early, or excessive daytime sleepiness. These findings suggest that perimenopause or postmenopause are not strong predictors of specific sleep complaints.

The use of HT as a means of reducing the risk of a complaint of insomnia is generally supported by data.[6,7,9] In cross-sectional observational samples, it appears that women who are taking HT are at higher risk for a complaint of insomnia. This unexpected association in these observational studies could be due to a possible confounding effect of women with more severe symptoms being more likely to be prescribed HT. In a longitudinal study, however, it was observed that there was an increased risk for insomnia only in those women who became menopausal without HT. Several trials of HT compared to placebo have been reported and the consensus from

KEY POINT

The recent Women's Health Initiative Study observed that the women assigned to hormone therapy (HT) had a lower risk for insomnia than those assigned to a placebo.

these studies is that the complaint of sleep disturbance is reduced with HT. The recent Women's Health Initiative Study observed that the women assigned to HT had a lower risk for insomnia than those assigned to a placebo at year 1 but not at year 3.[10]

Depressive symptoms appear to be associated with perimenopause, especially in women with vasomotor symptoms.[11] It has also been observed that women with a lifetime history of major depression tend to have an earlier decline in ovarian function.[12] Finally, treating perimenopausal women with psychotherapy or antidepressants combined with HT have been shown to be effective.[13] These data strongly suggest that the increased complaints of sleep disturbance in menopausal women may be associated with increased mood disturbances.

Objective Sleep Disturbance

It is commonly observed that the ability to sleep weakens with increasing age. Recently, we evaluated sleep patterns in a subset of 1324 adults aged 20–100 years without a complaint of a sleep disorder from the Penn State Cohort of the general public who were evaluated in the sleep laboratory.[14] In this subsample we observed that the ability to sleep worsened with age. This decrease in the ability to sleep with age included both the amount of sleep as well as sleep stage patterns (e.g., amounts of deep sleep and rapid eye movement [REM] sleep). Recently, Vgontzas has reported a possible mechanism for this decrease in sleep efficiency with increasing age.[15] Both stress hormones, corticotrophin-releasing hormone (CRH) and cortisol, are known to stimulate arousal wakefulness and inhibit slow-wave sleep. In a sample of young and middle-aged men, he injected a bolus of CRH after sleep onset and observed the anticipated increase of cortisol in both groups. However, it was only in the middle-aged group that an increase in wakefulness compared to the young group was observed indicating that the middle-aged group was much more sensitive to the arousal effects of CRH and/or cortisol.

KEY POINT

Both stress hormones, CRH and cortisol are known to stimulate arousal wakefulness and inhibit slow-wave sleep.

In the subsample of normal sleepers from the Penn State Cohort, we also evaluated the effects of gender on polysomnographically-recorded sleep.[14] We observed that women compared to men tended to sleep better in terms of both sleep efficiency as well as sleep stage patterns. This improved sleep occurred primarily between the ages of 45–70 years. A similar lack of objective sleep disturbance associated with perimenopause or menopause was observed in the subsample of women from the Wisconsin Sleep Cohort.[8] Thus, objective polysomnographic data do not support the assumed increase of sleep deterioration associated with menopause. There are, however, some objective data that would support the observation that the presence of hot flushes may be associated with some degree of sleep disturbance.[14]

KEY POINT

Estrogen does have sleep improving effects.

There are limited polysomnographic data available that support the efficacy of HT in terms of improving sleep.[6–8] It appears that estrogen does have sleep improving effects. Progesterone in the doses employed does not seem to add much in terms of sleep efficiency, even though in higher doses it has a marked sedative effect.

It would appear that the increased prevalence of a complaint of insomnia in women is incompatible with the observation that women tend to sleep better than men.[12] However, this apparent inconsistency can at least partially be understood in terms of the strong relationship between insomnia and depression.[1] Because women have an increased risk for depression, the complaint of insomnia may be more strongly associated with mood than actual time asleep. We have evaluated this question directly in the Penn State Cohort.[3] A subsample ($N = 1741$) was randomly selected for a single-night sleep laboratory polysomnographic evaluation from a larger random sample of the general public ($N = 16{,}583$), ranging in age from 20 to 100 years. The prevalence of chronic insomnia (duration 1 year) was 7.5%, while the prevalence of difficulty sleeping was another 22.4%. A multivariate logistic regression analysis indicated that depression was the single strongest factor followed by female gender for both chronic insomnia as well as difficulty sleeping. Another important observation was that the final model did not include menopause or HT status as well as age or BMI or any sleep laboratory findings. This finding strongly supports the position that mood variables would be the primary factor associated with difficulty sleeping in midlife women.

KEY POINT

Depression was the single strongest factor followed by female gender for both chronic insomnia as well as difficulty sleeping.

The available data support the association between complaints of sleep disturbance and perimenopause or menopause. When age is controlled, the association of menopause with specific sleep complaints is weakened. There does not appear to be any support for objective sleep disturbance associated with the onset on menopause. Thus, underlying sleep or mood disorders should be ruled out first before attributing a complaint of insomnia primarily to menopause.

Sleep Apnea

KEY POINT

Prevalence of sleep apnea peaks in the sixth decade for men and for women in the seventh.

Until very recently, it was assumed that sleep apnea was primarily associated with men. Several recent studies have demonstrated that the M:F ratio of sleep apnea is in the range of 2:1 to 4:1.[17–19] It was also originally assumed that the prevalence of sleep apnea increased linearly with age, i.e., the elderly were most at risk. In the Penn State Cohort, we observed that the prevalence of sleep apnea peaks in the sixth decade for men and for women in the seventh.[19,20] We also observed that the severity of sleep apnea decreased with age, which would be consistent with a possible genetic contribution.[20]

It has been demonstrated that menopause is a risk factor for sleep apnea when controlling for the relevant confounding factors by the Penn State Cohort[19] and confirmed by the Wisconsin Sleep Cohort.[21] In addition, a recent study observed that the M:F ratio of the incidence of sleep apnea declines with age, again suggesting that menopause is a risk factor for sleep apnea.[22] It has also been demonstrated in the Penn State Cohort and confirmed in the Sleep Heart Health Study, that HT use in postmenopausal women continued the protection from sleep apnea observed in premenopausal women.[19,23] This protective effect of HT for sleep apnea does appear to be limited in duration, i.e., women older than 70 years appeared to no longer be protected.[23]

In patients with significant central obesity (BMI >40 kg/m^2), there is approximately a 40% incidence of sleep-disordered breathing. In women, a neck circumference of 16 in. or greater is also a risk factor for sleep apnea.

Current studies have observed that metabolic factors play an important role in sleep apnea.[24] Specifically, there is a strong association between sleep apnea, type 2 diabetes, and insulin resistance, all factors of the metabolic syndrome. Women with polycystic ovary syndrome, which is the most common endocrine disorder in premenopausal women, are at high risk for sleep apnea and we speculate that this may at least partially account for premenopausal women with sleep apnea.[25]

KEY POINT

Hypertension is considered a major risk of sleep apnea.

Hypertension is considered a major risk of sleep apnea. There are currently four epidemiologic studies that have demonstrated that sleep apnea makes an independent contribution to the presence of hypertension when controlling for relevant confounding factors.[26–29] One of these studies established sleep apnea as an independent risk factor for hypertension after only a 4-year follow-up.[28] Gender appeared to be a contributing factor in only one of these studies.[27] The Sleep Heart Health Study observed that the fully adjusted model of the association between sleep apnea and hypertension remained significant for men but not for women. It must be remembered, however, that this study was based on an older cohort (mean age = 63 years) and the prevalence of sleep apnea would be expected to begin declining at about the mean age of this cohort. Thus, power may have been an issue. It has also been demonstrated in two of these studies that the strength of the association between sleep apnea and hypertension decreases with age (i.e., the association between sleep apnea and hypertension is weakest in the elderly).[27,29]

KEY POINT

Menopause is a strong independent risk factor for sleep apnea.

Data obtained from several epidemiologic studies have demonstrated that menopause is a strong independent risk factor for sleep apnea. Age is a confounding factor, as the prevalence of sleep apnea increases until about the age of 60 years and then declines. In postmenopausal women who use HT, the risk for sleep apnea appears to remain low at premenopausal levels, in spite of the increased age of these women. The major risk associated with sleep apnea is hypertension and other cardiovascular events. Thus, postmenopausal women who use HT appear to be at reduced risk for sleep apnea and thus at reduced risk for hypertension associated with sleep apnea.

Sleep Disorders Management

The two most frequent sleep disorders that perimenopausal and menopausal women present to their primary care physician or gynecologist are insomnia and sleep apnea.

Insomnia

Insomnia is manifested as difficulty falling asleep, difficulty staying asleep, early morning awakening, or a combination of the above. In a woman that experiences hot flushes, which are associated with a surge of sympathetic activity, difficulty falling or staying asleep may be a frequent complaint. While many menopausal women with insomnia report previous transient difficulties with sleep or that they have been "light" sleepers throughout life, some report onset of the sleep difficulty that coincides with the physiological changes associated with menopause, e.g., hot flushes. In all insomnia cases, it is important to obtain information about 24-hour sleep and wake patterns, including daytime fatigue and napping, mood swings, depression, and anxiety (see Table 5-1). Also, a history of substance abuse, such as alcohol or smoking cigarettes, family history of sleep and psychiatric disorders, as well as previous interventions for sleeplessness are an important element of the evaluation of this disorder. In the case of a preexisting insomnia that was exacerbated during menopause, psychiatric and emotional problems are frequent, thus, a psychiatric referral for outpatient pharmacotherapy and psychotherapy is warranted. If the onset of insomnia is placed around perimenopause or menopause, physiological changes may be primary causative factors, and sleep hygiene measures, appropriate exercise and diet, reassurance, and supportive therapy by the primary care physician are usually sufficient. Also, the short-term use of benzodiazepines, or sedative antidepressants (trazodone [Desyrel], nefazodone [Serzone], mirtazapine [Remeron]) if there is an indication for longer use, may be helpful.

A general outline of strategies to improve sleep hygiene is provided in Table 5-2. If the symptoms persist for more than 6 months and there is evidence of associated psychopathology, a referral to

Table 5-1. **SLEEP HISTORY SCREENING QUESTIONS**

What is your usual sleep routine?
- Focus on regular sleep/wake schedule
- Time spent in bed
- Other activities other than sleeping in bed

How long do you sleep every night?
Do you nap?
Do you wake up refreshed?
Are you tired during the daytime hours?
What are the potential lifestyle activities that may affect sleep?
- Caffeine
- Nicotine
- Late night exercise

Do you use medications to assist in getting to sleep
- Alcohol
- Over-the-counter medications
- Prescription medications
- Alternative medications

***Table 5-2.* SLEEP HYGIENE**

Optimal amount of sleep
7–8 hours usually adequate
Avoid extremes in duration
Do not force sleep
Regular schedules
Stabilize time to awaken
Set time to bed based on optimal amount of sleep
Maintain schedule 7 days a week
Avoid daytime naps
If you cannot sleep, get up and do something relaxing
Sleep environment
Control light, noise, temperature, and humidity
Improve bed comfort
Exercise
Establish regular exercise
Incorporate exercise into daily activities
Gradually increase exercise
Nutrition
Regularize eating habits
Avoid extreme weight changes
Light snack before bed may be helpful
Manage stress
Be aware of effects of age
Recognize association with stressful events
Tolerate occasional sleepiness
Relaxation exercises may help
Avoid drug-induced sleep disturbances
Minimize caffeine and cigarettes
Recognize that alcohol may disturb sleep
Assess role of stimulant or other medication on sleep

Source: Kales A, Kales D. *Evaluation and Treatment of Insomnia.* New York: Oxford University Press; 1984.

a psychiatrist or a sleep specialist should be considered. HT should be reserved for the more severe refractory cases of insomnia that are associated with persistent and more serious physiological changes such as sweats and hot flushes. HT should be considered for a specific period of time and after weighing the pros and cons of this intervention.

Sleep Apnea

It is now established that menopause is a risk factor for developing sleep-disordered breathing. Usually there are complaints by the bed partner of snoring or worsened snoring and nocturnal breath cessations. The patient subjectively may report daytime sleepiness and fatigue and occasionally waking up at night gasping for air or for unknown reasons. Usually the nighttime awakenings in an apneic person are brief compared to someone who suffers from insomnia. Other signs associated with increased risk of sleep-disordered breathing include weight gain, particularly from young age to middle age, or, after menopause, development of hypertension or other cardiovascular problems and diabetes as well as a family history of the latter conditions. In the presence of fatigue, routine laboratory work such as complete blood count with differential, urinalysis, erythrocyte sedimentation rate, fasting blood sugar, serum creatinine, and thyroid hormone levels is necessary to exclude secondary causes. If sleep apnea is suspected on clinical grounds, a referral to a sleep center and a standard polysomnogram is the next step. Although HT appears to play a protective role in sleep-disordered breathing in women, there is no evidence that it can improve or cure already existing sleep-disordered breathing. In addition to continuous positive airway pressure, which is the standard treatment for patients with sleep–disordered breathing, general lifestyle measures, such as weight loss and exercise, are important to improve sleep-disordered breathing, decrease fatigue, and enhance the feeling of well-being. If the sleep test is negative for sleep apnea, other disorders associated with fatigue should be considered, such as depression, obesity, diabetes, or autoimmune disorders such as fibromyalgia. Finally, the possibility of primary hypersomnia as a result of a significant drop of estrogen and progesterone levels should be considered and referral to a sleep center for further evaluation and treatment is warranted.

Discussion of Cases

CASE 1

A 47-year-old married woman complains of increasing difficulties with falling asleep and that she wakes up "not rested." She reports increasing intervals between her menstrual periods and hot flushes. She has tried over-the-counter *hypnotics* without significant relief. Her past history includes transient episodes of sleeplessness during periods of stress. She reports a mild degree of anxiety and "mood swings" but denies symptoms and signs of major depression or suicidality. She reports mild weight gain and an increase in her smoking from 5 to 10 cigarettes daily. She has been treated for hypothyroidism for many years. Her medical examination is unremarkable and routine blood tests are negative for abnormal findings. The patient is prescribed a relatively low dose of a sedative antidepressant and several sleep hygiene measures, such as quitting smoking, regular exercise, and avoiding staying in bed if not sleepy. She also attends "stress management" classes at a local fitness center. The patient experiences significant relief from her insomnia and continues the same regimen for 6 months. A follow-up visit indicates that both hot flushes and sleeplessness have subsided and she is recommended a gradual discontinuation of the low-dose antidepressant.

Case 2

A 53-year-old woman presents with a complaint of fatigue for the last several years. The onset of her fatigue appears to correlate with perimenopausal changes. The patient reports frequent brief awakenings at night and has been told that she snores loudly. She is not sure whether she stops breathing at night. She denies difficulty falling asleep or early morning awakening. She denies the auxiliary symptoms of narcolepsy, i.e., cataplexy, hypnagogic hallucinations, or sleep paralysis. Her past history is significant for chronic migraines, hypothyroidism, and hereditary hyperlipidemic syndrome. Her medical examination is negative for abnormal findings and routine blood work. Complete blood count (CBC), thyroid-stimulating hormone (TSH), sedimentation rate, creatinine, and fasting blood sugar are within normal limits. The patient denied having feelings of depression or anxiety. Also, there is no history of substance abuse. The patient's primary care physician prescribed trials on benzodiazepine hypnotics (i.e., flurazepam [Dalmane], estazolam [ProSom], triazolam [Halcion], zaleplon [Sonata], and zolpidem [Ambien]) and sedative antidepressants (i.e., tricyclic antidepressants, trazodone, and nefazodone). These medications reduced the number of nocturnal awakenings but did not decrease her daytime sleepiness. The patient was referred to a sleep center for sleep laboratory testing to rule out sleep apnea. Findings were negative for sleep-disordered breathing or nocturnal myoclonus. There were a moderate number of arousals, which, however, did not affect her sleep efficiency or sleep structure. A trial of trazodone did not improve her daytime sleepiness. A repeat nocturnal sleep testing associated with multiple sleep-onset latency test (the amount of time that it takes to fall asleep) showed sleep latencies that were in the pathologic range (<5 min). The patient was diagnosed with hypersomnia not otherwise specified (NOS) and was placed on stimulants which improved her daytime sleepiness.

References

1 Kales A, Kales D. *Evaluation and Treatment of Insomnia.* New York: Oxford University Press; 1984.

2 American Psychiatric Association. *Diagnostic and Statistical Manual of Mental Disorders Fourth Edition DSM-IV.* Washington, DC: American Psychiatric Association; 1994.

3 Bixler EO, Vgontzas AN, Lin H-M, et al. Insomnia in Central Pennsylvania. *J Psychosom Res.* 2002;53:589–592.

4 Lugaresi E, Cirignotta F, Zucconi M, et al. Good and poor sleepers: an epidemiological survey of the San Marino population. In: Guilleminault C, Lugaresi E, eds. *Sleep/Wake Disorders: Natural History, Epidemiology, and Long-Term Evolution.* New York: Raven Press; 1983.

5 Brugge KL, Kripke DF, Ancoli-Israel S, et al. The association of menopausal status and age with sleep disorders. *Sleep Res.* 1989; 18:208.

6 Shaver JLF, Zenk SA. Sleep disturbance in menopause. *J Women's Health Gend Based Med.* 2000;9:109–118.

7 Bixler EO, Vgontzas AN, Lin H-M, et al. Women and sleep related disorders. *Eur Respir Mon.* 2003;25:204–218.

8 Young T, Rabago D, Zgierska A, et al. Objective and subjective sleep quality in premenopausal, perimenopausal, and postmenopausal women in the Wisconsin Sleep Cohort study. *Sleep.* 2003;26: 667–672.

9 Manber R, Armitage R. Sex, steroids, and sleep: a review. *Sleep.* 1999; 22:540–555.

10 Hays J, Ockene JK, Brunner RL, et al. Effects of estrogen plus progestin on health-related quality of life. *N Engl J Med.* 2003;348: 1839–1854.

11 Joffe H, Hall JE, Soares CN, et al. Vasomotor symptoms are associated with depression in perimenopausal women seeking primary care. *Menopause.* 2002;9:392–398.

12 Harlow BL, Wise LA, Otto MW, et al. Depression and its influence on reproductive endocrine and menstrual cycle markers associated with perimenopause. *Arch Gen Psychiat.* 2003;60:29–36.

13 Anarte MT, Chadros JL, Herrera J. Hormonal and psychological treatment: therapeutic alternative for menopausal women? *Maturitas.* 1998;29:203–213.

14 Bixler EO, Vgontzas AN, Lin HM, et al. Normal sleep and sleep stage patterns: effects of age, BMI and gender. *Sleep.* 2003;26:A61.

15 Vgontzas AN, Bixler EO, Wittman AM, et al. Middle-aged men show higher sensitivity of sleep to the arousing effects of corticotropin-releasing hormone than young men: clinical implications. *J Clin Endocrinol Metab.* 2001;86:1489–1495.

16 Woodward S, Freedman RR. The thermoregulatory effects of menopausal hot flashes on sleep. *Sleep.* 1994;17:497–501.

17 Young T, Palta M, Dempsey J, et al. The occurrence of sleep-disordered breathing among middle-aged adults. *N Engl J Med.* 1993;328: 1230–1235.

18 Redline S, Kump K, Tishler PV, et al. Gender differences in sleep disordered breathing in a community-based sample. *Am J Respir Crit Care Med.* 1994;149:722–726.

19 Bixler EO, Vgontzas AN, Lin H-M, et al. Prevalence of sleep-disordered breathing in women: effects of gender. *Am J Respir Crit Care Med.* 2001;163:608–613.

20 Bixler EO, Vgontzas AN, Ten Have T, et al. Effects of age on sleep apnea in men: I. Prevalence and severity. *Am J Respir Crit Care Med.* 1998;157:144–148.

21 Young T, Finn L, Austin D, et al. Menopausal status and sleep-disordered breathing in the Wisconsin Sleep Cohort Study. *Am J Respir Crit Care Med.* 2003;167:1181–1185.

22 Tishler PV, Larkin EK, Schluchter MD, et al. Incidence of sleep-disordered breathing in an urban adult population: the relative importance of risk factors in the development of sleep-disordered breathing. *JAMA.* 2003;289:2230–2237.

23 Shahar E, Redline S, Young T, et al. Hormone replacement therapy and sleep-disordered breathing. *Am J Respir Crit Care Med.* 2003;167:1186–1192.

24 Vgontzas AN, Bixler EO, Chrousos GP. Metabolic disturbances in obesity versus sleep apnea: the importance of visceral obesity and insulin resistance. *J Int Med.* 2003;254:1–13.

25 Vgontzas AN, Legro RS, Bixler EO, et al. Polycystic ovary syndrome is associated with obstructive sleep apnea and daytime sleepiness: role of insulin resistance. *J Clin Endocrinol Metab.* 2001;86:517–520.

26 Young T, Peppard P, Palta M, et al. Population-based study of sleep-disordered breathing as a risk factor for hypertension. *Arch Intern Med.* 1997;157:1746–1752.

27 Nieto FJ, Young TB, Lind BK, et al. Association of sleep-disordered breathing, sleep apnea, and hypertension in a large community-based study. *JAMA.* 2000;283:1829–1836.

28 Peppard PE, Young T, Palta M, et al. Prospective study on the association between sleep-disordered breathing and hypertension. *N Engl J Med.* 2000;342:1378–1384.

29 Bixler EO, Vgontzas AN, Lin H-M, et al. Association of hypertension and sleep disordered breathing. *Arch Intern Med.* 2000;160: 2289–2295.

6 Perimenopause and Sexuality

Sheryl A. Kingsberg

Introduction

Fact or fiction: Perimenopause is highly correlated with an increase in sexual dysfunctions. At face value, this statement would seem relatively simple to confirm or deny. Upon a more rigorous investigation, this statement is not simple at all.

One reason this question is so difficult to answer is that the variables in question (perimenopause and female sexuality) are multifactorial and difficult even to define much less delineate to determine causality. Furthermore, if there are increased problems in sexual functioning during perimenopause, the question arises whether this is due specifically to the physiologic events we define as perimenopause (although the Stages of Reproductive Aging Workshop [STRAW] conference[1] now designates *menopausal transition* as a more accurate term, for the purposes of this chapter and ease of use, I will continue to use the term perimenopause) or to other things happening to women at this time (age-related changes and psychosocial factors). In other words, which comes first, the chicken or the (aging) egg(s)? Female sexuality, not just perimenopausal sexuality, is complex. Scientific research to understand the intricacies of female sexual physiology and the exact nature of the female sexual response is still in early stages as are the clinical trials to assess pharmacologic and psychotherapeutic treatment approaches to female sexual problems.

This chapter is not designed to provide an absolute answer to the initial question posed, but rather to review the factors specific to perimenopausal women that may impact their sexual health. It is neither sufficient nor all that useful to focus only on the science underlying our attempts to understand the basic mechanisms of female sexual functioning. We must also incorporate women's *experience* of sexuality. With this integrated conceptual framework in mind, this chapter is written with the goal of providing a practical guide for clinicians in the assessment and treatment of the sexual concerns of perimenopausal women. In order to provide these women effective medical care, particularly with regard to sexual health, clinicians must be able to understand the etiology of presenting problems in such a way as to distinguish what is physical, what is psychosocial, and what is the interaction of the two.

What is Sexual Health and Why Should Clinicians Consider It Important?

Most adults, including aging women, consider sexuality to be an important component of perceived quality of life.[2–4] In addition to the importance of sexuality to patients' quality of life, maintaining sexual health falls under the purview of physicians, particularly those who specialize in reproductive medicine. In 2000, the World Health Organization (WHO) in conjunction with the Pan American Health Organization (PAHO) organized an international meeting that resulted in the publication of a document entitled *Promotion of Sexual Health.*[5] This document includes the current accepted definition of *sexual health.*

Sexual Health is the experience of the ongoing process of physical, psychological, and sociocultural well-being related to sexuality. Sexual health is evidenced by the free and responsible expressions of sexual capabilities that foster harmonious personal and social wellness, enriching individual and social life. It is not merely the absence of dysfunction, disease, and/or infirmity. For sexual health to be attained and maintained, it is necessary that the sexual rights of all the people be recognized and upheld.

The promotion of sexual health document also provides recommendations for training physicians in sexual health. It specifically identifies health professionals specializing in reproductive health programs as requiring adequate training in human sexuality. "Due to the obvious connection between reproductive health and human sexuality, it is often assumed that taking care of the reproductive aspects of health will be enough to satisfy the needs posed by the right to Sexual Health, but this assumption is incorrect. Health professionals specializing in reproductive health should have a more in-depth training in human sexuality issues than the general health practitioner".[5]

Changes in Sexual Activity in Aging Adults

Although most national and international surveys on sexual activity confirm that the frequency of sexual activity does decline with age while the frequency of sexual problems increases (e.g., Refs. 6–8, just to name a few), these population surveys in no way indicate that aging marks the end of sexuality or sexual satisfaction. For example, the 1998 National Council on Aging survey of 1300 older Americans (age 60 and older) found that sexual activity plays an important role in relationships among older men and women.[9] Almost 50% reported engaging in sexual activity at least once per month. Of these sexually active respondents, 79% of men and 66% of women considered sex to be an important component of their relationship with their partner. With regard to the issue of sexual satisfaction remaining intact in older people, 70% and 74% of the sexually active women and men, respectively, reported being as satisfied or even more satisfied with their sexual lives as compared to when they were in their forties.

The Pfizer Global Study of sexual attitudes and behaviors[10] also supports the belief that older adults remain sexually active and consider sex to be important to their quality of life. This study looked to assess the importance of sex and intimacy in men and women ages 40–80 across 29 countries. More than 26,000 men and women were surveyed either in person, by telephone, or by mail-in questionnaire depending on the country. Subjects were asked their level of agreement with a variety of statements regarding sexual beliefs and behaviors. In response to the statement "older people no longer want sex," 64% of the males and 56% of the females strongly disagreed while only 17% of the males and 24% of the females agreed. In response to the question "How important is sex in your overall life?" 83% of men and 63% women said very or at least moderately important. 65% of the males and 58% of the females disagreed with the statement "older people no longer have sex." When asked if they had intercourse in the last year, 82% of men and 64% of women said yes. In a more specific question regarding frequency of sexual activity within the past year, 57% men and 51% women answered at least one to six times per week. These results suggest that older adults continue to value and enjoy sexual activity.

KEY POINT

Almost 50% of patients in a gynecology practice will experience a sexual problem at some point in their adult life.

The Pfizer Global Study is even more striking when put in a broader context. The fact is that sexual dysfunction is highly prevalent in both men and women. The National Health and Social Life Survey (NHSLS)[11] surveyed 1410 men and 1749 women between the ages of 18 and 59 and reported that 31% of men and 43% of women had experienced a sexual dysfunction. However, the NHSLS, similar to the Pfizer Survey, also noted that the prevalence of sexual dysfunction in women, unlike that in men, tends to decline with age. The most often cited population study of men is the Massachusetts Male Aging Study.[12] This was a community-based random sample observational survey of men 40–70 years old conducted from 1987 to 1989. The results showed that age alone was the single variable most strongly associated with erectile dysfunction and the prevalence of complete (vs. minimal and moderate) erectile dysfunction tripled from 5% to 15% between the 40- and 70-year-old subjects.

Age-Related Factors That Impact Sexual Functioning

Although the results from the Pfizer Global Study indicate that the only female sexual problem that consistently increases with age is difficulty with lubrication, and other studies have reported that female sexual satisfaction does not decline appreciably with age[11,13], research on the impact of menopause and sexual functioning has produced inconsistent and equivocal results, partially related to disagreements as to appropriate outcome measures. Avis et al. evaluated studies on postmenopausal sexual functioning and found wide variations in the kind of sexual functioning questions asked, the time frames studied, the inclusion of women without partners, and the nature of study samples.[13] Very diverse outcome measures were also found, including satisfaction, frequency of activity, desire, sexual thoughts/fantasies, arousal, beliefs/attitudes, pain, and anorgasmia. Furthermore, only a few large, general population-based studies have evaluated the impact of menopause on sexuality.[8,13–15] Of these, only one—the

Massachusetts Women's Health Study[13]—evaluated North American women. In this study, menopause (but not serum estrogen levels) was found to be significantly associated with several sexual function measurements, including lower sexual desire, a belief that interest in sexual activity declines with age, and women's reports of decreased arousal compared with their forties. The investigators also evaluated the impact of several other variables including sociodemographic variables, health, psychological variables, partner variables (particularly partner health or sexual problems), and lifestyle variables. Their results suggest that these other factors have a greater impact on sexual functioning than does menopausal status, underscoring the importance of the need to understand the context of women's lives when studying sexuality.

The Melbourne Women's Midlife Health Project[8,16] was specifically designed to address the methodological flaws in the earlier population-based studies. This was a decade long longitudinal study of 2100 premenopausal women between 45 and 55 years of age at baseline. A smaller prospective substudy with this population ($n = 438$) was designed to assess whether changes (declines) in sexual functioning are related to menopausal status or age. The investigators found that many aspects of female sexual functioning declined with the menopausal transition and concluded that while menopausal status was more relevant than age, the causes were multifactorial (i.e., hormonal changes, health status, or psychosocial factors related to menopause).

The high prevalence of sex in older people is even more striking when you look at the results of the National Survey of Sex in America.[11] This is the famous and often quoted survey of almost 1800 women and 1400 men, who are a much younger sample—from the ages of 18–59. As you can see, 43% of women in this sample and 31% of the men reported having had a sexual dysfunction at some time in their life.

For women, regardless of age, the most prevalent sexual dysfunction is hypoactive sexual desire disorder and this is the dysfunction most often assumed to go hand in hand with menopause. But this is the most prevalent sexual dysfunction regardless of age.

However, HSDD is not the only female sexual dysfunction and clinicians must be able to identify and try a first-line treatment for all the female sexual dysfunctions. Therefore, before reviewing

HSDD, a review of the other female sexual dysfunctions is necessary.

The Diagnostic and Statistical Manual of Mental Disorders—Fourth Edition (DSM–IV) lists six female sexual dysfunctions[17]:

- Hypoactive sexual desire disorder
- Sexual aversion disorder
- Female sexual arousal disorder (FSAD)
- Female orgasmic disorder
- Dyspareunia
- Vaginismus

Sexual aversion disorder is an often misunderstood sexual dysfunction diagnosis. Based on the symptoms, it could be considered an anxiety disorder, and was only classified as a sexual disorder with the publication of the DSM-III-R.[18] Since then there has been relatively little written on the etiology and treatment of sexual aversion. The criteria for sexual aversion disorder overlap with both panic disorder and hypoactive sexual desire disorder, which makes it difficult for many clinicians, even experts in treating sexual disorders, to diagnose sexual aversion.[19]

DSM-IV-TR *Criteria for Sexual Aversion Disorder* (302.79)

- Persistent or recurrent extreme aversion to, and avoidance of, all (or almost all) genital sexual contact with a sexual partner.
- The disturbance causes marked distress or interpersonal difficulty.
- The sexual dysfunction is not better accounted for by another Axis I disorder (except another sexual dysfunction).

Sexual aversion can be expressed as simple avoidance of partnered sexual behavior as well as a panic response to engaging in partnered sexual activity and the DSM-IV criteria do not require the physiologic responses that clinicians often associate with aversion (e.g., nausea and revulsion). Beyond the scope of sexuality, aversion implies more than simply phobic avoidance and is typically characterized by nausea, vomiting, and tremendous disgust. However, researchers in sexual aversion maintain that it is better equated with a phobia with the essential diagnostic feature of persistent fear and avoidance.[20]

Sexual aversion is often misdiagnosed as hypoactive sexual desire disorder because the persistent avoidance may be perceived (by the patient, partner, and even clinician) as lack of interest. However, women with sexual aversion may have significant sexual drive and engage in masturbation on a relatively frequent basis. On the other hand, hypoactive sexual desire disorder may also be mistaken for sexual aversion if sexual disinterest evolves into anger or agitation over years of feeling pressure to perform. However, this presentation would be about the fear and anxiety response to sexual activity.

Treatment typically follows a cognitive behavioral model that is used for deconditioning phobic and avoidant behavior patterns. For example, treatment may include the creation of a hierarchy of aversion and anxiety-provoking images, ranging from the least anxiety provoking (e.g., masturbation), to the most revolting or anxiety provoking (e.g., intercourse). Patients are then taught diaphragmatic deep breathing and autogenic relaxation techniques. Relaxation is then paired in a stepwise fashion with these images and then subsequently approached in vivo. Although this treatment appears to be relatively straightforward, sexual aversion is often difficult to treat and rarely abates on its own. Avoidance behavior is not easy to extinguish because individuals learn that avoidance prevents the elicitation of fear and if fear is not elicited, it cannot be extinguished (in this case in the presence of partnered sexual activity).[19]

Female Sexual Arousal Disorder

FSAD is defined in the DSM-IV as persistent or recurrent inability to maintain until completion of the sexual activity, an adequate lubrication-swelling response of sexual excitement. In this case, arousal is a physical response and has a behavioral manifestation of vaginal lubrication and swelling and increased heart rate. More recent discussions on this diagnosis support the idea of further dividing the disorder into women who have subjective arousal but have no physiologic arousal, such as lubrication or vaginal swelling, and women who have physiologic arousal but no perception of this. And this does not mean they do not have desire—they just have no subjective perception of their body's arousal. The diagnosis should only be made if it is determined that the patient experiences sufficient desire that would be expected to result in arousal and that there is adequate physical stimulation to elicit a physical response.

In addition, it is important to distinguish between women who have no arousal or perception of arousal and those who perceive their arousal but do not like it (in this case the more likely disorder would be hypoactive desire or sexual aversion).

The treatment for FSAD will depend on the subcategory of the disorder and the etiology. The etiology of FSAD is typically physiologic with the potential sources categorized as neurogenic (e.g., spinal cord injury, multiple sclerosis, peripheral neuropathies, and stroke), endocrine (e.g., diabetes, thyroid disorders, and adrenal disorders), hormonal (e.g., estrogen or androgen insufficiency), gynecologic (e.g., postsurgical effects particularly after hysterectomy with or without bilateral oophorectomy, recurrent cystitis), and medication side effects (e.g., antidepressants, antipsychotics, anticholinergics, antihistamines, and antihypertensives).[21–24]

Since the phosphodiesterase (PDE 5) inhibitors have become the sexual salvation for men with erectile dysfunction, the question of their effectiveness in women has naturally been raised. The PDE 5 inhibitors work by blocking the breakdown of cyclic guanosine monophosphate (cGMP) in the genitals, which causes smooth muscle relaxation and increased vasodilation. For women, the goal of increased vasodilation would be that increased blood flow leads to increased vulvar congestion, which leads to increased sensation. To date, the success of the PDE 5 inhibitors (sildenafil has been the only one of them with published data using double-blind placebo controlled trials) has been quite limited with most studies showing no improvement in comparison to placebo.[25] There are a few possible reasons for this. First, FSAD is not as prevalent a disorder in women as erectile dysfunction is in men. Second, and related to the first reason, is that many women with FSAD either have HSDD as a comorbid disorder or their FSAD is actually better accounted for as a symptom of HSDD. In fact, the most recent published study of Sildenafil in women showed a significant effect when they eliminated women with HSDD from their subject pool.[26] Third, even when vasoactive agents are used, the subjective sensation may be limited.[25,27]

Female Orgasmic Disorder

Female orgasmic disorder is the inability to experience orgasm following a normal sexual excitement phase with adequate time, intensity, and stimulation and the problem causes marked distress or interpersonal difficulty. A diagnosis should only be made when there is *personal* distress.

The DSM in a previous version to IV did emphasize in its criteria for inhibited orgasm that the absence of orgasm during intercourse represents a normal variation of the female sexual response and does not justify a diagnosis of inhibited orgasm.

Despite its importance in our lives, orgasm is simply a reflex. Orgasm is a reflex whose lowest neural center is probably located in the lumbosacral spinal cord. And similar to reflex centers serving other functions, the orgasmic reflex center is subject to multiple inhibitory and facilitory influences from direct sensory input and higher neural centers. It may be helpful to view orgasmic attainment in women as a normal distribution.

This distribution reflects women who have no physical problems that might interfere with achieving orgasm. On the left are women who have never experienced orgasm. The best estimate places this prevalence at about 10%. Similarly on the other end of the curve are those fortunate women who can experience orgasm under almost any circumstance including fantasy without any physical stimulation. This prevalence is also about 10%. The rest of the population falls somewhere in between.

A large percentage of women are *situationally* orgasmic; that is, they can achieve orgasm readily and reliably with some particular forms of stimulation but not others. Often women are reliably orgasmic with masturbation or oral sex but not with intercourse. Recall this is considered a normal variation in female sexual functioning.

It is important to recognize that intercourse is one of the most difficult ways for a woman to reliably achieve an orgasm. Only about 25–50% of women can achieve orgasm reliably by intercourse alone.

The cause of orgasmic difficulties is likely multifactorial and different for each woman. Many women develop performance anxiety around having an orgasm with a partner. If they start to worry that they are taking too long or will look funny when they do orgasm, anxiety and distraction creep in and desire and arousal are lost.

With appropriate information, guidance, and reading, most women are able to become orgasmic.

Dyspareunia

Dyspareunia is defined as pain or discomfort that occurs during or as a result of intercourse. Pain may be experienced as pressure, aching, tearing, friction, rubbing, or burning. The pain may be localized to the vulvovaginal region (superficial dyspareunia) or to the pelvis or lower abdomen (deep dyspareunia). Controversy remains as to what degrees of pain constitutes a diagnosis of dyspareunia. However, it would be prudent medical practice to define dyspareunia as coital pain that patients report is a problem.

The prevalence of dyspareunia in the general population is approximately 20% with increasing prevalence as women age and experience genital atrophy. The most important take home message about dyspareunia is to consider it as a symptom rather than a diagnosis and to focus on assessing and treating the underlying etiology.

VAGINISMUS

Vaginismus is defined as involuntary, recurrent, and persistent spasm of the outer-third of the vaginal muscles making penetration of the vagina impossible.[17] It is not technically a pain disorder because women may not feel pain. However, it is often the result of pain or may coexist with dyspareunia. Women can still enjoy sexual activity and be orgasmic despite having vaginismus; only penetration is not possible.

It is also important to note that for some women vaginismus is limited to sexual activity and therefore have little difficulty with pelvic examinations. Similarly some women have no difficulty with intercourse but have vaginismus related to fear of pelvic examinations. And of course, many women have vaginismus that is generalized to both circumstances.

Returning to my topic of the day—aging and sexuality, there are some sexual changes that are a direct result of aging.

Physiologic Factors of Aging That Impact Sexual Functioning

For women, the major problem, as shown from the Pfizer Global Study,[10] is difficulty with lubrication. Age itself does not necessarily increase other female sexual dysfunctions. Perimenopause is associated with a decline in estrogen levels. The changes in the epithelial lining of the vagina occur relatively rapidly as estrogen levels decline. Subsequent vascular, muscular, and connective tissue changes occur over time. Decreased vascularization starves the surrounding tissues of nutrients and makes it more difficult for engorgement and lubrication. The vagina also loses its elasticity and narrows, which can cause significant discomfort during sexual penetration. Additionally, the uterus typically contracts with orgasm, and with advancing age, those contractions may become painful.

The clitoris is also affected by aging. Clitoral changes include shrinkage, a decrease in perfusion, diminished engorgement during sexual arousal, and a decline in the neurophysiological response, including slowed nerve impulses and a decrease in touch perception, vibratory sensation, and reaction time. Decreased muscle tension may increase the time it takes for arousal to lead to orgasm, diminish the peak of orgasm, and cause a more rapid resolution. However, while all this sounds pretty ominous for older women, the actual perception of sexual satisfaction does not necessarily change.

Perimenopause and the Role of Androgens

While decreased estrogen is responsible for most of these physical changes, testosterone, too, can play an important role in midlife sexual changes affecting women.

Although this book includes a chapter devoted specifically to the role of androgens in perimenopause, they must be included in any discussion of female sexuality, particularly in perimenopausal women.

KEY POINT

Testosterone levels begin to decline as early as a woman's late-twenties.

Testosterone is necessary for a normal sex drive in both men and women, playing a role in motivation, desire, and sexual sensation. Women achieve peak androgen production in their mid-twenties. Beginning in their early thirties, they gradually lose testosterone in an age-related fashion. By the time most women reach their 60s, their testosterone levels are half of what they were before age 40.[22] During perimenopause, as estrogen levels are declining, women also experience a decrease in sex hormone-binding globulin (SHBG), which binds both estrogen and testosterone and, in fact, tends to bind testosterone more than it does estrogen. Some perimenopausal women will notice an increase in sexual desire and activity, perhaps because the declining levels of SHBG free up more testosterone. Women who take oral estrogen increase their SHBG levels and lower their free testosterone levels and may notice a decrease in sexual desire. Women who have had an oophorectomy are more likely to experience a decline in sexual drive—possibly because it is a sudden loss and we know that the ovaries are responsible for producing 50% of circulating testosterone and possibly because in some naturally post-menopausal women, the ovaries are still producing some level of testosterone.

The role of androgens in female sexuality has become the current hot topic for debate as to whether the relatively newly named syndrome called female androgen insufficiency (FAI) is a valid medical syndrome or a pharmaceutical marketing manager's sexual fantasy.

FAI is defined as a pattern of clinical symptoms in the presence of decreased bioavailable testosterone and normal estrogen status. The clinical symptoms include impaired sexual function, mood alterations, and diminished energy and well-being.[28] Braunstein[28] has developed a useful algorithm to help in the assessment of FAI (Fig. 6-1).

The reason it is insufficiency and not deficiency is because we do not yet know enough about normal levels of androgens in women to be able to state what is considered a deficiency. There are no consistent lab assessments. Most commercially available methods are inaccurate or unreliable. Treatment often involves replacing testosterone—in physiologic amounts. Currently, there are no FDA-approved androgen replacement treatments for women. However, clinical trials are well underway in this area. For example, Procter and Gamble is conducting Phase III trials of their 300 μg testosterone patch in naturally and surgically menopausal women with HSDD.

One of my own concerns about the potential overuse of FAI is that it is much too comfortable a diagnosis to provide physicians with. Health-care providers are very happy when there is a very simple biologic factor that is responsible for a specific problem. Unfortunately, this is not the case with regard to any female sexual dysfunction and this is particularly true with regard to aging women and decreased sexual desire. Female sexuality and hypoactive desire disorder are very complicated and cannot be summed up by a simple biologic theory.

Now I would like to return to the topic of hypoactive sexual desire disorder—the sexual dysfunction that is most often associated with perimenopause.

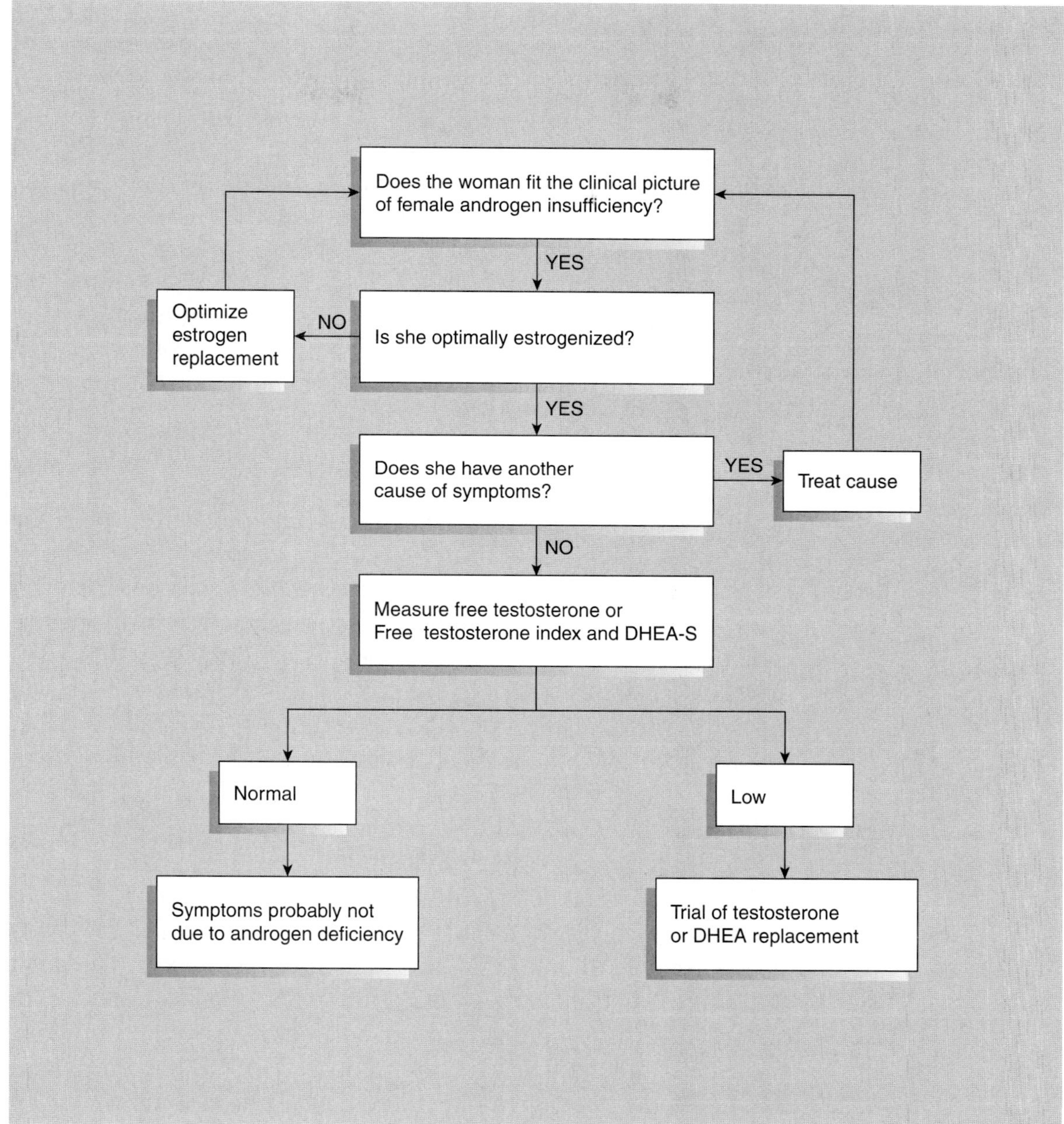

Figure 6-1: Algorithm for the diagnosis and treatment of androgen insufficiency syndrome. [*Source*: Braunstein GD. Androgen insufficiency in women: summary of critical issues. Fertil Steril 2002; 77(Suppl. 4): S94–S99.]

Decline in Drive

One of the most significant and universal changes that occurs with age is a decline in the drive component of sexual desire. Desire refers to one's interest in being sexual and is determined by the interaction of three related but separate components: drive, beliefs/values/expectations, and motivation.[29]

Drive is the biologic component of desire. It is the result of neuroendocrine mechanisms and is experienced as spontaneous, endogenous sexual interest. Drive is typically manifested by sexual thoughts, feelings, fantasies or dreams, increased erotic attraction to others in proximity, seeking out sexual activity (alone or with a partner), and genital tingling or increased genital sensitivity. Although we still do not fully understand the exact neuroendocrine mechanisms that are responsible for drive, we do know that drive declines in both men and women as a function of aging. For some women declining levels of free testosterone, related to declining ovarian function, will result in a noticeable decrease in sexual drive. The sudden decrease in free testosterone as a result of surgical menopause may also result in a noticeable decrease in sexual drive for some women. The second component of desire reflects an individual's expectations, beliefs, and values about sexual activity. The more positive the person's beliefs and values are about sexuality, the greater the person's desire to behave sexually. The third component of desire is the psychological and interpersonal motivation. Motivation is driven by emotional or interpersonal factors and is characterized by a willingness of a person to behave sexually with a given partner. This component tends to have the greatest impact overall on desire and is the most complex and elusive.

This distinction between drive and desire is absolutely essential for any physician assessing or treating sexual problems, because treatment is vastly different based on which component or components of desire have declined. For example, a woman might have a very strong sexual drive but if she is not motivated to be sexual, say if she is angry with her partner, dealing with a stressful work problem, or suffering from depression, she will not act on the drive. In fact, it is virtually wiped out. On the other hand, if a woman has lost some of her drive but remains motivated to be close and intimate with her partner, then despite having little physical cues or interest, she still enjoys the sexual experience.

This differentiation of drive from desire is particularly important to the understanding of female sexuality and points out some of the gender differences in prevalence of particular sexual problems. It also underscores the relative gender differences in the sexual response cycle itself and reminds us of the most important of heterosexual dilemmas: Men tend to use sex as stress reliever while women need stress relief to want sex.

For many women, particularly postmenopausal women, drive decreases and is no longer the initial step in the response cycle. The classic Masters and Johnson model first developed in 1966 suggested a progressive linear model of the sexual response cycle—desire leading to arousal and plateau then to orgasm and resolution.[30] While they believed that this linear model was universal and unchanging for both genders, they were very clear that despite this order of response, there was a significant gender difference; that is, for men, the response was always the same—never varying except for duration. However, for women, there is an infinite variety of responses.

KEY POINT

A woman's sexual response is often different than a man's and does not follow a linear model.

Although Masters and Johnson can be credited for their pioneering work to empirically study the female sexual response, their linear model of response does not appear to fit our modern conceptualization of the multifactorial nature of women's sexual response. Instead, Rosemary Basson offers an alternative model.[31] She suggests that women's responses are not so linear and that for many women, desire comes after arousal and that many women begin from a point of sexual neutrality. Arousal may come from a conscious decision or as a result of seduction or suggestion from a partner. This is an important distinction to make for patients because you can then normalize this reality for your patients who have come to believe that because their initial drive has diminished, they are no longer sexual beings.

Age-Related Factors: The Impact of Partner Sexual Dysfunction

In keeping with the model of looking at the context to understand female sexuality, one of the most significant psychosocial or contextual variables that affect women is the impact of their partner having a sexual dysfunction.

Although sexual drive does decline with age in both men and women, many older heterosexual couples cease being sexual because the male partner's interest declines, usually due to his experiencing erectile dysfunction. Erectile dysfunction is a major source of poor body image and resulting low desire for men. Many postmenopausal women are abstinent because of their male partner's erectile difficulties or his decline in drive.

While the PDE 5 inhibitors (e.g., Viagra, Cialis, and Levitra) are tremendously helpful to men in overcoming erectile dysfunction, a problem to recognize is that their efficacy may now cause a shift in a couple's sexual equilibrium. As women first adjusted to the sexual equilibrium of abstinence due to their partner's dysfunction, now they must once again accommodate to another change in equilibrium. This creates a challenge. Older people not only require a longer adjustment period to make the necessary accompanying cognitive shift, but older women definitely need time for their bodies to readjust to a partnered sexual life.[32] Unfortunately if he and his female partner have not had intercourse for a long time, her aging vagina has likely narrowed and atrophied and may not comfortably accommodate a penis without risking pain and/or injury. This may lead to a secondary female sexual dysfunction of dyspareunia or vaginismus. For heterosexual postmenopausal women who have been sexually abstinent a long time, physicians *must* remember this and first guide women to resume sexual activity slowly and by gradually stretching and "exercising" their vaginas. Women should be instructed to begin by penetration with a finger or dilator and gradually stretch the vagina to accommodate a penis.

Translating Theory into Practice: How to Efficiently Assess and Treat Sexual Problems

In order for any physician to be able to treat a sexual problem, they must be able to ask about them. You cannot treat a problem if you do not know it exists. Physicians do not need to be trained as sex therapists to effectively address many of the sexual problems of you peri/postmenopausal patients. Instead, physicians just need to minimally expand what you are already trained to do: first, assess and evaluate and second, treat and/or refer.

Simply initiating a discussion of sexual concerns is the most valuable treatment component for both men, women, and couples.

By asking about sexuality, the health-care provider informs the patient that it is appropriate to discuss sexual problems in that setting and validates an older person's self-perception as a sexual being.

What to Include in a Sexual History and How to Ask

The most important component of taking a sexual history is not the information you collect—it is the opening of the door to the topic of sexuality! By asking, even briefly, about sexual functioning or history, you have indicated to the patient that it is safe and appropriate to bring up sexual concerns in your office. Even if they do not say anything during that visit, or the next two after that, they know they can.

The most basic of sexual assessments includes the following three questions:

- Are you currently involved in a sexual relationship?
- Are you sexually involved with men, women, or both?
- Do you or your partner have any sexual problems or concerns.

A more thorough assessment would include a review of the sexual response cycle (desire-arousal-orgasm-satisfaction) and a further assessment of specific problems as:

- Primary versus secondary
- General versus specific
- Etiology: psychogenic, organic, mixed, idiopathic

Clinicians may find two algorithms, the second developed by Rosemary Basson[25] particularly helpful when assessing sexual problems in patients (Figs. 6-2 and 6-3).

Move to next algorithm for further assessment or explain the importance of conducting a thorough assessment and the need to schedule a follow-up appointment or refer to specialist.

Of course, it is important to review safer sex practices—no matter what age and to review contraceptive options with your heterosexual patients. In addition, knowledge of patients' past sexual history can be very useful when diagnosing current sexual dysfunctions.

A detailed sexual history would include gathering information listed in Table 6-1.

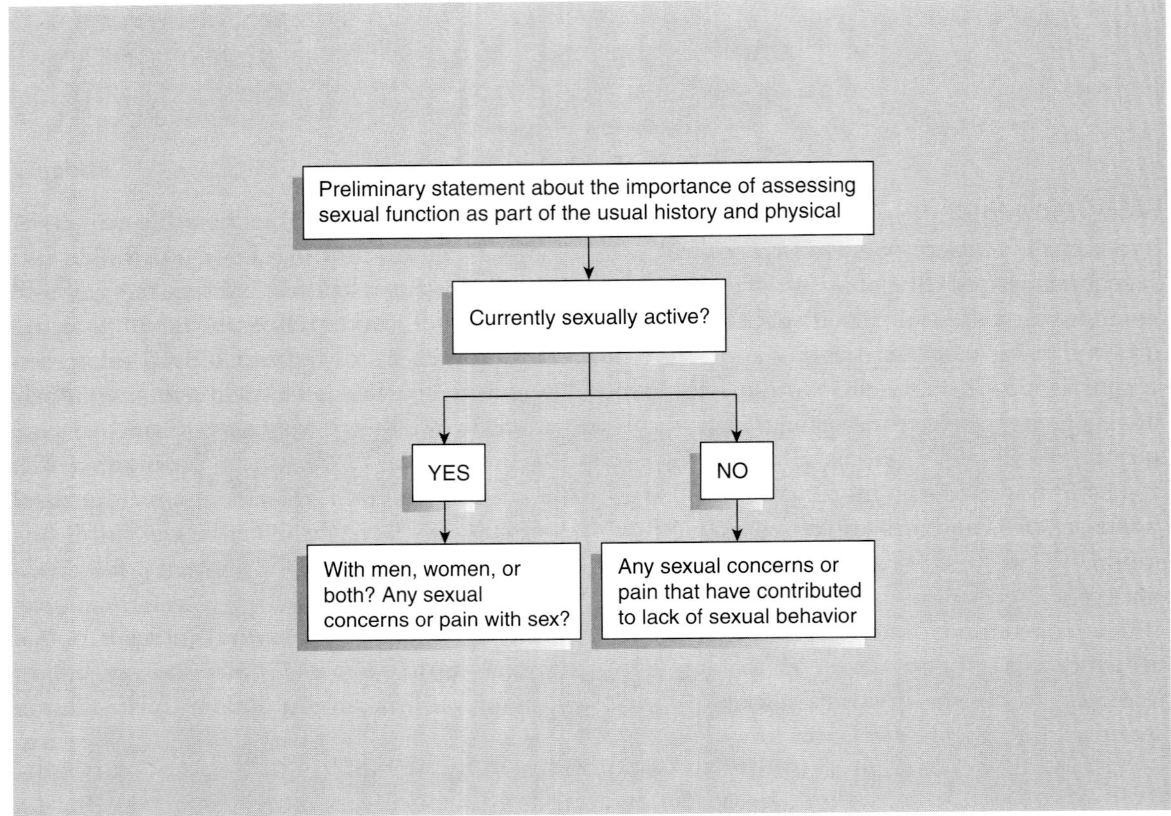

Figure 6-2: Algorithm for a basic screen of sexual functioning.

Guiding Questions

- Which aspect(s) of the sexual response is/are impacted?
- Why are you presenting now?
- Do you experience any spontaneous sexual thoughts/dreams, genital tingling (drive)?
- Do you have any religious or cultural beliefs that might interfere with your enjoyment of your sexual life?
- Are you motivated to be sexually intimate with your partner (regardless of spontaneous drive)?
- Once you are aware of desire are you able to become physiologically aroused as evidenced by vaginal lubrication and genital swelling?
- Are you able to subjectively perceive this arousal?

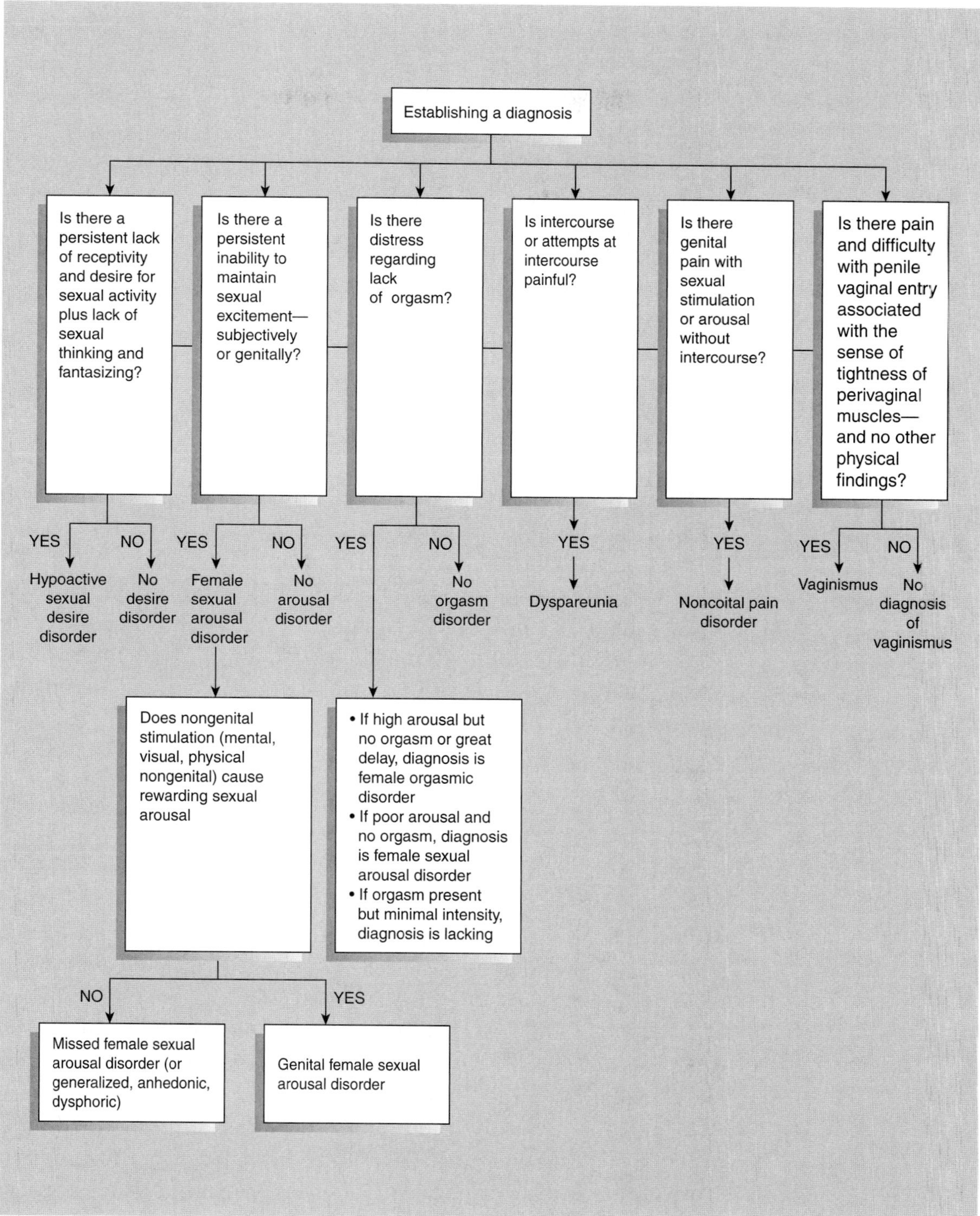

Figure 6-3: Algorithm to establish a sexual dysfunction diagnosis.

Table 6-1. INFORMATION TO BE INCLUDED AS PART OF A DETAILED SEXUAL AND REPRODUCTIVE HISTORY

First sexual experiences
Approximate number of lifetime sexual partners
Sexually transmitted diseases and reproductive history including number of pregnancies and/or terminations and gynecologic surgeries
Sexual or physical abuse history
Any use of prescribed or over-the-counter medications or treatments that may impact sexual functioning

- If adequately aroused, are you able to experience orgasm in a reliable way with any particular kind of stimulation (normalize that intercourse if often not a reliable method)?
- When did this problem begin?
- Has it been lifelong or did it develop after a period of healthy sexual functioning?
- Is it generalized to all sexual activity and partners or is it specific to one activity or one particular partner?
- Have you ever sought treatment for this problem before?
- If so, what treatments were attempted and did they help?
- Are there other psychosocial factors that may be contributing to or exacerbating the presenting problem?

Conclusions

The sexual health of perimenopausal women falls within the responsibility of the gynecologist. The topic of female *sexuality,* not just sexual *function,* has entered the spotlight of our media and society. This is either the cause or the effect of a frenzy of research attempting to better understand women's sexuality and to find psychological and medical treatments for women's sexual dysfunctions. At present, there are no universal truths to make the practice of sexual medicine easy for gynecologists who may not feel adequately trained in this area in the first place. This chapter is meant to convey that your sense of uncertainty is not due to lack of basic knowledge or skill but rather similar to the question of recommending hormone therapy (HT), each woman is different and treatment must be individualized. Effective communication with patients about sexual health is necessary and the most important skill that gynecologists must master to sufficiently meet the needs of their perimenopausal patients.

What's the Evidence?

OLDER ADULTS CONTINUE TO VALUE AND ENJOY SEX The Pfizer Global Study of more than 26,000 men and women indicated that 57% of men and 51% of women have sexual relations at least one to six times per week. The 1998 National Council on Aging survey of adults age 60 and older showed that 50% of respondents engaged in sexual activity at least once per month.

THERE IS A HIGH PREVALENCE OF SEXUAL DYSFUNCTION Results of the National Survey of Sex in American[11] indicate that 31% of men and 43% of women report having sexual dysfunction at some time in their life. The most common sexual dysfunction in women is hypoactive sexual desire disorder.

Discussion of Cases

CASE 1

Maureen

Maureen is a 47-year-old Caucasian homemaker referred to a sex therapist by her gynecologist with a chief complaint of loss of sexual interest.

Perimenopausal Status

Maureen reports regular menstrual cycles but notes that her bleeding pattern has been changing over the past year. She is not on any birth control since her husband, Richard, had a vasectomy.

Psychosocial and Sexual History

Maureen has been married 21 years. Richard is 52 and is a very successful consultant. They have a 19-year-old son and two daughters, aged 11 and 14 years, respectively.

Maureen reports that the onset of her loss of sexual interest became noticeable 6 months back but may have been developing gradually over the past 12 months. She first realized it as a major problem when she and her husband went on their annual tropical vacation a month ago and she had no sexual interest. This was the event that convinced her to seek help because, she says, although she has always had a relatively low drive (her highest drive in young adulthood was twice a month), she could always count on having interest in sex on that particular vacation. She has had no desire since then.

Maureen states that Richard has always had a higher drive than she, preferring to have sex at least three times a week. Richard travels for work quite a bit. Therefore, frequency of sex is often "all or nothing." When Richard is away, Maureen is not anticipating being sexual or feeling pressured to be sexual. As soon as she anticipates Richard's return, she feels some anxiety in knowing that he will want to be sexual fairly soon after he arrives. Maureen reports that when she does have drive, it is usually higher in the mornings. However, she states that her husband gets up too early to make use of this interest.

Sexual Response Cycle

Given Maureen's chief complaint of loss of desire, a primary focus of assessment was on the components of sexual desire, drive, expectations/beliefs/values (i.e., cognitive component), and motivation:

- Drive:Prior to 6 months ago, her drive was twice per month for most of her adult life. Currently, she has no drive.
- Cognitive: Maureen's beliefs and values are consistent with the wish to be sexual with Richard. She considers sex to be healthy and appropriate for a 47-year-old wife and mother. She does not feel that menopause reflects a loss of femininity or sexuality.
- Motivation: Maureen is very happily married. She loves her husband, is very attracted to him, and has no underlying issues regarding their relationship. Her mental health is good; there is no evidence of an underlying depression, anxiety disorder, or any other clinical or subclinical problem. Maureen has no history of any sexual or physical abuse or difficulties with sexuality in the past. However, because of her lifelong low drive, Maureen has a long-standing self-perception of being relatively asexual. Now that she has no drive, her identity as a sexual being is even more negative. In addition, given the long-standing discrepancy in drive levels, Maureen has always felt that she has engaged in sexual activity more frequently than she would have otherwise chosen. Behaviorally, this has manifested as Richard always being the initiator of sexual activity. Since Maureen assumed that Richard was always interested in having sex, she would just wait for his initiation instead of ever initiating first. Her reasoning was that if she would initiate on the infrequent occasions when she did feel drive, this would only add to the total frequency of sexual activity that Richard would want or expect. This was problematic, because it resulted in Maureen ignoring and suppressing her own drive when it would arise. In addition, given that sex did not often occur when she was feeling the drive, the experience was not going to be as passionate, exciting, or stimulating as it would have been with the added element of spontaneous physiologic drive. This suppression of her own drive has likely contributed to her feeling asexual and interfered with perceived sexual satisfaction. The couple's sexual script had been unsatisfying but tolerable for both for years. Her loss of the little drive she had altered the script enough to cause her to seek treatment.

With regard to the rest of Maureen's sexual response, once sex is initiated, she does perceive both genital and subjective arousal, she lubricates sufficiently, and experiences genital stimulation as pleasing. Orgasm is difficult and unreliable, but this has been a consistent problem throughout her sexual life. This has resulted in Maureen experiencing some performance anxiety—the more she worries about whether she will achieve orgasm, the less likely it is to occur. But it had not been a significant enough problem to warrant the diagnosis of anorgasmia nor was it a source of avoidance. She enjoys intercourse and a variety of other sexual activities and is willing to try new activities/positions. She is most reliably orgasmic with manual stimulation with or without vaginal penetration.

Partner's Sexual Health

Despite Richard's age of 52, his drive has remained consistent at about three times per week and he as not evidenced any decline in his erectile functioning. Maureen denies that Richard has any current or prior sexual problems or concerns.

Treatment

At first glance, treatment might seem quite obvious. Maureen had a fairly rapid loss of what sexual drive she did have and this loss corresponded in time to her changing menstrual cycle. The rapid loss of drive with perimenopause is certainly suggestive of a hormonal cause for what appears to be simply a *drive* problem. Therefore, first-line treatment might be to assess Maureen's total and free testosterone levels and if they appear low (acknowledging we do not yet have accurate measures of what constitutes normal and low levels) and prescribing testosterone replacement. However, given the couple's past sexual life and equilibrium, replacing testosterone as the only treatment, without also addressing the prior difficulties which were now exacerbated by loss of all Maureen's drive, might be a setup for failure. Her sexual history makes it difficult to be certain that the loss of desire is purely a drive and thus a hormonal problem. This is a critical issue. If only the drive component of desire is addressed (by replacing testosterone), it may not be sufficient and then two problems will arise. First, testosterone replacement will be incorrectly seen as a failure, when in conjunction with other treatment it might otherwise have worked. Second, by only treating one component of the desire problem, a woman or couple will not feel sufficiently improved. This leads patients to assume their gynecologist or sex therapist cannot solve their problem, they then feel hopeless, give up, and drop out of treatment.

Therefore, in Maureen's case, instead of prescribing testosterone replacement as the *first* treatment intervention, brief psychotherapy, consisting primarily of education and behavior modification was indicated. First, treatment addressed Maureen's self-perception as asexual and her beliefs about sexuality in general and her own sexuality and sensuality in particular. She learned that regardless of how much physiologic drive she has, if her *belief* is that she is not a sexual person and she does not see herself as sensual and desirable, she will have low *desire*.

In order to accomplish this treatment goal, therapy focused on challenging and altering Maureen's perception about her sexual identity. She learned that drive was only one component to desire and even if it was low, it did not necessarily reflect her identity and could be compensated for. She learned how to put more emphasis on her psychological motivation to be sexual and intimate with Richard instead of relying on her drive as the only signal to initiate sexual activity. Maureen also learned that she could play a stronger role in determining sexual frequency and that she could initiate without feeling the pressure that this would mean having more sex than she wished. As a result, sexual activity would no longer be perceived as a chore or obligation and she could maximize her enjoyment by having sex when her body was most physically receptive.

With regard to sexual response, therapy also addressed Maureen's difficulty with orgasm. Again, she was educated about the female sexual response. For example, she learned that many women are not reliably orgasmic, particularly with intercourse, and that this does not reflect an inadequacy but rather reflects the normal variation within women's sexual responses. In addition, she learned to use masturbation to help discover what kinds of stimulation worked most effectively for her to experience the most pleasure and what were the most reliable ways to achieve orgasms. This also helped with her performance anxiety. Maureen no longer felt pressured to have an orgasm every time she had sex. In contrast, she learned how to relax in Richard's presence and developed confidence to teach him how to effectively stimulate her. She also stopped her frequent worry that she was taking too long, a worry that almost always resulted in a self-fulfilling prophecy.

It was after these goals were accomplished that the timing was most appropriate to address the loss of drive. Now the other problematic components of desire would not sabotage the effectiveness of testosterone replacement. Instead, her improvement in beliefs and motivation set the stage to make the most effective use of her improved drive.

Treatment was successful within three sessions spaced 4 weeks apart. Maureen reported significant improvement in all three components of desire and ultimately sexual satisfaction. Using a testosterone cream preparation twice a week that was prescribed by her gynecologist, Maureen reported that within 2 weeks she noticed an increase in sexual thoughts, feeling more physically sensual, increased genital sensation, and more intense orgasms. She admitted that although she still had difficulty reaching orgasm, it was an improvement from baseline and was not a deterrent to her enjoyment of sex or to her sexual self-perception.

This case illustrates the importance of taking a careful sexual history in addition to a thorough physical examination and evaluation of menopausal status. This history should include an assessment of the three components of desire with regard to past and current functioning. It should also include an assessment of a patient's sexual equilibrium with her partner if there is one. Even when the source of the problem is physiologic in etiology, it is important not to ignore the other psychological factors that coexist or that may have resulted from the physiologic problem (e.g., men develop performance anxiety if they have a problem with gaining/keeping an erection).

References

1. Soules MR. Executive summary: stages of reproductive aging workshop (STRAW). Park City, UT, July, 2001. *Menopause.* 2001;8(6):402–405.
2. Kingsberg SA. Maintaining and evaluating quality of life after menopause. *The Female Patient.* 1996;(Suppl. 21):19–24.
3. Utian WH, Janata JW, Kingsberg SA, et al. The Utian Quality of Life (UQOL) Scale: development and validation of an instrument to quantify quality of life through and beyond menopause. *Menopause.* 2002;9:402–410.
4. Gelfand MM. Sexuality among older women. *J Womens Health Gend Based Med.* 2000;9(Suppl. 1);200:S-15-S-20.
5. World Health Organization (2000). *Education and Treatment in Human Sexuality: The Training of Health Professionals.* Report of a WHO Meeting. Q Corporation, 49 Sheridan Avenue, Albany, NY 12210.
6. Janus SS, Janus CL. *The Janus Report on Sexual Behavior.* New York: John Wiley & Sons; 1993.

7 Brecher E. *Love, Sex and Aging: A Consumer's Union Survey*. Boston, MA: Little, Brown and Co; 1984.

8 Dennerstein L, Dudley E, Burger H. Are changes in sexual functioning during midlife due to aging or menopause? *Fertil Steril.* 2001;76(3):456–460.

9 *The National Council on Aging (1998, September).* Healthy sexuality and vital again. Retrieved from *www.cin-ncoa.org/love/natural.part.htm.*

10 Pfizer, Inc. *The Pfizer Global Study of Sexual Attitudes and Behaviors (2003).* Retrieved from *www.pfizerglobalstudy.com.*

11 Laumann EO, Paik MA, Rosin R. Sexual dysfunction in the United States: prevalence and predictors. *JAMA.* 1999;281:537–544.

12 Feldman HA, Goldstein I, Hatzichristou DG, et al. Impotence and its medical and psychosocial correlates: results of the Massachusetts Male Aging Study. *J Urol.* 151:54–61.

13 Avis NE, Stellato R, Crawford S, et al. Is there an association between menopause status and sexual functioning? *Menopause.* 2000;7: 297–309.

14 Hällström T. Sexuality in the climacteric. *Clin Obstet Gynecol.* 1977;4:227–239.

15 Køster A, Garde K. Sexual desire and menopausal development. A prospective study of Danish women born in 1936. *Maturitas.* 1993;16:49–60.

16 Dennerstein LL. The sexual impact of menopause. In: *Handbook of Clinical Sexuality for Mental Health Professionals.* Levine SB, ed. New York: Brunner-Routledge; 2003:187–198.

17 American Psychiatric Association. *DSM-IV-TR: Diagnostic and Statistical Manual of Mental Disorders, 4th edition, Text Revision.* Washington, DC: American Psychiatric Press; 2000.

18 American Psychiatric Association. *DSM-III-R: Diagnostic and Statistical Manual of Mental Disorders, 3rd edition-revised.* Washington, DC: American Psychiatric Press; 1987.

19 Kingsberg SA, Janata JW. Sexual aversion. In: *Handbook of Clinical Sexuality for Mental Health Professionals.* Levine SB, eds. New York: Brunner-Rutledge; 2003:153–166.

20 Katz RC, Jardine D. The relationship between worry, sexual aversion, and low sexual desire. *J Sex Marital Ther. 1999;25:*293–296.

21 Phillips NA. Female sexual dysfunction: evaluation and treatment. *Am Fam Physician.* 2000;62:127–136.

22 Davis SR. Testosterone treatment: psychological and physical effects in postmenopausal women. *Menopausal Med.* 2001;9(2):1–6.

23 American College of Obstetricians and Gynecologists. *Issues in Women's Health*.Washington, DC: Office of Public Information; 1992.

24 Heiman JR, Meston CM. Evaluating sexual dysfunction in women. *Clin Obstet Gynecol*. 1997;40(3):616–629.

25 Basson R. *Clinical Updates in Women's Health Care: Sexuality and Sexual Disorders*. Vol 2, No. 2. Washington, DC: The American College of Obstetricians and Gynecologists; Spring 2003.

26 Berman JR, Berman LA, Toler SM, et al. Sildenafil Study Group. Safety and efficacy of sildenafil citrate for the treatment of females sexual arousal disorder: a double-blind, placebo controlled study. *J Urol*. 2003;170(6, pt 1):2333–8.

27 Basson R, Brotto LA. Sexual psychophysiology and effects of sildenafil citrate on oestrogenized women with acquired genital arousal disorder and impaired orgasm: a randomized controlled trial. *Br J Obstet Gynaecol*. 2003;110(11):1014–1024.

28 Braunstein GD. Androgen insufficiency in women: summary of critical issues. *Fertil Steril*. 2002;77(Suppl. 4):S94–S99.

29 Levine SB. *Sexual Life*. New York: Plenum Press; 1992.

30 Masters WH, Johnson VE. *Human Sexual Response*. Boston, MA: Little Brown & Co; 1966.

31 Basson R. The female sexual response. A different model. *J Sex Marital Ther*. 2000;26:51–65.

32 Kingsberg SA. The impact of aging on sexual function in women and their partners. *Arch Sex Behav*. 2002;31(5):431–437.

Headache Management

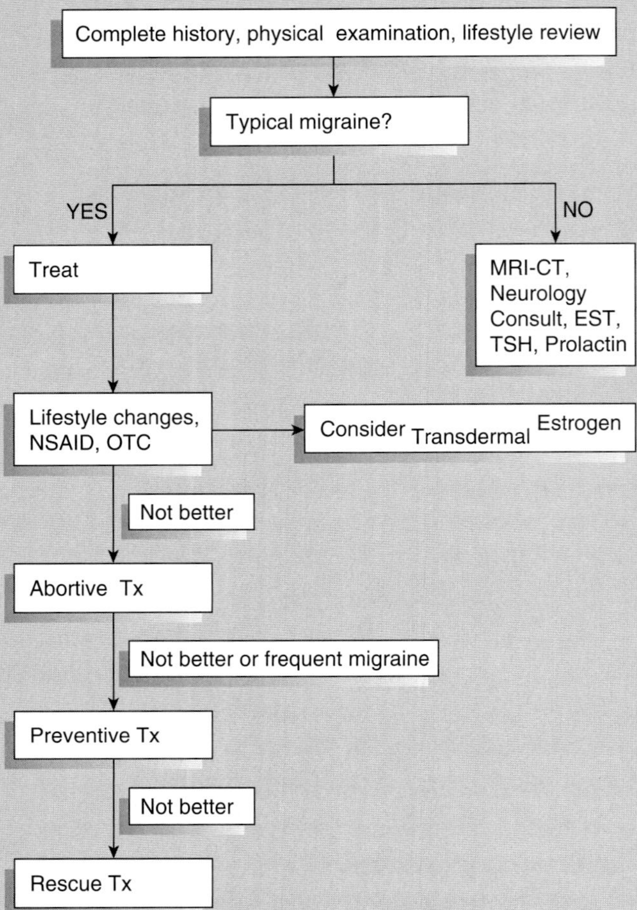

7 Migraine Headaches

Ken N. Muse

Introduction

Migraine headaches and related phenomena are some of the most common reasons perimenopausal women seek medical help. At any given time, approximately 18% of women and 6% of men suffer from migraine headaches, with a peak incidence during the reproductive years in women, particularly during the time of perimenopause. The 3:1 female:male ratio is thought to reflect the exacerbating effects of estrogen on the disease process, especially during times of changing estrogen levels, such as menstrual cyclicity, perimenopause, and starting or stopping estrogenic medications.

Migraine patients miss one day of work or school each month due to their symptoms, on average, and generate over a billion dollars of health-care bills in the United States each year. Despite the significant negative impact migraines have on a patient's quality of life, it is estimated that only half of such patients seek medical attention, with the rest being self-diagnosed and self-treated with over-the-counter medications.

Pathophysiology

KEY POINT

The etiology and pathophysiology of migraine headaches are still not completely understood.

Despite recent advances, little is known about the cause or mechanism of migraine. The disorder has a strong genetic component, with 90% of patients having at least one first-degree relative with similar symptoms. There is a racial predilection, with migraines most common in Whites and least common in African Americans. There is an inverse association between migraine prevalence and socioeconomic class. Migraines are more common in the obese, those with sedentary lifestyles, smokers, and certain neuropsychiatric conditions (epilepsy, depression, mania, premenstrual dysphoric disorder).[1]

The simple concept of the past in which migraine was thought to be the result of regional cerebral vasoconstriction followed by reactive vasodilation, has been replaced by a more complex model. Advanced neuroimaging techniques have revealed the initial event to be a dysfunction or depression of the activity of cortical neurons, which spreads across the cortex at a rate of 2–3 mm per minute. This process seems to cause the "aura" in patients with this phenomenon. Subsequently, there are alterations in cerebral blood flow (first decreased, then increased), extravasation of proteins and cytokines, and changes in inflammatory markers and the activity of certain brainstem regions, particularly the locus ceruleus and areas where serotonin receptors predominate. The pain of the headache derives from these and other processes, and is transmitted centrally via the trigeminal nerve roots.[2]

KEY POINT

Migraine symptoms vary but commonly include fatigue, neck pain, difficulty concentrating, and impaired functioning.

Clinically, the migraine symptoms are divided into sequential, and perhaps overlapping, phases: premonition, aura, headache, and resolution. Approximately one-third of patients report premonitory symptoms, which last from hours to several days before the actual headache. The nature of the symptoms varies from patient to patient, and most commonly includes a generalized decrease in functioning, fatigue, difficulty concentrating, and neck pain.

The symptoms of the aura phase develop over several minutes and typically last up to an hour. They can include a variety of neurologic processes, most commonly visual (flashing lights, jagged lines, grid-like patterns, scotomata, tunnel vision), but less commonly other sensory, motor, and complex manifestations can occur.

KEY POINT

Most migraineurs have some degree of nausea and one-third experience vomiting.

The headache phase symptoms are the most distressing, and are also quite variable. A *textbook* migraine headache starts early in the morning, slowly builds to a peak, and then subsides, lasts 4–72 hours, is unilateral, throbbing, and associated with photophobia, phonophobia, and nausea. The headache pain is usually worse with motion. It can be felt in all areas of the head, however, and start at any time of the day, including during sleep. Almost all patients have some level of nausea, and about one-third have vomiting as well. It is important to point out that not all patients with aura will go on to have headaches, and not all headaches are preceded by auras. The resolution phase is marked by fatigue, mood changes, and inability to concentrate in many, but not all migraineurs.

The International Headache Society has established research criteria for defining and classifying migraine headaches, other types of headaches, and their subtypes. Although invaluable for research, these schemes have little clinical utility as few patients have a "classic" presentation of any one type of headache. Also, the various headache categories are, to a great extent, similarly treated.

KEY POINT

An individual migraine patient tends to have a predictable pattern of symptoms.

Although the variation in symptoms between patients is large, a given patient tends to have a pattern of symptoms that is both repetitious and predictable. Most women migraineurs begin having symptoms soon after puberty, and quickly learn their own pattern of symptoms and frequency of migraine attacks. This is especially true of migraine *triggers*, things that tend to cause migraines to occur for that person. The most common triggers are dietary: alcohol intake, caffeine, and certain foods (especially those containing tyramine, nitrates, and monosodium glutamate). Alterations in daily habits (sleep patterns, meal times, and so forth) and emotional stress are also common triggers. Many patients have environmental triggers such as bright or flashing lights, or certain noises. Some prescription medicines can precipitate migraines, particularly nitrates and antihypertensives.

Role of Estrogen

KEY POINT

Fluctuations in estrogen levels are a common trigger for migraines. This phenomenon may be responsible for the exacerbation of migraines in perimenopause.

In the most general sense, estrogen is the most common migraine trigger for female migraineurs. The rise in estrogen at puberty is thought to initiate the problem in most women with migraines, and the threefold higher rate of migraines in reproductive-age women is attributed to the estrogen fluctuations seen during menstrual cyclicity. Approximately 20–25% of patients have *menstrual migraines*, in which most (but not all) of their migraines occur from the day before menses to the 4 days after the onset of menstruation. Migraine attacks seem to rise during perimenopause, perhaps due to the more erratic and unopposed estrogen secretion during that time, and to fade in frequency and severity after the menopausal transition is over. Migraines are relatively rare (prevalence less than 3%) in women over 65 years of age who are not taking estrogen therapy.[3]

Early pregnancy, a time when estrogen levels rise, is a time of migraine exacerbation for 25% of migraineurs; in the last two trimesters of pregnancy, a time of relatively high and constant estrogen concentrations, most patients have fewer attacks. When hormone levels fall precipitously postpartum, migraine attacks tend to rebound in frequency and severity. Breast-feeding may prolong this problem until estrogen levels stabilize.

Women with migraines who undergo surgical menopause (bilateral oophorectomy, usually at the time of hysterectomy) should be told that, in about one-third of cases, migraine headaches will increase in frequency and severity temporarily. This is attributed to the relatively sharp drop in estrogen seen after the ovaries are removed, and applies especially to the majority of women who do not pursue hormone replacement therapy after surgery.[4]

KEY POINT

Oral contraceptives can induce menstrual migraines similar to those seen with naturally occurring menses.

The use of oral contraceptives is also a common trigger for many female migraineurs. This is especially so during the hormone-free interval at the end of each cycle, mimicking the *menstrual migraine* pattern found in spontaneously cycling women, in whom the strongest migraine trigger is seen when estrogen levels are falling quickly.

Patient Evaluation

The evaluation of a perimenopausal woman with presumptive migraine headaches begins with a careful history taking and physical examination. A family history of migraine is important to note. All the features of the headache attacks should be noted, including the typical onset and duration of pain, the location and severity, the presence of aura and any associated symptoms, such as nausea or neurological deficits. Factors, which worsen the attacks (triggers; bright lights, sounds, and so forth) should be noted, as should factors that lessen the headache and the associated symptoms. Lifestyle issues in terms of sleep, exercise, and dietary patterns should be reviewed. Most patients will have already treated their symptoms with home remedies, over-the-counter medications, and perhaps alternative medicine therapies; these measures should be investigated carefully and their effectiveness noted.

KEY POINT

To diagnose migraines, the patient's symptoms and pattern of headaches should be consistent with the current description of migraine headaches.

Patients should be encouraged to record their symptoms prospectively in a daily headache diary, which serves several

KEY POINT

A headache diary provides validation and understanding of the patient's condition as well as a comparison for the efficacy of therapy.

valuable functions upon review with the health-care provider. The diary will verify and enlarge upon the history previously obtained. It will often reveal new features of the problem to both the patient and the clinician. In doing so, the patient gains a feeling of understanding her problem more comprehensively. Most importantly, when the diary is continued after therapy begins, it will allow an accurate assessment of the effectiveness of the therapy, where a retrospective, global patient assessment is often less than ideal.

DIFFERENTIAL DIAGNOSIS

The main goal of the patient evaluation process is to recognize that a headache is a symptom, not a diagnosis, and that it is important to identify patients with serious problems who require different therapies. Most patients with typical histories of migraine headaches, with patterns of attacks largely unchanged for years, beginning in the teen years, can be confidently diagnosed with migraine headaches and no further evaluation is needed.

It is very rare for a migrainous process to begin later in life, however, especially after 50 years of age. A headache history starting after age 50 should initiate a search for another, perhaps organic, cause. Neuroimaging (magnetic resonance imaging or computerized tomography) of the head and neck should be done to rule out a tumor, stroke, subdural hematoma, or other lesion. Thyroid-stimulating hormone and prolactin levels should be measured to help assess thyroid status and the possibility of a pituitary lesion.

KEY POINT

New onset headaches and headaches atypical for migraines require further evaluation.

A Westergren erythrocyte sedimentation rate should be done to rule out the elevation seen in giant cell arteritis, which is often described as headache associated with muscle and joint pain, visual loss, fever, weight loss, and night sweats. Tenderness over the temporal artery is a key diagnostic clue, and a temporal artery biopsy is the ideal form of diagnosis.

Another frequent cause of headache in the elderly is medications, such as nitrates for heart disease and antihypertensives.

Tension headaches are usually described as band- or vise-like, variable in timing and severity, and relatively frequent. They are not associated with aura or premonitory symptoms. They are best treated with physical therapy and analgesic medications.

Cluster headaches are very severe, unilateral headaches centered on the eye or nearby area, which are associated with tearing or sinus drainage on the affected side. They last 15–180 minutes and occur in *clusters*, interspersed with relatively long symptom-free intervals.

Therapies

General Therapies

KEY POINT

Lifestyle modifications can also lead to an improvement in migraines.

Most migraine patients in the perimenopausal years have already undergone extensive headache evaluation, but some have not. It is important to begin therapy in a logical, stepwise fashion without omitting necessary steps such as educating the patient about her disease process in a way that opens avenues for therapy. The initial step involves lifestyle modifications. Patients should be instructed to develop regular sleep habits, waking and going to sleep as much as possible at the same time each day. Likewise, regular meals should also be encouraged, stressing the importance of not skipping meals. Known food triggers should be avoided, taking special care when dining in restaurants. If obese, weight loss should be encouraged as part of this regimen and smoking cessation should always be encouraged. The patient's medications should be reviewed to determine if they could be contributing to her headaches. Regular aerobic exercise is an integral part of therapy, and efforts at stress reduction should be vigorous and ongoing. Cognitive therapies, relaxation therapies, biofeedback, and similar treatments may be of benefit, but are beyond the scope of most clinicians.

Estrogen Maneuvers

Perimenopausal headache patients are particularly appropriate for consideration of estrogen manipulation as part of their therapy. The marked fluctuations in estrogen levels of the menopausal transition, may be contributing to their symptoms. However, estrogen therapy and estrogen-progestin therapy, may also cause or contribute to perimenopausal headaches.

What's the Evidence?

In the Women's Health Initiative study, the largest randomized controlled trial of hormone therapy in menopausal women, about half of women initially complaining of *headaches or migraines* at baseline had improvement on hormone therapy when evaluated both 1 and 3 years later; however, so did those randomized to placebo therapy. Of women not complaining of headaches or migraines initially, 5.8% at year 1 and 7.5% at year 3, had headaches on combined hormone therapy, compared to 4.7% and 10.4% randomized to placebo. At year 1, headaches were significantly higher in women on hormone therapy, and at year 3, they were significantly lower.[6] One can conclude that hormone therapy has no predictable effect in the general population of menopausal women on headaches, but changes in individual women are, of course, quite possible.

Any form of estrogen therapy can be used, with the goal being a stable serum estrogen level. The dose of estrogen will often be determined by other endpoints, such as efficacy in treating vasomotor symptoms or estrogen therapy side effects. All routes of administration may be efficacious in treating perimenopausal headaches, but transdermal administration by patch or cream, with its more constant serum levels and fewer hepatic effects, would seem preferable.

KEY POINT

When using estrogen therapy, the goal is to achieve very stable serum estrogen levels.

Women with migraines who fear getting pregnant during perimenopause may wish to use oral contraceptive pills for migraine suppression. This is a reasonable request as long as it is understood that some women will see improvement, especially those with predominantly *menstrual migraine* symptoms, and some women will experience a worsening of their headaches. A key to successful treatment is prescribing the oral contraceptives continuously, with no hormone-free interval. Patients should be instructed to discard the placebo pills which comprise the last week of the pack. Once again, the goal is to keep estrogen levels constant by avoiding the fall normally seen at the end of the cycle. Alternatively, the hormone-free week could be included every 2, 3, or 4 months, or low-dose estrogen supplementation could be given during the otherwise hormone-free week. There are several small reports of this type of maneuver being helpful in migraineurs, but no large trial has been done.

The risk of stroke using oral contraceptives is of special concern in migraine. A recent large review found that in general migraineurs (with or without aura) have an approximate twofold increase risk of stroke, and those using oral contraceptives have an eightfold risk.[7,8] Thus, caution should be exercised in this setting, and an oral contraceptive trial should be used only when patient and physician believe benefits outweigh risks. Smokers and those with hypertension should be excluded.

ACUTE THERAPIES

Acute (also called *abortive*) therapies are those that are used to treat a headache when it is starting or beginning to start. They are given on an as-needed basis, and are divided into nonspecific and specific treatments. Nonspecific therapies include analgesics and nonsteroidal anti-inflammatory drugs (NSAIDs); alternative medicine therapies could also be used here, perhaps. Be aware that overuse of some of these agents may lead to rebound headaches afterward.

KEY POINT

Acute therapies are used to abort an incipient migraine attack.

Specific therapies are those which are only used to treat migraine headaches; they comprise the ergot and triptan family of medications. The latter have revolutionized the treatment of migraine and should be considered the first-line therapy for women with serious, frequent migraine attacks (Table 7-1).[9,10]

PREVENTIVE THERAPIES

KEY POINT

Preventive therapies are indicted for patients with frequent headaches or for patients who fail to respond adequately to acute therapies.

Preventive therapies are indicted for patients with frequent headaches or for patients who fail to respond adequately to acute therapies. They are given chronically, with the idea that the frequency and severity of attacks will be lessened. Beta-blockers, antidepressants, calcium channel blockers, and anticonvulsant medicines comprise this group of therapies. Clinicians often select the agent to be used by the patient's comorbidities; patients with hypertension may benefit by being placed on a beta-blocker or antihypertensive, and those with depression or related symptoms may benefit from being on an antidepressant (Table 7-2).

RESCUE THERAPIES

KEY POINT

Most patients respond very well to triptans and standard analgesics, but even the best patient needs rescue therapy availability for the inevitable breakthrough migraine.

Despite the efficacy of the above agents, some patients may not be able to use the agent in a timely fashion, or on occasion the response to the agent is suboptimal. For these occasions, *rescue therapies* should be made available to the patient. Opioid analgesics will provide significant, but nonspecific pain relief. Unlike the other therapies, which aim to allow the patient maximal normal activity, the use of rescue agents may impair normal function. Thus, they should not be first-line therapy nor should they be used frequently. The patient is allowed to medicate herself at these times in order to prevent a visit to the emergency room and to allow her to sleep during the night.

WHEN TO REFER

Even when these detailed algorithms are carefully pursued, a sizeable minority of women will fail to respond adequately to treatment. Referral to a neurologist or headache specialist may be of benefit

Table 7-1. ACUTE THERAPIES FOR MIGRAINE HEADACHES, INCLUDING RESCUE MEDICATIONS

SPECIFIC THERAPIES		
Triptans		
Almotriptan (Axert)	6.25, 12.5 mg PO	May repeat in 2 hours
Eletriptan (Relpax)	40–80 mg PO	May repeat in 2 hours
Frovatriptan (Frova)	2.5 mg PO	May repeat in 2 hours
Naratriptan (Amerge)	2.5 mg PO	May repeat in 2 hours
Rizatriptan (Maxalt)	5, 10 mg PO	May repeat in 2 hours
Sumatriptan (Imitrex)	25, 50, 100 mg PO 5, 10, 20 mg IN 6 mg SQ	May repeat in 2 hours
Zolmitriptan (Zomig)	2.5, 5 mg PO	May repeat in 2 hours
Ergots		
Tablets (Cafergot)	1 mg, 100 mg caffeine	2 now, 1–2 q 30–60 minutes
Ergotamine suppositories (Cafergot)	2 mg, 100 mg caffeine	
Intranasal (Migranal)	4 mg IN	Repeat in 1 hour
NONSPECIFIC THERAPIES		
Simple Analgesics		
Acetaminophen (Tylenol)	325 mg	
Aspirin	325 mg	
Aspirin/caffeine/butalbital (Fiorinal)	325/40/50 mg	
Acetaminophen/aspirin/caffeine (Excedrin)	250/250/65 mg	
Acetaminophen/aspirin/butalbital (Fioricet, Esgic)	325/40/50 mg	
Nonsteroidal anti-inflammatory drugs		
RESCUE MEDICATIONS		
Opioids		
Butorphanol (Stadol)	1 mg IN, IV, IM	
Hydromorphone (Dilaudid)	1, 4 mg PO	
Meperidine (Demerol)	50, 100 mg PO	
Morphine (MS Contin)	20, 60 mg PO	

when this occurs by allowing more exhaustive evaluation or more aggressive management. Similarly, referral is indicated when a patient has features suggesting that the patient may have a diagnosis other than routine migraine headache: headache with onset late in life, headache with neurologic deficits, or multiple comorbid conditions.

Table 7-2. **PREVENTIVE THERAPIES FOR MIGRAINE HEADACHES**

Preventive Therapies	
Anticonvulsants	
Gabapentin (Neurontin)	500–3000 mg PO
Topiramate (Topamax)	15–25 mg PO qhs
Valproic acid (Depakote)	500–3000 mg daily
Antidepressants	
Nortriptyline (Aventyl)	10–100 mg daily
Amitriptyline (Elavil)	25–75 qhs
Doxepin (Sinequan)	10–150 mg daily
Fluoxetine (Prozac)	10–80 mg daily
Beta-Blockers	
Atenolol (Tenormin)	50–150 mg daily
Metoprolol (Lopressor, Toprol))	100–200 mg daily
Nadolol (Corgard)	40–240 mg daily
Propranolol (Inderal)	40–120 mg bid
Timolol (Blocadren)	10–30 mg daily
Calcium Channel Blockers	
Verapamil (Calan)	160–320 mg daily
Nifedipine (Procardia)	30–180 mg daily
Diltiazem (Cardizem)	120–360 mg daily

Guiding Questions

Is This A Typical Migraine Headache Patient?

- Is there a history of many years of similar headaches?
- Is there a history of aura, and/or typical visual changes?

Is This A Patient Who Might Respond To Altering Estrogen Therapy?

- Is she having symptoms suggesting catamenial, perimenopausal, or menopausal, changes (hot flashes, vaginal dryness, and so forth)?
- Is she taking estrogen therapy now?
- Did she have a poor reaction to estrogen treatment in the past?

Should This Patient Be Referred?

- Onset of headaches late in life?
- Atypical symptoms present such as neurologic deficits or multiple comorbid conditions.

Discussion of Cases

CASE 1

A 50-year-old woman initially presents complaining of severe headaches perimenstrually. The headaches are absent at other times, are preceded by aura and are accompanied by visual changes. She has regular spontaneous menses, takes no medications except ibuprofen and aspirin that "haven't helped the headaches," and has no vasomotor symptoms. She wants stronger pain medicine. The rest of her history and physical examination is unremarkable.

Would you recommend further testing at this point?

No, a diagnosis of menstrual migraines can be confidently made.

What treatment should be done?

She has failed lesser treatments, so a triptan trial could be prescribed for use as needed. Alternatively, she could be given estrogen cream or an estrogen patch to wear during the time of expected menses, to see if estrogen supplementation would be sufficient.

Anything else?

A oral opioid *rescue* medication could be prescribed; also, she should start keeping a headache diary.

CASE 2

A 55-year-old woman has done well on combination estrogen-progestin hormone replacement therapy for 8 years, without menopausal symptoms; however, for the first time in her life she's developed severe headaches, centered on her left eye, with associated tearing and runny nose. She denies aura or other symptoms, but the headaches are frequent, several times in the past week. Her history and physical examination are otherwise normal.

What should be done next?

A new onset of headache after menopause is concerning. Her history strongly suggests cluster headache, and opioid analgesics could be given. Because the headache is of new onset, a neurologic consultation should be obtained and neuroimaging should be considered.

REFERENCES

1 Goadsby PJ. Migraine pathophysiology. *Headache.* 2005;45(Suppl. 1): S14–S24.

2 Goadsby PJ, Lipton RB, Ferrari MD. Migraine—current understanding and treatment. *N Engl J Med.* 2002;346:257–270.

3 Johnson CJ. Headache in women. *Prim Care Clin Office Pract.* 2004;31:417–428.

4 MacGregor EA. Oestrogen and attacks of migraine with and without aura. *Lancet Neurol.* 2004;3:354–361.

5 Silberstein SD. Migraine. *Lancet.* 2004;363:381–391.

6 Barnabei VM, Cochrane BB, Aragaki AK, et al. Menopausal symptoms and treatment-related effects of estrogen and progestin in the Women's Health Initiative. *Obstet Gynecol.* 2005;105:1063–1073.

7 Etminan M, Takkouche B, Isosrna FC, et al. Risk of ischaemic stroke in people with migraine: systematic review and meta-analysis of observational studies. *Br Med J.* 2005;330:63–66.

8 Kurth T, Slomke MA, Kase CS, et al. Migraine, headache, and the risk of stroke in women. A prospective study. *Neurology.* 2005;64: 1020–1026.

9 Ferrari MD, Roon, KI, Lipton RB, et al. Oral triptans (serotonin 5-HT1B/1D agonists) in acute migraine treatment: a meta-analysis of 53 trials. *Lancet.* 2001;358:1668–1675.

10 Loder E, Biondi D. General principles of migraine management: the changing role of prevention. *Headache.* 2005;45(Suppl. 1):S33–S47.

8 Impact of Perimenopause on Physical Appearance and Reproductive Tissues

James H. Liu

Introduction

A number of changes in physical appearance have been associated with the perimenopausal transition. These changes include a gradual increase in skin wrinkling, an increase in body weight, abdominal fat, and adipose tissue in the buttocks and thighs, a decrease in breast density, and a slight thinning of scalp hair. Are these changes due to aging, a gradual loss of estrogen production from the ovaries, or just genetics? The purpose of this chapter will be to review alterations in skin and connective tissue, reproductive tissues, body composition, and body mass that may occur during the perimenopausal transition. The impact of aging and the linkage between these physical changes and the overall hormonal environment will be discussed.

Skin and Underlying Connective Tissues

In many cultures, women are often judged by their external appearance, especially the appearance of the skin on the face, neck, and hands. The importance of this part of a woman's physical appearance is reflected by the increasing sales of skin care products and the growing demand for cosmetic plastic procedures over past decade.

KEY POINT

With aging, there is atrophy of the skin, decrease in collagen elasticity, and loss of subcutaneous tissues.

The structure of the skin is organized into several layers consisting of the epidermis, dermis, and subcutaneous fat and connective tissues. The changes in the skin associated with aging occur gradually over a 20–40-year time frame and are impacted adversely by smoking and sun exposure. In older women, the skin becomes thinner, more dry, wrinkly, and unevenly pigmented. There is an increased incidence of proliferative-type lesions such as basal cell carcinoma. In elderly women, the macroscopic appearance of the skin becomes shiny, thin, and translucent because of progressive atrophy of the epidermis, dermis, and the underlying subcutaneous fat. On a microscopic level, the epidermis has decreased keratinocyte cell volume, flattening of the dermal papillae with disappearance of the rete pegs, decreased melanocyte density, and a decrease in epidermal macrophages (Langerhans cells). Overall collagen content is reduced in the subcutaneous tissues and there is increased brittleness of collagen fibers because of increased collagen cross-linking and a reduction in vascularity.

Dermatologists have classified wrinkles into two types. In sun-exposed areas, such as the neck and face, permanent wrinkles may develop and do not disappear when the skin is stretched. This is due to a permanent indentation of the epidermis forming a wrinkle furrow. The second type of wrinkle is called a shallow or temporary wrinkle. These are usually localized to sun-protected areas and these wrinkles disappear when the skin is stretched.

KEY POINT

The skin responds to changes in estrogens and androgens.

The skin is an endocrine responsive organ containing both androgen and estrogen receptors.[1,2] In addition, the skin and the adipocyte cells in the subcutaneous fat contain the aromatase enzyme which convert androgens to estrogens.[3] The highest concentration of aromatase activity is in the thighs, abdomen, and buttocks.

It is difficult to differentiate the effects of skin aging from hormonal effects, genetic factors, and sun exposure. Most of the evidence for a favorable effect of systemic estrogen and/or estrogen/progestin use has been derived from observational, cross-sectional studies. These studies suggest that HT users are less likely to have facial wrinkling, dry skin, and loss of elasticity when other variables such as sun exposure and smoking are taken into account.[4–6]

There have been only two small randomized trials that have studied the impact of systemic estrogen therapy on skin. Maheux and coworkers randomized 60 subjects to either conjugated equine estrogens (CEE) 0.625 mg or placebo for 12 months and examined skin changes by skin biopsy.[7] There was an increase in skin thickness as measured by ultrasound and an increase in dermis thickness by skin biopsy. In a similar study design, Sauerbronn et al. randomized 21 menopausal subjects to estradiol valerate/ cyproterone acetate and 20 women to placebo for 6 months.[8] Treated subjects had a significant increase in the amount of collagen fibers but no significant changes in skin thickness. These studies suggest that estrogen therapy may have a beneficial role on the overall skin thickness and collagen content, but does not specifically address facial wrinkles.

Topical application of estrogen applied locally to the skin may have some benefits without significant elevations in blood levels of estrogen. Two studies have examined the impact of locally applied estrogens. Assessment of these local sites show increases in collagen content where the skin is directly exposed to estrogens.[9,10] At present, there is insufficient evidence to recommend the routine use of systemic or topical estrogens for the prevention and treatment of wrinkles or to delay skin aging.

Genitourinary Tract Changes

The female genital and urinary tracts are exquisitely sensitive to estrogens and progestins due to the high concentrations of estrogen and progesterone receptors.[11,12] With the onset of the perimenopause transition and the decline in estrogen, the vaginal blood flow to the mucosa decreases, there is loss of rugated folds, and the vaginal mucosa changes from a purple-red color to a pale-pink, shiny appearance . At the cellular level, the squamous epithelia shift from a superficial cell morphology to a greater percentage of basal and parabasal cells. The vaginal bacterial flora is shifted such that growth of *Lactobacillus* is no longer supported and vaginal pH becomes more neutral.

Vaginal Atrophy

In menopausal women, the incidence of vaginal dryness has been reported to range from 17% to 43%[13,14] while the incidence of urinary incontinence and recurrent urinary tract infections have been reported to increase.[15] Are these urinary tract changes strictly due to estrogen deficiency or does aging play a major role and thus urinary tract infections and incontinence will improve over time?

KEY POINT

Both systemic and locally applied estrogens are effective for the treatment of vaginal atrophy.

In randomized controlled trials to study the treatment of vaginal atrophy, replacement with systemic CEE at 0.3, 0.45, or 0.625 mg either alone or in combination with medroxyprogesterone acetate (MPA) shifted the vaginal epithelial cells toward a superficial phenotype that more closely resembled reproductive-aged women.[16] Topical application of vaginal estradiol tablets (25 μg daily for 2 weeks, then twice weekly) was also effective in treating vaginal atrophy.[17]

The use of selective estrogen receptor modulators such as tamoxifen is also associated with estrogenic effects on vaginal mucosa. Vaginal smears generally demonstrate an increase in superficial cells and a shift to a more acidic vaginal pH.[18] Raloxifene, another selective estrogen receptor modulator, has not been reported to change preexisting vaginal atrophy or increase vaginal discharge.[19] In a small, randomized placebo-controlled trial, pelvic organ prolapse appeared to be greater in women randomized to raloxifene or tamoxifen when compared to placebo or the estrogen groups.

Soy supplements also appear to have minimal estrogenic effects on vaginal maturation indices.[20] These studies are limited by the small numbers of participants, differences in the soy preparations, and the variation in bioavailability of isoflavones in these preparations.

Urinary Incontinence and Urinary Tract Infections

KEY POINT

HT increased the incidence of urinary incontinence and frequency of urinary tract infections.

In the Women's Health Initiative (WHI) randomized placebo-controlled trials, menopausal hormone therapy (HT) increased the incidence of all types of urinary incontinence at 1 year among women who were continent at baseline. The risk was greatest for stress urinary incontinence (CEE + MPA: relative risk [RR], 1.87 [95% confidence interval [CI], 1.61–2.18] and CEE alone: RR, 2.15 [95% CI, 1.77–2.62]). The frequency of general urinary incontinence worsened in both trials (CEE + MPA: RR, 1.38 [95% CI, 1.28–1.49]; CEE alone: RR, 1.47 [95% CI, 1.35–1.61]).). Based on these findings in over 25,000 menopausal women, "conjugated equine estrogen with or without progestin should not be prescribed for the prevention or relief of urinary incontinence."[21]

The frequency of urinary tract infections was investigated in the Heart Estrogen/Progestin Replacement Study (HERS). In this randomized trial of over 2700 women, there was a slight increase in frequency of urinary tract infections in the group receiving HT (odds ratio [OR] 1.16, 95% CI, 0.99–1.37).[22] Other controlled trials and a meta-analysis suggest that in women with *recurrent* urinary tract infections, estrogen may be beneficial compared to placebo.[23]

Body Mass and Composition

In the United States, there is a trend toward increasing body mass throughout adult life for both men and women.[24] Body composition also changes with a decrease in the fat-free mass component (i.e., muscle mass) and a progressive increase in visceral fat stores until approximately age 70 years. Thereafter, there is a gradual decrease in body mass index (BMI) with further aging. Although the concept is intuitively obvious, the biggest factor for weight gain in adults is physical activity. Increases in parity are also associated with progressive weight gain.[25] In the United States, lifestyle factors such as the increased use of the automobile and the reduced frequency of physical activity such as walking has created a growing population of overweight adults. These lifestyle factors have resulted in a nation of adults with increased visceral fat, increased insulin resistance, increased prevalence of Type 2 diabetes, and a greater incidence of metabolic syndrome (see Table 8-1).[26,27] It is estimated that overweight (BMI 25–29 kg/m^2) and obese adults (BMI ≥ 30 kg/m^2) now constitute over 39% of adults in the United States. This disturbing trend in conjunction with the increased

Table 8-1. **CHARACTERISTICS OF THE METABOLIC SYNDROME IN WOMEN**

Waist circumference > 35 in. or 88 cm
Serum triglycerides ≥ 150 mg/dL
Serum HDL < 50 mg/dL
Blood pressure ≥ 130/85 mmHg
Fasting plasma glucose ≥ 110 mg/dL

incidence of adults diagnosed with metabolic syndrome and its adverse health consequences will become our greatest burden for future health-care expenditures.

Impact of Physiological Hormonal Changes on Body Composition

KEY POINT

With onset of menopause, there is a shift in the androgen:estrogen ratio.

Current evidence suggests that most of the changes in body composition are related to aging and not the menopausal transition; however, changes in circulating estrogens and androgens can influence muscle mass, fat composition, and fat distribution. During the perimenopause, there is a relative decline in circulating estradiol levels and a maintenance of testosterone production from the ovaries.[28] This combination of factors leads to a physiological shift in the androgen:estrogen ratio. The overall androgen predominance can result in increased scalp hair loss or thinning in scalp hair and the occurrence of facial acne. The reduction in estrogen levels will also decrease overall breast density with fat replacing much of the glandular tissue network.

More importantly, this shift in the androgen:estrogen ratio will significantly modify liver metabolism. As a consequence, there is a decrease in sex hormone-binding globulin concentrations, reduced high-density lipoprotein (HDL), increased low-density lipoprotein (LDL), and increased triglycerides levels. The implications of these lipoprotein changes on long-term cardiovascular risk are not clear.

With normal aging, circulating levels of the adrenal steroid dehydroepiandrosterone (DHEA) and its stable conjugate DHEA sulfate decline progressively to low levels while cortisol production appears to be maintained.[29,30] The physiological decrease in DHEA sulfate can be as much as 70–80% and has been attributed to a reduction in 17,20-desmolase activity within the adrenal cortex.[31] Although the physiological role of DHEA remains to be defined, it can be conceptually considered a prohormone that is converted peripherally to androgens and estrogens. The metabolic consequences of these changes would suggest that these subsequent shifts in androgen levels contribute to the decline in fat-free mass. Short-term replacement with exogenous DHEA at doses of 25–50 mg/day in pilot studies has been purported to increase lean body mass, modestly elevate circulating androgens and estrogens levels without stimulation of significant endometrial growth.[32] In small prospective studies,

DHEA administration has been reported to improve insulin sensitivity,[33] sexual arousal,[34] reduce vasomotor symptoms,[35] increase bone density,[36] improve vaginal maturation index,[12] and improve cognitive performance.[37] However, long-term randomized trials to assess the risk:benefit ratio of DHEA administration have not been conducted.

Reduced growth hormone (GH) secretion is also observed with aging.[38] The nocturnal increases in GH secretion associated with sleep become more modest. This reduction in mean GH levels leads to an overall decline in insulin-like growth factor I (IGF-1) levels and is associated with decreases in muscle mass and increased body fat. Short-term replacement with GH or IGF-1 in older men and women appear to reverse some of these changes in body composition but the long-term benefits and risks with this approach are not known.[39]

Although hypothyroidism is more frequently diagnosed in older women, the levels of circulating thyroid-stimulating hormone (TSH) do not appear to change with aging. Women receiving thyroid hormone replacement should have monitoring of their TSH levels when starting or stopping HT so that thyroid replacement can be adjusted.

Hormone Therapy: Impact on Body Composition

There is a common perception that HT is a cause for weight gain. A number of observational trials suggest that HT use is associated with a decreased waist:hip ratio,[2] decreased BMI,[40,41] and reduced abdominal weight gain relative to nonusers.[42] These observations may be subject to healthy user's bias in the study volunteers since women who take HT have been purported to have a healthier lifestyle than nonusers. The preponderance of randomized clinical trials indicates that short and long-term administration of HT does not alter body weight, body composition, or fat distribution to any significant degree.[43]

Leptin is a peptide hormone that is synthesized by the adipocyte and has been implicated as a mediator for satiety.[44] Although leptin levels decrease with aging, there are no studies that implicate a direct role for leptin in weight changes or body composition.[45] There is no information available regarding the role of ghrelin with aging. Ghrelin is a peptide hormone produced by the gastric mucosa that is responsible for appetite stimulation.

Treatment Approaches

KEY POINT

The initial treatment approach for obesity should be exercise and dietary modification.

The first-line treatment for obesity is lifestyle changes, mainly diet modification and regular exercise. Dietary interventions should focus on calorie restriction. It is estimated that a 500–1000 kcal/day reduction from the usual daily intake will result in a weight loss of 1–2 lb a week.[46] To increase activity levels, an exercise program of at least 30 minutes of moderately intense exercise should be undertaken at a minimum of three times per week.[47]

Which diets are best? Current evidence suggests that low carbohydrate diet results in greater weight loss at 6 months when compared to a low fat diet in a randomized controlled trial.[48] However, by 12 months, participants in both diets achieved the same weight loss. Comparison of effectiveness of Weight Watchers to other popular diets such as Atkins, Ornish, and Zone indicates that all have similar results in weight reduction over a 1-year period.[49] As with many chronic diseases, these lifestyle changes must be maintained or weight gain will recur. The overall success rates for lifestyle changes indicate a lack of compliance and weight regain in 60–86% of patients within 3 years.[50]

KEY POINT

Medical treatment for obesity should be reserved until after lifestyle modification has been initiated.

Medical treatment of obesity has also met with limited success. This approach should not be recommended until patients have participated in at least a 6-month effort in lifestyle modifications. Therapy should be considered in those with BMI $\geq$ 30 kg/m^2 or those with risk factors with a BMI of $\geq$ 27 kg/m^2.[51] Evaluation of single-agent pharmacotherapy suggests that no single drug or class of drugs demonstrated superiority. Table 8-2 lists the available single agents in use in the United States. A meta-analysis of weight loss trials shows that the average weight loss subtracted from the placebo group ranged from 2 to 4 kg in trials that ranged from 7 to 48 weeks.[52]

Bariatric surgical approaches have dramatically increased for the treatment of morbid obesity ($\geq$40 kg/m^2). These operations can be classified into restrictive type or combined restrictive/malabsorptive procedures. The restrictive type procedures generally involve decreasing the size of the stomach with either stapling the stomach so that only a small pouch remains or by banding the stomach with a mechanical device leading to early satiety. These types of procedure have demonstrated short-term efficacy but long-term response are less encouraging.[53] Malabsorptive procedures involve

Table 8-2. **MEDICAL THERAPY FOR WEIGHT LOSS**

Medication	*Dose*	*Mechanism of Action*	*Weight Loss in Excess of Placebo*	*Cost Per Month*
Phentermine	30 mg/day	Enhances norepinephrine levels centrally inducing satiety	8.1 kg	$60
Sibutramine	15 mg/day	Inhibits norepinephrine and serotonin reuptake	5.0 kg	$116
Orlistat	120 mg/day	Binds intestinal lipase to prevent hydrolysis of dietary fat in GI tract	3.4 kg	$119
Metformin	1500–2000 mg/day	Reduces hepatic glucose output and reduces insulin levels	Not known	$52
Herbal supplements containing Ephedra*	Variable	Ephedra increases heart rate and accelerates basal metabolism	Not known	Variable

Abbreviation: GI, gastrointestinal.

*Food and Drug Administration (FDA) has banned Ephedra-containing supplements.

bypassing a portion of the small bowel thereby reducing the surface area of absorption and increasing food transit time. This may lead to diarrhea and decrease absorption of vital nutrients such as vitamins as well as electrolyte abnormalities. The gastric bypass (Roux-en-Y gastric bypass), which is a largely restrictive, mildly malabsorptive procedure is performed most commonly (65.1%). Other procedures such as biliopancreatic diversion, vertical banded gastroplasties, and laparoscopic adjustable banding are less popular.[54] Overall mortality with experienced surgical groups has been reported to be less than 1% and weight loss of 20–40 kg have been maintained for up to 10 years.[55] It is important to emphasize that the surgical approach is to be reserved for those that are morbidly obese.

What's the Evidence?

- **Both systemic and topically-applied estrogens can increase skin thickness and reduce wrinkles.** Observational and cross-sectional studies suggest that estrogen users have less facial wrinkling and less loss in skin elasticity relative to nonusers.[4,5,56] Only two, small randomized trials have shown that estrogen or estrogen/progestin use may increase skin thickness or improve the underlying collagen matrix.[7,8] Because of the small number of participants, these studies by themselves are insufficient evidence to propose estrogen as a treatment to retard skin aging.

- **Vaginal atrophy and vaginal dryness can be treated with either low-dose systemic estrogen or vaginally-applied estrogens.** Randomized placebo-controlled trials indicate that low-dose systemic estrogen such as CEE at a dose of 0.3 mg[16] or vaginally-applied estradiol at a dose of 25 μg twice per week[17] are effective treatments for vaginal atrophy and dryness.
- **Urinary incontinence and urinary tract infections appear to be increased with HT.** The WHI hormone trials show an increased incidence of urinary incontinence in both the estrogen-only and estrogen-progestin groups compared to baseline.[21] These findings confirm previous reports from smaller, prospective studies. The HERS trial showed an increased frequency of urinary tract infections with estrogen-progestin therapy. However, this was not statistically significant.[22]
- **HT is associated with increased weight gain.** Randomized clinical trials suggest that all women gain weight with aging, however, in estrogen users, weight gain tended to be less than that with placebo groups.[41]
- **Contrary to public perception, the caloric restriction principle is more important than the type of diet (Atkins, Ornish, Zone) utilized for treatment of obesity.** In controlled trials, weight reduction was similar among the four dietary approaches evaluated: Atkins, Ornish, Zone, and Weight Watchers.[49]

References

1 Schmidt JB, Lindmaier A, Spona J. Hormone receptors in pubic skin of premenopausal and postmenopausal females. *Gynecol Obstet Invest.* 1990;30:97–100.

2 Hasselquist MB, Goldberg N, Schroeter A, et al. Isolation and characterization of estrogen receptor in human skin. *J Clin Endocrinol Metab.* 1980;50:76–82.

3 Simpson ER, Mahendroo MS, Means GD, et al. Aromatase cytochromeP450, the enzyme responsible for estrogen biosynthesis. *Endocr Rev.* 1994;15:342–355.

4 Castelo-Branco C, Figueras F, Martinez de Osaba MJ, et al. Facial wrinkling in postmenopausal women: effects of smoking status and hormone replacement therapy. *Maturitas.* 1998;29:75–86.

5 Dunn LB, Damesyn M, Moore AA, et al. Does estrogen prevent skin aging? Results from the First National Health and Nutrition Examination Survey (NHANES I). *Arch Dermatol.* 1997;133:339–342.

6 Henry F, Pierard-Franchimont C, Cauwenbergh G, et al. Age-related changes in facial skin contours and rheology. *J Am Geriartr Soc.* 1997;45:220–222.

7 Maheux R, Naud F, Rioux M, et al. A randomized, double-blind, placebo-controlled study on the effect of conjugated estrogens on skin thickness. *Am J Obstet Gynecol.* 1994;170:642–649.

8 Sauerbronn AV, Fonseca AM, Bagnoli VR, et al. The effects of systemic hormonal replacement therapy on the skin of postmenopausal women. *Int J Gynaecol Obstet.* 2000;68:35–41.

9 Schmidt JB, Binder M, Demschik G, et al. Treatment of skin aging with topical estrogens. *Int J Dermatol.* 1996;35:669–674.

10 Varila E, Rantala I, Oikarinen A, et al. The effect of topical oestradiol on skin collagen of postmenopausal women. *Br J Obstet Gynaecol.* 1995;102:985–989.

11 Rizk DE, Raaschou T, Mason N, et al. Evidence of progesterone receptors in the mucosa of the urinary bladder. *Scand J Urol Nephrol.* 2001;35:305–309.

12 Copas P, Bukovsky A, Asbury B, et al. Estrogen, progesterone, and androgen receptor expression in levator ani muscle and fascia. *J Women's Health Gend Based Med.* 2001;10:785–795.

13 Dennerstein L, Dudley EC, Hopper JL, et al. A prospective population-based study of menopausal symptoms. *Obstet Gynecol.* 2000;96: 351–358.

14 Stadbert E, Mattson LA, Milsom I. The prevalence and severity of climacteric symptoms and the use of different treatment regimens in a Swedish population. *Acta Obstet Gynecol Scand.* 1997;76:442–448.

15 Molander U, Arvidsson L, Milsom I, et al. A longitudinal cohort study of elderly women with urinary tract infections. *Maturitas.* 2000;34:127–131.

16 Utian WH, Shoupe D, Bachmann G, et al. Relief of vasomotor symptoms and vaginal atrophy with lower doses of conjugated equine estrogens and medroxyprogesterone acetate. *Fertil Steril.* 2001;75: 1065–1079.

17 Notelovitz M, Funk S, Nanavati N, et al. Estradiol absorption from vaginal tablets in postmenopausal women. *Obstet Gynecol.* 2002; 99(4):556–562.

18 Miodrag A, Ekelund P, Burton R, et al. Tamoxifen and partial oestrogen agonism in postmenopausal women. *Age Ageing.* 1991;20:52–54.

19 Vardy MD, Lindsay R, Scotti RJ, et al. Short-term urogenital effects of raloxifene, tamoxifen, and estrogen. *Am J Obstet Gynecol.* 2003; 189:81–88.

20 Baird DD, Umbach DM, Landell L, et al. Dietary intervention study to assess estrogenicity of dietary soy among postmenopausal women. *J Clin Endocrinol Metab.* 1995;80:1685–1690.

21 Hendrix SL, Cochrane BB, Nygaard IE, et al. Effects of estrogen with and without progestin on urinary incontinence. *JAMA.* 2005;293(8): 935–948.

22 Brown JS, Vittinghoff E, Kanaya AM, et al. Urinary tract infections in postmenopausal women: effect of hormone therapy and risk factors. Heart and Estrogen/Progestin Replacement Study Research Group. *Obstet Gynecol.* 2001;98:1045–1052.

23 Cardozo L, Lose G, McClish D, et al. A systematic review of estrogens for recurrent urinary tract infections: third report of the Hormones and Urogenital Therapy (HUT) committee. *Int Urogynecol J Pelvic Floor Dysfunct.* 2001;12:15–20.

24 Guo SS, Zeller C, Chumlea WC, et al. Aging, body composition and lifestyle: the Fels Longitudinal Study. *Am J Clin Nutr.* 1999;70: 405–411.

25 Den Tonkelaar I, Seidell JC, van Noord PA, et al. Fat distribution in relation to age, degree of obesity, smoking habits, parity and estrogen use: a cross-sectional study in 11,825 Dutch women participating in the DOM-project. *Int J Obes.* 1990;14:753–761.

26 Reaven GM. Banting lecture 1988. Role of insulin resistance in human disease. *Diabetes.* 1988;37:1595–1607.

27 Eckel RH, Gundy SM, Zimmet PZ. The metabolic syndrome. *Lancet.* 2005;365:1415–1428.

28 Longcope C, Franz C, Morello C, et al. Steroid and gonadotropin levels in women during the peri-menopausal years. *Maturitas.* 1986; 8:189–196.

29 Orentreich N, Brind JL, Rizer RL, et al. Age changes and sex differences in serum dehydroepiandrosterone sulfate concentrations throughout adulthood. *J Clin Endocrinol Metab.* 1984;59:551–555.

30 Laughlin GA, Barrett-Connor E. Sexual dimorphism in the influence of advancing aging on adrenal hormone levels: the Rancho Bernardo study. *J Clin Endocrinol Metab.* 2000;85:3561–3568.

31 Liu CH, Laughlin GA, Fischer UG, et al. Marked attenuation of ultradian and circadian rhythms of dehydroepiandrosterone in postmenopausal women: evidence for a reduced 17,20 desmolase enzymatic activity. *J Clin Endocrinol Metab.* 1990;71:900–906.

32 Genazzani AD, Stomati M, Bernardi F, et al. Long-term low-dose dehydroepiandrosterone oral supplementation in early and late postmenopausal women modulates endocrine parameters and synthesis of neuroactive steroids. *Fertil Steril.* 2003;80:1495–1501.

33 Lasco A, Frisina N, Morabito N, et al. Metabolic effects of dehydroepiandrosterone replacement therapy in postmenopausal women. *Eur J Endocrinol.* 2001;145:457–461.

34 Hackbert L, Heiman JR. Acute dehydroepiandrosterone (DHEA) effects on sexual arousal in postmenopausal women. *J Womens Health Gend Based Med.* 2002;11:155–161.

35 Morales AJ, Nolan JJ, Nelson JC, et al. Effects of replacement dose of dehydroepiandrosterone in men and women of advancing age. *J Clin Endocrinol Metab.* 1994;78:1360–1367.

36 Labrie F, Diamond P, Cusan L, et al. Effect of 12 month dehydroepiandrosterone replacement therapy on bone, vagina, and endometrium in postmenopausal women. *J Clin Endocrinol Metab.* 1997;82:3498–3505.

37 Hirshman E, Merritt P, Wang CCL, et al. Evidence that androgenic and estrogenic metabolites contribute to the effects of dehydroepiandrosterone on cognition in postmenopausal women. *Horm Behav.* 2004;45: 144–155.

38 Degli Uberti EC, Ambrosio MR, Cella SG. Defective hypothalamic growth hormone-releasing hormone activity may contribute to declining GH with age in man. *J Clin Endocrinol Metab.* 1997;82: 2885–2888.

39 Blackman MR, Sorkin JD, Munzer T, et al. Growth hormone and sex steroid administration in healthy aged women and men: a randomized controlled trial *JAMA.* 2002;288:2282–2292.

40 Matthews KA, Abrams B, Crawford S, et al. Body mass index in midlife women:relative influence of menopause, hormone use, and ethnicity. *Int J obes Relat Metab Disord.* 2001;25:863–873.

41 Kritz-Silverstein D, Barrett-Connor E. Long-term postmenopausal hormone use, obesity, and fat distribution in older women. *JAMA.* 1996;275:46–49.

42 Kahn HS, Tatham LM, Heath CW Jr. Contrasting factors associated with abdominal and peripheral weight gain among adult women. *Int J Obes Relat Metab Disord.* 1997;21:903–911.

43 Norman RJ, Flight IHK, Rees MCP. Oestrogen and progestogen hormone replacement therapy for peri-menopausal and post-menopausal women: weight and body fat distribution (Cochrane Review). In: The Cochrane Library, Issue 2, 2000. Oxford:Update Software.

44 Friedman JM. The function of leptin in nutrition, weight, and physiology. *Nutr Rev.* 2002;60:S1–S14.

45 Hadji P, Gorke K, Hars O, et al. The influence of hormone replacement therapy (HRT) on serum leptin concentration in postmenopausal women. *Maturitas.* 2000;37:105–111.

46 Clinical Guidelines on the Identification, Evaluation, and Treatment of Overweight and Obesity in Adults-The Evidence Report. National Institutes of Health. *Obes Res.* 1998;6 (Suppl. 2):51S–209S.

47 Pate RR, Pratt M, Blair SN, et al. Physical activity and public health. A recommendation from the Centers for Disease Control and Prevention and the American College of Sports Medicine. *JAMA.* 1995;273: 402–407.

48 Foster GD, Wyatt HR, Hill JO, et al. A randomized trial of a low-carbohydrate diet for obesity. *N Engl J Med.* 2003;348:2082–2090.

49 Dansinger ML, Gleason JA, Griffth JL, et al. Comparison of the Atkins, Ornish, Weight Watchers, and Zone diets for weight loss and heart disease risk reduction. *JAMA.* 2005;293:43–53.

50 Bray GA. Uses and misuses of the new pharmacotherapy of obesity. *Ann Med.* 1999;31(1) 1–3.

51 Yanovski SZ, Yanovski JA. Obesity: drug therapy. *N Engl J Med.* 2002;346:591–602.

52 Haddock CK, Poston WSC, Dill PL, et al. Pharmacotherapy for obesity: a quantitative analysis of four decades of published randomized clinical trials. *Int J Obes.* 2002;26:262–273.

53 Maggard MA, Shugarman LR, Suttorp M, et al. Meta-analysis: surgical treatment of obesity. *Ann Intern Med.* 2005;142:547–559.

54 Buchwald H, Williams SE. Bariatric surgery worldwide 2003. *Obes Surg.* 2004;14:1157–1164.

55 Buchwald H, Avidor Y, Braunwald F, et al. Bariatric surgery: A systematic review and meta-analysis. *JAMA.* 2004;292:1724–1737.

56 Wolff EF, Narayan D, Taylor HS. Long-term effects of hormone therapy on skin rigidity and wrinkles. *Fertil Steril.* 2005;84:285–290.

PATHOPHYSIOLOGY

9 Abnormal Uterine Bleeding: Evaluation, Diagnosis, and Treatment

James H. Liu

Introduction

KEY POINT

AUB is defined as uterine bleeding that occurs at unexpected times or uterine bleeding that is abnormal in duration or amount.

Abnormal uterine bleeding (AUB) is one of the most common gynecologic complaints of women during the perimenopausal transition. AUB can be defined as uterine bleeding that occurs at unexpected times or bleeding that occurs at the expected time but is of abnormal duration or amount. It must be emphasized that this definition is a symptom and not a diagnosis. Excessive menstrual bleeding accounts for over 60% of the hysterectomies performed each year[1] as well as a significant number of diagnostic procedures such as dilatation and curettage (350,000 per year) and hysteroscopy.[2]

History

The etiology for AUB varies with the age of the patient, but for the purposes of this chapter, the focus will be on the late reproductive-aged and menopausal woman (see Fig. 9-1).

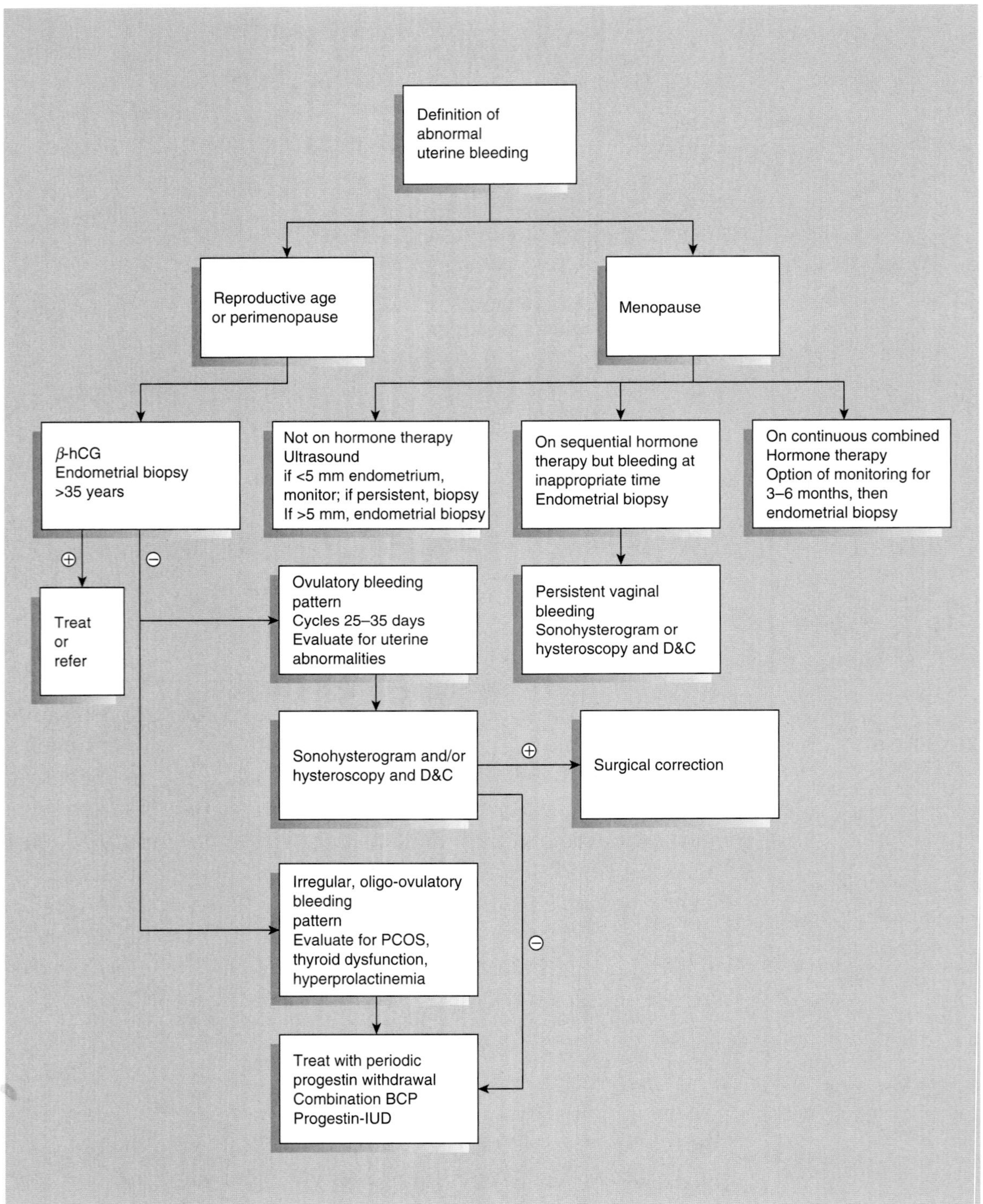

Figure 9-1: Algorithm for evaluation and treatment of abnormal uterine bleeding in the late reproductive-aged, perimenopausal, and menopausal woman. PCOS, polycystic ovarian syndrome.

In the late reproductive-aged individual, AUB can be divided into two broad general categories, ovulatory and anovulatory menstrual bleeding. A careful history of the age of menarche, regularity of cycles, duration of bleeding pattern, and a prospective menstrual calendar will help differentiate whether the bleeding is associated with ovulation. A history of the use of contraception will help to identify those women at risk for pregnancy-associated bleeding. Patients may have previously been placed on hormonal contraception to induce regular withdrawal menstrual flow thus obscuring the signs of AUB. Inadvertent skipping of hormonal doses can trigger episodes of uterine bleeding. A history of excessive bleeding with childbirth, nosebleeds, or heavy menstrual flow during early reproductive years is suggestive of an underlying coagulation disorder such as von Willebrand's disease.[3]

KEY POINT

Abnormal bleeding can be associated with either ovulatory or anovulatory menstrual cycles.

In the ovulatory, reproductive-aged woman, menses occur at 25–35-day intervals with the duration of menstrual flow of 2–8 days. During typical menses, the average blood loss is generally less than 80 mL. Menstrual blood loss greater than 80 mL is considered abnormal and is descriptively termed menorrhagia. The amount of menstrual bleeding can be prospectively documented utilizing standardized pictorial scales that quantitatively estimate the amount of blood loss based on the appearance sanitary protection used for a given cycle (Fig. 9-2).[4] In addition, women with menorrhagia will often have associated iron-deficiency anemia and require iron supplementation.

Women with irregular menstrual cycles most likely have anovulatory uterine bleeding or dysfunctional uterine bleeding. This menstrual pattern may be longstanding or may have occurred more recently such as during the perimenopausal transition. The characteristic symptoms associated with progesterone are missing (i.e., breast tenderness, mood changes, and pelvic bloating). In general, this type of bleeding is a result of a disruption of the normal physiological hypothalamic-pituitary-ovarian relationships.

Differential Diagnosis and Evaluation

OVULATORY BLEEDING Pregnancy-related disorders should be excluded in any woman of reproductive age with AUB irrespective of the type of bleeding. This can usually be accomplished with a sensitive urine pregnancy test or a serum β-hCG level. In this age group, new-onset diagnosis

Patient diary with blood loss, discharge, and pain assessments

Month: ______ Initials: ______ SCN: ______ Brands/absorbency of pad: ______

Brands/absorbency of tampon: ______

1. Pad	1	2	3	4	5	6	7	8	9	10	11	12	13	14	15
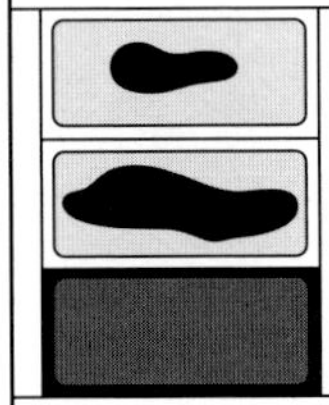															
Clots/flooding															
2. Tampon	1	2	3	4	5	6	7	8	9	10	11	12	13	14	15
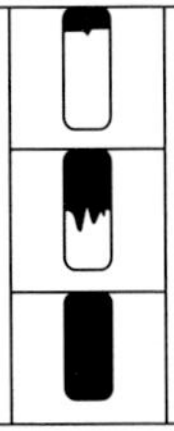															
Clots/flooding															
3. Discharge															
4. Assessment of premenstrual and menstrual pain_															

¯Rating scale: 0 = no symptom; 1 = mild; 2 = moderate; 3 = severe

☐ I did not have any bleeding this month

Figure 9-2: A pictorial menstrual diary for assessment of menstrual blood loss.

of coagulation disorders (von Willebrand's disease) or platelet dysfunction (Factor XI deficiency, thrombocytopenia) is unusual given that these individuals would have experienced increased bleeding with childbirth or previous operative interventions. Patients on chronic anticoagulant therapy for disorders such as atrial fibrillation will be at risk for increased menstrual bleeding.

Patients who are taking hormonal medications such as progestins or low-dose contraceptive pills can experience endometrial breakdown because of endometrial atrophy in response to a prolonged progestational effect. Perimenopausal women taking low-dose hormone therapy for control of vasomotor symptoms may occasionally have an unexpected menses because of spontaneous ovulation since menopausal hormone therapy does not effectively suppress the hypothalamus-pituitary unit.

KEY POINT

In women with ovulatory cycles, excessive bleeding is often associated with uterine abnormalities such as uterine fibroids and endometrial polyps.

The major causes of regular, excessive uterine bleeding (menorrhagia) or intermenstrual spotting in ovulatory women are uterine abnormalities such as uterine fibroids, endometrial polyps, and adenomyosis. Uterine fibroids and polyps can be detected by transvaginal ultrasound imaging. For more detailed imaging of the uterine cavity, a saline-contrast transvaginal ultrasound (sonohysterography) can be performed. This additional technique will approach 100% sensitivity in detecting submucous fibroids (see Chap. 10) and endometrial polyps. This diagnostic approach is similar in sensitivity to the *gold standard* hysteroscopy,[5] a more expensive diagnostic procedure.

Anovulatory Bleeding

KEY POINT

In women with anovulatory cycles, excessive bleeding can be associated with systemic disorders such as thyroid dysfunction, hyperprolactinemia, or polycystic ovarian syndrome.

Women with anovulatory bleeding may have new-onset abnormal bleeding or a lifelong history of irregular bleeding. Individuals who are excessively thin, exercise to excess, or who are under chronic stress may be at risk for hypothalamic-associated anovulation. In these individuals, the normal pattern of gonadotropin-releasing hormone is disrupted leading to low or low-normal follicle-stimulating hormone (FSH) and luteinizing hormone (LH) levels. These women will also have signs of hypoestrogenism without hot flushes. Thyroid-stimulating hormone (TSH) and prolactin levels will be in the normal or low range. Individuals with thyroid dysfunction such as hypo- or hyperthyroidism will also be at risk for ovulatory dysfunction and associated abnormal bleeding patterns.

Women with hyperprolactinemia will also have anovulatory bleeding. Prolactin elevations may be due to a pituitary adenoma, a psychotropic medication, or an occult central nervous system (CNS) lesion. Individuals that have a long history of irregular menstrual bleeding may have polycystic ovarian syndrome. If these individuals are obese, they may also be at risk for metabolic syndrome or adult-onset diabetes. For women with longstanding anovulation with continued estrogen production, an endometrial biopsy should be performed to exclude development of endometrial hyperplasia or endometrial cancer.

KEY POINT

In postmenopausal women with uterine bleeding, the most common finding is endometrial atrophy.

Postmenopausal women on sequential hormone therapy may experience vaginal bleeding at unexpected times. Because this is *not* related to estrogen withdrawal bleeding, an endometrial biopsy to assess endometrial pathology should be performed. Postmenopausal women on continuous estrogen-progestin therapy may experience vaginal spotting during the first 3–4 months of therapy. This type of bleeding can be managed expectantly. However, if bleeding persists beyond 6 months, an endometrial biopsy should be done. The most common pathological finding in this situation is endometrial atrophy.

Vaginal bleeding in postmenopausal women who are not on hormonal therapy can be evaluated with an endometrial biopsy. However, if the pelvic examination is normal and the patient is at low risk for endometrial cancer, a transvaginal ultrasound can be performed to assess endometrial thickness. If the endometrium is <5 mm, there is excellent sensitivity for excluding endometrial cancer (96%) or other endometrial pathology.[6] Bear in mind that this approach is not 100% sensitive and continued vaginal bleeding requires a full diagnostic evaluation.[7]

Treatment

KEY POINT

Acute uterine bleeding can usually be managed with high-dose estrogen-progestin therapy.

For acute, severe vaginal bleeding, the diagnostic evaluation can be deferred until the bleeding is controlled and the patient is hemodynamically stable. For the individual with severe anemia who is hemodynamically unstable, blood transfusion may be required. Medical therapy with use of high-dose estrogen followed by progestin to stabilize the endometrium is usually effective in controlling endometrial bleeding within 48 hours. Several medical regimens have been described. For example, a monophasic oral contraceptive pill containing 30–35 μg of ethinyl estradiol can be administered every 6 hours until the bleeding stops. The dose can then be reduced to two tablets per day for 1 week followed by one tablet daily for 3 weeks. An estrogen withdrawal flow will occur within 3 days of discontinuing the birth control pill. This strategy is effective in stabilizing the endometrium; however, endometrial shedding will occur at a later and planned occasion. The diagnostic evaluation can then be completed during this nonbleeding phase.

For patients who fail medical therapy, a dilatation and curettage and/or hysteroscopy should be performed. If these fail to control the hemorrhage, then tamponade of the uterine cavity with a large intrauterine Foley balloon or an emergency hysterectomy may become necessary.

Long-term management of AUB requires clinical judgement and is dependent on the underlying etiology (Fig. 9-3). For patients with anovulatory bleeding, correction of the primary defect (e.g., hypothyroidism) would be indicated. For chronic conditions, such as polycystic ovary syndrome or perimenopausal transition, hormonal manipulation of the endometrium has been highly successful. A variety of approaches have been used. These include long-term progestin therapy with either Depo-Provera, norethindrone (1–2.5 mg), or insertion of a progestin-containing intrauterine device (IUD). Cyclic progestin therapy administered on calendar days 1–12 every other month has also been used. However, patients may have an intervening bleeding episode if ovulation should occur during the nontreatment months. Low-dose oral contraceptives can be used and are highly effective provided that the patient does not have contraindications (i.e., smoking and hypercoagulable states).[8] The use of nonsteroidal anti-inflammatory agents with onset of uterine bleeding is efficacious in further reducing the amount of bleeding.[9]

For ovulatory bleeding secondary to submucous uterine fibroids or endometrial polyps, hysteroscopic resection is the treatment of choice. The use of oral contraceptives with nonsteroidal anti-inflammatory agents may also be effective in some patients. In the presence of larger uterine fibroids, a number of conservative techniques have been developed to selectively target and destroy the myomas. These include uterine artery embolization,[10] magnetic resonance imaging (MRI)-directed focused ultrasound, ultrasound-guided cryoprobe, electrocautery, and traditional myomectomy. It must be emphasized that these conservative procedures only target

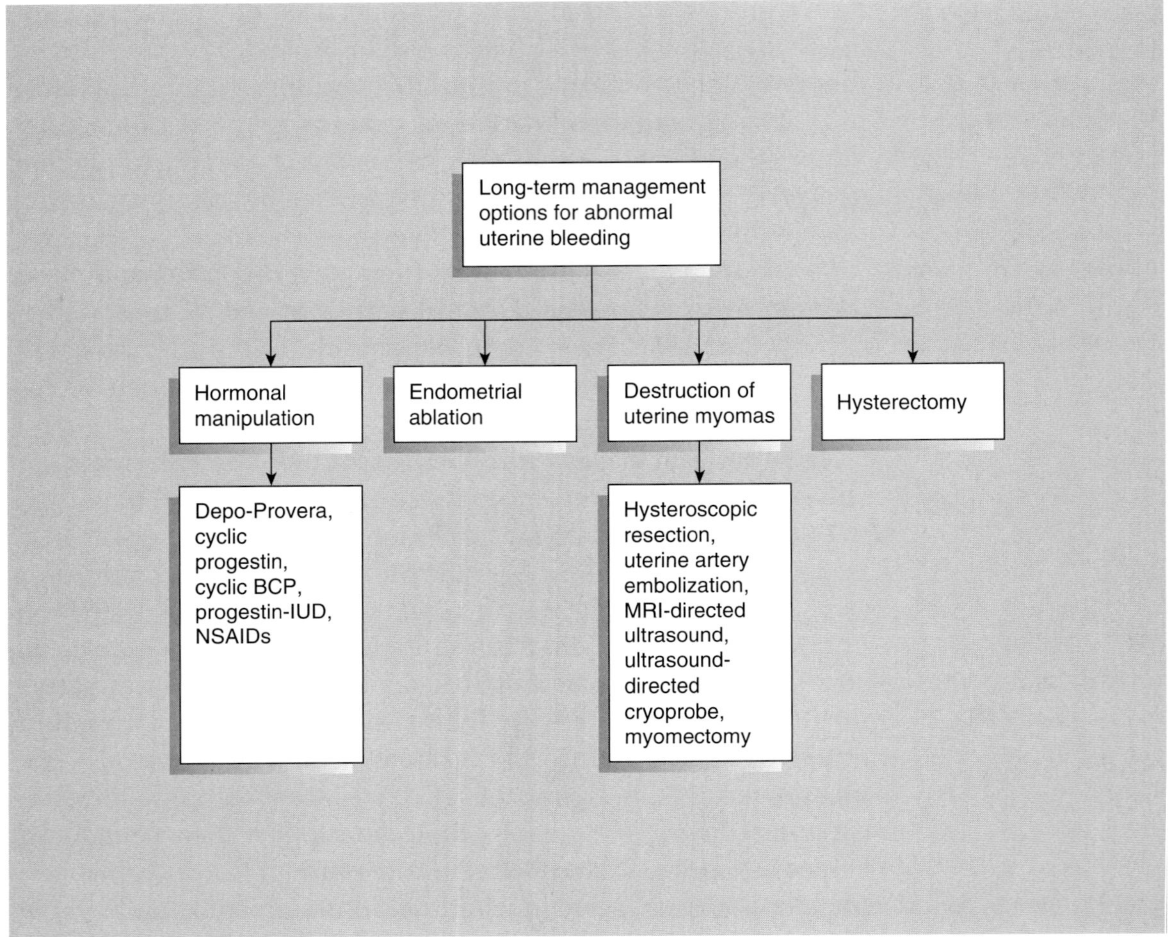

Figure 3: Algorithm for long-term management of abnormal uterine bleeding.

the myomas that are present and are not effective if new myomas develop several years later. Thus, conservative procedures are usually best suited for those women who are close to menopause. For definitive therapy, hysterectomy remains the most effective option.

In the absence of any significant uterine abnormalities, global surgical destruction of the endometrium (endometrial ablation) can be accomplished with a variety of devices[11] (i.e., NovaSure and ThermaChoice), which will reduce menstrual bleeding or induce amenorrhea.[12] The incidence of complications with this approach is low[13] and these predominantly involve uterine perforation and cervical trauma.[14]

Summary

The diagnostic evaluation of AUB relies on the history, endometrial biopsy, and pelvic ultrasound imaging studies. In most cases, AUB can be managed medically with hormonal manipulation or with conservative surgical techniques. It is estimated that only 1–2 % of women presenting with AUB will require hysterectomy. This option should be considered after medical therapy has failed and the patient has documented anemia.

What's the Evidence?

- For the individual with anovulatory AUB, hormonal therapy to control the growth and development of the endometrium should be a first-line treatment. The use of combination oral contraceptives has been recognized as an effective means to decrease menstrual flow.[15] In those who cannot take estrogen, the use of progestins can also be effective in controlling AUB. These include norethindrone (1–2.5 mg/day), medroxyprogesterone acetate (5–10 mg/day), and micronized progesterone (200 mg/day). For individuals with a normal uterine cavity, a progestin-containing IUD (Mirena) is also highly effective and can reduce blood loss by up to 90%.[16]
- For the patient with ovulatory AUB and a normal uterine cavity, the use of oral contraceptives alone or in combination with NSAIDs, antifibrinolytics[17] or progestin-releasing IUDs[18] are effective options. Destruction of the endometrium is another conservative approach. Endometrial ablation is now performed with a variety of new devices utilizing electrocautery, heated liquids, cryotherapy, and microwave.[19] Patient satisfaction with this technique is in the 90% range.[20] However, longitudinal follow-up suggests that the reoperation rate for endometrial ablation steadily increases to approximately 40% by 4 years.[21] In patients with submucous myomas or large intramural myomas, selective destruction of the myomas will reduce the uterine bleeding (see Chap. 10). Conservative procedures such as uterine artery embolization and MRI-focused ultrasound have become increasing popular. Long-term follow-up to assess whether these treated patients require additional future procedures is still not yet available.

Discussion of Cases

CASE 1

Vignette

A 46-year-old woman (G2P2,) presents with a complaint of 6 weeks of intermittent vaginal bleeding and spotting. She had regular menstrual cycles at 30-day intervals but over the past year, her cycles have decreased to 22–25 days. She also reports that hot flushes during her menses have become more intense but do not affect her daily activities. She is sexually active and her husband had a vasectomy. She does not smoke and drinks socially. On physical examination, she is 5 ft 5 in. and weighs 155 lb. Her general examination is unremarkable. On pelvic examination, there is a brownish-red mucus discharge in the vaginal vault; normal parous cervix; normal-sized, mobile uterus; and no adnexal masses. An endometrial biopsy is performed with a large amount of tissue obtained. Pathology reveals abundant proliferative endometrium with occasional early secretory endometrium. No endometrial hyperplasia is identified.

Discussion

The above clinical vignette in this late reproductive-aged patient is consistent with an anovulation perhaps secondary to the perimenopause. During this transitional phase, there is continued estrogen production from the ovaries, however, ovulation may not consistently occur giving rise to cycles with progesterone deficiency. This condition is usually associated with an estrogen-primed endometrium (proliferative changes) without a marked progesterone effect (secretory changes). Treatment options for this condition include expectant management, cyclic progestin therapy, or low-dose oral contraceptives until menopause. In this particular situation, the patient chose to start oral contraceptive pills. A TSH and prolactin level should be performed before starting therapy.

CASE 2

Vignette

A 48-year-old P3 woman is seen in the hospital ER for severe vaginal bleeding for the past 4 days. She reported using a sanitary pad and tampon together with pad changes every 3–4 hours. She has always had irregular cycles. Prior to this bleeding episode, she had been amenorrheic for the past 8 months. She was not on any medications and was sexually active without using contraception. A urine pregnancy test is negative. Vital signs were stable without orthostatic changes. She has a body mass index (BMI) of 31 kg/m^2. Her blood pressure was normal. She did not have acne or increased facial hair. The abdominal examination shows white striae and a palpable, firm midline mobile mass just above the symphysis. Pelvic examination revealed a male pattern escutcheon, small clots in the vagina, a normal cervix, and a 14 weeks gestation-sized uterus without discernable adnexal masses. Her hematocrit was 28.

Discussion

This individual has anovulatory AUB on the basis of her historical menstrual pattern and significant obesity. Contributing factors to her AUB may be an enlarged uterus secondary to uterine fibroids. Because she appeared hemodynamically stable, an endometrial biopsy to exclude endometrial carcinoma or hyperplasia should be performed. If the biopsy results in additional bleeding, she would be in the ideal setting for additional intervention. A pelvic ultrasound to evaluate uterine abnormalities would also be prudent. She should be evaluated for polycystic ovarian syndrome with a prolactin, testosterone, dehydroepiandrosterone (DHEA) sulfate, and 17-OH progesterone level. Assuming that the endometrial biopsy does not show endometrial carcinoma, this individual would be a candidate for hormonal manipulation with either cyclic progestin therapy, low-dose oral contraceptives, or a progestin-containing IUD. She should also be screened for metabolic syndrome and adult-onset diabetes. Iron supplementation should be encouraged.

References

1 Oehler MK, Rees MC. Menorrhagia: an update. *Acta Obstet Gynecol Scand.* 2003;82(5):405–422.

2 Ownings MF, Kozak LJ. Ambulatory and inpatient procedures in the United States, 1996. *Vital Health Stat.* 1998;13:1–127.

3 Strickland JL, Wall JW. Abnormal uterine bleeding in adolescents. *Obstet Gynecol Clin North Am.* 2003;30(2)321–335.

4 Higham JM, O'Brien PM, Shaw RW. Assessment of menstrual blood loss using a pictorial chart. *Br J Obstet Gynecol.* 1990;97(8): 734–739.

5 Farquhar C, Ekeroma A, Furness S, et al. A systematic review of transvaginal ultrasonography, sonohysterography and hysteroscopy for the investigation of abnormal uterine bleeding in premenopausal women. *Acta Obstet Gynecol Scand.* 2003;82(6):493–504.

6 Granberg S, Wikland M, Karlsson B. Endometrial thickness as measured by endovaginal ultrasonography for identifying endometrial abnormality. *Am J Obstet Gynecol.* 1991;164:47–53.

7 Persadie RJ. Ultrasonographic assessment of endometrial thickness: a review. *J Obstet Gynecol Can.* 2002;24(2):131–136.

8 Davis A, Godwin A, Lippman J, et al. Triphasic norgestimate-ethinyl estradiol for treating dysfunctional uterine bleeding. *Obstet Gynecol.* 2000;96:913–920.

9 Nonsteroidal anti-inflammatory drugs for heavy menstrual bleeding. *Cochrane Database Syst Rev.* 2000;(2):CD000400.

10 Worthington-Kirsch RL, Siskin GP. Uterine artery embolization for symptomatic myomata. *J Intensive Care Med.* 2004;19(1):13–21.

11 Cooper J, Gimpelson R, Laberge P, et al. A randomized, multicenter trial of safety and efficacy of the NovaSure system in the treatment of menorrhagia. *J Am Assoc Gynecol Laparosc.* 2002; 9(4):418–428.

12 McGurgan P, O'Donovan P. Endometrial ablation. *Curr Opin Obstet Gynecol.* 2003;15(4):327–332.

13 Overton C, Hargreaves J, Maresh M. A national survey of the complications of endometrial destruction for menstrual disorders: the MISTLETOE study. Minimally Invasive Surgical Techniques—Laser, Endothermal, or Endoresection. *Br J Obstet Gynecol.* 1997;104: 1351–1359.

14 Jansen FW, Vredegoogd CB, Van Ulzen K, et al. Complications of hysteroscopy: a prospective multicenter study. *Obstet Gynecol.* 2000;96:266–270.

15 Jensen JT, Speroff L. Health benefits of oral contraceptives. *Obstet Gynecol Clin North Am.* 2000;27(4):705–721.

16 Barrington JW, Arunkalaivanan AS, Abdel-Fattah M. Comparison between the levonorgestrel intrauterine system (LNG-IUS) and thermal balloon ablation in the treatment of menorrhagia. *Eur J Obstet Gynecol Reprod Biol.* 2003;108(1):72–74.

17 Bonnar J, Sheppard BL. Treatment of menorrhagia during menstruation: randomized controlled trial of ethamsylate, mefanamic acid, and tranexamic acid. *BMJ.* 1996;313:579–582.

18 Crosignani PG, Vercellini P, Mosconi P, et al. Levonorgestrel-releasing intrauterine device versus hysteroscopic endometrial resection in the treatment of dysfunctional uterine bleeding. *Obstet Gynecol.* 1997;90:257–263.

19 Brzozowski P, Liu JH. Four global ablation devices: efficacy, indications, and technique. *OBG Manage.* 2004;7:15–24.

20 Lethaby A, Hickey M. Endometrial destruction techniques for heavy menstrual bleeding: a Cochrane review. *Hum Reprod.* 2002;17(11): 2795–2806.

21 Aberdeen Endometrial Ablation Trials Group. A randomized trial of endometrial ablation versus hysterectomy for the treatment of dysfunctional uterine bleeding: outcome at four years. *Br J Obstet Gynecol.* 1999;106:360–366.

10 Clinical Management of Uterine Myomas

Karen L. Ashby

Introduction

Uterine leiomyomas, or fibroids, are the most common benign pelvic tumors. The incidence in women may be as high as 35% in White women, and up to 80% in African American women.[1] Additionally, African American women tend to be younger at the time of diagnosis and tend to have larger fibroids.[2] While leiomyoma or myoma is the correct term for these pelvic tumors, for the purpose of this discussion, uterine fibroid is the terminology that the majority of patients and practitioners use.

KEY POINT

Clinical symptoms of myoma include pelvic pressure, painful menses, heavy menses, and associated anemia.

While most women with uterine fibroids are asymptomatic, many women will have significant pelvic pain, vaginal bleeding, and associated iron deficiency anemia. Although fibroids are benign in nature, they nevertheless account for the majority of hysterectomies performed. Despite technological advances, alternative treatments have not yet had an impact on the hysterectomy rate, which was about 5.6/1000 women, as of 1997.[3] This is largely because the factors that cause myoma formation and growth are complex and not entirely understood. To date, current therapies have not addressed etiology and are directed at controlling symptoms.

Biology of Myomas

Uterine fibroids are monoclonal tumors that arise from a single myometrial cell. Over time, a single myometrial cell grows by clonal expansion into a solitary tumor or uterine myoma. The initial inciting event responsible for abnormal growth is postulated to be a somatic mutation associated with chromosomal abnormalities or breaks found in many myoma specimens. It is also conceivable that clonal proliferation precedes any cytogenetic rearrangements.[4]

KEY POINT

Each myoma arises from the growth of a single tumor cell.

In addition to genetic and racial differences, there are numerous other factors that may affect fibroid growth. Medications, diet, smoking, and body weight are all purported to play a role in the growth of fibroids.

One common medication that has been postulated to affect fibroid growth is oral contraceptives. The widespread use of oral contraceptives, especially during teenage years, makes it important to understand the potential relationship between oral contraceptives and fibroids. Oral contraceptive use at a young age (ages 13–16) has been identified as a factor for the risk of developing fibroids.[5] The presence of fibroids, however, is not a contraindication to oral contraceptive use.

It is difficult to determine the relationship between diet and fibroid formation. Diets high in red meat are associated with an increase in fibroid formation, although it has not been proven that dietary modifications, once a woman has fibroids, are of any benefit. These data, however, are difficult to interpret. In the study by Chiaffarino, subjects recorded frequency of meat intake, but not the quantity of red meat consumed. Additionally, the control subjects did not receive ultrasound screening for fibroids such that the actual incidence of fibroids in the control group could be underestimated. Therefore, it is difficult to conclude that diets high in red meat contribute to fibroid formation. Is the steroid content in red meat a potential issue? Thus far, studies linking diet and fibroids have not examined this issue. In contrast, smoking is thought to decrease the relative risk of fibroid formation. It is not surprising that weight change, or weight since age 18 is also associated with a risk of fibroid formation.[6–8]

KEY POINT

Myoma growth is dependent on the estrogen and progesterone hormonal environment.

The hormonal environment or the presence of estrogen and progesterone, both endogenous and exogenous are critical factors for fibroid formation. Although estrogen is not believed to directly stimulate fibroid growth, progesterone appears to be a more critical factor than estrogen in the growth of fibroids. Both progesterone and progestins have been demonstrated to promote uterine myoma growth and proliferation. With onset of menopause and cessation of ovarian function, myoma growth will be limited and in many cases there will be a decrease in myoma size.

Managing perimenopausal women with symptomatic fibroids provides a unique challenge for the clinician, because as many women approach menopause, they often do not want aggressive treatments, such as a hysterectomy. Because fibroids are hormone dependent, some perimenopausal women with fibroids experience a reduction in symptoms as they approach menopause. Other women may experience worsening symptoms, especially if they begin to experience vasomotor symptoms, or hot flushes, in addition to anovulatory cycles. While anovulatory cycles tend to cause heavy irregular bleeding, regular heavy bleeding, or menorrhagia, is more commonly associated with fibroids. Clinical history alone may not distinguish between these types of bleeding patterns, and the assumption that abnormal uterine bleeding is strictly due to perimenopausal *hormone* changes should not be made. In general, with the decrease in myoma growth as a woman approaches menopause, it is less likely that intervention for fibroids will be needed.

Clinical Presentation

Fibroids may be asymptomatic or may result in significant lifestyle altering practices. Women with large fibroids may have dysmenorrhea, pressure upon urination, and difficulty with bowel movements. Surprisingly, many large fibroids (greater than 20 weeks size) may be asymptomatic. Initial symptoms usually occur during the reproductive years. Fibroids, however, are not believed to be a major cause of infertility, unless they are submucosal, obstruct the fallopian tubes, or protrude into the endometrial cavity.[9]

The most common bleeding pattern for women with symptomatic fibroids is menorrhagia, or heavy menstruation that occurs on a regular basis with flow greater than 7 days in duration or greater than 80 mL/cycle. Perimenopausal women, however, may also experience occasional anovulatory cycles, which can make the clinical picture more confusing. Consequently, prolonged menorrhagia may result in iron deficiency anemia. Generally, women will provide a history of using excessive sanitary protection like a pad and tampon simultaneously or changing sanitary protection every 2–3 hours during the heaviest days of menstrual flow. The onset of symptoms, however, may be very gradual. Many women complain only of fatigue and poor exercise tolerance, and do not relate these symptoms to their menstrual cycle.

Women with heart disease may have worsening of the cardiac symptoms such as shortness of breath or chest pain, secondary to anemia.

It has been postulated that submucosal fibroids are primarily responsible for symptoms of menorrhagia or heavy bleeding. Intramural fibroids within the wall of the uterus may become extremely large and may cause symptoms of pelvic pressure or fullness. These women may not experience heavy menstrual bleeding. Recent studies have demonstrated that women's perception of heavier bleeding correlated with the size of the fibroids regardless of location.[10]

Diagnostic Approaches

The presence of fibroids can be diagnosed on physical examination. The diagnosis can then be confirmed by abdominal and vaginal ultrasound. Ultrasound studies are important because physical examination may not be able to distinguish between uterine fibroids

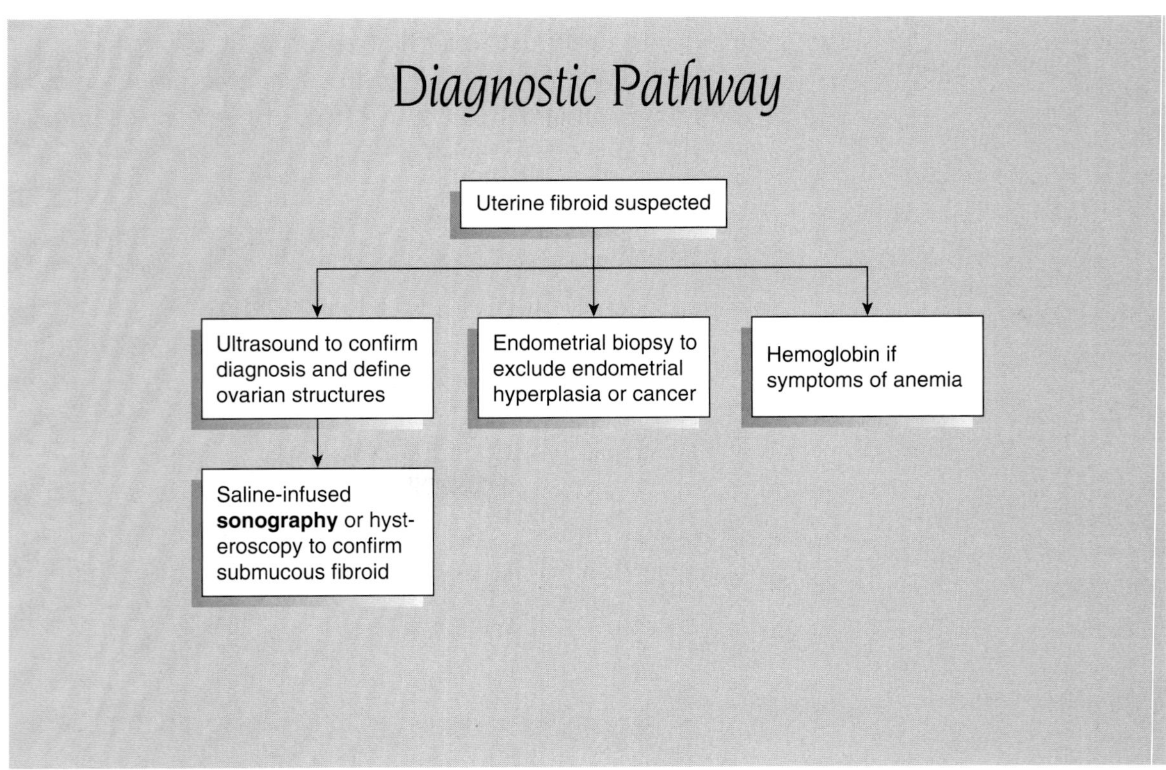

KEY POINT

The most useful diagnostic tests for evaluation of myomas are pelvic ultrasound and endometrial biopsy.

or ovarian mass or tumor. Further testing, such as saline-infused sonography (SIS), or office hysteroscopy, can further delineate the location of intracavity fibroids(see Fig. 10-1A and B). Menstrual history alone is not sensitive enough to exclude endometrial pathology. Therefore, an office endometrial biopsy should be performed to look for other endometrial pathology, such as hyperplasia or endometrial cancer. While uterine sarcoma is rare, it still must be included in the differential diagnosis. "Rapidly" growing leiomyoma are of particular concern, but it has been shown that the total incidence of uterine sarcoma (leiomyosarcoma, endometrial stromal sarcoma, and mixed mesodermal tumor) is extremely low in patients being operated on for uterine leiomyoma (0.23%).[11]

SIS is a particularly useful tool in triaging women with abnormal bleeding. Polyps can often be distinguished from submucous fibroids (see Fig. 10-1C). SIS is particularly useful when attempting to determine which women would benefit from operative hysteroscopy.

Office hysteroscopy is another tool that may ascertain the source of abnormal bleeding. A small 3-mm flexible hysteroscope can be inserted following a paracervical block and the endometrial cavity may be directly visualized in the office setting.

Figure 10-1: (A) Transvaginal ultrasound of the uterus suggesting an irregular-shaped mass within the body of the uterus. (B) Transvaginal ultrasound of the uterus in the same subject with saline contrast demonstrating an irregular-shaped myoma within the uterine cavity. (C) Transvaginal ultrasound of the uterus with saline contrast in a patient with heavy vaginal bleeding showing an intrauterine polyp.

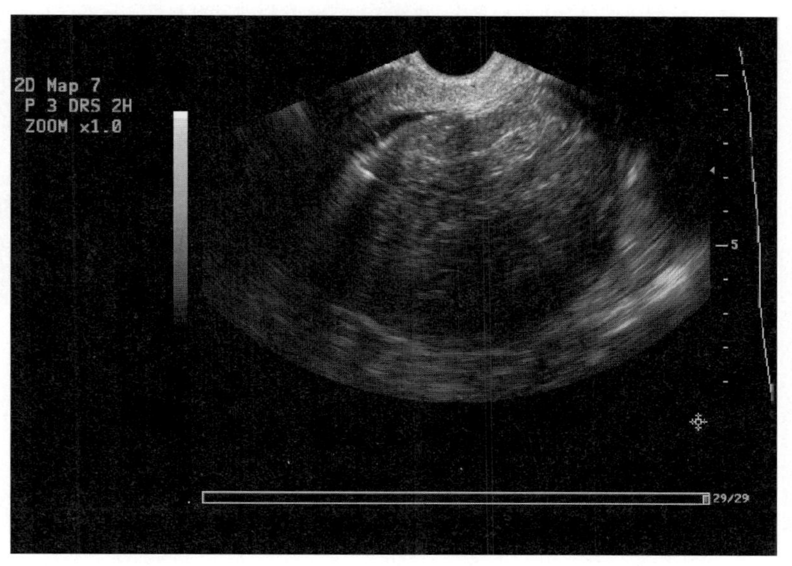

Figure 10-1: (*Cont.*)

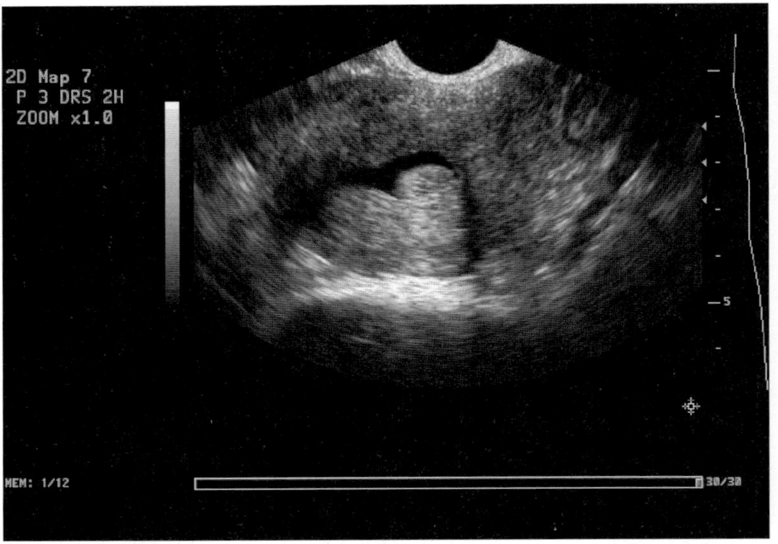

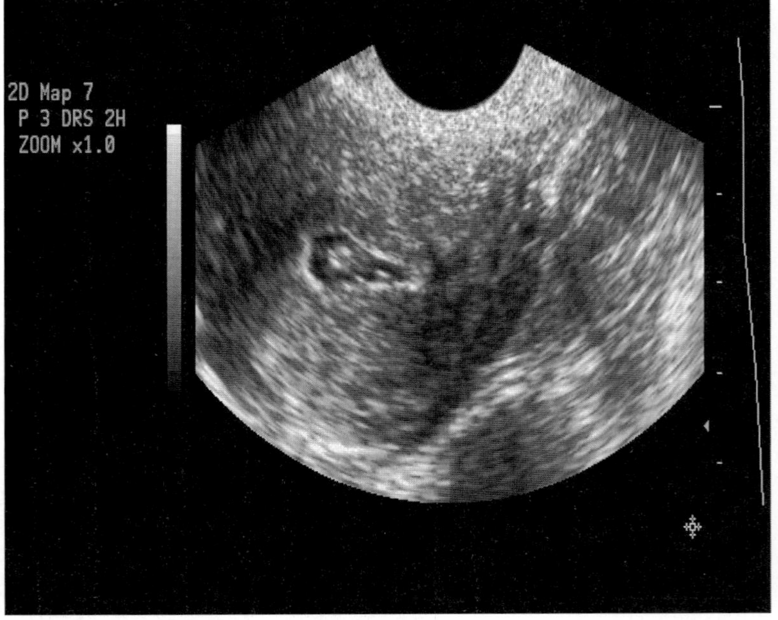

Surgical Management

Traditionally, surgical management has been the mainstay of treatment for uterine fibroids. Hysterectomy, at one time, was one of the most commonly performed operations and was sometimes performed for asymptomatic fibroids. For women with symptomatic fibroids who desire definitive treatment, abdominal or vaginal hysterectomy is a reasonable option (see Table 10-1). Highly skilled surgeons can remove large fibroids either vaginally or laparoscopically, which is an alternative to the traditional abdominal hysterectomy.

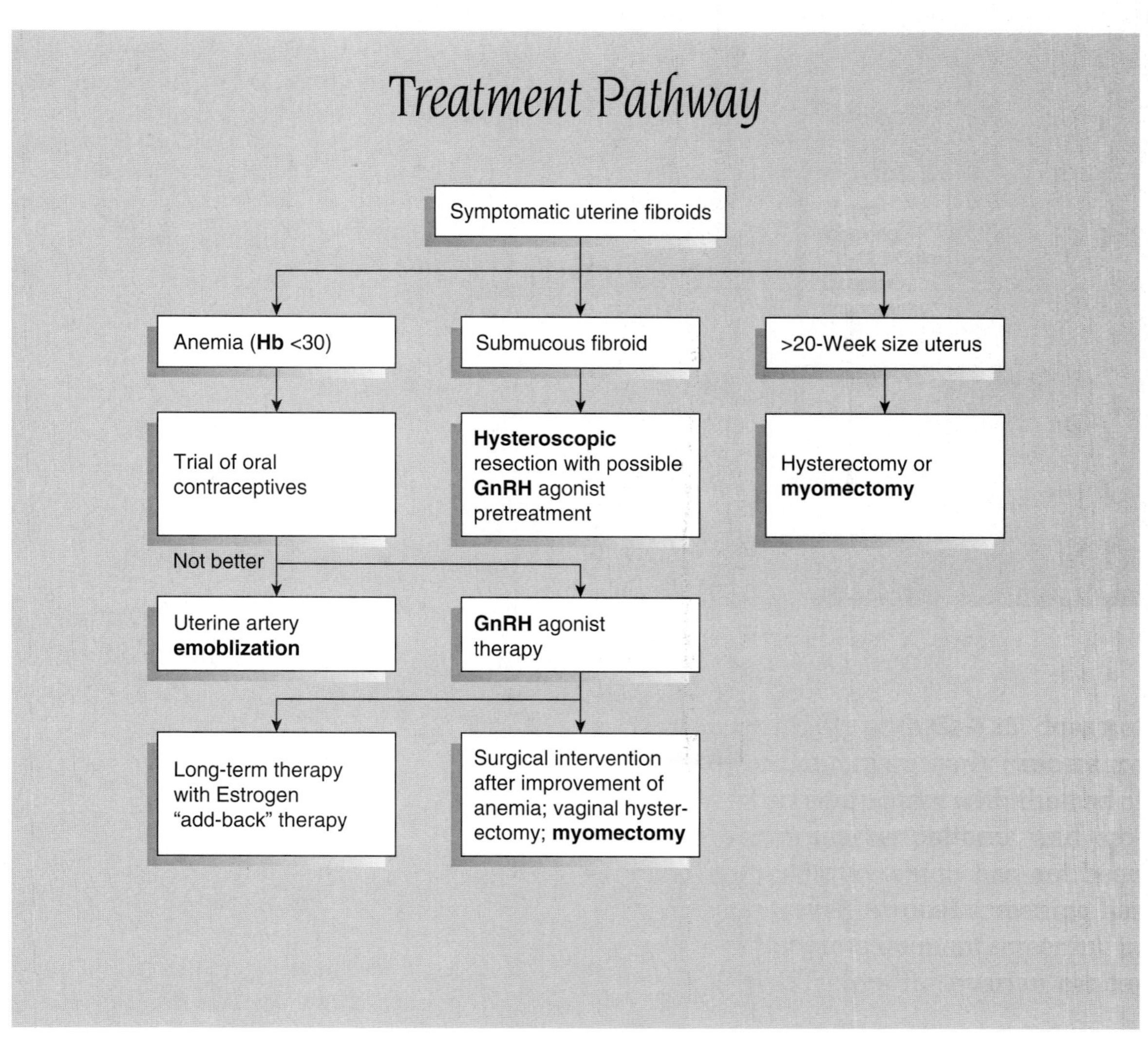

Table 10-1. TREATMENT OPTIONS

TREATMENT	ADVANTAGES	DISADVANTAGES AND SIDE EFFECTS
GnRH agonists	Induces amenorrhea Reduces fibroid volume; improves anemia	Vasomotor symptoms, bone loss >6 months of use, rapid regrowth after discontinuation, short-term treatment
GnRH agonists with "add-back" therapy	Reduces fibroid volume; improves anemia	Prolonged use may be costly, FDA approved
Mifepristone	Oral administration	Off-label use; difficult to obtain; possible risk of endometrial hyperplasia
Oral contraceptives	Can improve bleeding	Does not alter uterine fibroid volume
Uterine artery embolization	Can be definitive therapy; no surgery	Decrease in uterine volume is less predictable; pain management issues; may not preserve fertility
Hysterectomy and myomectomy	Definitive therapy	Major surgery requiring hospital stay and a 8–12-week recovery period
Hysteroscopic resection	Outpatient procedure	Not effective for intramural fibroids
Laparoscopic myomectomy	Outpatient procedure	Requires an experienced surgeon; may not be practical for multiple, small fibroids

Abbreviation: GnRH, gonadotropin-releasing hormone.

In general, vaginal hysterectomy and laparoscopic procedures have reduced postoperative recovery time, but there are no cost savings in operating time or hospitalization (see Table 10-2).

Myomectomy, which is a surgical removal of the fibroids and the preservation of the uterus, is often reserved for young women who wish to preserve fertility. There are, however, perimenopausal women who although not interested in fertility, still wish to retain

Table 10-2. TREATMENT COSTS

GnRH agonists	\$300–\$600/month
GnRH with "add-back" therapy	\$350–\$650/month
Mifepristone	Inexpensive, but not readily available
Oral contraceptives	\$4.00–\$30.00/month
Uterine artery embolization	Comparable to hysterectomy (\$10–\$15,000)

Abbreviation: GnRH, gonadotropin-releasing hormone.

KEY POINT

Hysterectomy or myomectomy are the two most common surgical options for treatment of symptomatic fibroids.

their uterus. A myomectomy may be performed abdominally, laparoscopically, and vaginally. Laparoscopic myomectomy is potentially a treatment option for women who may have one or two large fibroids, rather than multiple small ones. The postoperative recovery for women receiving an abdominal myomectomy is similar to those treated with abdominal hysterectomy.

For myomas that are located within the uterine cavity (submucosal or pedunculated myomas), hysteroscopic myomectomy can be accomplished using a specialized hysteroscope called the resectoscope (Fig. 10-2). This instrument is capable of shaving small fragments of the myoma using an electrocautery cutting loop. Alternatively, if fertility is not desired and the submucosal myomas are of small size, endometrial ablation can be performed

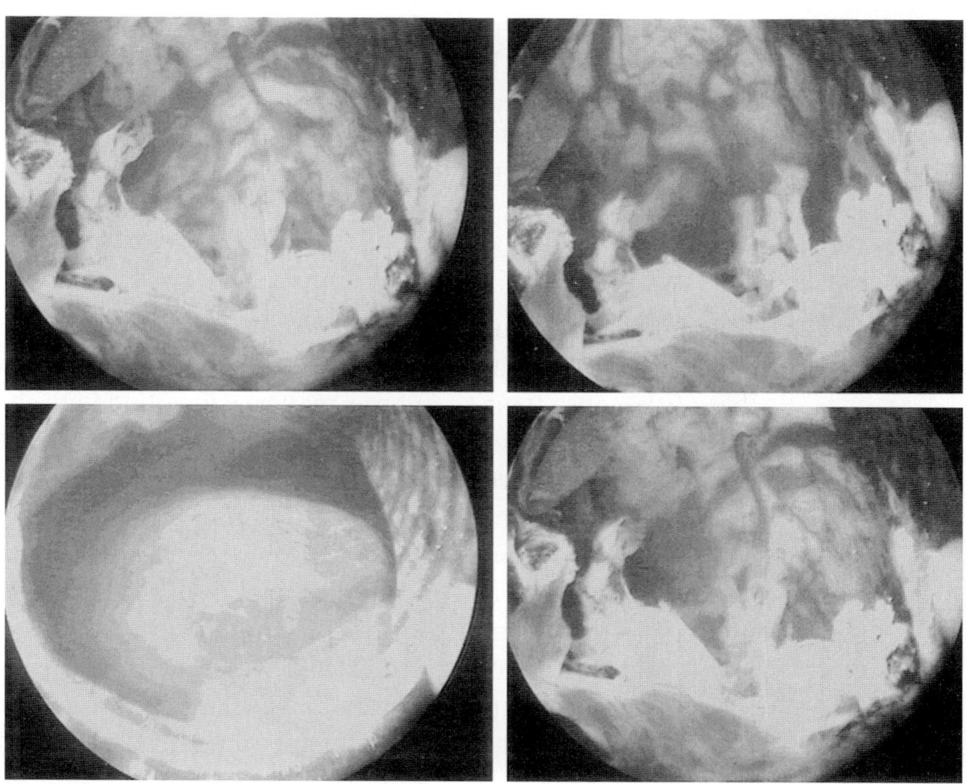

Figure 10-2. Hysteroscopic view of an intracavitary myoma before resection (bottom left panel) and following sequential resection (all remaining panels).

utilizing laser, thermal ablation, resection, and bipolar electrocautery devices.

Because new small fibroids may develop during the reproductive period, women who undergo myomectomy risk recurrence. However many women may not require further intervention. It is estimated that the risk of recurrence is approximately 10% in 5 years.[12] As a result, in younger women, the risk of reoperation is higher. In addition, small myomas, or nuclei, may be left behind during a myomectomy, regardless of the surgical approach.[13] When deciding upon a myomectomy, women should understand that they are unlikely to be totally free of their fibroids after surgery although their symptoms may improve.

Medical Treatment

Oral Contraceptives and Nonsteroidal Anti-Inflammatory Agents

For patients who present with heavy uterine bleeding in a regular or irregular pattern, oral contraceptive therapy is often a first choice. Low-dose oral contraceptives will induce a thinner endometrial lining and control the unpredictable uterine bleeding, secondary to ovulation abnormalities that are common in the perimenopausal years. Nonsteroidal anti-inflammatory agents, such as ibuprofen, will often reduce the painful uterine cramps and inhibit the vasodilatory prostaglandins resulting in a decrease in menstrual flow. A full discussion of this approach is in Chap. 9.

GnRH Agonists

Perimenopausal women with symptomatic fibroids are excellent candidates for gonadotropin-releasing hormone (GnRH) agonist therapy because their symptoms may be controlled for a short interval until natural menopause ensues. Unfortunately, current medical options to decrease myoma size and decrease symptoms are limited. GnRH agonist, or analogues, bind GnRH receptors at the level of the pituitary gland. With continued stimulation of the GnRH agonist over a 10–12-day period, a physiologic "down regulation" of the receptors occurs. LH and FSH secretion decrease to low levels and no longer stimulate ovarian activity. At this point, there may be an increase in hot flushes and vasomotor symptoms. Because the growth of fibroids is estrogen-progestin dependent, creating a hypoestrogenic environment, or a *pseudo-menopause*, is beneficial in reducing fibroid volume and decreasing uterine bleeding. Women who receive GnRH agonist therapy may benefit in several ways. First, treatment usually results in amenorrhea, which can improve anemia, especially in patients who may be contemplating surgical management. Second, GnRH agonists may also reduce fibroid volume, which can sometimes make a vaginal hysterectomy possible. In most clinical trials, GnRH agonists reduce fibroid size by 30–65% within 3 months.[14] Extending treatment beyond 3 months does not result in additional decrease in myoma size. GnRH agonists may also be useful preoperatively in patients undergoing hysteroscopic resection, making uterine cavity more atrophic, and enhancing visualization.

One disadvantage of GnRH agonists is that they must be given monthly or every 3 months by depot injection. In addition, drug cost is high ($300–$600/month, Table 10-2), especially for prolonged courses. Short-term side effects include vasomotor symptoms and sleep disruption. Discontinuation of GnRH agonist therapy can also lead to rapid regrowth of fibroids to the pretreatment size. Long-term side effects include bone loss after 6 months of use, which is a limitation for long-term therapy.

KEY POINT

Manipulation of the estrogen and progesterone environment with GnRH analogs will modify the growth pattern of fibroids and temporarily reduce the symptoms associated with myomas.

One method to "extend" the use of GnRH agonists is by utilizing *steroid add-back* therapy to reduce vasomotor symptoms and preserve bone density in the women requiring long-term treatment with GnRH agonists. This involves replacing or "adding back" small menopausal doses of estrogen and/or progesterone that will alleviate vasomotor symptoms, but will not stimulate additional fibroid growth. Several regimens have been studied. Initially, medroxyprogesterone acetate was used because of the hypothesis that estrogen would contribute to the growth of the fibroids and should be avoided. However, clinical studies have demonstrated that in women taking GnRH agonist therapy, progesterone inhibited the decrease in uterine and fibroid volume. In contrast, GnRH agonist therapy combined with low-dose estrogen and progesterone therapy decreases both bone reabsorption and vasomotor symptoms, and this regimen does not result in the increase of fibroid growth.[15]

In general, GnRH agonist therapy with add-back therapy (estrogen and progesterone), can be a costly treatment (Table 10-2), depending on the duration of treatment. In women near menopause with symptomatic fibroids, this approach may prevent the need for operative intervention.

Another alternative for steroid add-back therapy is the medication tibolone. Tibolone has not yet been approved for use in the United States. It is a synthetic steroid with estrogen, progesterone, and androgenic properties. Tibolone has been studied in both post- and premenopausal women. In women being treated with GnRH agonist therapy with addition of tibolone, bone density was preserved and vasomotor symptoms improved, as compared to GnRH agonist alone. The GnRH agonist reduction in fibroid volume was not affected by the addition of tibolone.[16]

GnRH antagonists have not been as extensively studied as GnRH agonists, and are not available in a long-acting formulation. GnRH antagonists have a theoretical advantage over GnRH agonists in that downregulaton of GnRH receptors is not necessary. Within minutes of GnRH antagonist administration, LH and FSH levels decrease to low levels and estrogen production from the ovaries falls precipitously.

Mifepristone

Because the stimulatory role of progesterone in fibroid growth is clear, compounds that block or reduce progesterone should decrease fibroid volume and reduce symptoms. Mifepristone, or RU-486, behaves as a progesterone and glucocorticoid receptor antagonist. It is synthesized from the precursor of norethindrone and is currently Food and Drug Administration (FDA)-approved in the United States for medical abortions. Doses between 5 and 15 mg have induced a significant reduction in fibroid volume. The usual response is approximately 48–49% reduction over 12 weeks. Like GnRH agonist therapy, women taking mifepristone will usually experience vasomotor symptoms. The lower doses of mifepristone demonstrate the same reduction in volume as the higher doses, but with fewer vasomotor side effects.[17] One concern regarding mifepristone use includes an observed increased incidence of endometrial hyperplasia. In these small studies with low-dose mifepristone endometrial biopsies were not performed prior to the study, so it could not be determined if endometrial hyperplasia was already present in these subjects. Another concern is that 8% of women taking mifepristone in this study also had elevation of hepatic enzymes. In summary, the long-term safety of mifepristone has yet to be established, but because of its antiprogestin effect and the significant reduction in fibroid volume, this compound may hold promise as a short-term therapy for fibroids.

Uterine Artery Embolization

In the search for nonsurgical treatment of fibroids, uterine artery embolization (UAE) has found a new role. UAE is not a new procedure and has been used in the past in some medical centers for controlling intractable postpartum hemorrhage. Ideally, perimenopausal women with symptomatic fibroids should be good candidates for UAE, because currently desired fertility is a contraindication. UAE is a procedure that is performed by interventional radiologists and is an alternative to hysterectomy for women with symptomatic fibroids.[18]

UAE is performed under local anesthesia and sedation in the angiography suite. A catheter is placed in the femoral artery, and with digital angiography, the appropriate uterine artery is identified on the side of the fibroid. Polyvinyl particles are then injected through the catheter. This obstructs the uterine artery causing ischemia and eventually tissue necrosis of the leiomyomas . This process is extremely painful and epidural analgesia is usually performed concurrently.

In women with very large fibroids and symptoms of pelvic pressure and fullness, the myoma volume may not decrease sufficiently to relieve their symptoms. Additionally, there is an incidence of premature ovarian failure in up to 15% of patients. Contraindications to UAE include current infection, allergy to contrast dye, and any possibility of malignancy.

KEY POINT

Uterine artery embolization should be performed by experienced interventional radiologists in collaboration with anesthesiologists and gynecologists.

Other potential complications of UAE include passage of submucous myomas, infection, groin hematoma, femoral artery injury, and postembolization syndrome. The postembolization syndrome is characterized by fever, nausea, vomiting, and leukocytosis. In general, the short-term complication risk is low and the morbidity is about 5%.[19] Pain management is another potential problem with UAE. The pain following UAE is usually significant and may require inpatient management with a combination of intravenous narcotics and nonsteroidal anti-inflammatory agents.

Other Nonsurgical Treatments

Focused ultrasound surgery (FUS) with magnetic resonance is another nonsurgical therapy for fibroid tumors that has recently been studied to treat symptomatic fibroids. This procedure involves delivery of an ultrasound beam that gives thermal energy to targeted areas to induce tissue necrosis. The treatment parameters are determined by the magnetic resonance imaging (MRI) images obtained at the time of the procedure. Treatment time is approximately 2 hours. Patients who received this treatment were all planning hysterectomy and had surgery after FUS. Pathology documented the effect of treatment, which is necrosis of the fibroids. FUS for the treatment of uterine fibroids is not a proven long-term solution for women with symptomatic fibroids, but may hold promise as a conservative, nonsurgical option.[20]

Future Treatments

In addition to progesterone receptor blockade and GnRH antagonists, the future of fibroid therapy most likely lies at the cellular level by modifying growth factors. Certain growth factors are expressed more in fibroids than in normal myometrium. Inhibition of these factors could prevent or decrease fibroid development. One such growth factor is transforming growth factor-β or (TGF-β), which has been shown to be overexpressed in fibroids.[21]

Additionally, basic fibroblast growth factor (bFGF) promotes new blood vessel formation and may also cause smooth muscle cell growth. In fibroids, bFGF has been demonstrated to be overproduced and stored. Blocking receptors for this protein may be a potential treatment.[22]

Discussion of Cases

Case 1

A 46-year-old, G2P2, African American woman presents complaining of heavy menses, lasting up to 1 week. She describes passing quarter-sized clots and having severe dysmenorrhea. Her menstrual pattern has changed in the last 18 months, and her cycles have become increasingly heavy and more irregular. She is currently using 10 super tampons a day in addition to pads. Her general medical history is remarkable for hypertension that is treated by a beta-blocker. Her only surgical procedure was a postpartum tubal ligation approximately 6 years ago.

On physical examination, she is a well-appearing woman in no acute distress. Her general physical examination is unremarkable. Her pelvic examination is remarkable for a 9–10-week sized, irregular-shaped uterus. Upon further questioning she does admit to having symptoms of fatigue and poor exercise tolerance, which she attributes to her smoking one pack of cigarettes daily. Hematocrit is 27. An ultrasound is performed and confirms the diagnosis of a multifibroid uterus, normal-sized ovaries, and an irregular uterine cavity with an endometrial thickness that measures 8 mm.

Discussion

What is the most likely diagnosis?

This patient does not have large fibroids, but does present significant anemia.

What diagnostic tests are necessary?

The first step in her evaluation would be to rule out any endometrial pathology, such as hyperplasia or endometrial cancer. This can be done with an office endometrial biopsy. Once it is determined that she does have benign pathology, it would be helpful to determine if she has a submucous myoma. This could be done with SIS.

What are the management options?

If she does have a submucous myoma, a hysteroscopic resection would be a good treatment option. If she does not have any submucous fibroids, then a trial of oral contraceptives may be indicated keeping in mind that she smokes and her blood pressure may increase after starting oral contraceptives. Alternatively, GnRH analog therapy with add back is another potential treatment, particularly given her age. After 6 months of therapy she may be close to natural menopause and her symptoms may abate. The effect of GnRH agonist lasts up to 10 weeks after the last injection.

Case 2

A 44-year-old, G3P3, presents for her annual examination. She has no medical problems and her only medication is a low-dose oral contraceptive. She complains of extreme pelvic pressure when she has to empty her bladder and worsening dysmenorrhea. She also notes that she seems to be gaining weight in her stomach. Her general physical examination is unremarkable, however, when her abdominal examination is performed, she is noted to have approximately 18–22-week sized mass that is consistent with an enlarged uterus. She reports no changes in her menstrual pattern, and she has been happy with her oral contraceptives. Because of her physical examination, an ultrasound is ordered and confirms the diagnosis of an enlarged 20-week sized fibroid uterus, with both ovaries being normal sized. She had a hemoglobin done 3 months ago by her primary doctor and it was normal.

Discussion

What diagnostic tests are warranted in this patient?

Endometrial sampling is probably not as critical in this patient because she is on oral contraceptives but it should be performed to exclude malignancy. She has symptoms of pelvic pressure without significant bleeding. If she feels that her symptoms are severe enough, a surgical option may be advisable.

Is conservative medical management an option for this patient?

She is probably not a candidate for prolonged GnRH agonist therapy because it may not reduce fibroid volume sufficiently to improve her symptoms. She is only 44-years-old, remote from menopause and could require a very long course of therapy, which is costly. UAE is another possibility, but, again, this may not reduce her fibroids significantly to give her symptomatic relief. She should be counseled carefully about the potential of having surgery and that a surgical procedure such as a simple hysterectomy may provide relief of her symptoms.

References

1 Marshall LM, Spiegelman D, Barbieri RL, et al. Variation in the incidence of uterine leiomyoma among premenopausal women by age and race. *Obstet Gynecol.* 1997;90(6):967–973.

2 Kjerulff KH, Langenberg P, Seidman JD, et al. Uterine leiomyomas. Racial differences in severity, symptoms and age at diagnosis. *J Reprod Med.* 1996;41(7):483–490.

3 Farquhar CM, Steiner CA. Hysterectomy rates in the United States 1990–1997. *Obstet Gynecol.* 2002;99(2):229–234.

4 Rein MS, Friedman AJ, Barbieri RL, et al. Cytogenetic abnormalities in uterine leiomyomata. *Obstet Gynecol.* 1991;77(6):923–926.

5 Marshall LM, Spiegelman D, Goldman MB, et al. A prospective study of reproductive factors and oral contraceptive use in relation to the risk of uterine leiomyomata. *Fertil Steril.* 1998;70(3):432–439.

6 Rein MS, Barbieri RL, Friedman AJ. Progesterone: a critical role in pathogenesis of uterine myomas. *Am J Obstet Gynecol.* 1995;172(1, pt. 1):14–18.

7 Chiaffarino F, Parazzini F, La Vecchia C, et al. Diet and uterine myomas. *Obstet Gynecol.* 1999;94(3):395–398.

8 Parazzini F, Negri E, La Vecchia C, et al. Uterine myomas and smoking. Results from an Italian study. *J Reprod Med.* 1996;41(5):316–320.

9 Pritts EA. Fibroids and infertility: a systematic review of the evidence. *Obstet Gynecol Surv.* 201;56(8):483–491.

10 Wegienka G, Baird DD, Hertz-Picciotto I, et al. Self-reported heavy bleeding associated with uterine leiomyomata. *Obstet Gynecol.* 2003;101(3):431–437.

11 Parker WH, Fu YS, Berek JS. Uterine sarcoma in patients operated on for presumed leiomyoma and rapidly growing leiomyoma. *Obstet Gynecol.* 1994;83(3):414–418.

12 Fauconnier A, Chapron C, Babaki-Fard K, et al. Recurrence of leiomyomata after myomectomy. *Hum Reprod Update.* 2000;6(6):595–602.

13 Rossetti A, Sizzi O, Soranna L, et al. Long-term results of laparoscopic myomectomy: recurrence rate in comparison with abdominal myomectomy. *Hum Reprod.* 2001;16(4):770–774.

14 Friedman AJ, Daly M, Juneau-Norcross M, et al. A prospective, randomized trial of gonadotrophin-releasing hormone agonist plus estrogen-progestin or progestin "add-back" regimens for women with leiomyomata uteri. *J Clin Endocrinol Metab.* 1993;76(6):1439–1445.

15 Friedman AJ, Daly M, Juneau-Norcross M, et al. Long-term medical therapy for leiomyomata uteri: a prospective, randomized study of

leuprolide acetate depot plus either oestrogen-progestin "add-back" for 2 years. *Hum Reprod.* 1994;9(9):1618–1625.

16 Gocmen A, Kara IH, Karaca M. The effects of add-back therapy with tibolone on myoma uteri. *Clin Exp Obstet Gynecol.* 2002;29(3): 222–224

17 Eisinger SH, Meldrum S, Fiscella K, et al. Low-dose mifepristone for uterine leiomyomata. *Obstet Gynecol.* 2003;101(2):243–250.

18 Pinto I, chimeno P, Romo A, et al. Uterine fibroids: uterine artery embolization versus abdominal hysterectomy for treatment – a prospective, randomized, and controlled clinical trial. *Radiology.* 2003;226(2):425–431.

19 Spies JB, Specto A, Roth AR, et al. Complications after uterine artery embolization for leiomyomas. *Obstet Gynecol.* 2002;100(5, pt. 1): 873–880.

20 Steward EA, Gedroyc WM, Tempany CM, et al. Focused ultrasound treatment of uterine fibroid tumors: safety and feasibility of a non-invasive thermoablative technique. *Am J Obstet Gynecol.* 2003;189(1): 48–54.

21 Sozen I, Arici A. Interactions of cytokines, growth factors, and the extracellular matrix in the cellular biology of uterine leiomyomata. *Fertil Steril.* 2002;78(1):1–12.

22 Anania CA, Stewart EA, Quade BJ, et al. Expression of the fibroblast growth factor receptor in women with leiomyomas and abnormal uterine bleeding. *Mol Hum Reprod.*1997;3(8):685–691.

11 Evaluation and Management of Pelvic Pain

Thomas Janicki

Introduction

Pain is an unpleasant multidimensional phenomenon involving sensory, affective, motivational, environmental, and cognitive components. Pain during perimenopause can be divided into three categories: acute, chronic, and chronic pain syndromes. Acute pain is characterized by a time-limited relationship to the noxious stimulus associated with tissue injury, e.g., inflammation or ischemia. Chronic pain in the pelvis contains elements of tissue injury and central nervous system (CNS) sensitization, which generally increases its intensity. Chronic pain syndrome does not reflect the degree of tissue damage. Key components of chronic pain syndrome include central and peripheral nervous system sensitization. This pain complex may occur without any obvious tissue injury and it can persist after removal or correction of initial pain source. Examples of chronic pain syndrome include complex regional pain syndromes and peripheral neuropathies.[1–3] In the case of chronic pelvic pain (CPP) and CPP syndrome, many women will exhibit multiple pain symptoms originating not only in their genital organs, but also related to their gastrointestinal (GI), urinary, musculoskeletal, and nervous systems. It is estimated that CPP consumes more than $3 billion in health resource dollars annually.[4,5]

Acute Pain

Acute pain conditions in perimenopause include most of the acute pain events throughout women's life. Most common conditions are shown in Table 11-1.

Table 11-1. VARIOUS CAUSES OF ACUTE PELVIC PAIN IN PERIMENOPAUSE

Acute pelvic inflammatory disease
Tubo-ovarian complex or abscess
Endometritis
Pregnancy-related events
Ectopic pregnancy
Spontaneous abortion
Degenerating leiomyomas
Ovarian cyst/ruptured ovarian cyst
Adnexal torsion
Cystitis
Nephrolithiasis
Acute urinary retention
Acute appendicitis
Diverticulitis
Bowel obstruction
Constipation

Treatment of acute pain states depends on the source of the pain and may include observation, surgical intervention, treatment of infection, and effective pain management including use of the opioids.

Chronic Pelvic Pain

KEY POINT

Chronic pain is non-menstrual-related pain that is at least 3 months in duration in women of reproductive age (18–50 years).

Chronic pain in the pelvis includes non-menstrual-related pain that is daily, reoccurs frequently or periodically for at least 3 months duration usually in women of reproductive age (18–50 years). This form of pain is more complex, as it contains elements of nociceptive impulses from the involved organ or area, as well as altered CNS processing of pain. The altered pain processing includes anticipation of pain based on previous experiences and sensitization of afferent neurons in certain areas of CNS leading to amplification of the pain impulses. It may also include degree of visceral hypersensitivity in which case pain can involve surrounding peritoneum and adjacent organs.

CPP can account for 2–10% of gynecologic office visits and 20% of all laparoscopies performed in the United States.[6,7] Women over the age of 35 have a lower incidence of CPP (odds ratio [OR] 0.72, 95% CI, 0.60–0.85).[6] Some of the examples of conditions associated with CPP are shown in Table 11-2.

Treatment of CPP includes treatment of the underlying condition, treatment of aggravating factors (menstruation, menstrual

Table 11-2. **CONDITIONS ASSOCIATED WITH CHRONIC PELVIC PAIN IN PERIMENOPAUSE**

Gynecologic
Endometriosis
Pelvic adhesions
Ovarian remnant syndrome
Adenomyosis
Uterine fibroids
Cervicitis and endometritis
Pelvic relaxation
Uterine malposition
Cancer
Musculoskeletal
Degenerative changes of vertebra and pelvic joints
Hernias
Gastrointestinal
Diverticulitis
Sprue
Inflammatory bowel disease
Cancer
Functional bowel disease (i.e., IBS)
Urinary System
Interstitial cystitis
Chronic calculi
Pain Processing disorders
Visceral hypersensitivity
Neuropathic pain
Fibromyalgia
Psychological factors
Sexual abuse
Depression
Somatization
Hypochondriasis

Abbreviation: IBS, irritable bowel syndrome.

irregularities, diet), as well as pain-modifying therapies and a comprehensive approach to restore or improve patient function. Separation of pain due to either a physical or mental etiology is not always helpful. Pain can be associated with psychological factors and can be modified by how the brain processes the pain stimulus as well as the duration of pain stimulus. A description of these treatment approaches is beyond the scope of this chapter but is summarized in Table 11-3. Only gynecological causes of CPP will be discussed in greater detail.

Table 11-3. EXAMPLES OF TREATMENT APPROACHES FOR NONGYNECOLOGIC CAUSES OF CPP

Condition	*Suggested Approaches*
Psychological-based	Psychotherapy, antidepressant medication
Pain-processing disorders	Tricyclics, cognitive behavioral therapy, acupuncture
Interstitial cystitis	Intravesical dimethylsulfoxide, pentosan polysulfate
Musculoskeletal	Surgical repair, anti-inflammatory medication

Treatment of Underlying Conditions

Endometriosis

Although often associated with younger women, endometriosis is one of the most common conditions associated with pelvic pain, dyspareunia, and dysmenorrhea. This condition should be considered also in the perimenopausal woman. It involves presence of active endometrium outside uterine cavity, mainly in the pelvis. The most popular theory regarding its etiology involves retrograde flow into the pelvis of the menstrual blood and endometrial fragments through fallopian tubes. Periodic presence of superficial endometrial implants in the pelvis can be confirmed pathologically in most of menstruating women, but most of them will not develop clinical endometriosis.[8] The exact mechanism of pain generation has not been established. Theories include inflammatory response, adhesions, neuronal involvement, and localized increased prostaglandin production.[9,10]

Medical management includes hormonal manipulation and antiprostaglandin agents. Continuous progestogens, gonadotropin-releasing hormone (GnRH) agonists (with or without add-back estrogen), and danazol (oral and recently vaginal administration) are the mainstay of hormonal manipulation used in treatment of pain symptoms. Surgical treatment includes conservative or extirpative surgery with removal of endometriotic implants including deep fibrotic retroperitoneal implants. Nonsteroidal anti-inflammatory drugs (NSAIDs) are helpful in controlling mild to moderate pain while opioids should be used sparingly for exacerbation of the pain. To date, short-term randomized trials comparing medical to surgical management have shown similar responses, however, no studies have addressed the optimal long-term strategies for control of pain from endometriosis. Continuous use of opioids in chronic pain states should be avoided due to risk of dependence and development of tolerance followed by loss of their pain-controlling ability.

Pelvic Adhesions–Including Ovarian Remnant Syndrome

The presence of intra-abdominal adhesions is often blamed as a cause of CPP. The data are not conclusive, as many women with extensive adhesions may not experience any pain. Laparoscopy is the preferred method for diagnosis as well as treatment as it potentially minimizes surgical trauma to intra-abdominal organs. Careful atraumatic dissection and proper hemostasis is an essential part of such surgery.

KEY POINT

Many women with extensive pelvic adhesions may not experience any pain.

For women who have had surgical removal of the ovaries for pelvic pain, ovarian remnant syndrome should be considered. Diagnosis of this disorder may require evaluation of serum estradiol levels, follicle-stimulating hormone (FSH), and pelvic ultrasonography. Removal of the ovarian remnant requires advanced surgical skills. Retroperitoneal dissection to identify the ureter and pelvic vessels is an essential part of this surgery and it allows the surgeon to safely remove entire ovarian remnant. Nonsurgical management of ovarian remnant syndrome includes hormonal suppression using continuous oral contraceptives, oral or intramuscular medroxyprogesterone, GnRH agonists, or low-dose radiation to the ovarian bed.

Adenomyosis

Adenomyosis is a condition caused by the presence of endometrial glands and stroma deep within the muscle of the uterus. Adenomyosis can produce intense uterine cramps due to periodic bleeding and release of prostaglandins within the myometrium during the menstrual cycle. This diagnosis is usually made clinically but can be confirmed by pelvic magnetic resonance imaging (MRI). Pain associated with adenomyosis is rarely seen in young adults and its incidence increases with age. Conservative treatment includes antiprostaglandins and hormonal suppression using continuous oral contraceptives, oral or intramuscular medroxyprogesterone, danazol, and GnRH agonists. Danazol or a progestin-releasing intrauterine device may offer another medical management alternative.[11,12] Patients who fail medical management may require total or supracervical hysterectomy to alleviate symptoms.

Uterine Fibroids Generally uterine fibroids are asymptomatic. On occasion they may produce pressure symptoms because of compression of adjacent organs (see Chap. 10). Occasionally degeneration of the fibroid due to diminished blood supply will be associated with varying degrees of discomfort or pain. This condition is self-limited and the symptoms will improve once degeneration is complete. Usually symptomatic treatment using NSAIDs and a short course of opioids will be sufficient. Rarely, torsion of a pedunculated fibroid will produce sufficient symptomatology to justify surgical intervention.

Chronic Cervicitis and Endometritis Chronic cervicitis and endometritis will occasionally produce CPP and dyspareunia. Presence of purulent cervical discharge and a tender cervix or uterus during bimanual examination should raise suspicion of an infectious process. Negative cervical cultures for gonorrhea and chlamydia do not exclude infection. If endometritis is suspected, an endometrial biopsy to determine presence of plasma cells may be useful. For endometritis, treatment with doxycycline or erythromycin for at least 2 weeks duration can be effective.

Pelvic Relaxation Pelvic relaxation increases in frequency and severity with age and parity. Numerous pelvic and lower back pain complaints can be linked to progressive prolapse of pelvic organs. A great variety of treatment options both surgical and nonsurgical exist and their detailed discussion is beyond scope of this chapter.

Uterine Malposition Uterine malposition, mainly in the form of severe retroflexion and retroversion of the uterus, may be associated with impact dyspareunia during deep thrusting and difficulties during defecation. Generally, accepted treatments include corrective pessaries and anterior uterine suspension via laparoscopy or mini-laparotomy.

Malignancy There is an increased incidence of malignancies involving genital organs, bowel, and urinary tract with aging. Pain symptoms can be nonspecific and confusing. The possibility of malignancy as a source of pain should always be excluded in patients suffering from any chronic pain, including CPP.

DEGENERATIVE CHANGES OF VERTEBRA AND PELVIC JOINTS

Arthritis, herniated vertebral discs, osteoporosis with vertebral fractures, and pelvic fractures can be a source of pelvic pain as well as referred pain in the pelvis. One key sign is that pain intensity will be affected by movement. Radiological studies of the pelvis and lumbosacral spine in addition to physical examination are useful diagnostic tools. Treatment depends on location and type of injury.

HERNIAS

Fascial planes in the pelvis and the lower abdomen contain several potential hernia openings. They include inguinal hernias both direct and indirect, femoral hernias, perineal hernias, obturator hernias, incisional hernias, and others. The diagnosis is made by physical examination and treatment usually involves surgical repair.

PAINFUL BOWEL CONDITIONS

KEY POINT

IBS is one of the common conditions associated with chronic pain and CPP syndromes.

Irritable bowel syndrome (IBS) is one of the conditions commonly associated with CPP and CPP syndromes.[13] Other painful bowel conditions include recurrent partial small-bowel obstruction, diverticulitis, and inflammatory bowel disease. Changes in bowel habits or abnormal bowel habits are the symptoms suggesting that GI tract may be contributing to patient pain symptoms. Imaging studies of small and large bowel as well as colonoscopy are helpful in evaluating the role of the bowel in pelvic pain. Celiac sprue is a condition that has been associated with CPP and its incidence has been grossly underestimated.

Close cooperation with a gastroenterologist is helpful in comprehensive management of these patients. Patients with constipation as the predominant form of IBS will usually respond to a comprehensive approach, which may include dietary modification, osmotic laxatives, magnesium sulfate, antispasmodics, tricyclic antidepressants, and selective serotonin reuptake inhibitors (SSRIs). Patients with diarrhea as the predominant form of IBS can be treated with loperamide, cholestyramine, antispasmodics, tricyclic antidepressants, and SSRIs. Two new preparations with action focused on enteric neuron serotonin receptors include alosetron hydrochloride and tegaserod maleate.[14–16] 5-hydroxytryptamine3 (5-HT3) receptors are non-selective cation channels extensively distributed on enteric neurons in the human GI tract, as well as other peripheral and central locations. Activation of these channels affects the regulation of visceral pain, colonic transit, and GI secretions. Selective 5-HT3 receptor antagonists inhibit activation of nonselective cation channels, which results in the modulation of the enteric nervous system. Alosetron hydrochloride is a selective 5-HT3 receptor antagonist. Alosetron is used primarily in diarrhea predominant form of IBS and its use is contraindicated in the constipation predominant form of IBS. Tegaserod maleate belongs to a new class of drugs called serotonin-4 receptor agonists (5-HT4 agonists). By activating 5-HT4 receptors, it stimulates the peristaltic reflex and normalizes impaired motility in the GI tract. It is used in constipation predominant form of IBS.

Interstitial Cystitis

Patients suffering from interstitial cystitis (IC) are commonly seen in a gynecologist's office because of pelvic pain and dyspareunia. IC is a chronic inflammatory condition of the bladder wall of unknown etiology. Symptoms of IC include urinary urgency and frequency, difficulty in urinating, small urine output, pain in the bladder and/or urethra that may be temporarily relieved by voiding. Urine cultures are usually negative. Pelvic examination is often significant for tenderness in the region of bladder and urethra. Cystoscopy and hydrodistention under general anesthesia reveal petechial hemorrhages or glomerulations in the bladder wall. In the minority of the patients, cystoscopy will reveal the presence of Hunner's ulcers.

KEY POINT

Interstitial cystitis is a condition that can be associated with chronic pain and CPP syndromes.

There is no standard effective treatment for IC.[17,18]. Consultation with a urologist in diagnosis and treatment is helpful. Treatment is prolonged and includes dietary modification, antihistamines, anti-inflammatory agents, sodium pentosan polysulfate, and anticholinergics. Additional treatment with intravesical administration of dimethyl sulfoxide (DMSO), hydrodistention of the bladder under general anesthesia, and implantable sacral nerve stimulators are used in resistant cases. Recent reports indicate relief of pain and urgency in patients who failed standard treatment of IC and were later treated with gabapentin.[19]

Neuropathic Pain

The process of labor and vaginal delivery is commonly associated with pudendal nerve injury. Usually patients suffer pain while sitting or walking. This pain is relieved by lying down or sitting on a toilet seat. Iliohypogastric and genitofemoral nerve injury can be associated with Pfannenstiel incision, use of retractors, or postoperative scaring. Pain is usually localized to the inguinal area, upper anterior and medial thigh. Similar pain can occur after ilioinguinal nerve injury associated with retropubic urethropexy. Other nerves that can produce sensory abnormalities in the pelvis include obturator, lateral femoral cutaneus, and femoral nerve. Nerve injury is commonly followed by centralization of the symptoms within CNS. If centralization has occurred, neurolysis is generally of limited value due to reoccurrence of the central pain after the procedure. Treatment generally includes pain medication on a time-contingent basis, therapeutic nerve blocks, and radiofrequency (RF) nerve ablation, gabapentin, tricyclic antidepressants, and physical therapy.

PAIN PROCESSING DISORDERS

There is a tremendous overlap among the pain processing disorders including fibromyalgia, chronic fatigue syndrome, depression, and somatization. The overall incidence of fibromyalgia is 2–8% of which 80% are females.[20] The criteria for fibromyalgia according to the American College of Rheumatology 1990 includes pain involving all four quadrants of the body including axial skeleton, tenderness at 11 of 18 specified sites, and inappropriate amplification of the pain.[21] These disorders should be part of the differential diagnosis of chronic pain and CPP syndromes.

Chronic Pelvic Pain Syndrome—Complex Visceral Pain Syndrome

CPP syndrome is one of the most challenging conditions that care providers face. Common characteristics of individuals that suffer from this disorder include (1) pain duration greater than 6 months, (2) significant impairment of daily activities, (3) incomplete pain relief with conventional treatments, (4) pain out of proportion to pathology, (5) signs of depression, and (6) presence of familial dysfunction. Many times, the patient will have a history of multiple surgeries and gradual removal of pelvic organs without improvement of the pain symptoms. This syndrome also includes patients who had multiple laparoscopies with negative or minimal findings. Pain is usually aggravated by stress, physical activity, intercourse, and menstruation.

One diagnostic modality is the use of laparoscopy under conscious sedation to map the location of the pain within the pelvis.[22] While doing pain mapping, one can reproduce severe pain by touching most of the normal-appearing areas in the pelvis indicating allodynia, hyperalgesia, and visceral hypersensitivity. In chronic pain syndrome, the relationship between the initial source of pain and the pain itself is lost. The pain will persist even if the initial source of pain has been removed. Theoretically, in these patients there is an imprint of the pain within the central, peripheral, and autonomic nervous system. These patients with chronic pain syndrome require a comprehensive therapeutic approach.

Treatment of Chronic Pelvic Pain

Complementary Medical Therapy for Chronic Pelvic Pain and Chronic Pelvic Pain Syndromes

As stated previously, chronic pain has components that go beyond the initial source and tissue injury. At present, there are no totally satisfactory analgesic drugs to control chronic pain of nonmalignant origin. The goal in the treatment of patients with CPP is different from the goal for patients with end-stage cancer. With CPP, the goal is to improve patient function and make pain as minimal as possible. That requires a comprehensive multidisciplinary approach available in pain clinics where there is access to psychologists, physical therapists, and anesthesiologists (Table 11-4).

Hormonal Manipulation

There is a significant difference in pelvic pain patterns in women before and after menopause. It has been postulated that estrogen is a pain sensitizer and most hormonal manipulation techniques involve decreasing estrogen levels or blocking estrogen receptors. Recent animal experiments have shown that in female rats, stress-induced visceral hypersensitivity is estrogen-dependent and involves tachykinin NK1 receptors.[23]

Table 11-4. **MODALITIES FOR TREATMENT OF CHRONIC PELVIC PAIN**

Hormonal manipulation
Drugs modifying pain perception
Psychotherapy
Physical therapy

Birth Control Pills, Progestagens Birth control pills are quite effective in the treatment of dysmenorrhea in ovulating women. Menstrual cramping is associated with the release of prostaglandins (mainly prostaglandin $F_{2\alpha}$) from breakdown of secretory endometrium. The level of prostaglandins in the endometrium increases by 300% in the luteal phase as compared with the early follicular phase. Birth control pills induce atrophy of decidualized endometrium, thus decreasing total prostaglandin production. Similarly, continuous use of progestogens will also induce decidualization and atrophy of the endometrium in the uterus and in some ectopic locations.

GnRH Analogs GnRH agonists (i.e., leuprolide acetate), produce pseudo-menopause including a significant drop in estrogen levels. These analogs reduce luteinizing hormone (LH) and FSH production by down regulation of pituitary GnRH receptors leading to a suppression of ovarian follicular growth and a reduction in estradiol levels that are in the menopausal range. The exact mechanism of pain relief is unknown, but it is possible that the decrease in sensitivity of visceral nociceptors rather than suppression of the growth of ectopic endometrium is a primary mode of action.

Danazol Danazol is an ethinyl testosterone derivative which can bind to androgen receptors. Danazol was the first effective drug used to treat endometriosis-related symptoms. Danazol induces amenorrhea, which is associated with a high androgen-low estrogen environment that does not support growth of endometriosis. Multiple side effects have limited its use in the recent decade. These include muscle cramps, decrease in breast size, oily skin, and hirsutism. Recent studies have demonstrated the effectiveness of danazol administered vaginally in treating pain associated with endometriosis without the amenorrhea or troublesome androgenic side effects.[24] The action mechanism of vaginal danazol seems to be related to its localized activity in the pelvis. In addition, in vitro studies of endometrial cultures indicates that danazol causes dose-dependent cell death.[25]

Drugs Modifying Pain Perception

It is possible that CPP patients experience more than one type of pain. This concept may explain why chronic pain usually requires the use of more than one drug to produce relief of symptoms.

At present there are no totally satisfactory analgesic drugs to control chronic pain of nonmalignant origin.

Anti-Inflammatory Drugs There are several classes of drugs that exhibit anti-inflammatory activity or inhibit prostaglandin synthesis.

Acetaminophen blocks prostaglandin synthesis in the CNS, but has no peripheral anti-inflammatory effect. It has analgesic and antipyretics effects (both centrally modulated). Prolonged use may be associated with liver and kidney damage.

Salicylates (i.e., aspirin) have broad central and peripheral antiprostaglandin activity with irreversible inhibition of the cyclooxygenase 1 (COX-1) and cyclooxygenase 2 (COX-2) enzymes responsible for prostaglandin synthesis. Prolonged use may be associated with increased risk of gastritis, gastric ulcers and GI bleeding.

NSAIDs: Selected subgroups are widely used in the treatment of visceral pain.

Propionic acids: Ibuprofen and naproxen inhibit prostaglandin synthesis centrally and peripherally, mainly by interaction with COX-1 and COX-2. Analgesic properties are attained at significantly lower levels than anti-inflammatory activity, which occurs at 3200 mg/day for ibuprofen and 1000 mg/day for naproxen. Prolonged use is associated with similar side effects as aspirin.

Anthranilic acids: Meclofenamate has a dual action, inhibiting prostaglandin synthesis and competitively binding to prostaglandin receptors. Long-term use is associated with similar side effects as aspirin.

COX inhibitors: Celecoxib (Celebrex), rofecoxib (Vioxx), and valdecoxib (Bextra) block selectively the COX-2 enzyme. Most of the side effects associated with aspirin-like drugs are due to blocking of COX-1 receptor. More recently, selective COX-2 inhibitors have been associated with increased risk of stroke and myocardial infarction in high-risk individuals.

Antidepressants Antidepressants are used in the treatment of chronic pain to alter pain perception by inhibition of neurotransmitter synaptic reuptake. The most commonly used are tricyclic antidepressants.

Tricyclic antidepressants: Amitriptyline and desipramine help patients sleep, reduce anxiety and depression, and can raise the pain threshold. The exact mechanism for increasing the pain threshold is unknown . One should evaluate their use for at least 1 month, starting at a low dose of 25 mg in the evening.

Serotonin and mixed serotonin and norepinephrine reuptake inhibitors: Sertraline (Zoloft), fluoxetine (Prozac), paroxetine (Paxil), and venlafaxine (Effexor) seem to be less effective and inconsistent as far as their effect on pelvic pain compared with older tricyclic antidepressants. In a small placebo-controlled study in women with CPP, the SSRI sertraline was not effective.[26] Coadministration of SSRIs with the newer mixed antidepressants (e.g., venlafaxine) can lead to serotonin syndrome, a potentially fatal manifestation of excess serotonin.

Anxiolytics: Diazepam (Valium), lorazepam (Ativan), flurazepam (Dalmane), and chlordiazepoxide (Librium), although quite useful in treatment of acute pain, are contraindicated in chronic pain because they may reduce the beneficial biogenic amine activity.

Opioids: Opioids are extremely useful in treatment of acute pain or pain associated with malignancy. The use of opioids in chronic pain is less desirable because of the tolerance phenomenon. Occasional use for exacerbation of pain should be considered on an individual basis.

Anticonvulsants Anticonvulsants have been used mainly in the treatment of neuropathic pain, postherpetic neuralgia, atypical fascial pains, and reflex sympathetic dystrophy. There are no data addressing their effectiveness in the treatment of CPP, but anecdotal reports are encouraging.

Clonazepam is used mainly in the form of a skin patch applied to a trigger point site.

Gabapentin has been used successfully in the treatment of chronic pain. It increases gamma-amino butyric acid (GABA), an inhibitory neurotransmitter and raises the threshold for synaptic transmission of the impulses. In patients with CPP who suffer from visceral hypersensitivity, it will theoretically decrease transmission of lesser impulses. To diminish side effects, one should start gabapentin at low dose (as low as 100 mg qhs) and advance it gradually until the desired effect is achieved.

Topiramate, or *levetiracetam,* can also be used in patients not responding to gabapentin.

Psychotherapy

By the time pelvic pain becomes a chronic condition, central processing of the pain involving emotions and cognition becomes one of the most important parts of pain perception. Virtually every patient with chronic pain will state that the pain gets worse during times of heightened stress. At the same time, constant pain produces increased stress by affecting the psyche, daily function, and interpersonal relationships. Patients who go to sleep in pain wake up in pain and suffer from pain every moment of the day, often lack coping skills to deal with this continuous burden. Such patients need trained help to develop new coping skills.

Psychotherapy by a trained therapist, regardless of any use of psychoactive drugs, is the most effective way to develop new coping skills for dealing with chronic pain and its exacerbations.

Physical Therapy

Evaluation and treatment by a physical therapist is an essential part of the management of patients with CPP. Patients with chronic pain will walk, sit, and sleep differently than patients without pain. These activities will create additional sources of pain, skeletal instability, and painful muscle contractions. A physical therapist with experience in treating CPP is an essential part of the team treating patients suffering from CPP.

Neuromodulating Techniques

Many patients with CPP will not achieve sufficient relief following surgical, medical, mental health, and physical therapy. For such patients, there are multiple noninvasive and invasive neuromodulatory techniques available.

These include transcutaneous nerve stimulators, diagnostic and therapeutic nerve blocks, cryo and radio frequency nerve ablation, and implantable spinal cord and peripheral nerve stimulation devices.

Key Issues

It is important to approach treatment of pelvic pain in a systematic manner. Figure 11-1 outlines a general diagnostic and treatment plan that can be applied to most of the patients suffering from pelvic pain. The following cases provide examples of evaluation and treatment in different clinical situations.

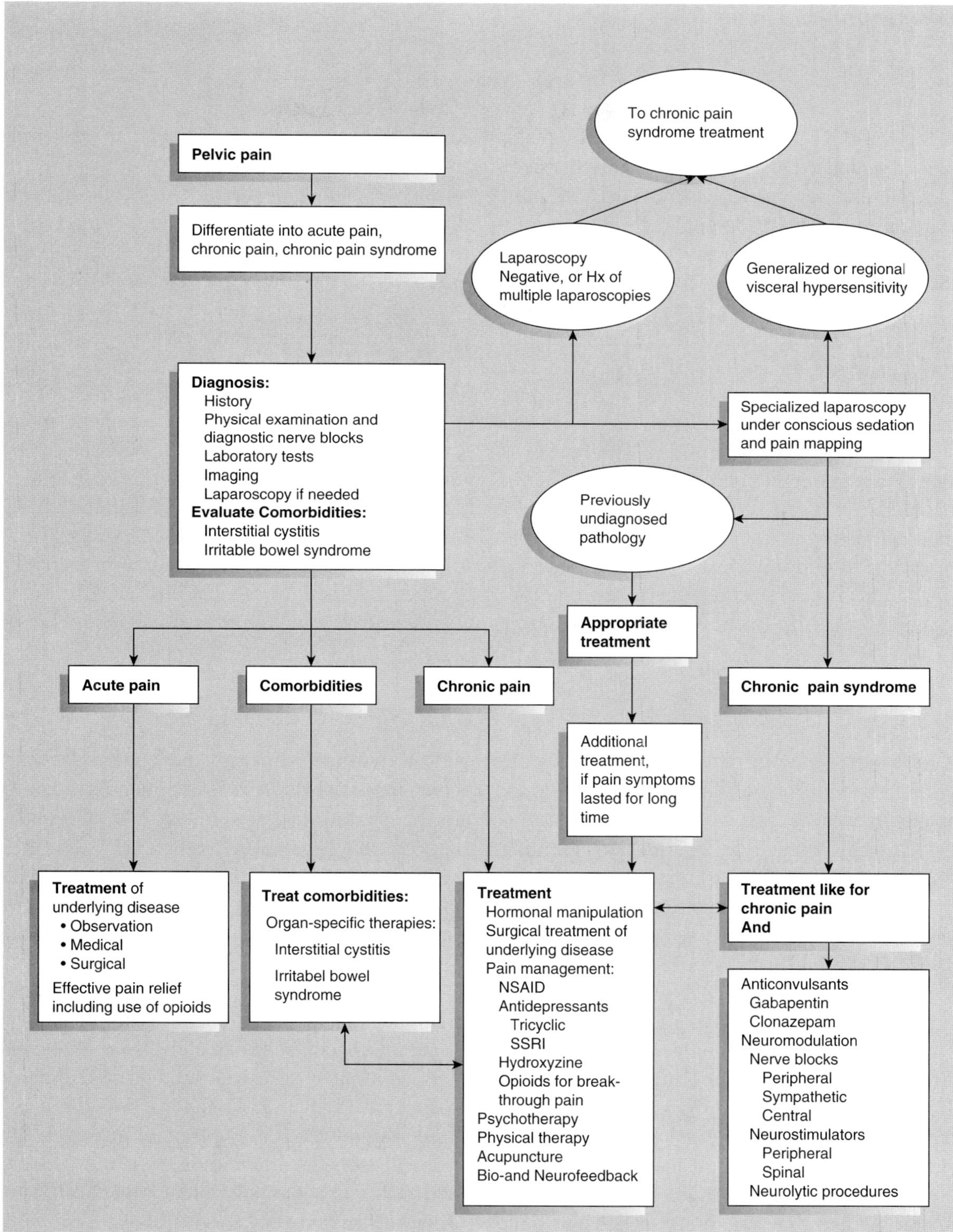

Figure 11-1: Pelvic pain. General diagnostic and treatment plan.

Discussion of Cases

CASE 1

A.K. is a 45-year-old gravida 2 para 2 female. She presented to her gynecologist's office because of acute and severe right lower quadrant pain starting the morning of her visit. Her periods were regular and generally painless; her last menstrual period was 3 weeks prior to her visit. She has been sexually active and she did not experience any dyspareunia since her laparoscopic surgery for endometriosis 6 years ago. For the last 2 months she noticed an occasional sharp right lower quadrant pain lasting a few seconds to a couple of minutes. The pain was significant enough to occasionally cause her to "double over". She thought it was gas. Her past medical history was significant for laparoscopic resection of endometriosis on the uterosacral ligaments and a postpartum tubal ligation. Physical examination revealed a slightly overweight woman in moderate distress laying on the table in fetal position. Her pulse was 90 and her blood pressure was 150/90. The abdomen was not distended and there were normal bowel sounds. She had significant guarding in the lower abdomen especially on the right but no peritoneal signs. Pelvic examination revealed moderate cervical motion tenderness and an exquisitely tender 7–8 cm right adnexal mass. Pelvic ultrasound showed 7 cm complex, solid/cystic adnexal mass, and moderate amount of free fluid in the cul-de-sac. To evaluate the adnexal mass further, color flow Doppler ultrasound was performed, which revealed a picture consistent with ovarian torsion. Appropriate surgical intervention is the proper treatment in this patient. Usually, there is no need for long-term medical therapy.

CASE 2

L.W. is a 44-year-old gravida 2, para 2 female with complaints of worsening right lower quadrant pain over the last 2 years. Her pain is aggravated by physical activity, voiding, and straining during defecation. Her past history is significant for two uncomplicated low transverse cesarian sections and an abdominal hysterectomy for uterine bleeding in her mid-thirties. One year ago she underwent laparoscopy because of right lower quadrant pain. Laparoscopic findings included anterior abdominal omental adhesions and small-bowel adhesions on the vaginal cuff. There was no evidence of endometriosis and both ovaries appeared normal and free of adhesions. Successful adhesiolysis was carried out laparoscopically, but during her 4 weeks postoperative visit the patient stated that her right lower quadrant pain was unchanged. She was given ibuprofen and acetaminophen/oxycodone for pain control, but she used it infrequently because they were not effective.

Important findings during physical examination included normal vital signs, no tenderness to palpation of the spinal column, costovertebral angles, back musculature, or sacroiliac joints. Bowel sounds were present and normal. Examination of the upper abdomen was unremarkable to superficial and deep palpation; lower abdomen and suprapubic area were quite tender to deep palpation. Right lower quadrant was the most tender area with some voluntary guarding. To further assess the origin of the pain and to separate the intra-abdominal content from the abdominal wall, patient was asked to elevate and hold both her legs 2 in. above the table. Palpation of lower abdomen was repeated and produced extreme pain in the right lower quadrant with its greatest intensity over right lateral aspect of her transverse laparotomy scar. Following examination of the abdomen, a single-digit pelvic examination was performed and it did not produce any pain; bimanual examination produced right lower quadrant pain, but there were no palpable pelvic masses. A provisional diagnosis was made that these findings represented iliohypogastric postsurgical neuralgia with the trigger point at transverse abdominal scar. A diagnostic trigger point injection of 5 cc of 0.25% Marcaine was performed at the site with complete relief of pain within 1 hour of injection. Total pain relief lasted for 4 days. The patient was then referred to the Pain Center for RF ablation of Iliohypogastric nerve. Since the pain has been present for 2 years, follow-up is needed because of the possibility of incomplete resolution or recurrence of the pain symptoms. In that event, aggressive treatment with low-dose desipramine, gabapentin, physical therapy, and psychotherapy are options.

CASE 3

D.C. is a 45-year-old gravida 1, para 1 with complaints of dyspareunia, abdominal and pelvic pain for over 10 years. Her past medical history is significant for endometriosis, adenomyosis, and reflex sympathetic dystrophy in her right foot. She also suffers from migraine headaches and allergies. At present, she is being treated for depression with Venlafaxine. She has had multiple surgeries for her pelvic pain including laparoscopic treatment of endometriosis, total abdominal hysterectomy, left salpingooophorectomy, appendectomy, cholecystectomy, and lysis of adhesions. Most of the surgeries were associated with modest relief of pain symptoms for up to 6 months. She is using NSAIDs and opioids for pain control. Physical examination reveals a middle-aged woman laying in fetal position on the examining table. Her blood pressure is 120/70 and her pulse is 76. Screening for fibromyalgia trigger points reveals some painful trigger points in abdominal area, but none above the diaphragm, the back, or the extremities. Examination of the abdomen shows presence of multiple surgical scars and brown mottling of the skin in the middle of the abdomen consistent with prolonged use of a heating pad. Palpation of the abdomen reveals moderate tenderness over the entire abdominal area; deep palpation induces voluntary guarding and severe pain without a particular epicenter. Elevation of the legs and reexamination of the abdominal wall reveals a trigger point in the right lower quadrant but the remainder of the abdominal wall was less painful.

The single-digit pelvic examination reveals tenderness at the introitus, tenderness and spasm of the pubococcygeus muscles, the urethra and the bladder. Palpation of the vaginal cuff, parametria, and the cul-de-sac produces extreme tenderness. Bimanual examination is difficult due to the patient's discomfort, but there are no obvious pelvic masses. The patient cannot tolerate a rectal examination. Pelvic ultrasound reveals a normal right ovary and no evidence of any unusual findings. In the light of previous multiple unsuccessful surgical procedures, the patient is offered laparoscopy and pain mapping under conscious sedation and she agrees to that plan.

Laparoscopy reveals the pelvic peritoneum to be hyperemic and to have diffuse superficial scaring in the sites of previous surgeries, but there is no evidence of endometriosis or pelvic adhesions. Pain mapping under conscious sedation using the Endometriosis USA pain mapping form was graded as moderate to severe in all areas examined. Discomfort associated with touching and moving of the right ovary and sigmoid colon were graded as moderate. The result of pain mapping was consistent with generalized visceral hypersensitivity.

In this situation there are two surgical options: (a) superior hypogastric plexus block using 2% lidocaine with repeating pain mapping to see if presacral neurectomy would reduce the pain, and (b) removal of the right ovary to diminish the level of estrogen and the monthly hormonal fluctuations. Regardless of the surgical procedure performed, the patient will require long-term management of her complex visceral pain syndrome. A comprehensive treatment program will have to include (1) psychotherapy to assist in developing new coping skills and to evaluate and manage depression, (2) physical therapy to evaluate and treat secondary neuromuscular dysfunction, and (3) medications to modulate pain perception and neuron to neuron transmission. Use of opioids should be limited to management of breakthrough pain. If the ovary is not removed, the patient may require hormonal manipulation to suppress ovarian function. Other potentially useful treatments include acupuncture, yoga, neuro- and biofeedback, and neuromodulating procedures.

References

1 Schwartzman RJ, Grothusen J, Kiefer TR, et al. Neuropathic central pain: epidemiology, etiology, and treatment options. *Arch Neurol.* 2001;58(10):1547–1550.

2 Janig W. Neurobiology of visceral afferent neurons: neuroanatomy, functions, organ regulations and sensations. *Biol Psychol.* 1996;42(1): 29–51

3 Janicki TI. Chronic pelvic pain as a form of complex regional pain syndrome. *Clin Obstet Gynecol.* 2003;46(4):797–803

4 Davies L, Granger KF, Drummond M, et al. The economic burden of intractable gynecological pain. *Obstet Gynecol.* 1992;12:S54.

5 Mathias SD, Kuppermann M, Liberman RF, et al. Chronic pelvic pain: prevalence, health-related quality of life, and economic correlates. *Obstet Gynecol.* 1996;87:321–327.

6 Reiter RC. A profile of women with chronic pelvic pain. *Clin Obstet Gynecol.* 1990;33:130–136.

7 Nolan TE, Elkins TE. Chronic pelvic pain: differentiating anatomic from functional causes. *Postgrad Med.* 1993;94:125–128.

8 Koninckx PR, Kennedy SH, Barlow DH. Pathogenesis of endometriosis: the role of peritoneal fluid. *Gynecol Obstet Invest.* 1999;47 (Suppl. 1): 23–33.

9 Anaf V, Simon P, El Nakadi I, et al. Hyperalgesia, nerve infiltration and nerve growth factor expression in deep adenomyotic nodules,

peritoneal and ovarian endometriosis. *Hum Reprod.* 2002;17(7): 1895–1900.

10 Dawood MY, Khan-Dawood FS, Wilson L. Peritoneal fluid prostaglandins and prostanoids in women with endometriosis, chronic pelvic inflammatory disease, and pelvic pain. *Am J Obstet Gynecol.* 1984;148(4):391–395.

11 Igarashi M, Abe Y, Fukada M, et al. Novel conservative medical therapy for uterine adenomyosis with a danazol-loaded intrauterine device. *Fertil Steril.* 2000;74:412–413.

12 Wildemeersch D, Schacht E, Wildemeersch P. Treatment of primary and secondary dysmenorrhea with a novel "frameless" intrauterine levonorgestrel-releasing drug delivery system: a pilot study. *Eur J Contracept Reprod Health Care.* 2001;6:192–198.

13 Longstreth G, Preskill D, Youkeles L. Irritable bowel syndrome in women having diagnostic laparoscopy or hysterectomy. Relation to gynecologic features and outcome. *Dig Dis Sci.* 1990;35(10): 1285–1290.

14 Chey W. Tegaserod and other serotonergic agents: what is the evidence? *Rev Gastroenterol Disord.* 2003;3(Suppl. 2):S35–S40.

15 Mertz HR. Irritable bowel syndrome. *N Engl J Med.* 2003;349(22): 2136–2146.

16 Shaath N, Whorwell P. 5-HT and the treatment of irritable bowel syndrome: a clinical perspective. *Drugs Today.* 2001;37(7):437–440.

17 Rovner E, Propert KJ, Brensinger C, et al. Treatments used in women with interstitial cystitis: the interstitial cystitis data base (ICDB) study experience. The Interstitial Cystitis Data Base Study Group. Urology. 2000;56:940–945.

18 Sant G, Propert KJ, Hanno PM, et al. A pilot clinical trial of oral pentosan polysulfate and oral hydroxyzine in patients with interstitial cystitis. *J Urol.* 2003;170(3):810–815.

19 Sasaki K, Smith CP, Chuang YC, et al. Oral gabapentin (neurontin) treatment of refractory genitourinary tract pain. *Tech Urol.* 2001;7(1): 47–49.

20 Clauw D, Chrousos GP. Chronic pain and fatigue syndromes: overlapping clinical and neuroendocrine features and potential pathogenic mechanisms. *Neuroimmunomodulation.* 1997;4:134–153.

21 Wolfe F, Smythe H, Yunus M, et al. The American College of Rheumatology 1990 Criteria for the Classification of Fibromyalgia. Report of the Multicenter Criteria Committee. *Arthritis Rheum.* 1990;33: 160–172.

22 Palter SF, Olive DL. Office microlaparoscopy under local anesthesia for chronic pelvic pain. *J Am Assoc Gynecol Laparosc.* 1996;3: 345–364.

23 Bradesi S, Eutamene H, Garcia-Villar R, et al. Stress-induced visceral hypersensitivity in female rats is estrogen-dependent and involves tachykinin NK 1 receptors. *Pain.* 2003;102(3):227–234.

24 Igarashi M, Iizuka M, Abe Y, et al. Novel vaginal danazol ring therapy for pelvic endometriosis, in particular deeply infiltrating endometriosis. *Hum Reprod.* 1998;13(7):152–156.

25 Taguchi M, Kubota T, Aso T. Direct effect of danazol on the DNA synthesis and ultrastructure of human cultured endometrial stromal cells. *Gynecol Obstet Invest.* 1995;39(3):192–196.

26 Engel CC Jr, Walker EA, Engel AL, et al. A randomized, double-blind crossover trial of sertraline in women with chronic pelvic pain. *J Psychom Res.* 1998;44:203–207.

12 Management of Cystic Ovarian Tumors in the Perimenopausal Woman

Fred R. Ueland
Paul D. DePriest
John R. van Nagell, Jr.

Introduction

KEY POINT

Three to five percent of asymptomatic perimenopausal women will have ovarian cysts on annual ultrasound screening.

With the increased use of transvaginal sonography (TVS) as part of an annual gynecologic examination, more perimenopausal women are being diagnosed with cystic ovarian tumors. In fact, 3–5% of asymptomatic perimenopausal women actually have ovarian cysts when screened annually by TVS.[1] Since the risk of malignancy in ovarian tumors increases significantly in women over the age of 50, it is important to develop evaluation and treatment algorithms for perimenopausal women with cystic ovarian neoplasms. Such algorithms should allow for prompt operative intervention in women with ovarian tumors at significant risk for malignancy while deferring surgery and providing periodic follow-up for lesions at minimal risk for neoplasia.

Evaluation

KEY POINT

A family history of ovarian or breast cancer in a first-degree relative will increase the lifetime risk of ovarian cancer from 1.2% to 5%.

Any patient referred for evaluation of suspected ovarian tumor should have a thorough history and physical examination, including a careful family history. A family history of ovarian cancer or breast cancer in a first-degree relative increases the lifetime risk of ovarian cancer from approximately 1.2% to 5%, and the presence of ovarian cancer in more than one primary or secondary relative further increases this lifetime risk to 7%. The patient should also be questioned concerning any change in bowel habits which might signify an occult colon or gastrointestinal cancer with spread to the ovary. Physical examination should include a careful pelvic examination to document the size and location of the ovarian tumor as well as a rectal examination with Hemoccult testing of the stool.

KEY POINT

Transvaginal ultrasound usually provides the most accurate imaging technique to assess ovarian volume and morphology.

The first step in the evaluation of a cystic ovarian tumor detected on pelvic examination is transvaginal (TVS) or transabdominal sonography (TAS). Since the distance between the vaginal transducer and the ovary is short, TVS usually provides the most accurate definition of ovarian tumor volume and morphology. TAS may be required to visualize extremely large ovarian tumors, and should also be considered if either ovary is not visualized by TVS. Once an accurate image of the tumor has been generated, every effort should be made to assess its risk of malignancy. Several methods are now available which help predict risk of malignancy in sonographically-confirmed cystic ovarian tumors. These include tumor morphology indexing, color Doppler analysis of ovarian tumor blood flow, serum marker analysis, and serum proteomic patterns.

Ovarian Morphologic Index

Although a number of investigators have proposed scoring systems relating tumor morphology to risk of malignancy, we prefer the morphologic index (MI) reported initially by DePriest and coworkers[2,3] and modified recently by Ueland and colleagues.[4] These investigators formulated an index related to tumor volume and morphologic complexity, since both of these variables are associated with risk of malignancy. Ovarian volume was calculated from sonographic measurements using the prolate ellipsoid formula (length × width × height × 0.523). Tumors were given a score of 0–5 in the categories of volume (cm^3) and structure, with total points varying between 0 and 10 (Table 12-1). Increasing tumor

Table 12-1. SONOGRAPHIC MORPHOLOGY INDEX FOR OVARIAN TUMORS

CATEGORY	0	1	2	3	4	5
Volume* (cm^3)	<10	10–50	>50–100	>100–200	>200–500	>500
Structure	Smooth wall, sonolucent	Smooth wall, diffuse echogenicity	Wall thickening, <3 mm fine septa	Papillary projection ≥3 mm	Complex, predominantly solid	Complex solid and cystic areas with extratumora fluid

*Calculated using prolate ellipsoid formula (L × H × W × 0.523).

morphologic complexity was defined by the presence of papillary projections on the cyst wall, solid areas within the cyst, and documentation of extratumoral free fluid (Fig. 12-1). Four hundred and forty-two tumors were evaluated using this morphology index. There was minimal interobserver variation in the interpretation of tumor volume and morphology, with 437 of 442 cases (98%) receiving the identical score from separate investigators. Risk of

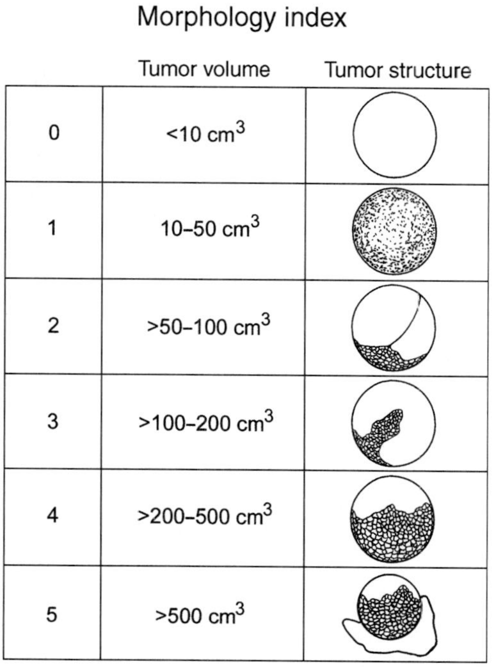

Figure 12-1: Morphology index relating tumor volume and structure to risk of malignancy.

Morphology index

	Tumor volume	Tumor structure
0	<10 cm^3	
1	10–50 cm^3	
2	>50–100 cm^3	
3	>100–200 cm^3	
4	>200–500 cm^3	
5	>500 cm^3	

malignancy in an individual tumor was related directly to the MI score. There was only one malignancy in 315 ovarian tumors (0.3%) with a MI <5 (Fig. 12-2). In contrast, there were 52 malignancies in 127 ovarian tumors (41%) with a MI ≥5 ($P < 0.01$) (Fig. 12-3). These findings are consistent with the observations of Bailey and coworkers,[1] who noted no malignancies in 45 unilocular cystic ovarian tumors <5 cm in diameter. In a later investigation,

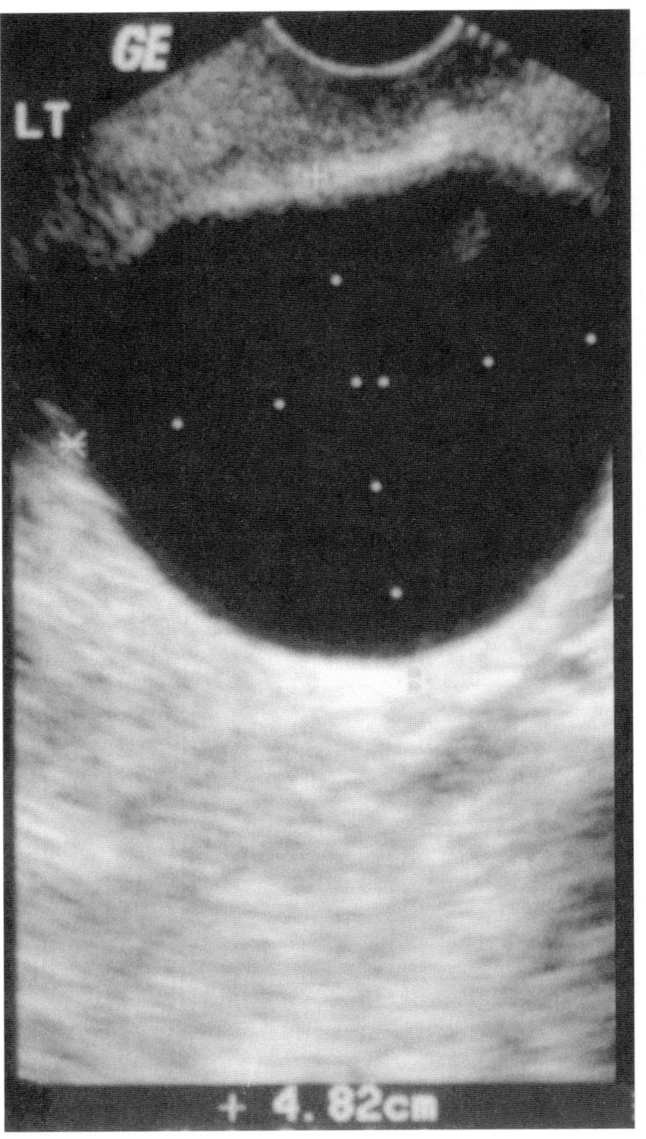

Figure 12-2: Unilocular cystic tumors in perimenopausal woman (morphology index = 1). Risk of malignancy essentially 0.

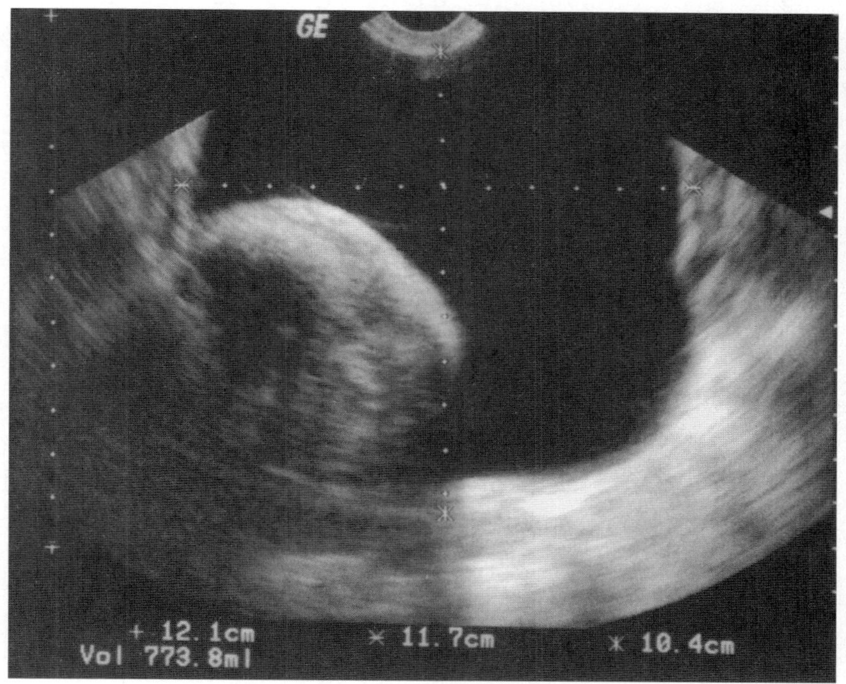

Figure 12-3: Complex ovarian tumor in perimenopausal woman (morphology index = 8). Risk of malignancy ≥75%.

KEY POINT

Small unilocular ovarian cysts (<5 cm) can be safely monitored without operative intervention.

Modesitt and colleagues[5] followed over 3000 unilocular ovarian cysts <10 cm in diameter with periodic ultrasound examinations at 4–6-month intervals, for an average of 6 years. Over two-thirds of these tumors resolved spontaneously, and there were no cases of ovarian cancer reported during the follow-up period. These authors concluded that small unilocular ovarian tumors could be safely followed without operative intervention even in postmenopausal women. Morphology indexing is a reliable and inexpensive method of assessing risk of malignancy in cystic ovarian tumors, and is now being used by an increasing number of physicians in their clinical practice.

Ovarian Blood Flow

The use of color Doppler evaluation of ovarian blood flow as a means to differentiate benign from malignant ovarian tumors is based on the observed difference in resistance to flow between vessels supplying normal ovarian tissue and those supplying ovarian malignancies. The vessels associated with neovascularization induced by tumor angiogenesis[6] often have little smooth muscle within their walls.[7] Consequently, resistance to blood flow in these vessels

KEY POINT

Blood vessels that supply malignant ovarian tumors have a lower resistance to blood flow.

is significantly lower than that found in normal vasculature. Vascular flow is quantitated by measuring the pulsatility index (PI), which is defined as the difference between peak-systolic and end-diastolic flow velocity divided by the mean flow velocity, and the resistive index (RI) defined as the difference between the peak-systolic and end-diastolic flow velocity divided by the peak systolic velocity. Early studies by Weiner and colleagues[8] indicated that vessels supplying malignant ovarian tumors had a PI ≤ 1.0 in over 95% of cases. Since that time, numerous investigations[9–11] have confirmed that the blood vessels supplying malignant ovarian tumors have a lower impedance to flow (PI < 1.0 and RI < 0.4) than those associated with benign ovarian tumors. However, there is an overlap in the PI and RI ranges between benign and malignant ovarian tumors such that no one cut-off value has both a high sensitivity and a high specificity for malignancy.[12,13] Therefore, Doppler flow studies can provide clinically useful data concerning risk of malignancy in ovarian tumors, but they cannot accurately identify ovarian cancer on an individual basis.

Serum Markers

KEY POINT

In Stage 1 ovarian cancers, less than 50% are associated with CA-125 elevations.

Serum marker values have also been evaluated as a means to predict risk of malignancy in sonographically-confirmed cystic ovarian tumors. Gaducci and coworkers[14] evaluated a panel of serum markers in 334 women undergoing exploratory laparotomy for a pelvic mass. Serum Ca-125 was the most useful marker in discriminating malignant from benign ovarian tumors. Using a serum Ca-125 level of 35 U/mL as indicative of malignancy, the sensitivity and specificity of this marker were 0.82 and 0.67, respectively. Unfortunately, the frequency of serum Ca-125 elevation in clinically diagnosed Stage I ovarian cancers is no higher than 50%, and is even lower in small ovarian malignancies detected sonographically.[15] In a more recent study, Skates and colleagues[16] reported that Ca-125 levels increase over time in women with ovarian cancer, as opposed to remaining stable or decreasing in women with benign ovarian lesions. They proposed that women with an elevated serum Ca-125 have a repeat marker determination over a short period of time in order to assess the rate of increase of serum Ca-125. This approach involving serial marker determinations increased the positive predictive value (PPV) of serum Ca-125 to 16%. In a related study, Wilder and coworkers[17] reported that progressively rising serum Ca-125 values even within the normal range (<35 U/mL) were universally predictive of recurrent disease in patients previously treated for ovarian cancer. The observation of rising serum Ca-125 values preceded clinical or radiographic evidence of recurrence by an average of 5 months. These two studies indicate that a pattern of progressively rising serum Ca-125 more accurately predicts the presence of ovarian malignancy than one elevated serum marker value.

PROTEOMICS

KEY POINT

Pilot studies suggest that ovarian cancers are associated with a specific proteomic pattern.

A relatively new research area which is being utilized in the identification of ovarian cancer is proteomics or the study of the protein environment of neoplastic cells. Two new technologies are being used to facilitate the study of tumor-specific proteins: matrix-assisted desorption/ionization time-of-flight mass spectrometry, and surface enhanced laser desorption and ionization (SELDI). Matrix-assisted desorption/ionization is a process by which a coprecipitate of an ultraviolet light absorption matrix and a specific protein is produced. The coprecipitate is then ionized using a laser, and the ionized particles are accelerated in an electric field. Ionized proteins are then separated according to their mass.[18] SELDI involves the capture and isolation of proteins on a resin chip based on charge.[18] These proteins are then analyzed using mass spectroscopy. Using this technology, Petricoin and colleagues[19] analyzed proteins from the sera of 50 ovarian cancer patients and 66 control patients. A specific proteomic pattern correctly identified all ovarian cancer cases including 18 patients with Stage I disease. Another approach has been to combine plasma proteomic profiles with serum Ca-125 as a means to identify ovarian cancer. Rai and colleagues[20] evaluated proteomics and serum Ca-125 from 43 ovarian cancer patients and 38 control patients without neoplastic disease. Two protein biomarkers were identified and compared to serum Ca-125. Individually, these markers did not perform better than Ca-125. However, their discriminatory power was complementary to serum Ca-125 and, when combined with serum Ca-125, improved the sensitivity of ovarian cancer detection from 81% to 94%. Clearly, proteomic technology offers hope for the identification of signature protein patterns or fingerprints which can discriminate malignant from benign ovarian tumors.

The algorithm used in the evaluation of patients with clinically detected ovarian tumors at the University of Kentucky Medical Center is illustrated in Fig. 12-4. First, every ovarian tumor is

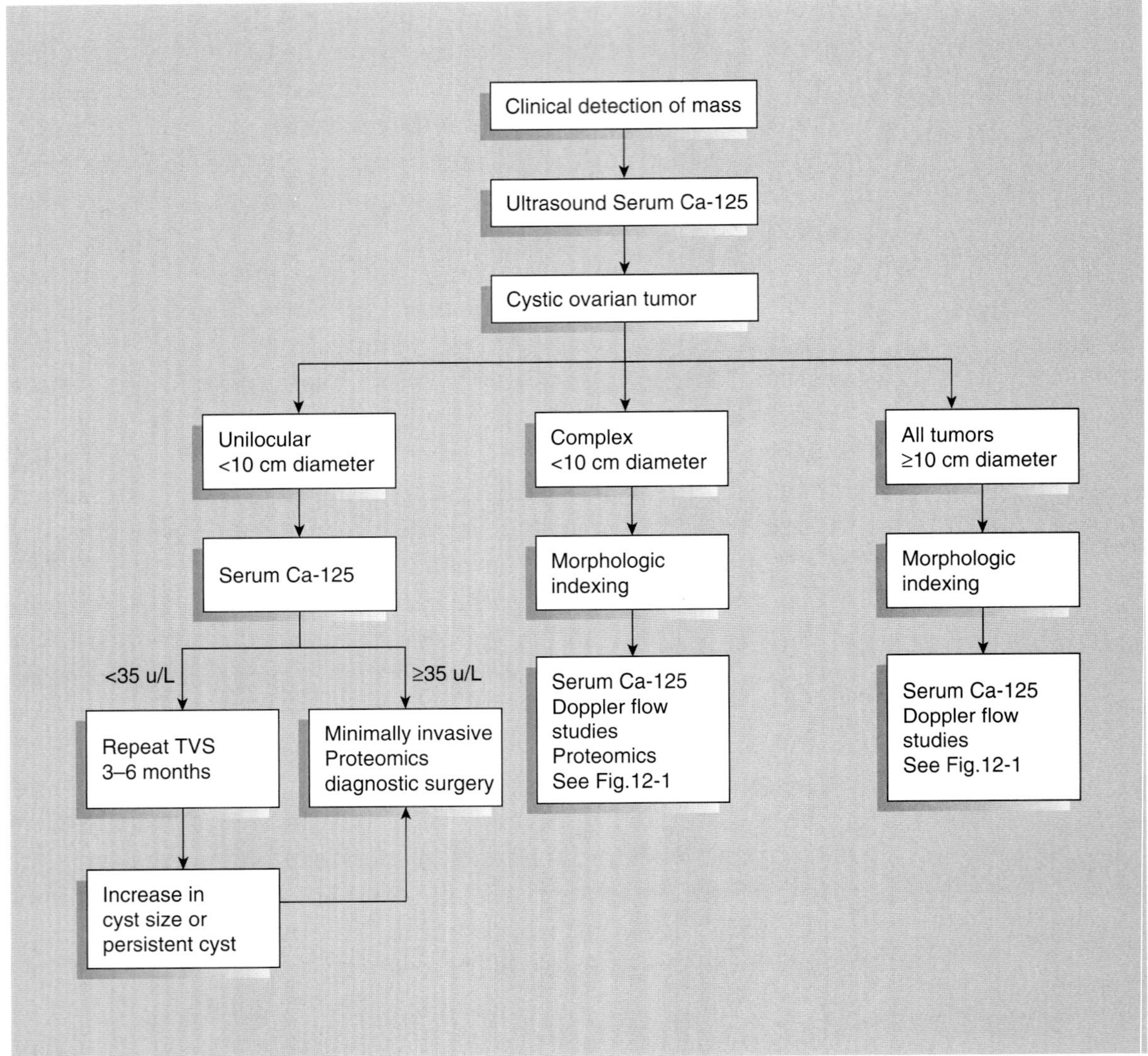

Figure 12-4: Evaluation algorithm for cystic ovarian tumors in perimenopausal women.

imaged sonographically to define its size and morphologic structure. In addition, a serum Ca-125 is obtained. The risk of ovarian malignancy in a patient with a unilocular ovarian tumor ≤10 cm diameter and a normal serum Ca-125 is extremely small. Therefore, no additional tests are performed immediately. Rather, a repeat ultrasound examination and serum Ca-125 is scheduled in 3–6 months. If a unilocular cyst persists or increases in size, minimally invasive diagnostic surgery may be performed. This involves the transvaginal insertion of a 2 mm endoscope with

KEY POINT

The risk of an ovarian malignancy, where there is a unilocular ovarian cyst of <10 cm diameter and a normal serum CA-125, is extremely small.

visualization of the ovarian tumor. A biopsy of the cyst wall is taken and the cyst fluid is aspirated. This fluid is analyzed for cytology, serum Ca-125, and protein markers. The risk of neoplasia in morphologically complex ovarian tumors is much greater than that in purely cystic tumors, and additional tests are utilized to help define this risk even in relatively small lesions. These include morphologic indexing, serum Ca-125, Doppler flow analysis of tumoral blood flow, and proteomics. The risk of malignancy in a patient with an ovarian tumor having a MI ≥ 5, a PI < 1.0, and a serum Ca-125 ≥ 60 U/mL is at least 30%.[4] Therefore, a patient with these findings may be referred to gynecologic oncologist for tumor excision, staging, and treatment.

Treatment

The treatment of a cystic ovarian tumor in a perimenopausal woman is based on its size and morphologic complexity (Fig. 12-5). As has been mentioned, the risk of malignancy in a unilocular cystic ovarian tumor ≤10 cm in a patient with a normal serum Ca-125 is so low that these tumors may be followed every 3–6 months by repeat TVS rather than removed surgically. Should tumor growth or a rise in serum Ca-125 be documented at the time of repeat sonography, operative intervention is indicated. Over two-thirds of unilocular cystic tumors will resolve spontaneously, and the majority will do so within 3 months. In selected patients, unilocular cysts may be aspirated under endoscopic guidance using minimally invasive technology.

KEY POINT

Two-thirds of unilocular cysts will resolve spontaneously usually within 3 months.

However, complex ovarian tumors <10 cm diameter are excised laparoscopically, placed in an endocatch bag, and removed after aspiration through a small subumbilical incision (Fig. 12-6). A frozen section histologic examination is then performed with the patient still anesthetized. If the tumor is benign, no further surgery is performed and the patient is discharged, usually on the evening of surgery. If the tumor is malignant, a full staging laparotomy is performed through a midline vertical incision. This may include a total abdominal hysterectomy, omentectomy, tumor debulking, and pelvic/para-aortic lymph node biopsies. In patients with larger tumors (≥10 cm diameter), an exploratory laparotomy with tumor removal and frozen section histologic evaluation is performed. The extent of surgery is determined by the cell type and stage of the lesion, and clinical characteristics of each patient.

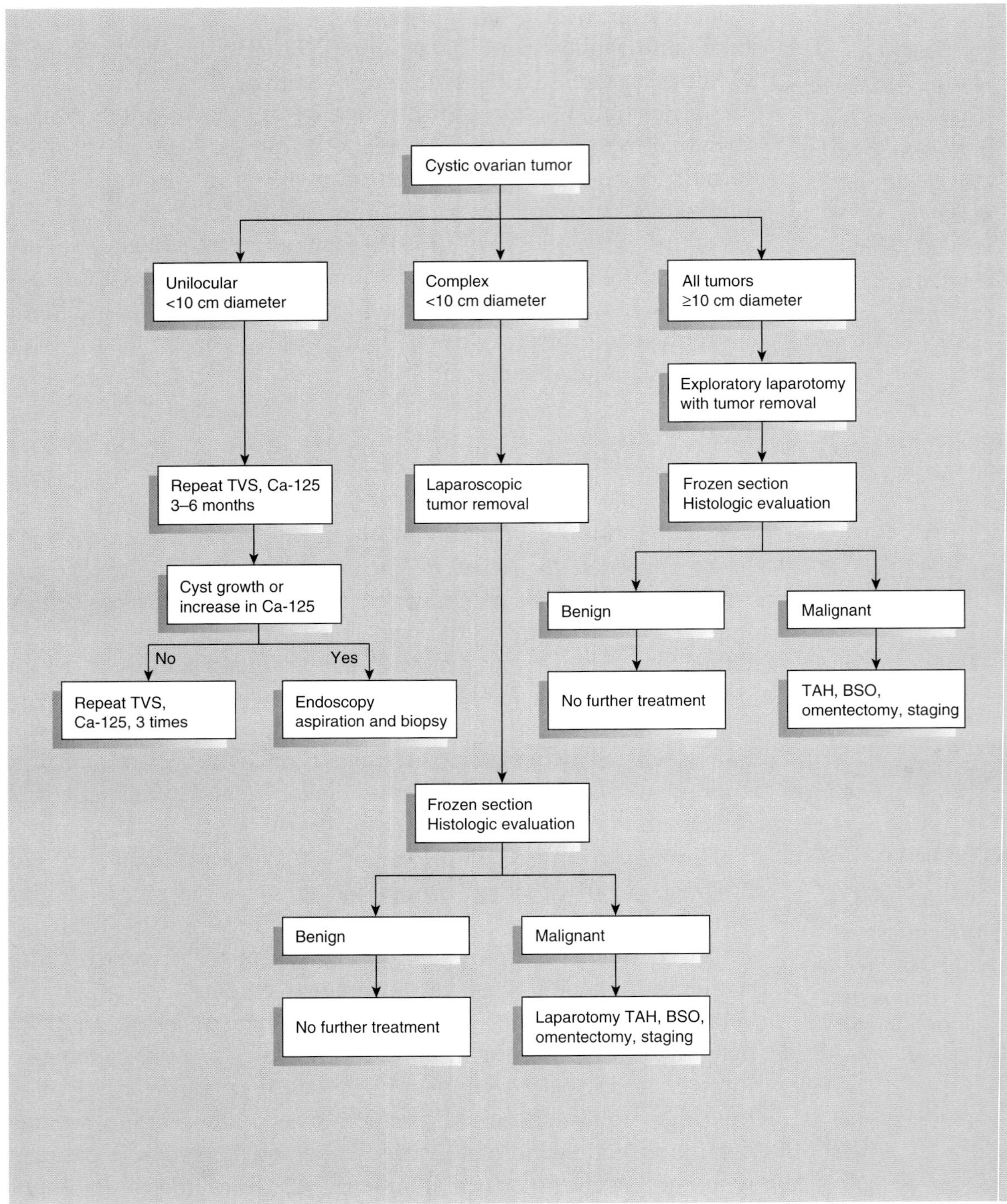

Figure 12-5: Treatment algorithm for cystic ovarian tumors in perimenopausal women.

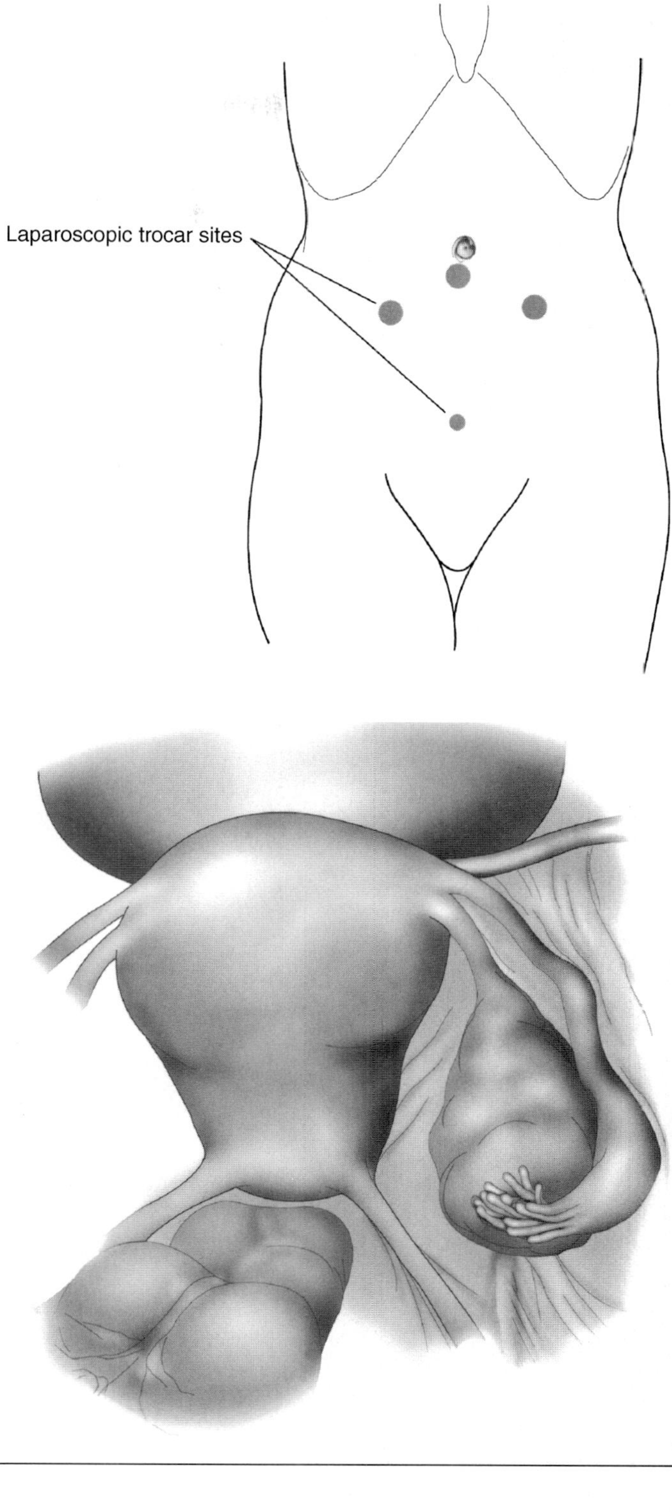

Figure 12-6: Laparoscopic tumor removal. This surgical approach is indicated in suspicious ovarian tumors <10 cm diameter.

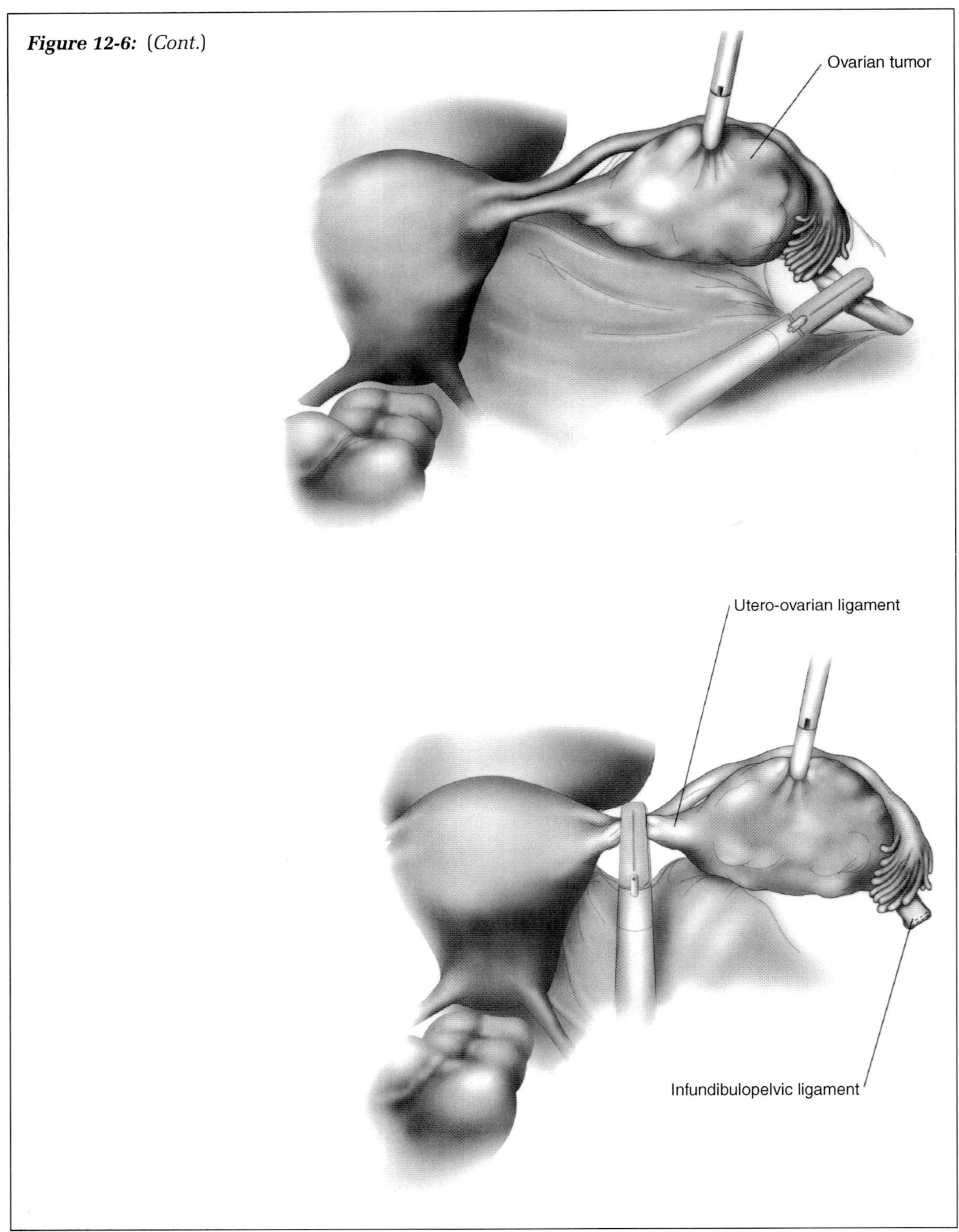

Figure 12-6: (*Cont.*)

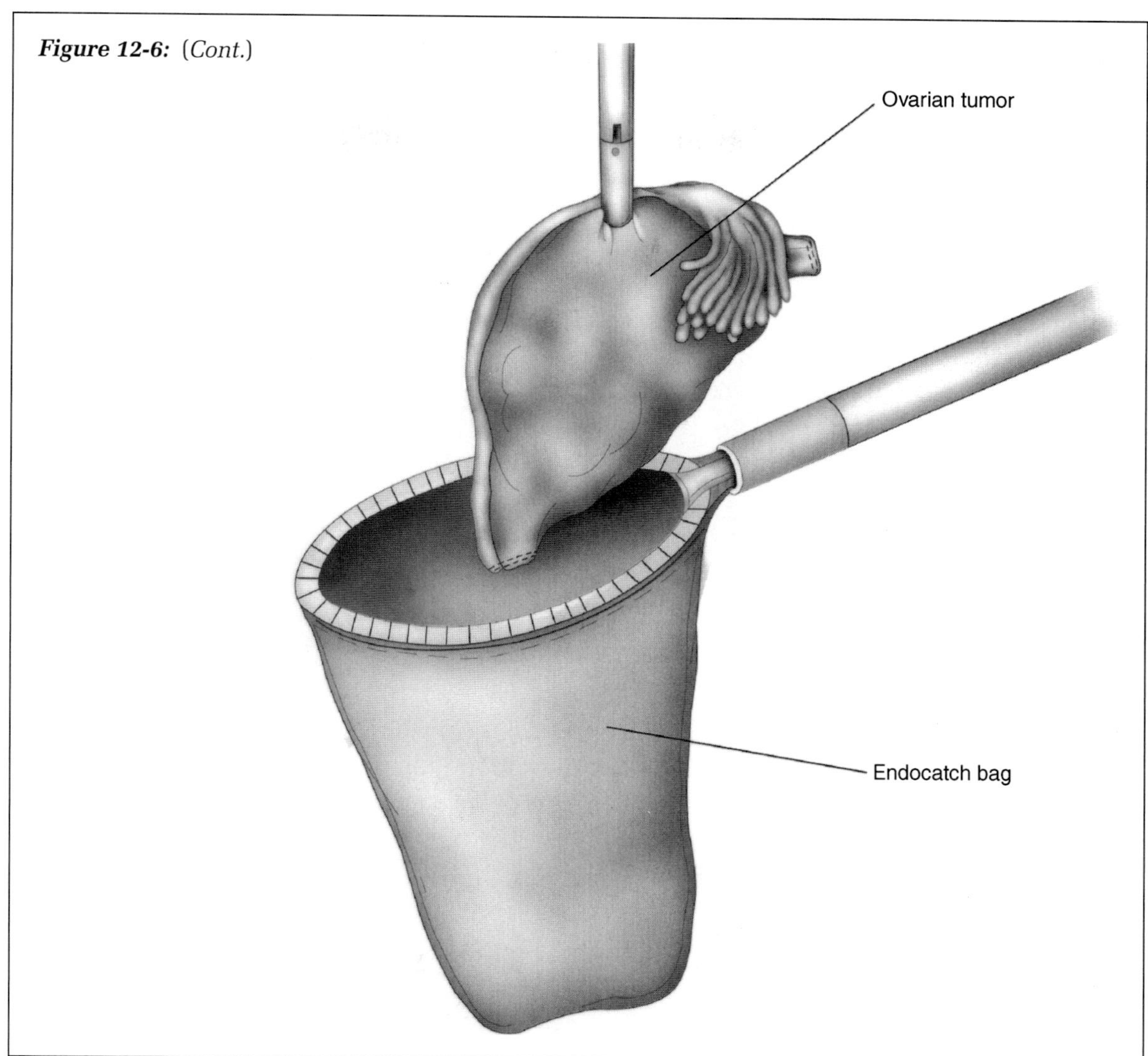

Figure 12-6: (*Cont.*)

Ovarian Cancer Screening

KEY POINT

Early stage ovarian cancer produces few specific symptoms.

Since early stage ovarian cancer produces few specific symptoms, most women continue to present with advanced stage disease. Radical surgery followed by combination of platinum-based chemotherapy has resulted in prolonged remission for selected patients. Nevertheless, resistance to chemotherapy often develops, resulting in tumor recurrence and limited survival. Since the best chance of cure occurs in women with cancer localized to the

Figure 12-6: (Cont.)

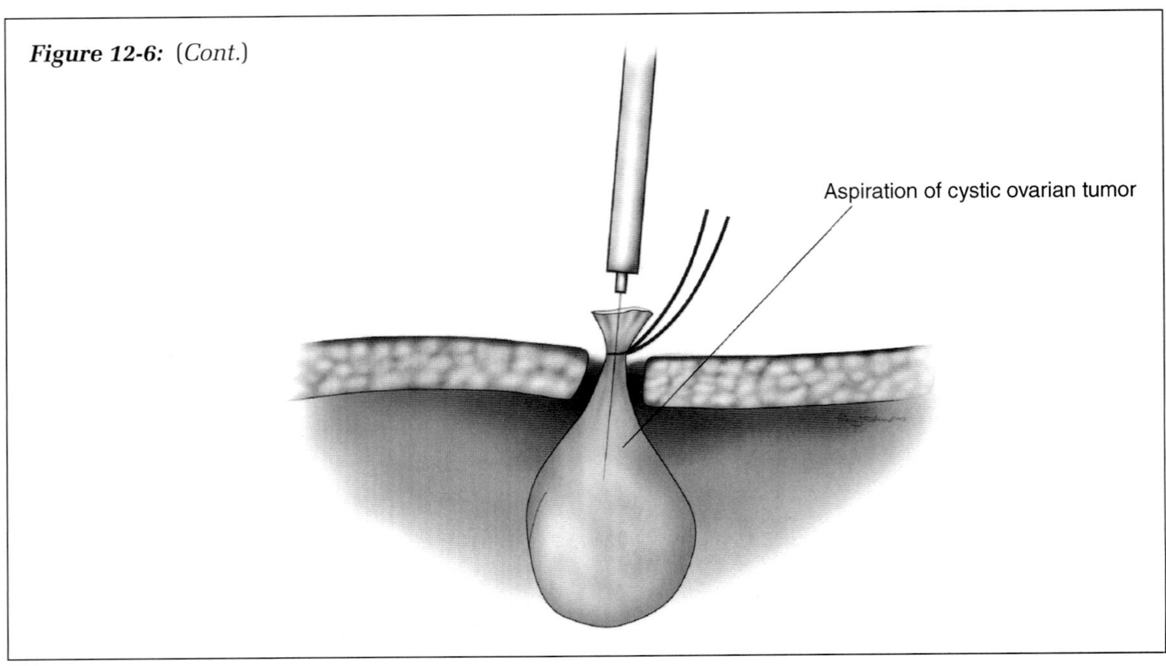

ovary, efforts at early detection have focused on screening asymptomatic women at high risk for developing the disease.

Rationale

In order to be amenable to screening, a disease should have the following characteristics.[21] First, it should be a major cause of mortality in the population. Second, it should be relatively curable at an early stage such that early detection would result in a survival benefit to those screened. Finally, the disease should be sufficiently prevalent in the population so that effective screening would identify a significant number of cases. Ovarian cancer meets these criteria in that it is the fifth leading cause of cancer death in American women. Also, it is highly curable if detected when cancer is confined to the ovary. The present 5-year survival of patients with Stage I ovarian cancer is over 90% in many institutions, which is significantly higher than that of symptomatic patients who present with clinical evidence of advanced ovarian cancer. Although ovarian cancer is not prevalent in the general population, it occurs more frequently in women over the age of 50 (50 cases/100,000 population), and in women with a family history of ovarian cancer (5% lifetime risk of the disease in patients with one primary degree relative with ovarian cancer). Therefore, these high-risk populations are most suitable for screening.

KEY POINT

Serum marker screening was not effective in reducing mortality rate from ovarian cancer.

A screening test must meet certain specific criteria to be effective. It should be time- and cost-efficient, easy to perform, and well-accepted by patients. Most important, it should be sensitive, specific, have a high PPV, and a high negative predictive value (NPV).[21] The statistical definitions used in ovarian cancer screening are presented in Table 12-2. An effective screening test will (1) lower stage at detection and (2) decrease case-specific mortality, and reduce site-specific mortality in the screened population.[22]

Basically, there have been two approaches in ovarian cancer screening. The first is to screen initially with a serum marker or combination of markers. Sonography is then performed to document the presence of an ovarian tumor in women with elevated serum marker levels. Using this methodology, Einhorn and coworkers[23] performed serum Ca-125 screening in 5550 apparently healthy Swedish women. Serum Ca-125 was elevated (>35 U/mL) in 175 of these women (3.1%), and 6 had ovarian cancer. Unfortunately, 4 of the 6 women with ovarian cancer had advanced stage disease at the time of detection. An additional 6 women with normal serum Ca-125 levels also were found to have ovarian cancer. In a larger controlled trial, Jacobs and colleagues[24] randomized 22,000 women to a screening group or a control group. Women in the screening group received three annual serum Ca-125 determinations. Pelvic sonography was performed if a patient's serum Ca-125 was >30 U/mL. Women with an elevated serum Ca-125 and an ovarian volume ≥8.8 cm^3 were referred for surgical evaluation.

Table 12-2. **STATISTICAL DEFINITIONS IN OVARIAN CANCER SCREENING**

Term	*Screen*	*Findings*
True positive (TP)	Positive	Histology confirms primary ovarian cancer
False positive (FP)	Positive	Benign ovarian histology
True negative (TN)	Negative	No evidence of disease 12 months following negative screen
False negative (FN)	Negative	Ovarian cancer diagnosed within 12 months of negative screen

NOTE: Sensitivity = TP/TP + FN; specificity = TN/TN + FP; positive predictive value = TP/TP + FP; negative predictive value = TN/TN + FN.

Elevated serum Ca-125 levels were observed in 468 women (4.3%) in the screened group, and 29 had an ovarian tumor confirmed on ultrasound. All 29 patients underwent surgery, and six had epithelial ovarian cancer (23 false positives). During a follow-up period of 7 years, 10 additional women in the screened group developed ovarian cancer, as compared to 20 new cancers diagnosed in the control group. The median survival of women whose cancers were detected in the screened group was longer than that of women who developed ovarian cancer in the control group (73 months vs. 41 months). However, there was no statistical difference in the mortality rate between the two groups.

KEY POINT

In this trial, survival of ovarian cancer patients for those screened with transvaginal ultrasound was 95% at 2 years and 88% at 5 years.

The second approach to ovarian cancer screening is to perform TVS as the initial screening test, followed by serum Ca-125, morphology indexing, and Doppler flow studies in women with persistent ovarian tumors confirmed sonographically. Using this methodology, Van Nagell and colleagues[15] performed annual TVS screening in 14,469 asymptomatic postmenopausal women (Fig. 12-7). All women with an abnormal TVS had a repeat sonogram in 4–6 weeks. Patients with a persisting abnormal second screen had a serum Ca-125, morphology indexing, Doppler flow sonography, and surgical excision of the tumor was recommended. Surgery was recommended in all patients with complex ovarian tumors on both screens. Exploratory laparoscopy or laparotomy was performed on 180 women (0.1%) with sonographically-confirmed ovarian tumors. Seventeen ovarian cancers were detected: 11 Stage I, 3 Stage II, and 3 Stage III. All patients with Stages I and II ovarian cancer were alive without evidence of recurrence: 1.9 years – 9.8 years (median 4.5 years) after diagnosis. Two of the three patients with Stage III ovarian cancer died of disease—one at 4.3 years and one at 7.7 years after detection. The survival of ovarian cancer patients in the annually screened population was 95% at 2 years and 88% at 5 years. This screening format decreased stage at detection and significantly increased ovarian cancer survival in women receiving annual screening.

At present, there are many questions remaining to be answered about ovarian cancer screening. Although TVS is highly sensitive in detecting ovarian tumors, it does not reliably differentiate benign from malignant lesions, and its PPV is low (~10%). On the other

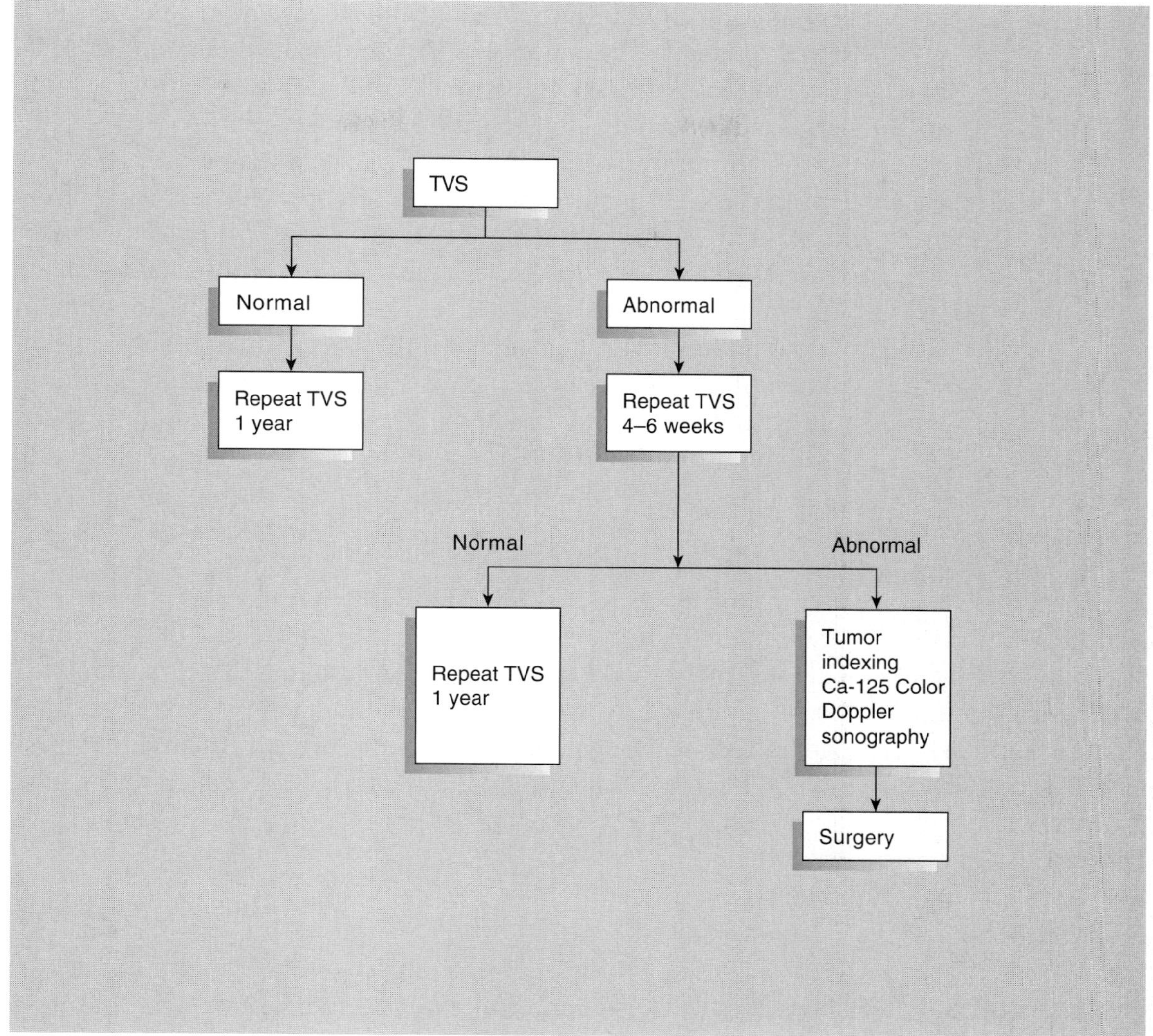

Figure 12-7: Ovarian cancer screening algorithm.

hand, serum marker screening, specifically with Ca-125, does not reliably detect Stage I ovarian cancers, and many early cancers are missed. We favor TVS as the initial screening test with the use of adjuvant morphology indexing, serum marker patterns, and proteomics to increase its PPV. Another issue which has not been resolved is the optimal screening interval. Annual screening has been recommended by convention, but more frequent screening in selected patients with increased risk factors for ovarian cancer may be indicated. Likewise, it may be beneficial to alternate TVS and serum marker screening every 6 months in certain populations. The answers to these questions will be answered by ongoing screening trials both in the United States and Europe.

Despite its imperfections, ovarian cancer screening is saving lives through early detection, and should be continued in carefully monitored research settings. If the percent of ovarian cancer patients detected with Stage I disease were increased from its present level of 25% to 75% through early detection, the number of deaths from ovarian cancer would be cut in half using present treatment methods. These early detection goals should be attainable with the discovery of more specific protein markers and the refinement of present screening protocols.

What's the Evidence?

Management of Ovarian Cysts in the Perimenopausal Patient Should be Based on Transvaginal Ultrasound Findings and Ca-125 Levels

Asymptomatic ovarian cysts are found in 3–5% of perimenopausal women.[1] If the cyst is unilocular and less than 5 cm in diameter, these can be safely monitored without operative intervention.[5] The risk of ovarian cancer in a patient with a unilocular cyst less than 10 cm and a serum Ca-125 less than 35 U/mL is very small.

Ovarian Blood Flow is a Useful Adjunct in Discriminating Benign versus Malignant Ovarian Tumors

The use of power Doppler ultrasound to evaluate ovarian blood flow is based on the rationale that blood vessels supplying the tumor have very little smooth muscle within the arterial walls.[7] Hence, the resistance to blood flow is significantly lower than in normal vasculature. This difference in blood flow characteristics is usually manifested by a low PI <1.0 and a low resistance index of <0.4.[8]

A Single Ca-125 Level is Inadequate as a Screening Tool for Ovarian Cancer

Although Ca-125 antigen levels can detect occult ovarian malignancies, the frequency of this finding in Stage 1 ovarian cancer is no greater than 50%.[15] Rising serum levels of Ca-125 more accurately predicts presence of ovarian cancer.[17]

Discussion of Cases

CASE 1

You are evaluating an asymptomatic perimenopausal patient who, on clinical examination, has a right adnexal mass approximately 5 cm in diameter.

What test, if any, would you recommend at this point?

- **A transvaginal sonogram reveals a unilocular right ovarian cystic tumor 5.0 cm × 4.6 cm × 5.2 cm (volume 62.5 cm^3).**
- **A serum Ca-125 is 10 U/mL.**

What is your initial management?

- **Operative intervention is not indicated at the present time. Rather, she should be scheduled for a repeat sonogram and serum Ca-125 in 3–6 months. Over two-thirds of unilocular cystic ovarian tumors will resolve spontaneously, and the majority will do so within 3 months.**
- **A repeat sonogram reveals that the unilocular right ovarian cystic tumor has decreased in size to 2.0 cm × 3.0 cm × 2.0 cm (volume 6.3 cm^3).**
- **A repeat serum Ca-125 is again 10 U/mL.**

What are your instructions to this patient concerning her follow-up?

- **This patient should be followed up at 6-month intervals with repeat sonography and serum Ca-125 testing until this cystic ovarian tumor has resolved spontaneously. Should the tumor develop solid components or increase in volume, operative removal should be considered. Likewise, a progressive rise in serum Ca-125 should mandate operative removal of this tumor.**

CASE 2

You are evaluating an asymptomatic perimenopausal patient with a solid ovarian tumor which on pelvic examination is approximately 7 cm in diameter. A transvaginal sonogram reveals a 6.5 cm × 7.0 cm × 7.5 cm (volume 178 cm^3) complex right ovarian tumor with solid and cystic components.

What additional studies should be performed to help assess the risk of malignancy in this tumor?

- **Morphology indexing reveals a MI of 6.**
- **Color Doppler evaluation of ovarian tumoral blood flow indicates a PI of 0.8 and a RI of 0.3.**
- **A serum Ca-125 is 50 U/mL.**

Is the risk of malignancy in this tumor nonexistent, or moderate?

Since the morphology index is >5, and the PI is <1.0, and serum Ca-125 is >35 U/mL, there is a moderate risk that this tumor is malignant.

What is the appropriate surgical approach in this patient?

- **Exploratory laparoscopy or laparotomy with ovarian tumor removal and frozen section histologic evaluation.**

If this tumor is an epithelial ovarian malignancy, is additional surgery indicated?

- **Any perimenopausal patient with an epithelial ovarian cancer should have complete surgical staging, including total abdominal hysterectomy, bilateral salpingo-oophorectomy, omentectomy, and appendectomy. Every effort should be made to remove all visible or palpable tumor prior to initiation of chemotherapy.**

CASE 3

A 51-year-old perimenopausal patient whose mother had ovarian cancer would like to have ovarian cancer screening.

Does this patient qualify as being in a high-risk group that should benefit from screening?

- **Since (1) the patient's mother had ovarian cancer, and (2) she is over the age of 50, she would be in a high-risk group and eligible for screening in a number of trials.**

Which tests are currently employed in screening algorithms?

- **TVS, serum Ca-125, Doppler flow analysis of tumoral blood flow, morphology indexing, and proteomics.**

In order for an ovarian cancer screening test to be effective, what statistical goals should it meet?

- **An effective ovarian screening test should be sensitive and specific. Also, it should have a high PPV and a high NPV.**

An effective ovarian screening test should:

- **decrease stage of ovarian cancer at detection.**
- **decrease case-specific mortality in women whose ovarian cancer is detected by screening.**
- **decrease site-specific ovarian cancer mortality in the screened population.**

References

1 Bailey CL, Ueland FR, Land GL, et al. Malignant potential of small cystic ovarian tumors in postmenopausal women. *Gynecol Oncol.* 1998;69:3–7.

2 DePriest PD, Shenson D, Fried A, et al. A morphology index based on sonographic findings in ovarian cancer. *Gynecol Oncol.* 1993;51:7–11.

3 DePriest P, Varner E, Powell J, et al. The efficacy of a sonographic morphology index in identifying ovarian cancer: A multi-institutional investigation. *Gynecol Oncol.* 1994;55:174–178.

4 Ueland FR, DePriest PD, Pavlik EJ, et al. Preoperative differentiation of malignant from benign ovarian tumors: the efficacy of morphology indexing and Doppler flow sonography. *Gynecol Oncol.* 2003;91:46–50.

5 Modesitt SC, Pavlik EJ, Ueland FR, et al. Risk of malignancy in unilocular ovarian cystic tumors less than 10 cm in diameter. *Obstet Gynecol.* 2003;102:594–599.

6 Folkman J, Watson K, Ingber D, et al. Induction of angiogenesis during the transition from hyperplasia to neoplasia. *Nature.* 1989;339:58–61.

7 Emoto M, Iwasaki H, Mimura K, et al. Differences in the angiogenesis of benign and malignant ovarian tumors, demonstrated by analyses of color Doppler ultrasound, immunohistochemistry and microvessel density. *Cancer.* 1997;80:899–907.

8 Weiner Z, Thaler I, Beck D, et al. Differentiating malignant from benign ovarian tumors with transvaginal color flow imaging. *Obstet Gynecol.* 1992;79:159–162.

9 Kurjak A, Zanid I, Alfirevic Z. Evaluation of adnexal masses with transvaginal color ultrasound. *J Ultrasound Med.* 1991;10:296–297.

10 Fleischer AC, Rogers WH, Rao BK, et al. Transvaginal color Doppler sonography of ovarian masses with pathological correlation. *Ultrasound Obstet Gynecol.* 1991;1:275–278.

11 Timor-Tritsch LE, Lerner JP, Monteagudo A, et al. Transvaginal ultrasonographic characterization of ovarian masses by means of color-flow-directed Doppler measurements and a morphologic scoring system. *Am J Obstet Gynecol.* 1993;168:909–913.

12 Brown DL, Frates MC, Laing FC, et al. Ovarian masses: can benign and malignant lesions be differentiated with color and pulsed Doppler US. *Radiol.* 1994;190:333–336.

13 Tekay A, Jouppila P. Controversies in assessment of ovarian tumors with transvaginal color Doppler ultrasound. *Acta Obstet Gynecol Scand.* 1996;4:316–329.

14 Gadducci A, Ferdeghini M, Prontera C, et al. The concomitant determination of different tumor markers in patients with epithelial ovarian cancer and benign ovarian masses: relevance for differential diagnosis. *Gynecol Oncol.* 1992;44:147–154.

15 Van Nagell JR, DePriest PD, Reedy MB, et al. The efficacy of transvaginal sonographic screening in asymptomatic women at risk for ovarian cancer. *Gynecol Oncol.* 2000;77:350–356.

16 Skates SJ, Zu FJ, Yu YH, et al. Toward an optimal algorithm for ovarian cancer screening with longitudinal tumor markers. *Cancer.* 1995;76 (Suppl.): 2004–2010.

17 Wilder JL, Pavlik EJ, Straughn JM, et al. Clinical implications of a raising Ca-125 within the normal range in patients with epithelial ovarian cancer. *Gynecol Oncol.* 2003;89:233–235.

18 Bandera CA, Ye B, Mok SC. New technologies for the identification of markers for early detection of ovarian cancer. *Curr Opin Obstet Gynecol.* 2003;15:51–55.

19 Petricoin EF, Ardekani AM, Hitt BA, et al. Use of proteomic patterns in serum to identify ovarian cancer. *Lancet.* 2002;359:572–577.

20 Rai AJ, Zhang Z, Rosenzweig J, et al. Proteomic approaches to tumor marker discovery. Identification of biomarkers for ovarian cancer. *Arch Pathol Lab Med.* 2002;126:1518–1526.

21 Prorok PC. Evaluation of screening program for the early detection of cancer. *Natl Cancer Inst Stat Textbk Monogr.* 1984;51:267–328.

22 Hulka, BS. Cancer screening: degrees of proof and practical application. *Cancer.* 1989;62:1776–1769.

23 Einhorn N, Sjovall K, Knapp RC, et al. Prospective evaluation of serum Ca-125 levels for early detection of ovarian cancer. *Obstet Gynecol.* 1992;80:14–18.

24 Jacobs IJ, Skates S, Davies AP, et al. Risk of diagnosis of ovarian cancer after raised serum Ca-125 concentration: a prospective cohort study. *BMJ.* 1996;313:1355–1358.

13 Breast Pain, Mass, or Discharge

Elizabeth A. Shaughnessy

Introduction

KEY POINT

The three common categories of breast complaints are breast pain, nipple discharge, and breast mass.

Women's breast complaints generally fall into three categories: breast pain, nipple discharge, and breast mass. These complaints are found in the perimenopausal population as well. The majority of complaints are not associated with malignancy, but rather with fibrocystic changes that are found in 50% of all American women according to autopsy studies. Since fibrocystic changes are affected by hormones, the fluctuations in hormone levels during the perimenopause may simply exacerbate a preexisting condition. In general, age and menopausal status have not been reported in the majority of studies addressing these issues; thus, specific changes in the breast associated with perimenopause have not been identified. However, the standard approach to all three of the complaints is as discussed below, and is not influenced by menopausal status. This chapter addresses these management issues given our current level of understanding.

Breast Pain

Breast pain, also called mastalgia or mastodynia, is one of the most frequent breast complaints that a primary care physician encounters.[1] The complaint was frequently dismissed or not addressed by physicians in the past, perhaps because early reports considered it to be psychosomatic.[2,3] Preece and colleagues attempted to address the psychosocial aspects of breast pain in a systematic fashion. Using a questionnaire to assess personality type, no significant differences were identified between women with mastalgia and those undergoing varicose vein surgery. However, they did identify a subgroup of patients with treatment-resistant pain who had personality characteristics similar to psychiatric patients.[4]

Most consider breast pain a disorder that has a hormonal basis.[5] No consistent abnormality of estradiol nor progesterone has been identified. Prolactin levels appear to be normal to slightly elevated in symptomatic women. Following domperidone stimulation to release prolactin, those women with mastodynia produced significantly higher levels of prolactin.[6] Determining the etiology of this prolactin response can be a challenge, as it may reflect increased pituitary response, a preexisting abnormality, a prolonged stress response, or a response from within the breast itself.[7]

KEY POINT

Most women with breast pain consult a breast specialist out of their concern about an underlying breast cancer.

In evaluating breast pain, it is important to identify whether the patient's concern is the pain and its treatment, or whether the concern stems mainly from fear of an underlying breast cancer. Certainly, most of the patients who present with breast pain are concerned that it may reflect more ominous breast pathology. Frequently, those who pursue consultation because of this concern are not interested in the treatment of the pain per se. It is helpful to differentiate cyclic versus noncyclic breast pain, whether noncyclic pain is solely associated with the chest wall or with the breast. A woman who is cycling may not have noted whether the pain seems worse relative to the onset of her menses. If it seems episodic, she may need to track her pain relative to her menstrual bleeding on her calendar. Use of a diary to determine if it is cyclic may be particularly helpful in those women who have undergone a previous hysterectomy.

A focused physical examination incorporates these concerns as well. Following visual inspection, the breast should be palpated, first gently over the entire area of both breasts, then more firmly, probing the site(s) indicated as painful. The texture of the breast may suggest the presence of fibrocystic breast changes or a focal pathology. Nodularity, ranging mild to coarse, may reflect a cystic process that tends to be diffusely painful. However, neither the extent of the nodularity nor the degree of coarseness correlates directly with the degree of pain experienced. Focal sites of tenderness that reproduce the pain are usually associated with either a chest wall etiology or a more focal disease process of the breast,

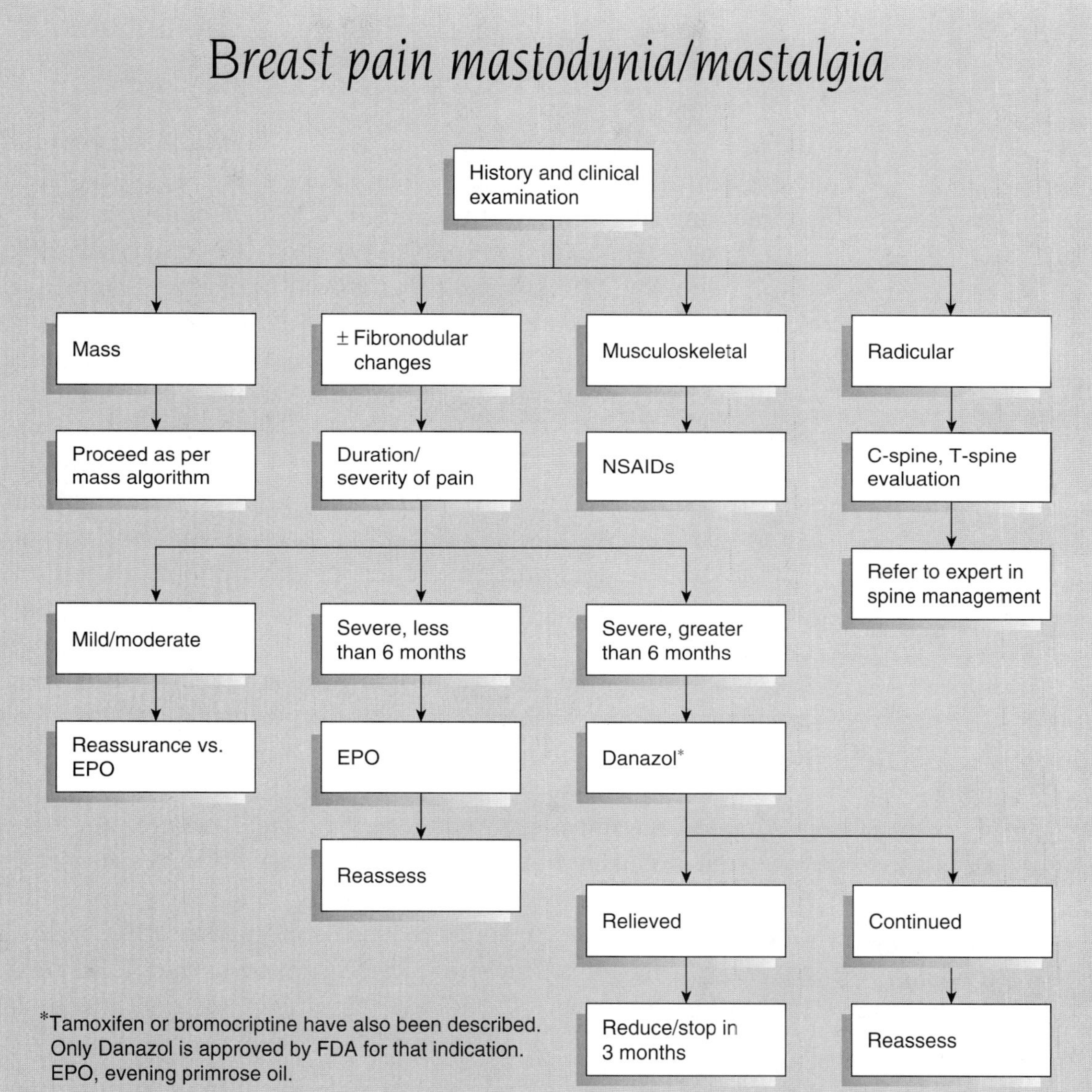

*Tamoxifen or bromocriptine have also been described. Only Danazol is approved by FDA for that indication. EPO, evening primrose oil.

such as a mass or induration. The latter should then be worked up appropriately (see section on Breast Mass).

After a thorough evaluation of the breast tissue, attention is given to the chest wall. This part of the examination can be facilitated by having the woman lie on her side so that the breast falls away from the lateral chest wall. The clinician palpates the underlying ribs and chest wall muscle. Occasionally, pain with a radicular distribution may indicate vertebral pathology. Cervical and thoracic spine films would be the next step in the patient's evaluation.

Mondor's disease is an uncommon cause of pain. It presents with focal and specific physical findings. The etiology of Mondor's disease is a thrombosis of the thoracoepigastric vein. The physical manifestations include a palpable cord that can be appreciated near the midinframammary fold. It may include some skin tethering in a linear fashion lateral to the areola and angling upward. Retraction is seldom present without a palpable cord. In one series of patients presenting with Mondor's disease, no underlying cause could be established in approximately half the patients.[8] Among those determined to have a cause, the most frequently cited associations were physical trauma (including surgery), inflammatory processes, or carcinoma. Mammography should be considered if indicated.

KEY POINT

A mammogram may be helpful in the evaluation of breast pain, but other imaging may be warranted.

Breast imaging is not mandatory in the evaluation of breast pain, but it can be helpful in specific cases. Should the patient have pain associated with a focal finding, a mammogram and/or ultrasound may be appropriate (see section Breast Mass). If the patient is due for a mammogram, it should be included in the evaluation. However, it is seldom employed solely to determine the source of pain.

For those with musculoskeletal pain reproducible by palpation over the ribs or muscle, nonsteroidal anti-inflammatory drugs are indicated. Those with radicular pain, i.e., along a nerve distribution, are more likely to have pain consequent to spinal or vertebral pathology. The treatment for this type of pain is complex and beyond the scope of this discussion. Determination of the source may include cervical and/or thoracic spine films, and possibly magnetic resonance imaging (MRI). However, therapy may be best managed by specialists in neurology or spine surgery.

The majority of trials for the treatment of breast pain come from Britain. Perhaps because of the influence of socialized medicine, treatment is seldom initiated until the symptoms have been present for 6 months. For those needing more than reassurance, an attempt to relieve the pain is in order. For those with cyclic pain, a nonendocrine or nonpharmacologic approach may be a reasonable starting point. Some investigators have described a role for fatty acids in cyclic pain. The imbalance in the ratio of saturated versus unsaturated fatty acids plays a role in the development of breast pain. Based on this theory, they advocate a long-term reduction in saturated fats in the diet to 15% of the total calories.[9] This approach requires significant counseling and education, and the long-term diet change may not be acceptable to the patient. Another approach is the addition of evening primrose oil (EPO) as a dietary supplement to increase the intake of unsaturated fatty acids relative to saturated fatty acids. Studies to support the use of EPO are not recent and their design not sufficient to draw strong conclusions. For those who respond, it may be sufficient to avoid medical management; however, it is unclear whether it constitutes a placebo effect. The mechanism behind the effect of unsaturated fatty acids on breast pain is unclear; experimental data support greater membrane fluidity and improved nerve conduction.[10] Even though the largest clinical trial performed had incomplete follow-up, EPO appears to have the greatest impact on those with cyclic pain.[11] A single 400 mg capsule taken once a day for 1–4 months is recommended over a single capsule three times a day with meals. A regimen of dosing three times a day may provide a more rapid improvement; however, there is concern that higher dosing may lead to a greater chance of fatty liver development. Thus, women should refrain from taking EPO at this higher dose after 4 months. Since EPO is a dietary supplement, it is not regulated by the Food and Drug Administration (FDA). Side effects are uncommon and are generally limited to nausea or vomiting. Trials using vitamin E, caffeine reduction, or reduction in smoking have had variable success and in general have shown no greater benefit than placebo.

KEY POINT

Vitamin E and EPO may be helpful for some women with cyclic breast pain.

Danazol, or danacrine, is an antigonadotropin that produces both androgenic and hypoestrogenic effects. It is the only drug approved by the FDA for the treatment of breast pain. Its efficacy is reported to be 90% or higher.[12,13] Dosing can begin at 50 mg twice daily and titrated up to 200 mg twice a day. However, given its androgenic properties, some women may experience male-pattern facial and body hair, as well as deepening of the voice that can be temporary or permanent. Other side effects may occur in up to two-thirds of the patients studied[14] and may prompt discontinuation or poor compliance. These symptoms include menstrual irregularities, acne, headaches, depression, and nausea.

The drug tamoxifen, approved for use in the treatment of breast cancer and breast cancer prevention, has also been studied in the treatment of breast pain. In a randomized, controlled trial, it appeared to have similar efficacy to that of danacrine,[14] but fewer individuals had side effects (approximately 50%). The most common side effect of tamoxifen is hot flushes, but rare side effects include an increased rate of uterine carcinoma and sarcoma, a risk that must be discussed with the patient. Starting doses to achieve pain relief begin at 10 mg a day for 3 months; if relief is achieved, reduction to 10 mg every other day for 3 months is recommended.

KEY POINT

Severe breast pain can be treated with danacrine for a short duration.

Breast Discharge

The secretory activity of the breast takes place throughout the reproductive years. The degree of activity varies according to hormonal and physical stimulation. The ongoing secretion in the nonlactating, nonpregnant woman is generally not appreciated because of keratotic plugs in the openings on the nipple. Frequent testing or squeezing of the nipple can dislodge these plugs, allowing for detection of *discharge*, which is rarely pathologic. However, spontaneous discharge is cause for greater concern. Discharge from the nipple accounts for 5–10% of referrals to a breast center.[15,16] The symptom is disconcerting, in part for the hygienic problem of stained clothing, but also because it raises the fear of cancer. In general, 95% are associated with a benign cause.[17]

Greater attention is being given to nipple discharge and its possible underlying pathology. Previously, algorithms based on small series dictated that only bloody discharge needed to be evaluated, since that was the subset associated with cancer. With the appearance of the newer techniques of ductal lavage, and the more experimental ductoscopy, changes are occurring in our current algorithms in managing nipple discharge. Newer evidence has demonstrated that even nonbloody discharge may be associated with malignancy.

KEY POINT

It is important to note whether nipple discharge is spontaneous or elicited, bilateral or unilateral.

In taking a history of nipple discharge, it is important to determine if the discharge is unilateral or bilateral, spontaneous or elicited, acute or persistent, and whether multiple ducts are involved. To be considered persistent, the discharge must be found on clothes or gown at least once a week for 1 month. The discharge should be characterized as to color (red/bloody, white, colorless, green, blue-black), turbidity (clear vs. cloudy or turbid), and consistency (thin, cheesy). Behavior that enhances the flow of discharge should be noted; e.g., sleeping on the side or abdomen, taking a shower, sexual stimulation to the nipple, or frequently checking the nipple for discharge. Inquire as to the frequency with which the patient checks for nipple discharge because serous fluid can be induced with frequent examination of the nipple.

The physical examination of the breast is very important because other sources of breast fluid could include Montgomery's glands and excoriations or ulcerations of the skin. Special note should be made as to whether the nipple is retracted or inverted. Retraction is an incomplete pulling of the nipple inward, often associated with chronic or repeated episodes of periductal mastitis, usually with a transverse folding of the areolar skin over the nipple. Inversion of the nipple means the whole nipple is drawn in. Notation should be made as to whether there is any associated underlying mass or nipple induration. Close inspection may reveal punctate erythema of a nipple duct, or more diffuse erythema, compared to the color of the contralateral nipple. As these infections are generally caused by skin organisms, the drugs of choice include dicloxacillin or amoxicillin/clavulanate administered for 2 weeks; in the case of penicillin-allergic individuals, erythromycin is the first choice. An abscess may also present with discharge. Usually there is erythema and mass with central fluctuance. Management includes aspiration, if small, or incision and drainage if larger. Since abscess may include anaerobic organisms, metronidazole can be added to the regimen.[18]

If the nipple does not have keratotic plugs, a small amount of fluid can be elicited with gentle pressure in nearly two-thirds of nonlactating women.[19] Generally, physiologic discharge is neither spontaneous nor bloodstained. Secretions pool within the lactiferous

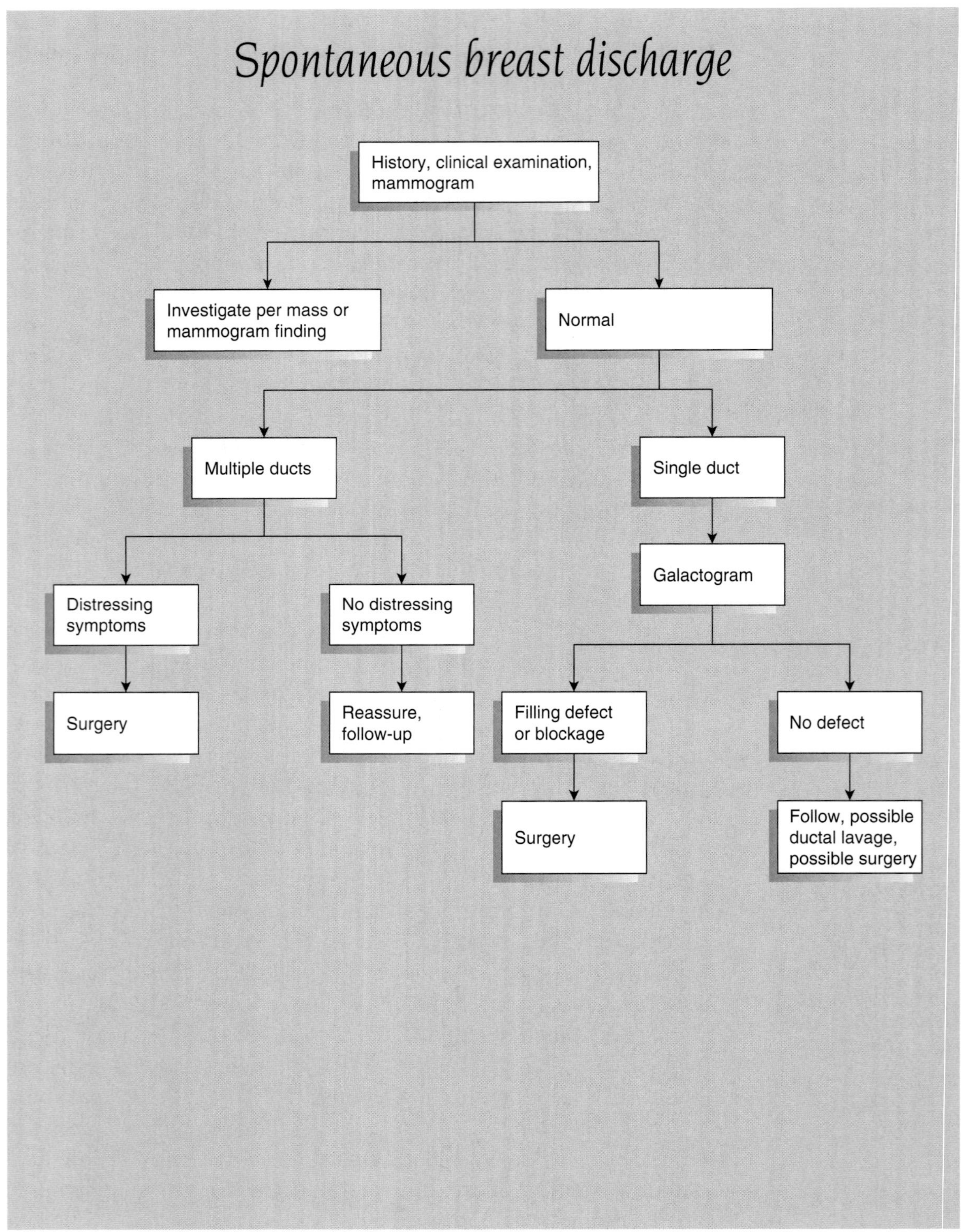
Spontaneous breast discharge
History, clinical examination, mammogram
Investigate per mass or mammogram finding
Normal
Multiple ducts
Single duct
Galactogram
Distressing symptoms
No distressing symptoms
Filling defect or blockage
No defect
Surgery
Reassure, follow-up
Surgery
Follow, possible ductal lavage, possible surgery

sinuses or cysts. These secretions can be from multiple ducts, and may vary in color. Ectatic ducts can have a range of discharge from thin to cheesy or viscous.

Should the discharge be bilateral, consideration should be given to a systemic cause such as hyperprolactinemia or a thyroid disorder. These two conditions may be a primary or secondary cause of the problem. Both hypothyroidism and hyperthyroidism have been reported as a potential cause of nipple discharge.[20] Antipsychotic drugs which block the dopaminergic D2 receptors, such as haloperidol, can elevate prolactin, and place the patient at risk for the development of galactorrhea. The galactorrhea may persist after discontinuation of the medication if the patient continues to actively check for nipple discharge. Breast manipulation stimulates prolactin release.

The treatment of nipple discharge begins with correction of the underlying disorder. Medical management can be used for most thyroid disorders. If primary hyperprolactinemia exists, medical therapy with bromocriptine mesylate or cabergoline is indicated. Surgical therapy is not indicated in vast majority of circumstances of bilateral discharge. If the galactorrhea is drug-associated, a change in medication should be considered. If no systemic cause can be identified, imaging should be pursued as long as there are no multiple ducts involved. When multiple ducts are involved, galactography should be performed only if there is a single, suspicious duct; otherwise, it would be considered physiologic.

In the context of breast discharge, imaging begins with a mammogram in an effort to identify a focal abnormality. If only one duct is suspicious, galactography is the diagnostic procedure of choice.[21,22] Galactography is highly sensitive for the detection of carcinomas, but has low specificity in that other abnormalities are detected as well.[22,23] The procedure can be hampered by filling defects, duct ectasia, or a blockage of the duct. Cytology of the fluid elicited demonstrates the reverse of these characteristics. It is highly specific[16,22] but not very sensitive. Consequently, a negative result should be interpreted with caution, and pursued further if there is sufficient concern for malignancy.[24]

When a defect is identified on galactography, it should be pursued surgically since the differential includes the possibility of carcinoma. Overall, a papilloma or inflammatory process is of greater likelihood. A microdochectomy, or nipple exploration

KEY POINT

Galactography is the most sensitive test for identifying the abnormality that causes a spontaneous discharge from a single duct, but lack of findings still warrant surgical exploration.

with duct excision, can be performed either through an incision along the periphery of the areola, or through a radial incision across the areola, through the duct. The majority of lesions are identified within the first 2–3 cm of the duct, and nearly all are within 5 cm.[18] Galactography does not always identify a lesion, even when only one duct is producing the discharge. In those instances where concern is high, *blind* surgical excision is performed; a lacrimal probe or blue dye is inserted into the affected duct to identify it intraoperatively prior to excision of the duct (microdochectomy). A generous length of duct is taken for evaluation. Any malignancy identified would be managed according to current protocols.

Smoking appears to be a risk factor for periductal mastitis, especially in these cases with recurrent periareolar abscesses and fistula formation.[25] The role smoking plays is not fully understood. Possible mechanisms include toxic metabolites,[26] microvascular changes,[27] as well as shifts in bacterial flora.[28] The association of periductal mastitis with duct ectasia is controversial. Direct ectasia may be the consequence of recurrent episodes of periductal mastitis,[29] but may also be an involutionary process that occurs with age. The associated thickened cheesy secretions are not felt to place the patient at risk of malignancy; however, they may cause distress from a hygiene perspective. If ectasia is related to a single duct, the duct can be surgically excised. If multiple ducts are involved, excision of all the ducts below the nipple should be considered. A significant length (2–5 cm) of duct should be removed. Perioperative antibiotics are advised because of the commonly associated bacterial colonization.

KEY POINT

The role of newer techniques such as ductal lavage and ductoscopy in evaluating breast discharge are yet to be defined.

The recent development of techniques such as ductal lavage and breast ductoscopy may lead to changes in the current management paradigm. When aspiration of a duct yields fluid, ductal lavage should be performed. The technique involves cannulation of the duct with flushing and aspiration.[30] The cells collected are sent for cytologic evaluation. Initially developed as a technique to assist in the earlier diagnosis of malignancy in high-risk women with a dense mammogram, the procedure may provide a greater sensitivity in cytologic evaluation than exfoliative cytology where superficial secretions are placed on a slide for evaluation. Breast ductoscopy is also a new technique under evaluation. The indications for its use are not yet defined; however, it appears to improve lesion localization for lesions deeper to the nipple and may facilitate ductal excisions previously performed "blindly."[31,32].

Breast Mass

A mass found by the patient or by the clinician generally provokes significant anxiety on the part of the patient. The diagnostic team is under pressure to remove an adequate amount of tissue to cure or provide accurate diagnosis while not removing so much that future treatment options are compromised or that cosmesis is a problem if the mass is benign.

As with the preceding two breast conditions, the practitioner should begin with both the history of the chief complaint and physical examination. Details specific to the mass should be addressed, such as when the mass was discovered, how the mass was discovered, and whether the mass is associated with any pain, tenderness, or discharge. It is important to know if the patient has had prior masses and if so, whether they were biopsied or aspirated, and what the diagnosis was. Has the size changed since its discovery? Does size or tenderness fluctuate with the patient's menstrual cycle? Is the patient having regular menstrual cycles? A full gynecologic history should be obtained to identify menstrual irregularities and risk factors associated with the development of breast cancer, such as age at menarche, parity, age at parturition of first full-term pregnancy, and age at menopause. It is important to note whether any family members, male or female, on both maternal and paternal sides of the family have had any cancers. Particular attention should be given to breast and ovarian cancers, because of the association with heritable breast cancer risk.

The pertinent physical examination should include examination of the breasts, axillae, and neck. Additional systems should be covered as indicated. Fibrocystic changes are common in the population, and the texture of the breast can vary with each patient. It will also vary with the hormonal milieu, whether endogenous and exogenous. Palpation technique varies according to the preference of the practitioner. No one technique has been shown to be superior. In performing the examination, attention is paid to focal change compared to the general texture.[33] A true mass is three-dimensional, distinct from the adjacent tissues, and usually asymmetric as compared to the contralateral breast. Characteristics associated with clinically suspicious masses include ill-defined or indistinct borders, fixation to the overlying skin or underlying muscle, irregularity of the border, and greater firmness relative to the adjacent tissues. Benign masses tend to be well circumscribed with smooth borders, mobile, and may either be of equal or greater firmness than the adjacent tissues. However, these two sets of descriptors are not mutually exclusive, and thus, further evaluation is necessary.

Confirmation of the mass by a clinician is preferred before proceeding with an evaluation; however, the increased density of the tissue during the premenstrual phase of the cycle can obscure the finding. A mammogram or ultrasound may be required to confirm a mass. If no mass is found by imaging or examination, a repeat examination in approximately 6 weeks is reasonable in order to reexamine the patient at a different time in her cycle. In the patient where the clinician feels the mass, the first step is to determine whether it is solid or cystic. Cysts are fluid-filled sacs thought to result from lobular involution.[34] Haagensen estimated the frequency of cysts with distinct physical findings as 7%.[35] Cysts are frequently incidental findings at biopsy. They can occur at any age, but are more common in premenopausal women over the age of 40. As cysts are hormonally related, a cyst in postmenopausal woman not receiving hormonal replacement should be regarded with suspicion.

KEY POINT

Cysts are more common in premenopausal women over 40.

Either ultrasound or fine needle aspiration can be used to determine if a mass is cystic. Cysts frequently present with pain, but not exclusively. Aspiration provides a more immediate answer unless the ultrasound unit is in the same room. If the mass fully resolves with aspiration and the fluid is not bloody, no further evaluation is necessary since the incidence of associated malignancy is less than 1%.[35,37] However, if the fluid is bloody, or the mass does not fully resolve, surgical excision is indicated because of the heightened risk of malignancy. The likelihood of the cyst recurring is greatest in cysts that were larger than 2 cm. Despite resolution of a cyst with aspiration, the patient should still be followed. Patients who present with a cystic recurrence after two aspirations have a higher risk of intracystic malignancy. Consequently, if the cyst returns after two aspirations, surgical excision is recommended.

KEY POINT

If the cyst returns after two aspirations, surgical excision is recommended.

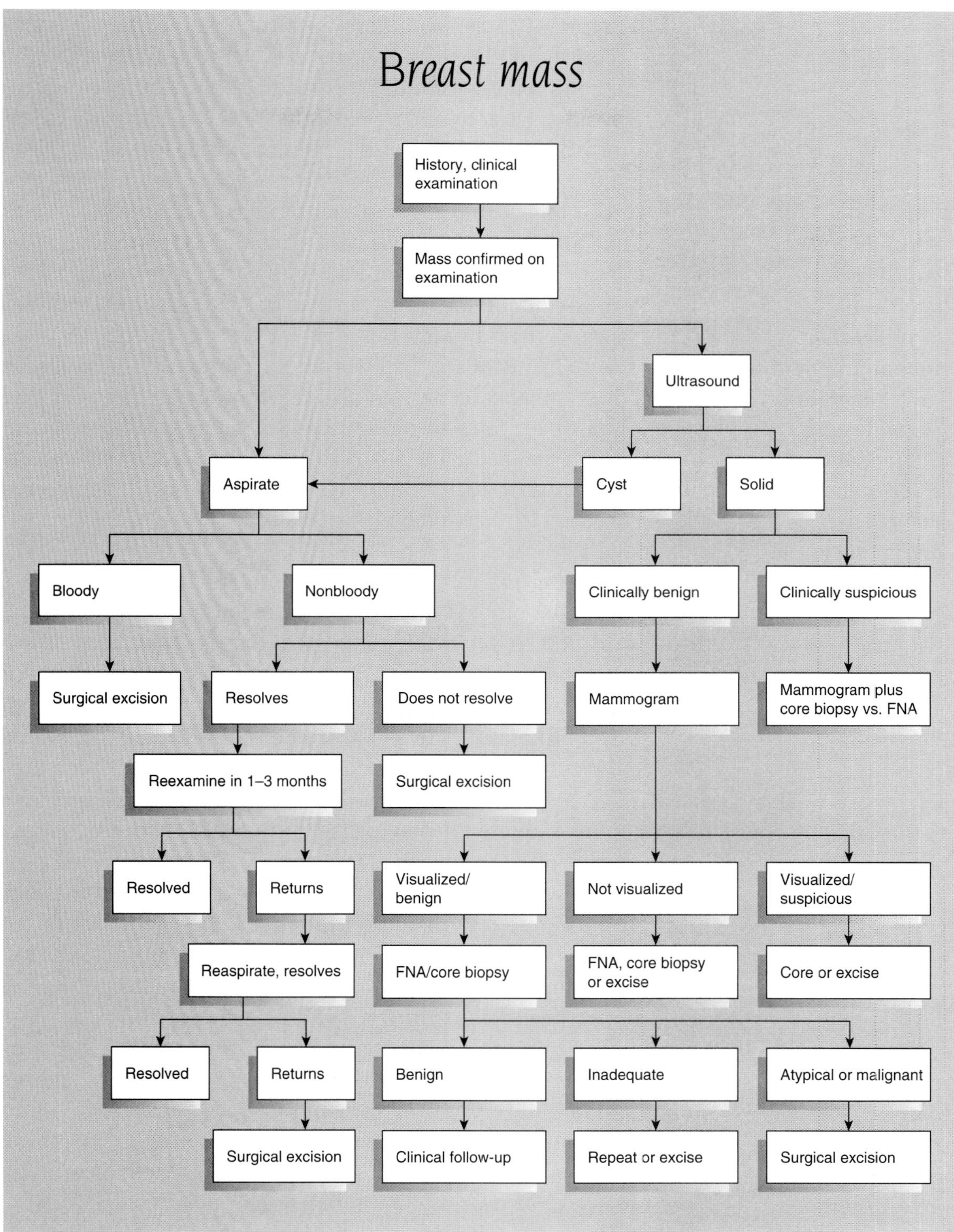
Breast mass
History, clinical examination
Mass confirmed on examination
Ultrasound
Aspirate
Cyst
Solid
Bloody
Nonbloody
Clinically benign
Clinically suspicious
Surgical excision
Resolves
Does not resolve
Mammogram
Mammogram plus core biopsy vs. FNA
Reexamine in 1–3 months
Surgical excision
Resolved
Returns
Visualized/ benign
Not visualized
Visualized/ suspicious
Reaspirate, resolves
FNA/core biopsy
FNA, core biopsy or excise
Core or excise
Resolved
Returns
Benign
Inadequate
Atypical or malignant
Surgical excision
Clinical follow-up
Repeat or excise
Surgical excision

If the attempt to aspirate fails to yield fluid, and the practitioner is confident that the mass was pierced with the needle, the mass is considered to be solid. Fine needle aspirate may yield sufficient cells for cytology to be performed. However, further imaging is indicated at this point. The combination of clinical examination, mammography, and fine needle aspirate is 95% sensitive in the detection of breast carcinomas.[18] A negative result should not lull the practitioner into a false sense of security. The result should always be interpreted in the clinical context, and if there is a lack of concordance, further tissue containing cellular architecture (core biopsy or excisional biopsy) should be obtained. Of note, the finding of atypical hyperplasia or papillomas on core biopsy, or atypical cells on fine needle aspirate can be associated with a significant false-negative rate, i.e., there can be adjacent ductal carcinoma in situ (DCIS) or invasive carcinoma that may be missed by sampling error.[38] Consequently, with these findings one should proceed to excisional biopsy despite the seemingly benign histology.

KEY POINT

Atypical cells or papillomas on needle biopsy (core or aspiration) should prompt full excision of the lesion because of the risk of sampling error in the detection of malignancy.

In the young patient with a mass that is consistent with a benign fibroadenoma on examination, the mass can be imaged by ultrasound first to avoid the effect of radiation on young, developing breast tissue. Should the findings on fine needle aspirate or core biopsy support the diagnosis of fibroadenoma, the mass can be followed clinically. The sensitivity of a biopsy in this setting is 86%.[39] If ultrasound is added, there is 95% sensitivity in differentiation between a benign and malignant lesion.[40] Should the biopsy be inadequate for diagnosis, a fine needle aspirate or core biopsy can be repeated or the mass excised. Often, when the mass is symptomatic, excision of the mass is preferred since there is a high likelihood of pain resolution. It should be emphasized that fine needle aspiration or core biopsy always has the risk of sampling error. Hence, if the mass is not removed, the patient's physical findings need to be followed with measurements of the mass to ensure that the mass remains stable. Intervals of 6 months or less are suggested, until the age of 35. As long as the mass remains stable, further intervention is generally not pursued. Before embarking on this path of expectant management, the small risk of a missed malignancy is discussed with the patient. Should the mass change or grow, excision is recommended.

KEY POINT

A mass that changes or grows, despite previous benign cytology or histology, needs to be excised.

Discussion of Cases

Case 1

A 55-year-old woman with a history of fibrocystic changes presents with bilateral breast pain. She underwent an excisional biopsy for microcalcifications 3 years ago. The pathology report was consistent with fibrocystic changes, including sclerosing adenosis associated with calcifications. Her pain is diffuse and bilateral, similar to the quality of pain she would experience when approaching the onset of her menses but more intense. Presently, her menstrual cycles are not regular, and her last menstrual period was 3 months ago. She is not sexually active, and notes no findings or changes in her self breast examination. Physical examination demonstrates the presence of a well-healed incision in the right breast, in the upper outer quadrant, with no skin changes, no nipple discharge or inversion. Upon palpation, her breast tissue is diffusely firm and dense.

What other testing would you recommend at this point, if any?

It would be prudent to make sure that she is current with annual mammographic screening. No specific imaging is indicated independent of this, given the diffuse nature of the pain.

What would you recommend for initial management?

I would recommend one EPO capsule daily or, one capsule three times a day for 1–4 months for more rapid resolution of the pain The fact that the EPO capsules are not pain relievers and may take time to have an effect should be explained to the patient. Compliance with the prescribed regimen is important for its efficacy. In follow-up, the response of her pain to the EPO should be evaluated.

Case 2

The patient is a 50-year-old woman who is mentally challenged but lives independently near her parents. She has a history of a left breast infection 6 months ago, which responded to dicloxacillin. She relates that she has had a long-standing left breast discharge, occasionally bloody, which occurs spontaneously at least once a week. She thought that the tissue deep to her left areola was a little lumpy, but not much different as compared to the contralateral side. She has a family history of breast cancer in a maternal aunt and a paternal grandmother, both diagnosed after the age of 70. The patient underwent menarche at the age of 13 years, and is nulliparous. Her last menstrual period was 1 year ago, and she is not on hormone replacement. A very small drop of bloody discharge could be elicited with massage of the breast superiorly, but not with gentle subareolar pressure.

What further testing, if any, would you recommend?

A diagnostic mammogram should be obtained to check for any focal abnormalities.

What further testing would you recommend?

Galactography is indicated, given that a single duct is associated with a bloody discharge.

Assume the procedure reveals partial filling of a rounded structure in the immediate retroareolar region associated with several smoothly enlarged ducts (Fig. 13-1). The mass demonstrates multiple filling defects, possibly related to an intracystic mass or debris.

Would you recommend any further management?

The patient should be referred to a surgeon for duct exploration and excision.

Figure 13-1

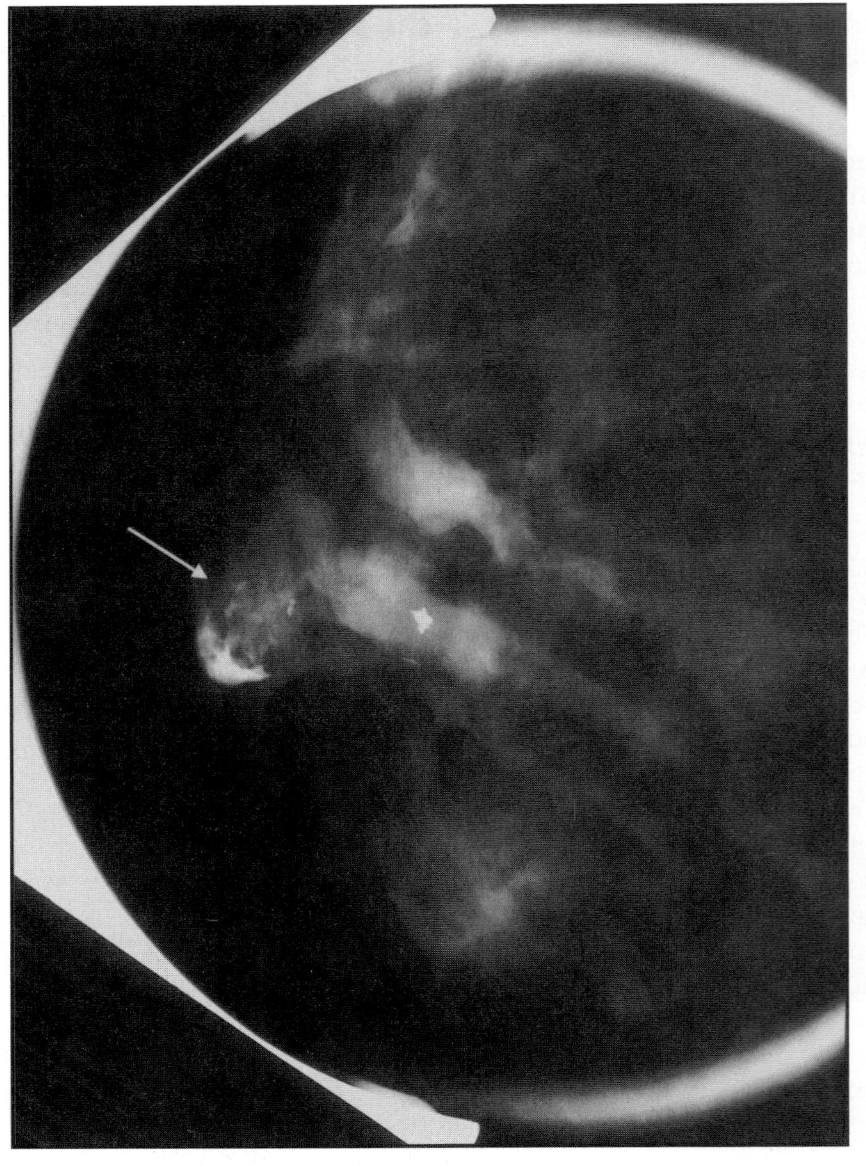

Case 3

The patient is a 52-year-old woman with a long-standing history of fibrocystic changes as evidenced by multiple cysts aspirated bilaterally in the past, all with resolution. When premenopausal, she had experienced cyclic mastodynia. Her last menstrual period was 6 months back, and she reports awakening to hot flushes during the night. Over the past weekend, she noted a new lump in the left breast in the upper outer aspect associated with tenderness but not pain. She notes no discharge or any other change in her self breast examination. She underwent menarche at the age of 13, and is gravida 2 para 2, with her first full-term pregnancy at the age of 23. She is currently self-medicating with phytoestrogens. She has no family history of breast cancer. Physical examination reveals a 3 cm mass, well circumscribed and mobile, in the upper outer quadrant of the left breast. It is slightly tender to palpation. Mammogram at this time demonstrated a markedly dense breast with no finding correlating with the palpable mass (Fig. 13-2).

What testing would you recommend, if any?

Fine needle aspiration is recommended, given her past history of cyst formation and a palpable mass with benign characteristics on examination. Aspiration results in 8 mL of a cloudy green fluid, with resolution of the mass.

Any further testing required?

As the aspirate is not frankly bloody, no further testing of the fluid is necessary.

What steps would be taken in further management?

The patient should return in 1–3 months for repeat examination to check for cyst recurrence. Should it recur, one additional aspiration is indicated; further recurrence should be managed by excision, as a recurring cyst is associated with an increased incidence of intracystic malignancy.

What's the Evidence?

Breast pain is seldom associated with malignancy, but can be when a tumor is in proximity to a nerve or when a nerve is entrapped in the tumor. Breast pain associated with malignancy is focal, if pain is present at all; focal pain is also associated with infection or inflammation. Thus, focal breast pain necessitates a thorough evaluation. The etiology of diffuse or cyclic breast pain is not well understood. Observation is acceptable or treatment can be addressed systemically using EPO capsules for milder symptoms. Treatment trials for more intense, chronic breast pain show improvement with use of danacrine or tamoxifen. These trials are based on patient self-reporting and the studies suffer from a high rate of participants who were lost to follow-up.

Figure 13-2

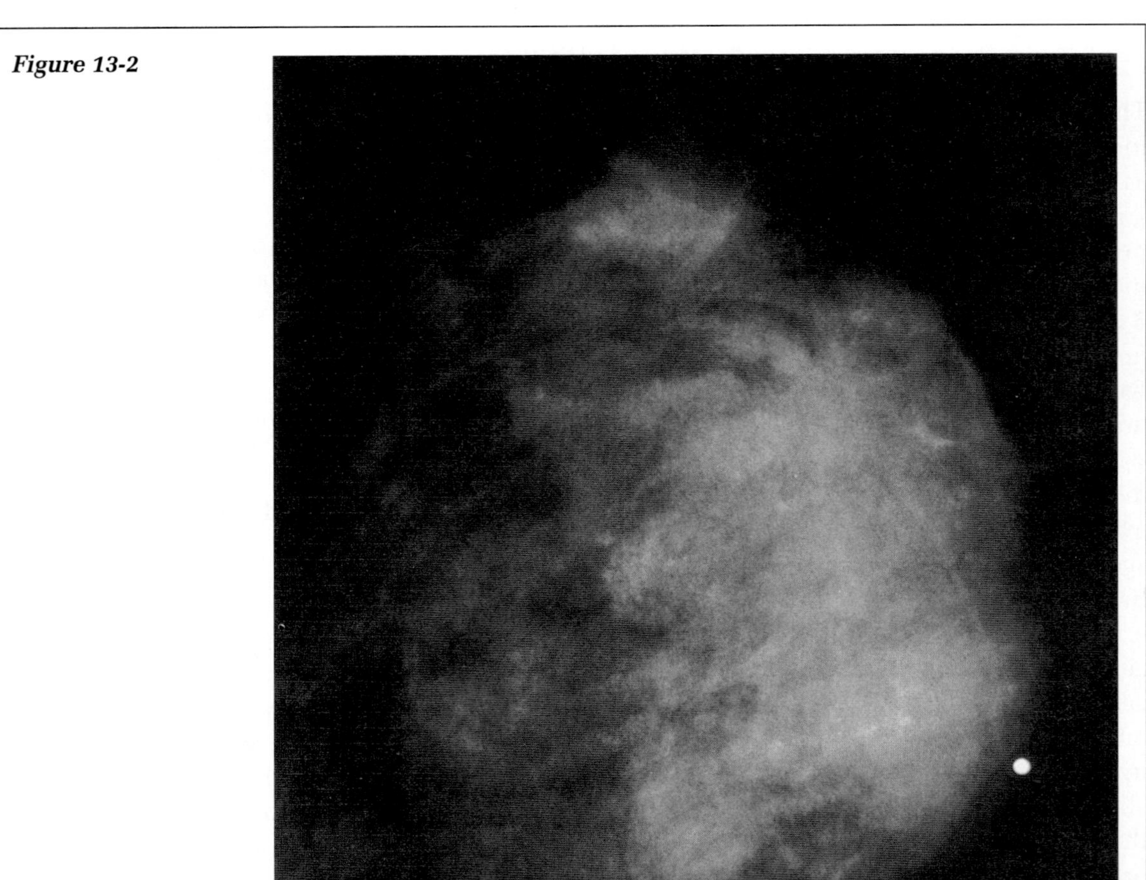

Tamoxifen is not approved by the FDA for use in treatment of breast pain in the United States. Reduction in caffeine intake or in smoking appears to be no better than placebo in treating this type of breast pain.

A nipple discharge is seldom associated with malignancy. Unfortunately, a discharge associated with a malignancy can look identical to a benign discharge After a standard mammogram, galactography should be utilized. The sensitivity of nipple aspirates in detecting malignancy is not as high as the galactogram (>90%). Drying artifact can lead to false positive cytology, which may prompt inappropriate surgical intervention. Because galactogram is not 100% sensitive, definitive duct excision is indicated if a unilateral discharge continues in the face of a negative galactogram.

The incidence of malignancy with a breast mass, given all types of biopsy methods, is approximately one in five patients. As long as there is concordance for benign disease using breast examination, mammogram (or ultrasound) and biopsy, there is less than a 5% chance of error. Because there can be error, a lack of concordance requires full excision for certainty in diagnosis. A benign solid mass, consistent with a fibroadenoma, can be followed clinically as long as it remains stable or gets smaller; most remain stable or resolve in about 5 years. Since the cell types identified in the fibroadenoma are seen in other more aggressive fibroepithelial variants (i.e., juvenile fibroadenoma, phyllodes tumor, and cystosarcoma phyllodes), continued growth of the mass raises concern for sampling error. The presence of atypical cells or papillomas within a core biopsy or fine needle biopsy necessitates full excision; 5–30% of these biopsies may have an adjacent malignancy that has been missed. Generally, a core biopsy has an accuracy of 96% and fine needle aspirate cytology, an accuracy of 94% with a reliable cytologist.

Management of breast problems continues to evolve. There is no evidence that the approaches described in this chapter are the final word in diagnosis and treatment, but they are currently accepted practice. The role of MRI, ductal lavage, and technologies yet to be discovered will continue to make this area a work in progress.

References

1 Millet AV, Dirbas FM. Clinical management of breast pain: a review. *Obstet Gynecol Surv.* 2002;57:451.

2 Atkins HJB. Chronic mastitis. *Lancet.* 1938;1:707.

3 Patey DH. Two common non-malignant conditions of the breast: the clinical features of cystic disease and the pain syndrome. *Br Med J.* 1949;1:96.

4 Preece PE, Mansel RE, Hughes LE. Mastalgia: psychoneurosis or organic disease? *Br Med J.* 1978;1:29.

5 Hughes LE, Mansel RE, Webster DIT. Aberrations of normal development and involution (ANDI): a new perspective on pathogenesis and nomenclature of benign breast disorders. *Lancet.* 1987;2: 1316.

6 Kumar S, Mansel RE, Hughes LE, et al. Prolactin response to thyrotropin-release hormone stimulation and dopaminergic inhibition in benign breast disease. *Cancer.* 1984;53:1311.

7 Zinger M, McFarland M, Ben-Jonathan N. Prolactin expression and secretion by human breast glandular and adipose tissue explants. *J Clin Endocrinol Metab.* 2003;88:689.

8 Catania S, Zurrida S, Veronesi P, et al. Mondor's disease and breast cancer. *Cancer.* 1992;69:2267.

9 Boyd NF, Shannon P, Kruikov V, et al. Effect of a low-fat high-carbohydrate diet on symptoms of cyclical mastopathy. *Lancet.* 1988;2:128.

10 Horrobin DF. Essential fatty acids in the management of impaired nerve function in diabetes. *Diabetes.* 1997;46(Suppl. 2):S90.

11 Preece PE, Hanslip JI, Gilbert L, et al. Evening primrose oil (Efamol) for mastalgia. In: Horrobin D, ed. *Clinical Uses of Essential Fatty Acids.* Montreal: Eden Press; 1982:45.

12 Mansel RE, Wisbey JR, Hughes LE. Controlled trial of the antigonadotropin Danazol in painful nodular benign breast disease. *Lancet.* 1982;1:928.

13 Doberl A, Tobiassen T, Rasmussen T. Treatment of recurrent cyclical mastodynia in patients with fibrocystic breast disease. *Acta Obstet Gynecol Scand.* 1984;123(Suppl.):177.

14 Powles TJ, Ford HT, Gazet J-C. A randomized trial to compare tamoxifen with Danazol for treatment of benign mammary dysplasia. *Breast Dis.* 1987;2:1.

15 Dixon JM, Mansel RE. Symptoms, assessment and guidelines for referral. ABC of breast diseases. *Br Med J.* 1987;309:722.

16 Simmons R, Adamovich T, Brennan M, et al. Nonsurgical evaluation of pathologic nipple discharge. *Ann Surg Oncol.* 2003;10:113.

17 Ambrogetti A, Berni D, Catarzi S, et al. The role of ductal galactography in the differential diagnosis of breast carcinoma. *Radiol Med.* 1996;91:198.

18 Dixon JM, Bundred NJ. Management of disorders of the ductal system and infections. In: Harris JR, Lippman ME, Morrow M, Osborne CK, eds. *Diseases of the Breast.* 2nd ed. New York: Lippincott Williams & Wilkins; 2000:47.

19 Wynder EL, Hill P, Laakso K, et al. Breast secretions in Finnish women. *Cancer.* 1981;47:1444.

20 State D. Nipple discharge in women: is it cause for concern? *Postgrad Med.* 1991;89:65.

21 Tabar L, Dean PB, Pentek Z. Galactography: the diagnostic procedure of choice for nipple discharge. *Radiology* 1983;149:31.

22 Funovics MA, Philipp MO, Lackner B, et al. Galactography: method of choice in pathologic nipple discharge? *Eur Radiol.* 2003;13:94

23 Cabioglu N, Hunt KK, Singletary SE, et al. Surgical decision making and factors determining a diagnosis of breast carcinoma in women presenting with nipple discharge. *J Am Coll Surg.* 2003;196:354.

24 Klimberg VS. Nipple discharge: more than pathologic. *Ann Surg Oncol.* 2003;10:98.

25 Schafer P, Furrer G, Mermillod B. An association of cigarette smoking with recurrent subareolar breast abscesses. *Int J Epidemiol.* 1988;17:810.

26 Petrakis NL, Maack CA, Lee RE, et al. Mutagenic activity of nipple aspirates of breast fluid. *Cancer Res.* 1980;40:188.

27 Bundred NJ. Surgical management of periductal mastitis. *Breast.* 1988;7:79.

28 Ertel A, Eng R, Smith SM. The differential effect of cigarette smoke on the growth of bacteria found in humans. *Chest.* 1991;100:628.

29 Dixon JM, Ravi Sekar O, Chetty U, et al. Periductal mastitis and duct ectasia: different conditions with different aetiologies. *Br J Surg.* 1996;83:820.

30 O'Shaughnessy JA, Ljung BM, Dooley WC, et al. Ductal lavage and the clinical management of women at high risk for beast carcinoma: a commentary. *Cancer.* 2002;94:292.

31 Dooley WC. Routine operative breast endoscopy for bloody nipple discharge. *Ann Surg Oncol.* 2002;9:920.

32 Dietz JR, Crowe JP, Grundfest S, et al. Directed duct excision by using mammary ductoscopy in patients with pathologic nipple discharge. *Surgery.* 2002;132:582.

33 Donegan WL. Evaluation of a palpable mass. *N Engl J Med.* 1992;327:937.

34 Dupont WD, Page DL. Risk factors for breast cancer in women with proliferative breast disease. *N Engl J Med.* 1985;312:146.

35 Haagensen CD. *Diseases of the Breast.* Philadelphia, PA: WB Saunders; 1986.

36 McSwain GR, Valicenti JF Jr, O'Brien PH. Cytologic evaluation of breast cysts. *Surg Obstet Gynecol.* 1978;146:921.

37 Smith DN, Kaelin CM, Korbin CD, et al. Impalpable breast cysts: utility of cytologic examination of fluid obtained with radiologically guided aspiration. *Radiology.* 1997;204:149.

38 Winchester DJ, Berstein JR, Jeske JM, et al. Upstaging of atypical ductal hyperplasia after vacuum-assisted 11-gauge stereotactic core needle biopsy. *Arch Surg.* 2003;138:619.

39 Fornage BD, Lorigan JF, Andry E. Fibroadenoma of the breast: sonographic appearance. *Radiology* 1989;172:671.

40 Greenberg R, Skornick Y, Kaplan O. Management of breast fibroadenomas. *J Gen Intern Med* 1998;13:640.

14 Hypercholesterolemia and Lipoprotein Disorders

Cynthia A. Stuenkel

Cardiovascular Disease in Women

KEY POINT

Cardiovascular disease, the primary killer of American women, is largely preventable with lifestyle choices and medical therapy of risk factors.

Cardiovascular disease (CVD) is the number one killer of American women claiming more lives than the next seven causes of death—accountable for more than one-half million deaths per year.[1] Women having a heart attack are more likely to die within a year than men, and twice as many women than men who survive the initial heart attack will have a second heart attack within the next 6 years.[1] For women aged 20–45 years, coronary heart disease (CHD) is rare, and usually occurs in the setting of familial hypercholesterolemia, heavy cigarette smoking, or diabetes.[2] For older women (>age 45 years), including those likely to be in the perimenopausal transition, CHD is usually delayed 10–15 years compared to men. Women who develop CHD are usually ≥65 years old; premature CHD is often related to multiple risk factors or the presence of the metabolic syndrome.[2]

Most CVD is preventable and related to lifestyle choices. In the Nurses Health Study, women who followed a healthy diet, did not smoke, exercised, maintained a desirable weight, and consumed a moderate amount of alcohol reduced their risk of heart disease by 83%.[3] Only 3% of participants incorporated all five components into their lifestyle. In updated evidence-based guidelines for CVD prevention in women, the American Heart Association (AHA) defines lifestyle interventions as smoking cessation, 30 minutes of moderate-intensity physical activity daily, an overall healthy eating pattern that includes a variety of fruits, vegetables, grains, low-fat or nonfat dairy products, fish, legumes, and sources of protein low in saturated fat, limitation of saturated fat intake to <10% of calories, limitation of cholesterol intake to <300 mg/day, and limitation of intake of trans fatty acids. Maintenance of a body mass index (BMI) between 18.5 and 24.9 kg/m^2 and a waist circumference <35 in. is also recommended.[4] These recommendations reflect the therapeutic lifestyle changes (TLC) endorsed by the National Cholesterol Education Program (NCEP) in their guidelines.[2] and should be reviewed with your patients at every visit.

Lipid Disorders

Lipid disorders are among the most prevalent risk factors for CVD and one of the most remedial to available therapies. Over 55 million adult women have cholesterol levels of ≥200 mg/dL (almost half of all women >20 years old), and almost 1 in 5 women over age 20 years have cholesterol levels ≥240 mg/dL.[1] The National Cholesterol Education Program Adult Treatment Program–III (NCEP ATP III) guidelines prioritize low-density lipoprotein cholesterol (LDL-C) as the target for therapy.[2] Non-high-density lipoprotein cholesterol (non-HDL-C) has been recognized as a measure of atherogenic lipoproteins and includes LDL-C, very low-density lipoprotein cholesterol (VLDL-C), and intermediate-density lipoprotein cholesterol (IDL-C). Non-HDL-C is calculated by subtracting HDL-C from total cholesterol (TC). Non-HDL-C is now a secondary target of therapy in patients with triglycerides (TG) >200 mg/dL.[5] Treatment goals are included in the NCEP guidelines for treatment of hypertriglyceridemia.[6]and incorporated into the AHA clinical recommendations for lipid therapy in women.[4]

KEY POINT

LDL-cholesterol, a significant risk factor for coronary heart disease is the primary target for lipid-lowering therapy.

The clinical approach to lipid management takes into consideration family and medical history, associated cardiovascular risk factors, concurrent medical conditions and therapies, and lifestyle choices. The AHA's evidence-based guidelines for prevention of CVD in women[4] incorporate and expand upon the NCEP ATP III guidelines for risk assessment.[2] In addition to providing algorithms for management of lipid disorders, the NCEP guidelines also accentuate the importance of the metabolic syndrome and approaches to modify associated cardiovascular risks.

The Metabolic Syndrome

The metabolic syndrome, a constellation of risk factors that places a woman at increased risk for CHD, includes dyslipidemia

Table 14-1. **CHARACTERISTICS OF THE METABOLIC SYNDROME IN WOMEN***

Risk Factor	*Defining Level*
Abdominal obesity (waist circumference)	>35 in.
TG	≥150 mg/dL
High-density lipoprotein cholesterol	<50 mg/dL
Blood pressure	≥130/85 mmHg
Fasting glucose	≥100 mg/dL

*Diagnosis of metabolic syndrome requires presence of ≥3 risk determinants (Ref. 2).

characterized by low HDL-C, increased TG, and small dense LDL particles in the face of normal or modest LDL-C elevations.[2] (Table 14-1). Other components not routinely measured include a proinflammatory state and a prothrombotic state.[7] In an analysis of the Third National Health and Nutrition Examination Survey (NHANES) from 1988 to 1994, approximately 20% of women aged 40–49 years and almost a third of women aged 50–59 years met criteria for the metabolic syndrome.[8] Identification and treatment of the metabolic syndrome has been designated by the NCEP as a secondary target for CHD risk reduction. Treatment is multifactorial and dependent upon the components of the metabolic syndrome present in any individual.[7]

Women with polycystic ovary syndrome (PCOS) share many characteristics of the metabolic syndrome, including dyslipidemia.[9] Not surprising then, subclinical cardiovascular atherosclerosis, as determined by coronary artery calcium score, was more prevalent in 30–45-year-old women with PCOS (39%) compared to lean age-matched women (10%; odds ratio [OR] 5.89; $P = 0.001$) or age and weight matched women (21%; OR 2.4; $P = 0.05$).[10] Increased carotid intima-media wall thickness, another measure of subclinical atherosclerosis, has also been reported in PCO women less than age 45 years.[11] Because of the increased CHD risk, women with PCO should be approached during (if not before) the menopause transition with a higher index of suspicion for CHD and possibly a lower threshold to treat CHD risk factors.

Risk Assessment

Coronary Heart Disease Risk

Risk factor assessment should begin at age 20 years and includes measurement of blood pressure, pulse, BMI, and waist circumference

KEY POINT

The absolute 10-year risk of CHD should be established for every woman by the age of 40 and reassessed at least every 5 years or when her risk factors change.

every 2 years and fasting lipid and glucose determinations at least every 5 years.[12] (Table 14-2). If a nonfasting sample is all that is available, the total and HDL-C can still be measured and non-HDL-C can be calculated. If TC is >200 mg/dL or HDL-C is <40 mg/dL, a follow-up fasting lipoprotein profile is required to determine LDL-C.[2] Optimal levels of lipids and lipoproteins have been established for women.[4] (Table 14-3).

By age 40, the absolute 10-year risk of CHD (Table 14-4) should be established for every woman, placed in her permanent medical record, and reassessed every 5 years (more often if risks change).[12] Thus, by the time a woman reaches the perimenopausal transition, she and her provider should have a reasonably clear idea of her

Table 14-2. **GUIDE TO PRIMARY PREVENTION OF CARDIOVASCULAR DISEASE AND STROKE: RISK ASSESSMENT[a]**

Risk Assessment	*Recommendations*
Risk factor screening	Risk factor assessment should begin at age 20 years
At every routine evaluation	Family history of CHD Smoking status Diet Alcohol intake Physical activity
At least every 2 years	Blood pressure BMI Waist circumference Pulse (screen for atrial fibrillation)
At least every 5 years[b]	Fasting serum lipoprotein profile (total and HDL if fasting is unavailable) Fasting blood glucose
Global risk estimation[c]	Every 5 years[d] all adults >40 years of age[e] should have their 10-year risk of CHD assessed with a multiple risk score[f]

[a] See Ref. 12.

[b] Should be measured according to patient's risk for hyperlipidemia and diabetes, respectively; if risk factors are present, measure every 2 years.

[c] See Tables 14-4 and 14-5.

[d] More frequently if risk factors change.

[e] Or those with ≥2 risk factors.

[f] The NCEP guidelines incorporate the Framingham Point Score. See Ref. 2.

Table 14-3.* OPTIMAL LEVELS OF LIPIDS AND LIPOPROTEINS IN WOMEN

LIPOPROTEIN	OPTIMAL LEVEL
LDL-C	<100 mg/dL
HDL-C	>50 mg/dL
TG	<150 mg/dL
Non-HDL-C†	<130 mg/dL

* See Ref. 4.

† Calculated as TC minus HDL-C.

current cardiovascular risk profile. The 10-year absolute CHD risk is determined by history of CVD and level of CHD risk factors.[6] A history of vascular disease, diabetes, or kidney disease places a woman in the high-risk group (>20% 10-year absolute risk of CHD) (Table 14-4). Relatively few women will present with a history of vascular disease during the perimenopausal transition, but some will have a diagnosis of diabetes, which also places them at high risk. For the majority of women, the Framingham Point Score should be used to calculate their 10-year absolute risk (Table 14-5). Determinants of risk include age, TC, smoking status, HDL-C, and systolic blood pressure. Once calculated, the 10-year absolute risk percent determines the target for LDL-C (Table 14-6).

INTERPRETING LIPID LEVELS

SECONDARY CAUSES OF DYSLIPIDEMIA Prior to initiating therapy for elevated LDL-C, screen for secondary causes of dyslipidemia: diabetes, hypothyroidism, nephrotic syndrome, obstructive liver disease, and chronic renal failure. These conditions can be ruled out by history and straightforward laboratory analysis: fasting blood glucose or glycosylated hemoglobin if diabetes is present, serum thyroid stimulating hormone (TSH), alkaline phosphatase (rule out obstructive biliary disease), and urinalysis for proteinuria. Drugs that increase LDL include progestins, anabolic steroids, corticosteroids, and protease inhibitors (treatment of human immunodeficiency virus [HIV] infections).[6]

THE PERIMENOPAUSAL TRANSITION In longitudinal studies of the menopausal transition, the lipid profile deteriorated over several

Table 14-4. SPECTRUM OF CARDIOVASCULAR DISEASE RISK IN WOMEN[a]

Risk Group	Framingham Global Risk (10-Year Absolute CHD Risk)	Clinical Examples
Very high risk (5)		Established cardiovascular disease AND Diabetes Currently smoking Poorly controlled high blood pressure Metabolic syndrome (especially dyslipidemia) Acute coronary syndromes
High risk	>20%	Established CHD Cerebrovascular disease[b] Peripheral arterial disease Abdominal aortic aneurysm Diabetes mellitus Chronic kidney disease[c]
Intermediate risk	10–20%	Subclinical CVD[d] (e.g., coronary calcification) Metabolic syndrome Multiple risk factors[e] Markedly elevated levels of a single risk factor[f] First-degree relative(s) with early-onset atherosclerotic CVD Age < 55 years in men Age < 65 years in women
Lower risk	<10%	May include women with multiple risk factors, metabolic syndrome, or one or no risk factors
Optimal risk	<10%	Optimal levels of risk factors and heart healthy lifestyle

Abbreviations: CHD, coronary heart disease; CVD, cardiovascular disease.

[a] See Ref. 4.

[b] Cerebrovascular disease may not confer high risk for CHD if the affected vasculature is above the carotids. Carotid artery disease (symptomatic or asymptomatic with >50% stenosis) confers high risk.

[c] As chronic kidney disease deteriorates and progresses to end-stage kidney disease, the risk of CVD increases substantially.

[d] Some patients with subclinical CVD will have >20% 10-year CHD risk and should be elevated to the high-risk category.

[e] Patients with multiple risk factors can fall into any of the three categories by Framingham scoring.

[f] Most women with a single, severe risk factor will have a 10-year risk <10%.

years and was characterized by a decrease in HDL-C and increase in LDL-C and TG.[13] In a cross-sectional study, smaller, denser (more atherogenic) LDL-C particles appeared early in the menopausal transition prior to changes in serum LDL-C.[14] The Women's Healthy Lifestyle Project provided evidence that women might be able to

Table 14-5. FRAMINGHAM POINT SCORE ESTIMATE OF 10-YEAR RISK FOR WOMEN*

Framingham Point Score
Estimate of 10-year Risk for Women

Age	Points
20–34	−7
35–39	−3
40–44	0
45–49	3
50–54	6
55–59	8
60–64	10
65–69	12
70–74	14
75–79	16

Total Cholesterol (mg/dL)	Age 20–39	40–49	50–59	60–69	70–79
	Points				
<160	0	0	0	0	0
160–199	4	3	2	1	1
200–239	8	6	4	2	1
240–279	11	8	5	3	2
≥280	13	10	7	4	2

Smoking	Age 20–39	40–45	50–59	60–69	70–79
	Points				
Nonsmoker	0	0	0	0	0
Smoker	9	7	4	2	1

HDL (mg/dL)	Points
≥ 60	−1
50–59	0
40–49	1
<40	2

Systolic BP (mmHg)	If Untreated	If Treated
<120	0	0
120–129	1	3
130–139	2	4
140–159	3	5
≥160	4	6

(*Continued*)

Table 14-5. **FRAMINGHAM POINT SCORE ESTIMATE OF 10-YEAR RISK FOR WOMEN*** **(*CONTINUED*)**

Framingham Point Score
Estimate of 10-year Risk for Women

Point Total	10-Year Risk (%)
≤9	<1
9	1
10	1
11	1
12	1
13	2
14	2
15	3
16	4
17	5
18	6
19	8
20	11
21	14
22	17
23	22
24	27
≥25	≥30

*See Ref. 2.

Source: A more precise method of calculating CHD risk in women is available online at http://www.nhlbi.nih.gov/guidelines/cholesterol/index.htm. Adapted from the Third Report of the National Cholesterol Education Program (NCEP) Expert Panel on Detection Evaluation, and Treatment of High Blood Cholesterol in Adults (Adult Treatment Panel III): Final Report. *Circulation.* 2002;106:3143–3421. Table III, 1-6, p 3231.

prevent the perimenopausal increase in LDL-C. In this randomized controlled trial, 535 women were assigned to placebo or lifestyle intervention during the menopause transition. After 54 months of follow-up, the perimenopausal increase in LDL-C was significantly less in women who ate a prudent diet, exercised, and as a consequence, gained less weight.[15]

Hormone Therapy and Selective Estrogen Receptor Modulators

Hormone therapy (HT) affects lipoprotein concentrations in postmenopausal women. In the Postmenopausal Estrogen and Progestin Intervention (PEPI) trial, oral HT with standard dose (at that time) conjugated equine estrogens and medroxyprogesterone acetate or micronized progesterone increased HDL-C, decreased LDL-C and TC, and increased TG concentrations.[16] Other oral

Table 14-6. **CLINICAL RECOMMENDATIONS FOR LIPID THERAPY**[*]

Diet therapy

In high-risk women or when LDL-C is elevated:

- Saturated fat intake should be reduced to <7% of calories
- Cholesterol intake reduced to <200 mg/day
- Trans fatty acid intake should be reduced

Pharmacotherapy

Very high-risk women

- Initiate statin therapy (unless contraindicated) in women with an LDL-C ≤100 mg/dL to achieve an LDL-C level of <70 mg/dL (a therapeutic option)[†]
- Initiate niacin or fibrate therapy when HDL-C is low[‡] or non-HDL-C elevated[§]

High-risk women (10-year absolute CHD risk >20%)

- Initiate LDL-C lowering therapy (preferably a statin) simultaneously with lifestyle therapy in women with LDL-C ≥100 mg/dL
- Initiate statin therapy (unless contraindicated) in women with an LDL-C ≤100 mg/dL; an LDL-C level goal of ≤70 mg/dL is a therapeutic option[†]
- Initiate niacin or fibrate therapy when HDL-C is low[‡] or non-HDL-C elevated[§]

Intermediate risk women (10-year absolute CHD risk 10–20%)

- Initiate LDL-C lowering therapy (preferable a statin) if LDL-C ≥130 mg/dL on lifestyle therapy
- If LDL-C is 100–129 mg/dL, consider initiating LDL-C lowering therapy to achieve a level of <100 mg/dL (a therapeutic option)
- Initiate niacin or fibrate therapy when HDL-C is low[‡] or non-HDL-C elevated[§] after LDL-C goal is reached

Lower risk women (10-year absolute CHD risk <10%)

- Consider LDL-C lowering therapy in low-risk women with 0 or 1 risk factors when LDL-C level is ≥190 mg/dL
- Consider LDL-C lowering therapy in low-risk women if multiple risk factors (≥2) are present when LDL-C is ≥160 mg/dL
- Consider niacin or fibrate therapy when HDL-C is low[*] or non-HDL-C elevated[**] after LDL-C goal is reached

[*] See Refs. 4 and 5.

[†] See Ref. 5.

[‡] Low HDL in women is < 50 mg/dL.

[§] If triglycerides >200 mg/dL, non-HDL-C is a secondary goal of therapy with a target non-HDL-C level 30 mg/dL higher than the identified LDL-C goal.

estrogen preparations have similar lipid effects. The degree that HDL increases with oral estrogen therapy appears to be under genetic control and related to specific alleles of the estrogen receptor-α[17] Different progestins can modify the lipid response; androgenic progestins reduce HDL-C.[18] Oral methyltestosterone therapy (given with oral esterified estrogens) decreases HDL and TG compared with estrogen alone. However, these changes may be beneficial and reflect a reduction in apoCIII, an emerging risk factor for CHD.[19] Transdermal preparations have less effect on lipid fractions.[18,20] Oral HT has been reported to increase small, dense LDL particles, rendering them more atherogenic.[21] In a head-to-head comparison trial, the deleterious changes in LDL particle size and TG elevation with 0.625-mg conjugated equine estrogen were not present in women assigned to a 0.3 mg dose.[22]

Both raloxifene[23] and tamoxifen[24,25] reduce total and LDL-C to a similar degree as oral estrogen therapy with little to no effect on HDL or TG. If women have recently started or stopped HT, testosterone supplementation, or selective estrogen receptor modulator (SERM) therapy, it makes sense to wait a month or two before checking lipid levels and if necessary, adjusting the dose of lipid-lowering therapy.

Management of Lipoprotein Disorders

Therapeutic Lifestyle Changes

A stepwise approach to managing hyperlipidemia is most practical. The first and universal step is lifestyle modification. TLC include reduced intakes of saturated fats and cholesterol, therapeutic dietary options to enhance LDL lowering (plant stanol/sterols and viscous fiber), weight control, and increased physical activity.[6] Lifestyle modifications are effective and should be encouraged, but success is challenging. A collaborative approach is best.

Medical Therapy for Hyperlipidemia

If TLC do not improve lipid levels to the expected goal after 3 months, if patients have marked hypercholesterolemia, or if cholesterol elevation is noted during hospitalization for an acute coronary event, medical therapy should be initiated promptly and targeted to the specific lipoprotein abnormality.[6] The average of two lipid determinations obtained several weeks apart (while the patient is taking a low-fat diet) should constitute the baseline determination in non-hospitalized patients.[6] The NCEP guidelines focus on LDL-C but also include recommendations for treating other lipid disorders.[2,6]

In this chapter, four categories of dyslipidemia are addressed, keeping in mind that overlap often exists in your patients: increased LDL-C (the primary focus of the NCEP), the syndrome of low HDL-C with elevated TG (characteristic of the metabolic syndrome), hypertriglyceridemia, and isolated low HDL-C. With an awareness of these four categories, the majority of dyslipidemias should be recognized and appropriate treatment initiated. Unless otherwise specified, recommendations are taken from the NCEP ATP III guidelines.[6] and the AHA evidence-based guidelines for CVD prevention in women[4]; evidence summary tables for lipid-lowering therapies can be viewed in an online-only Data Supplement at *http://www.circulationaha.org*. New recommendations for modifications to the ATP III treatment algorithm for LDL-C are also included.[5] For complex dyslipidemias or therapeutic dilemmas, referral is always appropriate.

KEY POINT

Following therapeutic lifestyle changes, statin therapy is the treatment of choice for lowering LDL cholesterol.

Elevated LDL *Statin therapy*: Statin therapy (3-hydroxy3-methyl-glutaryl-coenzyme A [HMG-CoA] reductase inhibitor) is the treatment of choice to lower LDL-C (except in pregnant and nursing women) (Table 14-7). Statins work by blocking the formation of cholesterol in the liver and increasing the production of hepatic LDL receptors enhancing hepatic LDL uptake. Depending upon the statin preparation and dose, LDL can be successfully lowered by 25–50%. When LDL-lowering therapy is used in high-risk or moderately high-risk persons, therapy should achieve at least a 30–40% reduction in LDL-C.[5] Statins are generally administered with the evening meal or at bedtime. After initiating therapy or increasing the dose, lipid levels should be rechecked in 6 weeks, and the dose increased if target goal has not been reached. For every doubling of the dose of statin, LDL levels fall by 6%. Once LDL-C goal has been reached, follow-up should be every 4–6 months with lipid levels measured at least annually. If after 12 weeks, goal has not been achieved, drug therapy can be intensified (increase dose or add another agent) or refer to a lipid specialist. With the availability of well-tolerated drugs such as ezetimibe, it may be more effective to add a second agent prior to increasing the dose of statin therapy—thereby increasing lipid-lowering effectiveness and minimizing side effects.

During the past decade, a number of randomized controlled trials have demonstrated a consistent 20–40% reduction in myocardial infarction, CHD death, and stroke with statin therapy, initially in men with high cholesterol[26] and more recently, in men and women with a history of CHD (Table 14-8). Women generally constitute ≤25% of participants enrolled in statin trials, as is the case with many other cardiovascular therapies.

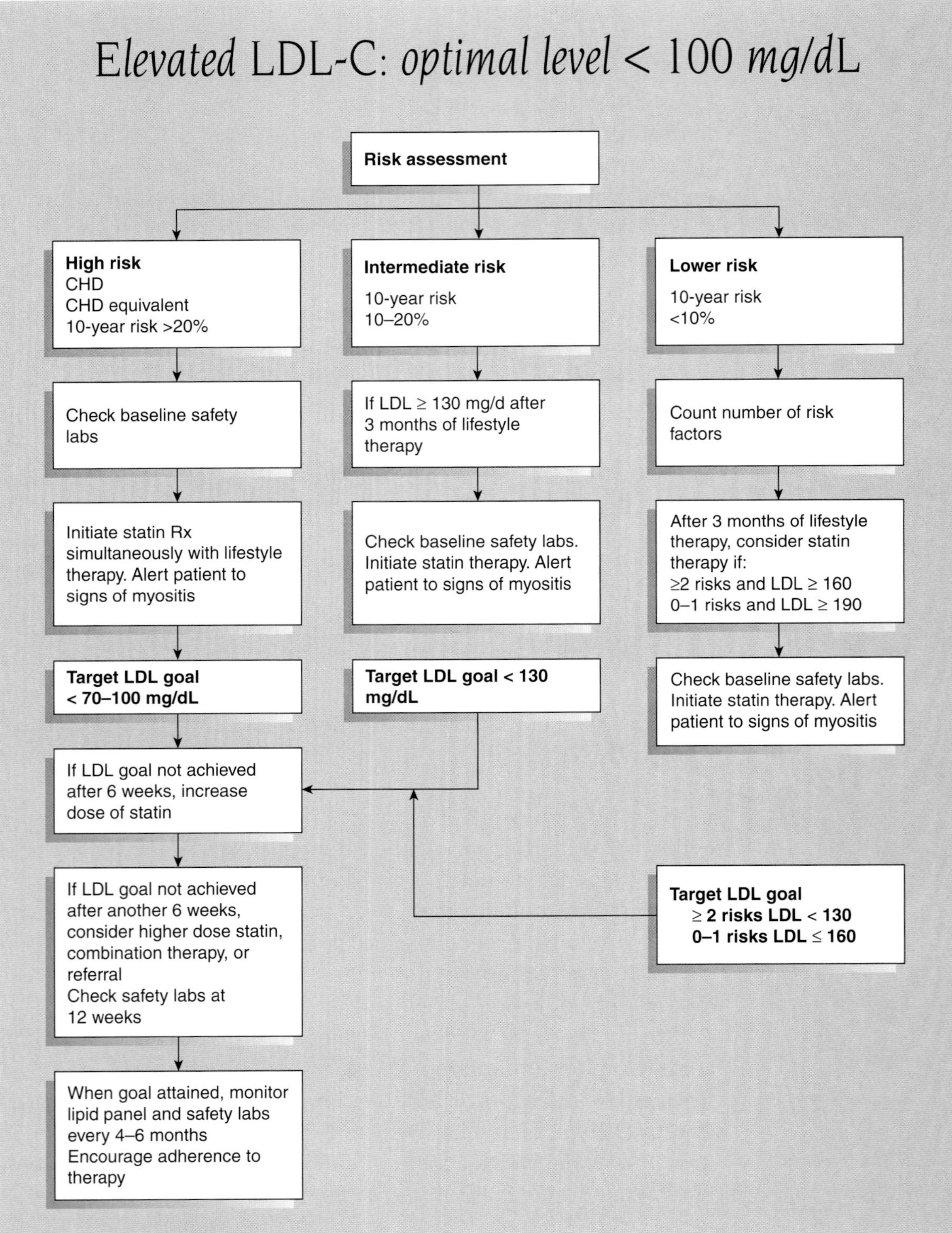
Elevated LDL-C: optimal level < 100 mg/dL
Risk assessment
High risk
CHD
CHD equivalent
10-year risk >20%
Intermediate risk
10-year risk
10–20%
Lower risk
10-year risk
<10%
Check baseline safety labs
If LDL ≥ 130 mg/d after 3 months of lifestyle therapy
Count number of risk factors
Initiate statin Rx simultaneously with lifestyle therapy. Alert patient to signs of myositis
Check baseline safety labs. Initiate statin therapy. Alert patient to signs of myositis
After 3 months of lifestyle therapy, consider statin therapy if:
≥2 risks and LDL ≥ 160
0–1 risks and LDL ≥ 190
Target LDL goal < 70–100 mg/dL
Target LDL goal < 130 mg/dL
Check baseline safety labs. Initiate statin therapy. Alert patient to signs of myositis
If LDL goal not achieved after 6 weeks, increase dose of statin
If LDL goal not achieved after another 6 weeks, consider higher dose statin, combination therapy, or referral
Check safety labs at 12 weeks
Target LDL goal
≥ 2 risks LDL < 130
0–1 risks LDL ≤ 160
When goal attained, monitor lipid panel and safety labs every 4–6 months
Encourage adherence to therapy

Table 14-7. **THERAPEUTIC AGENTS FOR LIPID LOWERING**

DRUG	AVAILABLE DOSAGE	MAXIMUM DOSAGE	DOSE TO ATTAIN
			30–40% LDL Reduction
HMG-CoA reductase inhibitors (statins)			
Atorvastatin	10–80 mg/day	80 mg	10 mg
Fluvastatin	20–80 mg/day	80 mg	40–80 mg
Lovastatin	10–40 mg/day	80 mg	40 mg
Pravastatin	10–80 mg/day	80 mg	40 mg
Rosuvastatin	5–40 mg/day	40 mg	5–10 mg
Simvastatin	5–80 mg/day	80 mg	20–40 mg
Absorption inhibitor			
Ezetimibe	10 mg/day	10 mg/day	
Nicotinic acid			
Crystalline	1.5–3 g/day	4.5 g/day	
Sustained release	1–2 g/day	2 g/day	
Extended release, Niaspan	1–2 g/day	2 g/day	
Fibrates			
Gemfibrozil	600 mg bid	600 mg bid	
Fenofibrate	200 mg/day	200 mg/day	
Clofibrate	1000 mg bid	2000 mg bid	
Bile acid sequestrants			
Cholestyramine	4–16 g/day	24 g/day	
Colesevelam	2.6–3.8 g/day	4.4 g/day	
Colestipol	5–20 g/day	30 g/day	
Combination therapy			
Extended-release niacin	500 mg–2 g/day	2 g/day	
and lovastatin	20–40 mg/day	40 mg/day	
Ezetimibe	10 mg/day	10 mg/day	10 mg/day
and simvastatin	10–80 mg/day	80 mg/day	20 mg/day

SOURCE: Adapted from Drug Update: Lipid modification for secondary prevention of coronary events. Cardiology News, February 2003, NCEP Guidelines, *Circulation.* 2002;106:3143, and Grundy SM, Cleeman JI, Bairey Merz CN, et al. Implications of recent clinical trials for the National Cholesterol Education Program Adult Treatment Panel III Guidelines. *Circulation.* 2004;110:227.

When women *without a history of CVD* were evaluated in a recent meta-analysis of randomized clinical trials of lipid-lowering therapy, total mortality or CHD mortality was not reduced.[39] The authors stated that, "Lipid lowering may reduce CHD events, but current evidence is insufficient to determine this conclusively." In three primary prevention trials (AFCAPS/TexCAPS: Air Force/Texas Coronary Atherosclerosis Prevention

Table 14.8 PIVOTAL RANDOMIZED CLINICAL TRIALS OF STATIN THERAPY WITH CORONARY HEART DISEASE EVENT END POINTS

TRIALS	ENTRY CRITERIA	SUBJECTS (N) TOTAL/WOMEN (%)	DRUG/DOSE	DURATION (YEARS)	RR (95% CI)* OVERALL	MEN	WOMEN
Primary Prevention Trials							
WOSCOPS(26)	High LDL-C	6,595/0 (0)	Pravastatin 40 mg	4.9	0.69 (0.57–0.83)	0.69 (0.57–0.83)	N/A
AFCAPs/ TexCAPS(27)	Low HDL-C	6,605/ 997 (15)	Lovastatin 20–40 mg	5.2	0.63 (0.50–0.79)	0.63 (0.5–0.7)	0.54 (NS)
ALLHAT-LLT(28)	Treated HTN and risks	10,355/2511 (49)	Pravastatin 40 mg	4.8	0.91 (0.79–1.04)	0.84 (0.71–1.00)	1.02(0.81–1.28)
ASCOT(29)	HTN and multiple risk factors	10,305/1942 (19)	Atorvastatin 10 mg	3.3	0.64 (0.50–0.83)	0.59 (0.44–0.77)	1.10 (0.57–2.12)
Secondary Prevention Trials							
4S (30,31)	High cholesterol	4,444/827 (19)	Simvastatin 20–40 mg	5.4	0.66 (.59–.75)	0.66 (0.58–0.76)	0.66 (0.48–0.91)
CARE (32)	Moderate cholesterol	4,159/576 (14)	Pravastatin 40 mg	5.0	0.76 (0.64–0.91)	0.79 (0.65–0.96)	0.57 (0.34–0.96)
LIPID(33)	Moderate cholesterol	9,014/1516 (17)	Pravastatin 40 mg	6.1	0.76 (0.68–0.85)	0.75 (0.65–0.83)	0.89 (0.67–1.18)
PROSPER(34)	Elderly with CVD & risks	5,804/3,000 (52)	Pravastatin 40 mg	3.0	0.81 (0.69–0.94)	0.74 (0.65–0.90)	0.90 (.65-1.18)
HPS(35)	TC > 135 mg/dL	20,536/5,082(24)	Simvastatin 40 mg	5.0	0.76 (0.72–0.8)	0.76 (0.68–0.84)	0.78 (0.70–0.90)
MIRACL(36)	Acute coronary syndrome	3,086/1,074 (35)	Atorvastatin 80 mg	16 week	0.74 (0.57–0.95)†	N/A‡	N/A
Head-to-Head Trials							
PROVE-IT§ (37)	Acute coronary syndrome	4,162/ 911 (22)	Atorvastatin 80 mg vs.Pravastatin 40 mg	2	0.84 (0.74–0.96)	0.87 (0.75–0.99)	0.76 (0.61–0.99)
TNT(38)	CHD	10,003/1902 (19)	Atorvastatin 80 mg vs. Atorvastatin 10 mg	5	trial in progress		

* Primary end point: Nonfatal myocardial infarction and fatal coronary heart disease (unless otherwise specified).

† Recurrent symptomatic muyocardial ischemia with objective evidence and emergency rehospitalization.

‡ Rates in men and women were not available, but no significant interactions between treatment assignment and baseline characteristics (including gender) were reported.

§ Primary end point of death from any cause or a major cardiovascular event. Results given as hazard ratio for the primary end point in the high-dose atorvastatin group as compared with the standard-dose pravastatin group.

WOSCOPS: West of Scotland Coronary Prevention Study Group (Ref. 26).

AFCAPS/TexCAPS: Air Force/Texas Coronary Atherosclerosis Prevention Study (Ref. 27).

ALLHAT-LLT: Antihypertensive and Lipid-Lowering Treatment to Prevent Heart Attack Trial-Lipid Lowering Trial (Ref. 28).

ASCOT: Anglo-Scandinavian Cardiac Outcomes Trial—Lipid Lowering Arm (Ref. 29)

4S: Scandinavian Simvastatin Survival Study (Refs. 30, 31).

CARE: Cholesterol And Recurrent Events (Ref. 32).

LIPID: Long-Term Intervention with Pravastatin in Ischaemic Disease (Ref. 33).

PROSPER: PROspective Study of Pravastatin in the Elderly at Risk (Ref. 34).

HPS: Heart Protection Study (Ref. 35), outcomes given by gender for Vascular Events.

MIRACL: Myocardial Ischemia Reduction with Aggressive Choesterol Lowering (Ref. 36).

PROVE-IT: Pravastatin or Atorvastatin Evaluation and Infection Therapy—Thrombolysis in Myocardial Infarction (Ref. 37).

TNT: Treatment to New Targets (Ref. 38 2004).

Study,[27] the Antihypertensive and Lipid-Lowering Treatment to Prevent Heart Attack Trial (ALLHAT-LLT),[28] and ASCOT: Anglo-Scandinavian Cardiac Outcomes Trial—Lipid Lowering Arm,[29] and two secondary prevention trials, LIPID: Long-Term Intervention with Pravastatin in Ischaemic Disease[33] and the Prospective Study of Pravastatin in Elderly at Risk (PROSPER),[34] CHD event reduction was not significant in women, though a trend to benefit was present, possibly because of the small number of women and few CHD events in some of these trials.

In the same meta-analysis, lipid-lowering therapy in women *with CVD* did not reduce total mortality, but did significantly reduce CHD mortality by 26%, nonfatal myocardial infarction (MI) by 29%, revascularization by 30%, and total CHD events by 20%.[39] The Scandinavian Simvastatin Survival Study (4S) (Scandinavian Simvastatin Survival Group),[30,31] Cholesterol and Recurrent Events (CARE)[32] and Heart Protection Study (HPS)[35] reported significant CHD risk reduction in women with a history of vascular disease (Table 14-8). In a post hoc analysis of the Heart and Estrogen/Progestin Replacement Study (HERS), nonfatal myocardial infarction or coronary heart disease death (relative hazard [RH] 0.79, 95% confidence interval [CI], 0.63–0.99; $P = 0.04$) and total mortality (RH 0.67, 95% CI, 0.51–0.87, $P = 0.003$) were reduced in women taking statin therapy at baseline.[40]

Statin therapy reduced CHD events when given to *high-risk* persons whose LDL-C was already at NCEP target level, challenging the dogma of an LDL-C target goal of 100 mg/dL. In the HPS, in which all participants had a history of vascular disease or diabetes, statin therapy reduced recurrent cardiovascular events regardless of the baseline lipid levels.[35] In three trials (Myocardial Ischemia Reduction with Aggressive Cholesterol Lowering [MIRACL],[36] Pravastatin or Atorvastatin Evaluation and Infection Therapy [PROVE-IT],[37] and Reversal of Atherosclerosis with Aggressive Lipid Lowering [REVERSAL]),[41] intensive LDL-C reduction to 60–70 mg/dL with atorvastatin 80 mg/day was accompanied by further reduction in hospitalizations for acute coronary syndromes (MIRACL), reduction of death or major cardiovascular events after hospitalization for acute coronary syndrome (PROVE-IT), and less progression of atherosclerosis measured by intravascular ultrasound (REVERSAL). While all three trials reported benefit in women, PROVE-IT and REVERSAL showed greater benefit in women than men. In the wake of these trials, the

NCEP ATP III has established a "therapeutic option" that endorses lowering LDL-C to <70 mg/dL in persons at very high risk (Table 14-4), consistent with the general trend of "tightening the belt" on cardiovascular risk factor management.[5] The 2001 NCEP goal of LDL-C <100 mg/dL has been retained as the formal "recommendation" for high-risk patients pending the outcome of ongoing trials.[5]

More data are forthcoming. The Beyond Endorsed Lipid-Lowering with EBT Scanning (BELLES) trial is a 1-year head-to-head trial comparing the effects of standard therapy (Pravastatin 40 mg) to intensive therapy (Atorvastatin 80 mg) on coronary artery calcium score in 600 women with positive coronary calcium scores at randomization who met 2001 NCEP guidelines for LDL-C lowering.[42] A number of clinical end-point trials, including Treating to New Targets (TNT), should further define the effects of aggressive lipid lowering.[38]

Women with LDL levels ≥190 mg/dL usually have a genetic form of hypercholesterolemia: monogenic familial hypercholesterolemia, familial defective apolipoprotein B, or polygenic hypercholesterolemia. Referral for family testing at the time of diagnosis to identify other affected members is important. Statin therapy alone may not be adequate to lower LDL levels to target, and combination therapy with another agent (intestinal absorption inhibitor, nicotinic acid, or bile acid sequestrant) might be required. It is important to realize, however, that when baseline LDL-C is >150 mg/dL, it may not be possible with currently available drugs to achieve an LDL-C <70 mg/dL in high-risk patients.[5] When LDL-lowering therapy is used in high-risk or moderately high-risk persons, however, therapy should achieve at least a 30–40 % reduction in LDL-C.[5]

Statin therapy is safe and well tolerated by most persons.[43] The most common side effects include liver function abnormalities and myopathy. Statin therapy is associated with a dose-dependent 0.5–2% risk per year of abnormalities of liver function characterized by increased hepatic enzymes. The incidence of clinically important (>3 times upper limit of normal) transaminase elevation in large statin trials was not increased compared to placebo, but was increased in head-to-head trials with high-dose statin therapy (PROVE-IT, MIRACL). It is a good idea to have a baseline set of liver enzymes prior to initiating therapy, check another value 6–12 weeks after starting therapy, increasing the dose, or adding a second lipid-lowering agent, and then checking biannually. If an elevation occurs, a decrease in dose or a change to a different statin is usually effective at normalizing enzymes, but occasionally statin therapy will have to be permanently discontinued. Statin therapy is contraindicated in persons with active or chronic liver disease.

Myalgia (muscle pain) is fairly common (5%) with statin therapy (but similar between placebo and drug in randomized trials). Women should be advised to report unexplained muscle pain, tenderness, or weakness, particularly if they also have malaise, fever, or brown urine. Determination of serum creatinine kinase (CK) at baseline and with the occurrence of symptoms will establish the diagnosis of myositis (muscle pain and increased CK) occurring <1/1000 treated persons. The risk of myositis can increase (1% incidence) when statin therapy is combined with gemfibrozil. Rhabdomyolysis, a much less common but potentially fatal side effect (<1 death/million prescriptions), leads to myoglobinuria and acute renal necrosis and is diagnosed by an increase (greater than tenfold) in circulating CK. Complex medical conditions and concurrent therapies (cyclosporine, gemfibrozil, niacin, macrolide antibiotics, certain antifungal drugs, and cytochrome P-450 inhibitors) also increase the risk of rhabdomyolysis. If myositis is present, the statin should be discontinued immediately. Overall, the benefits of statin therapy exceed the risks.[6,43]

Ezetimibe: Ezetimibe, an inhibitor of intestinal cholesterol absorption, reduces TC 13%, LDL 19%, and TG 8% while increasing HDL 3% compared to placebo (Ezetimibe package insert). Maximal response is generally achieved within 2 weeks. Ezetimibe, 10 mg/day, can be used as monotherapy for modest LDL lowering or as combination therapy with statins.[44] The combination of ezetimibe with a statin (Ezetimibe Add-on to Statin for Effectiveness, EASE trial) achieved an additional 23% reduction of cholesterol, a greater magnitude of cholesterol lowering than achieved with either drug alone or the anticipated 6–8% increase by doubling statin dose.[45] Initiating ezetimibe therapy prior to maximizing statin dose might achieve LDL-C goal with fewer side effects. The effects of ezetimibe on cardiovascular morbidity and mortality have not been established. In a study of 18 healthy adult females, coadministration of ezetimibe with oral contraceptives had no significant effect on the bioavailability of ethinyl estradiol or levonorgestrel. In general, ezetimibe has been well tolerated with a slight increase in transaminase elevation when combined with statin therapy. Cholestyramine may interfere with ezetimibe absorption and reduce efficacy. Because of insufficient safety data, use of ezetimibe with fibrates is not recommended at this time.

Nicotinic acid: Nicotinic acid can also be added to statin therapy, especially if increases in HDL and decreases in TG are desired. It is not usually used as monotherapy for LDL lowering, and in general, because of side effects, should be reserved for combination therapy in patients with CHD, CHD equivalents, or 10-year CHD risk of 10–20%. LDL-C will be reduced by 5–25%, HDL increased by 15–35%, and TG reduced by 20–50%. In clinical trials, nicotinic acid has been shown to reduce the risk of recurrent MI and progression of atherosclerosis in combination with other lipid-lowering therapies.[6] The major side effects include flushing, itching, hyperglycemia, hyperuricemia or gout, upper gastrointestinal distress, peptic ulcer, and hepatotoxicity (sustained release forms). Nicotinic acid is contraindicated in patients with chronic liver disease and severe gout. Relative contraindications include hyperuricemia and type 2 diabetes. Extended release nicotinic acid (Niaspan) is taken at bedtime, better tolerated, and has fewer side effects than other nicotinic acid preparations. For maximum benefit, if tolerated, nicotinic acid should be titrated to at least 2 g/day, starting at 500 mg/day.

Fibrates: Addition of a fibrate (fenofibrate) to statin therapy may be useful to lower LDL in select patients who have not tolerated other therapies or who have combined hyperlipidemia, even though the fibrates (gemfibrozil, fenofibrate, and clofibrate) are usually reserved for treatment of hypertriglyceridemia. Reduction of CHD death and MI has been observed in some but not all fibrate trials.[6] Because of the potential for increased risk of myopathy, combination therapy of fibrates with statins should be undertaken by those experienced in treating lipid disorders. Fenofibrate has less likelihood of side effects than gemfibrozil and is preferred in combination with statins. Fibrates may be associated with abdominal pain, headache, drowsiness, and increased risk of cholelithiasis.

Bile acid sequestrants: Bile acid sequestrants are powders that must be taken once or twice daily with meals. They lower LDL-C 15–30% and increase HDL-C by 3–5%. Added to a statin, sequestrants lower LDL another 12–16%. Clinical trials have demonstrated evidence of CHD risk reduction and lack of systemic toxicity.[6] Bile acid sequestrants can be used alone in younger persons, women contemplating pregnancy, and when only modest LDL lowering is necessary. In clinical trials, bile acid sequestrants did not demonstrate systemic toxicity. The most common complaints included inconvenience of administration and gastrointestinal symptoms, usually constipation. Bile acid sequestrants (except colesevalam) can interfere with absorption of concurrent medications (other drugs should be taken an hour before or 4 hours after). Bile acid sequestrants (except colesevelam) raise serum TG levels and should not be used in women with TG >400 mg/dL and with caution if TG >200 mg/dL. Because better medications are available, bile acid sequestrants are no longer commonly used.

Postmenopausal therapies: HT should not be initiated for lipid benefits. The NCEP guidelines from 2001 reverse their previous recommendations and state, "the favorable effects of statin therapy in women in clinical trials make a cholesterol-lowering drug preferable to hormone replacement therapy for CHD risk reduction."[2] Because of the lack of benefit and early harm in recent randomized clinical trials,[46–48] the AHA, in its evidence-based guidelines for CVD prevention in women, recommends that combined HT should not be initiated or continued to prevent CVD in postmenopausal women nor should unopposed estrogen be initiated or continued to prevent CVD in postmenopausal women.[4]

The effect of SERM therapy on CHD events is uncertain. In both the Breast Cancer Prevention Trial (BCPT) and the International Breast Cancer Intervention Study (IBIS-1) of healthy women with increased risks for breast cancer, tamoxifen neither increased nor decreased CHD events.[49,50] In a post hoc analysis of an osteoporosis treatment clinical trial, raloxifene reduced cardiovascular events by more than 40% in women with a history of CHD or CHD risk factors.[51] Unless cardiovascular benefit is conclusively demonstrated in the recently completed RUTH (Raloxifene Use for The

Heart) trial,[52] raloxifene should not be prescribed for treatment of hypercholesterolemia or CHD prevention.[51]

Decreased HDL and Increased TG (with or without Increased LDL) Any woman with low HDL-C (<50 mg/dL) and an elevated TG (≥150 mg/dL) should be carefully evaluated for other components of the metabolic syndrome, which includes a constellation of cardiovascular risk factors (Table 14-1). In the NCEP guidelines, lifestyle modification (weight loss and exercise to reduce insulin resistance) is the primary treatment recommended for patients with the metabolic syndrome.[2] In the Diabetes Prevention Program (consisting of 68% women), intensive lifestyle coaching enabled participants at risk for diabetes to reduce weight by 7% and increase exercise to 30 minutes five times a week. With this regimen, the incidence of new cases of diabetes was reduced by 58% over 2.8 years of follow-up, more than with metformin therapy (31% reduction).[53]

KEY POINT

The dyslipidemia of the metabolic syndrome is characterized by high triglycerides and low HDL-cholesterol.

Cardiovascular risk is increased in persons with the metabolic syndrome.[54–56] In an analysis of the placebo groups in the 4S and the AFCAPS/TexCAPS trials, patients with the metabolic syndrome showed increased risk of major coronary events regardless of their Framingham calculated risk score.[56] The NCEP guidelines do not provide clear targets for lipid therapy in patients with the metabolic syndrome except for treatment of LDL-C. If LDL-C is above target, statin therapy is the initial treatment choice. Statin therapy increases HDL-C by at least 5–10%, possibly more in women with the metabolic syndrome, and reductions in TG levels range from 7 to 30%.[6]

If LDL-C is <130 mg/dL in the face of low HDL and high TG, fibrate monotherapy could be the first choice.[57] Gemfibrozil increased HDL and reduced CHD events in men with low HDL and hypertriglyceridemia in the Helsinki Heart Study (primary prevention),[58] and in the secondary prevention Veterans Affairs High-Density Lipoprotein Cholesterol Intervention Trial (VA-HIT).[59] The Bezafibrate Infarction Prevention (BIP) Study, another secondary prevention trial, showed a 40% reduction in recurrent CHD in patients (92% men) with HDL ≤45 mg/dL and TG ≥200 mg/dL.[60] Fenofibrate is safer than other fibrates in combination with statin therapy because it does not interfere with statin metabolism and can be taken once a day.

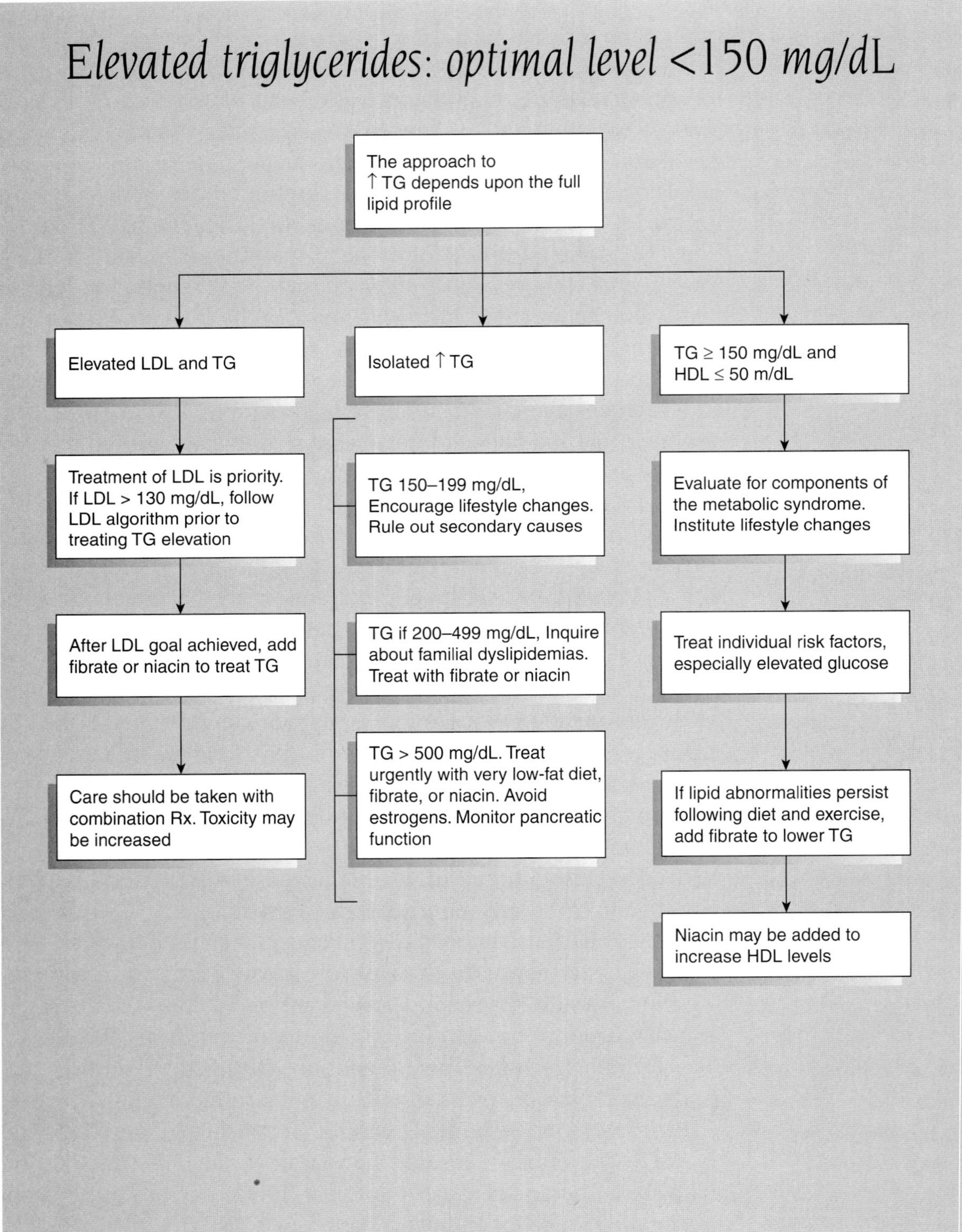
Elevated triglycerides: optimal level <150 mg/dL
The approach to ↑ TG depends upon the full lipid profile
Elevated LDL and TG
Isolated ↑ TG
TG ≥ 150 mg/dL and HDL ≤ 50 m/dL
Treatment of LDL is priority. If LDL > 130 mg/dL, follow LDL algorithm prior to treating TG elevation
TG 150–199 mg/dL, Encourage lifestyle changes. Rule out secondary causes
Evaluate for components of the metabolic syndrome. Institute lifestyle changes
After LDL goal achieved, add fibrate or niacin to treat TG
TG if 200–499 mg/dL, Inquire about familial dyslipidemias. Treat with fibrate or niacin
Treat individual risk factors, especially elevated glucose
Care should be taken with combination Rx. Toxicity may be increased
TG > 500 mg/dL. Treat urgently with very low-fat diet, fibrate, or niacin. Avoid estrogens. Monitor pancreatic function
If lipid abnormalities persist following diet and exercise, add fibrate to lower TG
Niacin may be added to increase HDL levels

Isolated Hypertriglyceridemia (with Normal HDL and LDL) Borderline high TG (between 150 and 199 mg/dL) usually reflect lifestyle (obesity, physical inactivity, cigarette smoking, excessive alcohol consumption, high carbohydrate diets >60% energy intake), and secondary causes (type 2 diabetes, chronic renal failure, and nephrotic syndrome, Cushing's disease, lipodystrophy, and drugs). In practice, the most common contributing factor to TG levels >150 mg/dL is insulin resistance and the metabolic syndrome.[6] If TG are borderline high (150–199 mg/dL), lifestyle changes may be adequate to reduce serum TG to <150 mg/dL. If LDL-C is also elevated, reduction of LDL with statin therapy should be the primary goal of therapy.

KEY POINT

Both niacin and fibrate therapy effectively reduce high triglyceride levels.

If the fasting triglyceride level is greater than 200 mg/dL, an inquiry should be made about family history of dyslipidemia, (familial combined hyperlipidemia, familial hypertriglyceridemia, and familial dysbetalipoproteinemia). In patients with high TG (200–499 mg/dL), LDL-C is still the primary target of therapy; non-HDL-C is the secondary target.[5] If LDL is elevated, statin therapy will also reduce TG by 20–40%. Once LDL goal has been achieved, elevated non-HDL-C should be treated by increasing the statin dose or by adding nicotinic acid or a fibrate.[6] Non-HDL-C goal is 30 mg/dL higher than LDL-C goal (Table 14-6).[6]

If LDL is within target from the onset, a specific triglyceride-lowering drug should be used to treat non-HDL-C. Nicotinic acid reduces TG by 30–50% and raises HDL by 20–30%. If nicotinic acid is not tolerated or contraindicated, fibric acid derivatives, such as gemfibrozil 600 mg twice daily or fenofibrate 200 mg once daily, will reduce TG by 40–60% and raise HDL by 15–25%. If LDL-C levels increase on fibrate therapy, a statin could be added. Another possible adjunct to statin therapy is supplements of long chain *n*-3 polyunsaturated fatty acids present in fish oil. A dose of 3 g/day reduces TG by 30%. Bile acid sequestrants are contraindicated as monotherapy because they raise TG.

If TG levels are very high (>500 mg/dL), urgent therapy to reduce the risk of pancreatitis is indicated. Therapy should include a very low-fat diet (<15% of total calories), weight reduction, increased physical activity, and drug therapy with nicotinic acid or a fibrate. When TG levels are reduced to <500 mg/dL, LDL again becomes the therapeutic target.[6] Because of the potential for oral estrogens to increase TG, care should be given when initiating estrogen therapy in women with elevated TG. Though rare, cases of pancreatitis have been associated with estrogen-induced hypertriglyceridemia.[61] If the fasting TG level is greater than 250 mg/dL, transdermal rather than oral estrogens should be cautiously considered. If estrogens are prescribed, fasting TG levels should be monitored within 2 weeks of starting therapy.[62] Because of the risk of pancreatitis, oral estrogens are contraindicated if the fasting triglyceride level is markedly elevated.[61] If a woman develops pancreatitis while taking estrogen, discontinue estrogen immediately. Women with a history of oral estrogen-induced hypertriglyceridemia should have TG monitored while taking raloxifene therapy.[63,64]

Low HDL (without Hypertriglyceridemia or Elevated LDL) Obesity, physical inactivity, metabolic syndrome, and genetic factors contribute to low HDL (<50 mg/dL) in women. Though low HDL is an independent CHD risk factor, the NCEP guidelines do not specify an HDL target for therapy.[5] Patients with CVD, the metabolic syndrome, or CHD risk equivalents with low HDL could be treated to raise HDL-C to >40 mg/dL.[57] Because lowering LDL may reduce risk, statin therapy may still be effective. In the AFCAPS/TexCAPS trial, healthy persons with low HDL (<40mg/dL) and LDL-C of 150 mg/dL randomized to statin therapy (which increases HDL 6–14%) had a reduction of first myocardial infarction.[27] Nicotinic acid is the most effective HDL-raising drug, and in combination with statin therapy, has additive effects.[65] In the HDL-Atherosclerosis Treatment Study (HATS) (13% of the 160 participants were women), combination therapy with niacin and simvastatin increased HDL by 26% and decreased CVD outcomes by 60%.[66] The effect of fibrate therapy on raising HDL is intermediate between the effects of niacin and statin. In clinical trials, experimental therapy with short-term HDL infusions reduced the volume of coronary atheromas on intravascular ultrasound,[67] and treatment with torcetrapib, a potent inhibitor of cholesteryl ester transfer protein, raised serum HDL-C levels by 60–100% when used as monotherapy or in conjunction with statin therapy.[68] Cardiac outcomes were not measured.

In women with isolated low HDL and no apparent risk factors, lifestyle improvements should be the cornerstone of therapy. Further delineation of risk with emerging risk factor analysis such as highly sensitive C-reactive protein or noninvasive measures of subclinical atherosclerosis (carotid intimal-medial thickness or coronary artery calcium scanning) might be helpful to define risk and justify therapy.

New and Emerging Cardiovascular Risk Factors

Our ability to identify persons at risk for CVD will be enhanced by exploration and refinement of new risk factors. For example, the new AHA recommendations for prevention of CHD in women assign positive coronary artery calcium determined by electron-computed tomography to the intermediate risk group with specific treatment implications. Levels of coronary calcium that imply increased risk are uncertain. Other risk factors such as high-sensitivity C-reactive protein, fibrinogen, lipoprotein(a), homocysteine, and LDL-C particle size and characteristics may become increasingly important in clinical assessment and identification of appropriate candidates for therapy.

High-sensitivity C-reactive protein (hs-CRP) is a marker of systemic inflammation that has received increasing attention as a possible independent risk factor for CHD,[69] and a possible indication for statin therapy. In AFCAPS/TexCAPS trial, statin therapy reduced cardiovascular events in participants with hs-CRP above the median (1.6 mg/L), even if the ratio of total to HDL-C was lower than the median.[70]

A statement from the Centers for Disease Control and Prevention and the AHA recommended against screening the entire population for hs-CRP and suggested that testing be reserved for individuals with intermediate risk (10-year CHD risk in the range of 10–20%) to increase motivation for lifestyle improvements or to justify more intense medical therapy.[71] Though the role of hs-CRP is considered controversial,[72] ongoing clinical trials will evaluate statin therapy in persons with elevated hs-CRP (but lipid levels that would not meet NCEP guidelines for therapy) to assess CHD benefit.[73]

Future Directions in Lipid Management

Since the publication of the NCEP ATP III guidelines, new clinical trial evidence in very high-risk persons shows added cardiovascular benefit when lower LDL-C (i.e., 60 or 70 mg/dL) levels are achieved. The benefits of raising HDL have also been highlighted by randomized clinical trials. The increasing prevalence of the metabolic syndrome will necessitate clear guidelines for risk management. Combination therapy will become the rule rather than the exception as fewer side effects and greater potency are demonstrated. Finally, accrual of clinical trial data in women will help to finesse recommendations specific to women for cholesterol lowering and heart disease prevention.

Guideline Questions

- What is the risk of coronary heart disease in your patient?
- If her lipid profile is abnormal, what other medical conditions might contribute to the dyslipidemia?
- At what level of LDL cholesterol should you institute medical therapy?
- How does the presence of hypertriglyceridemia alter your approach?
- What if the only abnormality is a low HDL cholesterol level?
- What are the risks of therapy for hyperlipidemia?
- When should you consider combination therapy?

Discussion of Cases

CASE 1

A 56-year-old postmenopausal woman on HT for the last 8 years is found to have an electrocardiogram (ECG) consistent with a silent myocardial infarction. She is an ex-smoker and denies a history of hypertension or diabetes. She exercises 30 minutes four times/week and follows a low-fat diet.

Her BMI is 27 kg/m^2, blood pressure is 128/75, no evidence of bruits or subcutaneous cholesterol deposits.

What is her absolute future risk of CVD?

Clearly this woman presents with a history of a myocardial infarction and meets criteria for being in a high-risk group as defined by the NCEP guidelines (10-year absolute risk of CVD >20%). She will therefore have the most aggressive targets for LDL lowering.

What laboratory evaluation do you want to pursue?

The lipid panel is critical to plan a treatment strategy. Her lipid levels after an overnight 12-hour fast reveal:

TC	**231 mg/dL**
HDL	**45 mg/dL**
LDL	**142 mg/dL**
TG	**220 mg/dL**

What other laboratory evaluation is important?

A measurement of TSH should be included to rule out hypothyroidism. Hypothyroidism commonly occurs in perimenopausal/ postmenopausal women and can contribute to dyslipidemia. Fasting blood glucose to rule out prediabetes or impaired glucose tolerance

is also reasonable in this woman with a history of premature CHD. Baseline safety labs can be ordered in anticipation of lipid therapy. Hepatic transaminases and creatinine are reasonable baseline safety labs. A creatinine phosphokinase (CK) measurement is also prudent to establish the baseline level prior to starting statin therapy.

Results:

- Normal fasting blood glucose
- Normal thyroid function tests
- Normal liver function tests (LFTs)
- Normal creatinine
- Normal creatine kinase (CK)

How should she be treated?

In the high-risk group (history of CVD), the LDL-C treatment goal is 100 mg/dL (with a therapeutic option of LDL-C <70 mg/dL). This patient's LDL is 142 mg/dL, which qualifies her for lipid-lowering therapy, preferably with a statin. Her baseline labs are normal. Any statin could be instituted depending upon the medical care plan, and so forth. A reasonable goal is to reduce her LDL-C by 30–40%.

It is also important to discuss with her the advisability of discontinuing HT. In the Women's Health Initiative (WHI), HT was associated with an increased risk of CHD, particularly in the first year of therapy, and an ongoing increased risk of stroke and venous thromboembolic events. In the HERS trial and other trials in women with a history of CHD, there was no cardiac benefit to continuing HT. Therefore, she should probably be advised to discontinue therapy. If she has persistent vasomotor symptoms, a lower dose of estrogen or other nonhormonal preparation could be initiated. Remember that her lipid profile might deteriorate slightly upon stopping the HT.

How should therapy be monitored?

Recheck her lipids and safety labs after 6–12 weeks of therapy. If the transaminases have increased more than threefold from baseline, reduce the dose of the statin and recheck transaminases in a few weeks. Another approach would be to switch to another statin preparation.

If she complains of muscle aches and pains, obtain another CK determination. If the CK is more than 10 times the upper limit of normal, discontinue therapy and repeat CK weekly until it normalizes. In the rare instance of marked CPK elevation, myoglobin released by damaged muscle can cause renal impairment. In that case, renal function should also be followed closely. For CK levels 3–10 times the upper limit of normal, follow symptoms and CK levels weekly until resolution occurs.

What else should be considered?

Statin therapy might reduce the LDL-C to expected level but the addition of ezetimibe can enable you to reach LDL goal at a lower statin dose, therefore, reducing the incidence of side effects associated with maximal dose therapy. It will be important to follow the HDL and TG levels. Recall that HDL in women should be >50 mg/dL and TG should be <150 mg/dL. If TG remains elevated in spite of statin therapy, fibrate therapy could be added. Be aware that combination statin/fibrate therapy carries a higher risk of side effects, though these are less common with fenofibrate than other fibrates. Addition of a fibrate would also raise HDL to some extent, though formal treatment goals have not been established. Monitoring of transaminases and CK should continue when new drugs are initiated or doses changed.

What's the Evidence?

What is the evidence that statin therapy reduces cardiovascular events in women? All secondary prevention trials, with two exceptions (LIPID and PROSPER), have demonstrated a significant reduction in cardiovascular end points in women (Table 14-8). Two recent head-to-head statin trials (PROVE-IT and REVERSAL) demonstrated comparable (or greater) reduction of acute coronary events and progression of atherosclerosis with aggressive lipid-lowering therapy in women with CHD compared to men. For primary prevention, three trials have included women. In the AFCAPS/TexCAPS trial, the effect of statin therapy on first acute major coronary events was greater in women (though not statistically significant) than in men, but the number of women in the trial and the number of events in women were small. In the ASCOT trial, no significant benefit was apparent among women. However, total cardiovascular events were reduced by 20% in women ($P = 0.17$) and total coronary events were reduced by 14% ($P = 0.56$). In neither trials was there a significant interaction between sex and the impact of statin on the primary end point of CHD death and nonfatal myocardial infarction. In ALLHAT-LLT, neither men nor women showed benefit with statin therapy. A recent meta-analysis of lipid-lowering clinical trials concluded that currently available evidence is insufficient to determine if lipid-lowering agents reduce CHD events in women with no previous history of CVD.[39]

What is the evidence that treating LDL-C is beneficial in persons with the metabolic syndrome? No randomized controlled trials examining statin effects on CHD events exclusively in patients with the metabolic syndrome have been conducted. In a post hoc analysis of the 4S trial, persons with the metabolic syndrome (HDL-C <39 mg/dL and TG >159 mg/dL) had the highest coronary event rate in the placebo group and the largest event reduction (52%) in the treatment group, a treatment effect more substantial than in the group with isolated increased LDL-C.[54] The subset of the 4S trial participants with metabolic syndrome, however, included only 458 persons, 93% of which were men. An analysis of the placebo group in AFCAPS/TexCAPS (1467 persons with metabolic syndrome, 22% women) showed similar increased CHD risks.[56] As stated in a recent Scientific Statement from the

AHA and the NHLBI, "No specific drugs are currently recommended for people with the metabolic syndrome independent of those agents most appropriate for specific, abnormal risk factors."[3]

References

1 American Heart Association. *Women, Heart Disease, and Stroke Statistics.* Dallas, TX: American Heart Association Web site, accessed January 27, 2004.

2 Expert Panel on Detection, Evaluation, and Treatment of High Blood Cholesterol in Adults: Executive summary of the third report of the National Cholesterol Education Program (NCEP) expert panel on detection, evaluation, and treatment of high blood cholesterol in adults (Adult Treatment Panel III). *JAMA.* 2001;285;2486.

3 Stampfer MJ, Hu FB, Manson JE, et al. Primary prevention of coronary heart disease in women through diet and lifestyle. *N Engl J Med.* 2000;343:16.

4 Mosca L, Appel LJ, Benjamin EJ, et al. Evidence-based guidelines for cardiovascular disease prevention in women. *Circulation.* 2004;109:672.

5 Grundy SM, Cleeman JI, Bairey Merz CN, et al. Implications of recent clinical trials for the National Cholesterol Education Program Adult Treatment Panel III Guidelines. *Circulation.* 2004;110:227.

6 National Cholesterol Education Program Expert Panel on Detection, Evaluation, and Treatment of High Blood Cholesterol in Adults (Adult Treatment Panel III). Final Report. *Circulation.* 2002;106:3143.

7 Grundy SM, Hansen B, Smith SC, et al. Clinical management of metabolic syndrome. Report of the American Heart Association/National Heart, Lung, and Blood Institute/American Diabetes Association conference on Scientific Issues Related to Management. *Circulation.* 2004;109:551.

8 Ford ES, Giles WH, Dietz WH. Prevalence of the metabolic syndrome among U.S. adults. *JAMA.* 2002;287:356.

9 Legro RS, Urbanek M, Kunselman AR, et al. Self-selected women with polycystic ovary syndrome are reproductively and metabolically abnormal and undertreated. *Fertil Steril.* 2002;78:51.

10 Christian RC, Dumesic DA, Behrenbeck T, et al. Prevalence and predictors of coronary artery calcification in women with polycystic ovary syndrome. *J Clin Endocrinol Metab.* 2003;88:2562.

11 Talbott EO,Guzick D, Sutton-Tyrell K, et al. Evidence for association between polycystic ovary syndrome and premature carotid atherosclerosis in middle-aged women. *Arterioscler Thromb Vasc Biol.* 2000;23:2414.

12 Pearson TA, Blair SN, Daniels SR, et al. AHA Guidelines for primary prevention of cardiovascular disease and stroke: 2002 update. *Circulation.* 2002;106:388.

13 Matthews KA, Kuller LH, Sutton-Tyrrell K, et al. Changes in cardiovascular risk factors during the perimenopause and postmenopause and carotid artery atherosclerosis in healthy women. *Stroke.* 2001; 32:1104.

14 Carr MC, Kim KH, Zambon A, et al. Changes in LDL density across the menopause transition. *J Investig Med.* 2000;48:245.

15 Kuller LH, Simkin-Silverman LR, Wing RR, et al. Women's Healthy Lifestyle Project: a randomized clinical trial. *Circulation.* 2001;103:32.

16 The Writing Group for the PEPI Trial. Effects of estrogen or estrogen/progestin regimens on heart disease risk factors in postmenopausal women. *JAMA.* 1995;273:199.

17 Herrington DM, Howard TD, Hawkins GA, et al. Estrogen-receptor polymorphisms and effects of estrogen replacement on high-density lipoprotein cholesterol in women with coronary disease. *N Engl J Med.* 2002;346:967.

18 Godsland IF. Effects of postmenopausal hormone replacement therapy on lipid, lipoprotein, and apolipoprotein (a) concentrations: analysis of studies published from 1974-2000. *Fertil Steril.* 2001;75:898.

19 Chiuve SE, Martin LA, Campos H, et al. Effect of the combination of methyltestosterone and esterified estrogens compared with esterified estrogens alone on apolipoprotein CIII and other apolipoproteins in very low density, low density, and high density lipoproteins in surgically postmenopausal women. *J Clin Endocrinol Metab.* 2004;89:2207.

20 Shifren JL, Braunstein GC, Simon JA, et al. Transdermal testosterone treatment in women with impaired sexual function after oophorectomy. *N Engl J Med.* 2000;343:682.

21 Wakatsuki A, Ikenoue N, Okatani Y, et al. Estrogen-induced small low density lipoprotein particles may be atherogenic in postmenopausal women. *J Am Coll Cardiol.* 2001;37:425.

22 Wakatsuki A, Okatani Y, Ikenoue N, et al. Effect of lower dose of oral conjugated equine estrogen on size and oxidative susceptibility of low-density lipoprotein particles in postmenopausal women. *Circulation.* 2003;108:808.

23 Walsh BW, Kuller LH, Wild RA, et al. Effects of raloxifene on serum lipids and coagulation factors in healthy postmenopausal women. *JAMA.* 1998;279:1445.

24 Love RR, Wiebe DA, Newcomb PA, et al. Effects of tamoxifen on cardiovascular risk factors in postmenopausal women. *Ann Intern Med.* 1991;115:860.

25 Love RR, Wiebe DA, Feyzi JM, et al. Effects of tamoxifen on cardiovascular risk factors in postmenopausal women after 5 years of treatment. *J Natl Cancer Inst.* 1994;86:1534.

26 Shepherd J, Cobbe SM, Ford I, et al. Prevention of coronary heart disease with pravastatin in men with hypercholesterolemia. West of Scotland Coronary Prevention Study Group. *N Engl J Med.* 1995;333:1301.

27 Downs JR, Clearfield M, Weis S, et al for the AFCAPS/TexCAPS Research Group. Primary prevention of acute coronary events with lovastatin in men and women with average cholesterol levels: results of AFCAPS/TexCAPS. *JAMA.* 1998;279:1615.

28 ALLHAT Officers. Major outcomes in moderately hypercholesterolemic, hypertensive patients randomized to pravastatin vs usual care. The Antihypertensive and Lipid-Lowering Treatment to Prevent Heart Attack Trial (ALLHAT-LLT). *JAMA.* 2002;288:2998.

29 Sever PS, Bahlof B, Poulter NR, et al. Prevention of coronary and stroke events with atorvastatin in hypertensive patients who have average or lower-than-average cholesterol concentrations, in the Anglo-Scandinavian Cardiac Outcomes Trial—Lipid Lowering Arm (ASCOT-LLA): a multicentre randomized controlled trial. *Lancet.* 2003;361:1149.

30 Scandinavian Simvastatin Survival Group. Randomised trial of cholesterol lowering in 4444 patients with coronary heart disease: the Scandinavian Simvastatin Survival Study (4S). *Lancet.* 1994;344:1383.

31 Miettinen TA, Pyorala K, Losson AG, et al. Cholesterol-lowering therapy in women and elderly patients with myocardial infarction or angina pectoris: findings from the Scandinavian Simvastatin Survival Study (4S). *Circulation.* 1997;96:4211.

32 Lewis S, Sacks FM, Mitchell JS, et al. for the CARE Investigators. Effects of pravastatin on cardiovascular events in women after myocardial infarction: the Cholesterol and Recurrent Events (CARE) Trial. *J Am Coll Cardiol.* 1998;32:140.

33 The Long-Term Intervention with Pravastatin in Ischemic Disease (LIPID) Study Group. Prevention of cardiovascular events and death with pravastatin in patients with coronary heart disease and a broad range of initial cholesterol levels. *N Engl J Med.* 1998;339:1349.

34 Shepherd J, Blauw GJ, Murphy MB, et al. Pravastatin in elderly individuals at risk of vascular disease (PROSPER): a randomized controlled trial. *Lancet.* 2002;360:1623x.

35 Heart Protection Study Collaborative Group. MRC/BHF Heart Protection Study of cholesterol-lowering with simvastatin in 20 536 high risk individuals: a randomised placebo-controlled trial. *Lancet.* 2002;360:7.

36 Schwartz GG, Olsson AG, Ezekowitz MD, et al. Myocardial Ischemia Reduction with Aggressive Cholesterol Lowering (MIRACL) Study

Investigators. Effects of atorvastatin on early recurrent ischemic events in acute coronary syndromes: the MIRACL study: a randomized controlled trial. *JAMA.* 2001;285:1711.

37 Cannon CP, Braunwald E, McCabe CH, et al. for the Pravastatin or Atorvastatin Evaluation and Infection Therapy—Thrombolysis in Myocardial Infarction 22 Investigators. Intensive versus moderate lipid lowering with statins after acute coronary syndromes. *N Engl J Med.* 2004;350:1495.

38 Waters DD, Guyton JR, Herrington DM, et al. Treating to New Targets (TNT) Study: does lowering low-density lipoprotein cholesterol levels below currently recommended guidelines yield incremental clinical benefit? *Am J Cardiol.* 2004;93:154.

39 Walsh JME, Pignone M. Drug treatment of hyperlipidemia in women. *JAMA. 2004*;291:2243.

40 Herrington DM, Vittinghoff E, Lin F, et al. Statin therapy, cardiovascular events, and total mortality in the Heart and Estrogen/Progestin Replacement Study (HERS). *Circulation.* 2002;105:2962.

41 Nissen SE, Tuzcu EM, Schoenhagen P, et al. REVERSAL Investigators. Effect of intensive compared with moderate lipid-lowering therapy on progression of coronary atherosclerosis: a randomized controlled trial. *JAMA.* 2004;291:1071.

42 Raggi P, Callister TZ, Davidson M, et al. Aggressive versus moderate lipid-lowering therapy in postmenopausal women with hypercholesterolemia: rational and design of the Beyond Endorsed lipid Lowering with EBT Scanning (BELLES). *Am Heart J.* 2001;141:722.

43 Pasternak RC, Smith SC Jr, Bairey-Merz CN, et al. American Heart Association; National Heart, Lung and Blood Institute. ACC/AHA/NHLBI Clinical Advisory on the use and safety of statins. *Circulation.* 2002;106:1024.

44 Gagne C, Bays HE, Weiss SR, et al. for the Ezetimibe Study Group. Efficacy and safety of ezetimibe added to ongoing statin therapy for treatment of patients with primary hypercholesterolemia. *Am J Cardiol.* 2002;90:1084.

45 Pearson T, Denke M, McBride P, et al. Ezetimibe added to statin therapy reduces LDL-C and improves goal attainment in patients with hypercholesterolemia. March 7–10, 2004, American College of Cardiology, New Orleans.

46 Writing Group for the Women's Health Initiative. Risks and benefits of estrogen plus progestin in healthy postmenopausal women. *JAMA.* 2002;288:321.

47 Manson JE, Hsia J, Johnson KC, et al. Estrogen plus progestin and the risk of coronary heart disease. *N Engl J Med.* 2003;349:523.

48 The Women's Health Initiative Steering Committee. Effects of conjugated equine estrogen in postmenopausal women with hysterectomy. The Women's Health Initiative Randomized Controlled Trial. *JAMA.* 2004;291:1701.

49 Reis SE, Costantino JP, Wickerham DL, et al. Cardiovascular effects of tamoxifen in women with and without heart disease: breast cancer prevention trial. National Surgical Adjuvant Breast and Bowel Project breast Cancer Prevention Trial Investigators. *J Natl Cancer Inst.* 2001;93:16.

50 Cuzick J, Forbes J, Edwards R, et al. First results from the International Breast Cancer Intervention Study (IBIS-I): a randomized prevention trial. *Lancet.* 2002;360:817.

51 Barrett-Connor E, Grady D, Sashegyi A, et al. for the MORE Investigators. Raloxifene and cardiovascular events in osteoporotic postmenopausal women: four-year results from the MORE (Multiple outcomes of Raloxifene Evaluation) randomized trial. *JAMA.* 2002; 287:847.

52 Mosca L, Barrett-Connor E, Wenger NK, et al. Design and methods of the Raloxifene Use for The Heart (RUTH) study. *Am J Cardiol.* 2001;88:392.

53 Knowler WC, Barrett-Connor E, Fowler SE. Reduction in the incidence of type 2 diabetes with lifestyle or metformin. *N Engl J Med.* 2002;346:393.

54 Ballantyne CM, Olsson AG, Cook TJ, et al. Influence of low high-density lipoprotein cholesterol and elevated triglyceride on coronary heart disease events and response to simvastatin therapy in 4S. *Circulation.* 2001;104:3046.

55 Vega GL, Ma PT, Cater NB, et al. Effects of adding fenofibrate (200 mg/day) to simvastatin (10 mg/day) in patients with combined hyperlipidemia and metabolic syndrome. *Am J Cardiol.* 2003;91:956.

56 Girman CJ, Rhodes T, Mercuri M, et al., the AFCAPS/TexCAPS Research Group. The metabolic syndrome and risk of major coronary events in the Scandinavian Simvastatin Survival Study (4S) and the Air Force/Texas Coronary Atherosclerosis Prevention Study (AFCAPS/TexCAPS). *Am J Cardiol.* 2004;93:136.

57 Toth PP. High-density lipoprotein and cardiovascular risk. *Circulation* 2004;109:1809.

58 Frick MH, Elo MO, Haapa K, et al. Helsinki Heart Study. primary-prevention trial with gemfibrozil in middle-aged men with dyslipidemia: safety of treatment, changes in risk factors, and incidence of coronary heart disease. *N Engl J Med.* 1987;317:1237.

59 Rubins HB, Robins SJ, Collins D, et al. Gemfibrozil for the secondary prevention of coronary heart disease in men with low levels of high-

density lipoprotein cholesterol. Veterans Affairs High-Density Lipoprotein Cholesterol intervention trial Study Group. *N Engl J Med.* 1999;341:410.

60 BIP Study Group. Secondary prevention by raising HDL cholesterol and reducing triglycerides in patients with coronary artery disease: the Bezafibrate Infarction Prevention (BIP) Study. *Circulation.* 2000;102:21.

61 Glueck CJ, Lang J, Hamer T, et al. Severe hypertriglyceridemia and pancreatitis when estrogen replacement therapy is given to hypertriglyceridemic women. *J Lab Clin Med.* 1994;123:59.

62 Stone NJ. Estrogen-induced pancreatitis: a caveat worth remembering. *J Lab Clin Med.* 1994;123:18.

63 Mosca L, Harper K, Sarkar S, et al. Effect of raloxifene on serum triglycerides in postmenopausal women: influence of predisposing factors for hypertriglyceridemia. *Clin Ther.* 2001;29:1552–1565.

64 Evista. In: *Physicians' Desk Reference.* 58th ed. Montvale, NJ: Thomson PDR; 2004:1804.

65 Bays HE, Dujovne CA, McGovern ME, et al. Comparison of once-daily, niacin extended-release/lovastatin with standard doses of atorvastatin and simvastatin, the Advicor Versus Other Cholesterol-Modulating Agents Trial Evaluation (ADVOCATE). *Am J Cardiol.* 2003;91:667.

66 Brown BG, Zhao XQ, Chait A, et al. Simvastatin and niacin, antioxidant vitamins, or the combination for the prevention of coronary disease. *N Engl J Med.* 2001;345:1583.

67 Nissen SE, Tsunoda T, Tuzcu EM, et al. Effect of recombinant ApoA-1 Milano on coronary atherosclerosis in patients with acute coronary syndromes: a randomized controlled trial. *JAMA.* 2003;290:2292.

68 Brousseau ME, Schaefer EJ, Wolfe ML, et al. Effects of an inhibitor of cholesteryl ester transfer protein on HDL cholesterol. *N Engl J Med.* 2004;350:1505.

69 Ridker PM, Buring JE, Shih J, et al. Prospective study of C-reactive protein and the risk of future cardiovascular events among apparently healthy women. *Circulation.* 1998;98:731.

70 Ridker PM, Rifai N, Clearfield M, et al. Air Force/Texas Coronary Atherosclerosis Prevention Study Investigators. Measurement of C-reactive protein for the targeting of statin therapy in the primary prevention of acute coronary events. *N Engl J Med.* 2001;344:1959.

71 Pearson TA, Mensah GA, Alexander RW, et al. Markers of inflammation and cardiovascular disease. Application to clinical and public health practice. A statement for healthcare professionals from the Centers for Disease Control and Prevention and the American Heart Association. *Circulation.* 2003;107:499.

72 Tall AR. C-Reactive protein reassessed. (ed.) *N Engl J Med.* 2004; 350:14.

73 Ridker PM, JUPITER Study Group. Rosuvastatin in the primary prevention of cardiovascular disease among patients with low levels of low-density lipoprotein cholesterol and elevated high-sensitivity C-reactive protein: rationale and design of the JUPITER trial. *Circulation.* 2003;108:2292.

15 Depression, Moodiness, and Premenstrual Syndrome

Lesley M. Arnold

Introduction

Although the menopausal transition is not associated with depression for most women, some women are vulnerable to experiencing the onset or exacerbation of mood disturbances during this phase of life. Similarly some women develop marked mood changes during the premenstrual phase of the menstrual cycle. Reproductive hormonal fluctuations that occur during the menstrual cycle and perimenopause may trigger the onset of mood disorders by a mechanism that is not fully understood. This chapter reviews the clinical characteristics and treatment of premenstrual dysphoric disorder (PMDD) and perimenopausal mood symptoms that range in severity from mild, subsyndromal depressive symptoms to major depressive disorder.

Perimenopausal Depression

Epidemiology

The perimenopause is associated with an increased risk of depressive symptoms.[1] In longitudinal, community-based studies, up to 10% of women report perimenopausal mood disturbances.[2] Similarly, a higher than expected prevalence of depressive symptoms has been found in perimenopausal women attending gynecology clinics.[2] In studies of perimenopausal women using structured diagnostic interviews to assess the prevalence of mood disorders, 29–45% of women attending gynecology clinics had a current depressive disorder.[3,4]

Clinical Characteristics and Course

Perimenopausal mood disturbances, including feeling tense, depressed, and irritable,[5] are frequently associated with sleep disturbance, anxiety, fatigue, lack of concentration, and memory complaints.[6] Women may also report discrete episodes of tearfulness, apathy, specific food cravings, and weight gain along with the distinguishing physical concomitants of the perimenopause such as hot flushes, vaginal dryness, dyspareunia, and loss of libido.[2] Vasomotor symptoms that occur with changing estrogen levels during perimenopause (e.g., hot flushes) are strongly associated with mood disturbances.[7] In one recent study, perimenopausal women who had vasomotor symptoms were four times more likely to have depressive symptoms than perimenopausal women without vasomotor symptoms.[8]

KEY POINT

Perimenopausal depression ranges in severity from mild symptoms to major depressive disorder.

Depression during perimenopause ranges in severity from minor depressive symptoms to more severe forms of major depressive disorder as defined by the Diagnostic and Statistical Manual for Mental Disorders, Fourth Edition (DSM-IV).[9] Although depressive symptoms are often part of the clinical presentation of perimenopause and are usually not severe enough to warrant a diagnosis of major depressive disorder, the symptoms may contribute to substantial distress and social or occupational dysfunction.[2]

In a large, prospective study, the rate of depressive symptoms decreased as women progressed from the perimenopausal to postmenopausal status.[10] Cross-sectional community studies also indicate that depressive symptoms are less in postmenopausal women compared with perimenopausal women.[1] In clinic settings, perimenopausal women are significantly more symptomatic than postmenopausal women.[11] These findings suggest that, for many women, the depressive symptoms that occur during the perimenopause are transitory and resolve once they reach the postmenopausal state. However, depression may be more severe and enduring for a subset of women.[7] Epidemiological surveys of major depressive disorder indicate that women who have the onset of this disorder during midlife have a poorer outcome and more chronic course than depressed men.[12]

Risk Factors and Etiology

The mechanism by which the perimenopause is associated with increased affective vulnerability is unknown.[13] Although some women may develop depressive symptoms in response to vasomotor symptoms and sleep disruption,[14] these problems do not fully explain the presence of depressive symptoms in many perimenopausal women.[7,8] Women who have an underlying vulnerability to mood disorders may be sensitive to the perimenopausal fluctuations in reproductive hormone levels, which affect central neurotransmitters involved in mood regulation.[1,15] Indeed, women with prior depressive episodes, a family history of mood disorders, or a history of mood disorders at other times of hormonal change such as postpartum depression and premenstrual syndrome (PMS) have an increased risk of developing perimenopausal depressive symptoms.[6,16,17] Furthermore, women who have been exposed to the changing hormone levels through a long perimenopausal period (at least 27 months) are also at increased risk for depression.[10] The postmenopausal phase, when women are no longer experiencing shifts in hormone levels, is associated with a decline of depressive symptoms in many women.

Some women may also be vulnerable to the development of depressive symptoms during the perimenopausal years because of increased psychosocial stressors at this phase of life. These stressors may include health problems, changing interpersonal roles in the family, loss of a significant others by death, or divorce, and other age-related changes.[1,6]

What's the Evidence?

TREATMENT

HORMONAL THERAPY

Estrogen Monotherapy Estrogen may enhance mood through its stimulatory effects on neurotransmitters involved in mood regulation.[15] In nondepressed women, estrogen therapy has been associated with an increased sense of well-being.[6] Some, but not all, trials have reported a positive effect of estrogen therapy on depressive symptoms in perimenopausal women.[2] Comparisons across multiple studies of perimenopausal depression have been hampered by heterogeneity of methods to define and assess perimenopause, lack of control for the presence or severity of vasomotor symptoms, lack of standard assessment and diagnosis of the mood disturbance, variable levels of depression severity, and differences in the estrogen preparation and dose.[13] A meta-analytic research review of 26 studies of the effect of hormone therapy (HT) on mood in peri- and postmenopausal women concluded that estrogen therapy (mostly conjugated equine estrogens 0.625 or 1.25 mg/day) exerted a moderate to large effect on depressed mood that was greater among perimenopausal than postmenopausal women.[18] However, most of the subjects included in the studies were not depressed or had only mild depression and the results may not apply to women with moderate to severe major depressive disorder.

Recent studies of well-defined perimenopausal women in whom the depression status was well-characterized and assessed found that oral or transdermal 17β-estradiol was effective in the treatment of syndromal and subsyndromal depressive disorders.[19–22] The antidepressant benefit associated with estrogen therapy was independent of improvement in vasomotor symptoms, suggesting that estrogen's effect on depression is not solely related to a reduction in the distress of hot flushes.[19,20,22] These results are encouraging for the potential use of estradiol (particularly transdermal estradiol) in the treatment of perimenopausal depression. Transdermal administration of estradiol, which results in a rapid rise in serum levels of estradiol and provides nearly constant serum levels, may be more effective than other estrogen delivery systems in treating depressed mood.[13,23] However, these studies were limited by short duration of treatment, small sample sizes, and relatively few women with major depressive disorder.[13] Furthermore, the risks associated with long-term use of unopposed estrogen in women with an intact uterus (e.g., uterine cancer) might outweigh the potential benefit of estrogen monotherapy on mood.

Estrogen and Progestogen Combination Therapy Because unopposed estrogen increases the risk of endometrial proliferation, progestogen is coadministered with estrogen in women with an intact uterus. Progestogen use is associated with symptoms of dysphoria, irritability, and mitigation of the mood-enhancing effects of estrogen.[1,15] Few studies have examined the impact of combined estrogen and progestogen regimens on perimenopausal women with depressed symptoms. In studies of peri- and postmenopausal women with mild depressive symptoms, the addition of progestogen diminished the positive treatment effects of estrogen on mood.[18] By contrast, in one study of transdermal estradiol in perimenopausal women with depressive symptoms, the addition of medroxyprogesterone acetate for 1 week to precipitate progestogen withdrawal-induced menstruation was not associated with a significant worsening of mood.[19] However, these results should be interpreted with caution because of the short duration of progestogen treatment. Repeated cyclic progestogen regimens might also precipitate symptoms associated with PMS. More studies are needed to investigate the long-term effects of estrogen and progestogen combination therapy on perimenopausal women with depressive symptoms or major depressive disorder. Strategies to reduce the negative impact of progestogen on mood include increasing the estrogen/progestogen dose ratio,[24] using continuous rather than cyclic progestogen regimens to reduce cyclic mood changes, or switching to other estrogen or progestogen formulations.

Androgens Androgens, such as testosterone, androstenedione, dehydroepiandrosterone (DHEA), and DHEA sulfate have modulatory effects on mood through biotransformation into estrogen or direct effects on brain function.[13] Recent evidence for mood-enhancing effects of testosterone comes from studies of women who have undergone oophorectomy. For example, depressive and anxiety symptoms associated with decreased testosterone levels in women after oopohorectomy,[25,26] were alleviated with testosterone supplementation.[27] In another recent double-blind, placebo-controlled study, women on oral conjugated estrogens following hysterectomy and oophorectomy, received either transdermal testosterone containing 150 or 300 µg/day or placebo patches for 12 weeks. Women who received testosterone reported greater psychological well-being and significant improvement in mood and anxiety compared with placebo recipients.[28] However, more study is needed to clarify the role of androgens in the development of mood dysfunction during perimenopause and to determine the potential efficacy of androgen therapy in the treatment of perimenopausal depression.

Nonhormonal Therapy

Antidepressants Risks associated with long-term and relatively short-term use of combination therapy with estrogen (conjugated equine estrogen 0.625 mg/day) and progestogen (medroxyprogesterone acetate 2.5 mg/day) revealed by the recent findings from the Women's Health Initiative Study,[29] may outweigh any beneficial effects of HT on mood for many women. Although it is unclear whether estrogen alone or other hormone formulations are associated with similar risks, it is important to identify alternatives for the treatment of perimenopausal mood symptoms.

Most studies do not support the use of estrogen as a treatment for major depressive disorder, and trials of estrogen treatment of perimenopausal depression are mostly limited to women with less severe forms of depression, as reviewed previously. Therefore, antidepressants should be considered for perimenopausal women who present with major depressive disorder. While there are many antidepressants with diverse mechanisms of action available, there is evidence that women may be more responsive to the selective serotonin reuptake inhibitors (SSRIs) for the treatment of major depressive disorder.[30] Table 15-1 describes the SSRIs in addition to venlafaxine, which predominately inhibits serotonin reuptake at lower doses and is a dual serotonin and norepinephrine reuptake inhibitor at higher doses. However, there are few studies examining the efficacy of antidepressant treatment of major depressive disorder specifically during perimenopause. A recent open trial of citalopram monotherapy resulted in remission of major depression in 13 out of 15 (86.6%) peri- and postmenopausal women.[31]

In addition to the treatment of major depressive disorder, antidepressants would likely alleviate subsyndromal perimenopausal depressive symptoms. Menopausal vasomotor symptoms and related distress may also be responsive to antidepressant treatment. Studies of venlafaxine, fluoxetine, and paroxetine in women with a prior history of breast cancer demonstrated that antidepressants that inhibit serotonin reuptake may significantly reduce vasomotor symptoms associated with menopause.[32–34] One study has evaluated the efficacy of an SSRI (paroxetine controlled release [CR]) in the treatment of menopausal vasomotor symptoms in women who were not primarily breast cancer survivors.[35] In this randomized, double-blind, placebo-controlled, parallel group study, hot flushes were reduced over a 6-week period by 62.2% in those receiving 12.5 mg/day and 64.6% in those receiving 25 mg/day of paraoxetine CR compared with 37.8% in the placebo group. These results are similar to those for fluoxetine (50% reduction over 4 weeks at 20 mg/day) and venlafaxine (61% reduction

Table 15-1. SELECTED SEROTONERGIC ANTIDEPRESSANTS

Drug	Usual Adult Dose Range (mg/day)	Elimination Half-Life (Hours)	Comments
Fluoxetine	20–80	48–144 (active metabolite 7–15 days)	Long half-life of parent compound and active metabolite helpful for noncompliant patients or for those who have had difficulty with SSRI discontinuation symptoms; potential for clinically relevant drug interactions;* may have relatively more stimulatory effects
Sertraline	50–200	26	Low potential for drug interactions;* SSRI discontinuation symptoms
Paroxetine controlled release	25–62.5	15–20	Sedative effects; SSRI discontinuation symptoms; potential for clinically relevant drug interactions*
Citalopram	20–40	35	Low potential for drug interactions;* discontinuation symptoms may be less problematic
Escitalopram	10–20	27–32	The more potent *S*-enantiomer of citalopram
Fluvoxamine	150–250	15–26	Potential for clinically relevant drug interactions;* SSRI discontinuation symptoms
Venlafaxine extended release	75–225	5 (active metabolite 11 hours)	Low potential for drug interactions;* low risk of weight gain (and possibly weight loss); potential for dose-related increase in blood pressure; SSRI discontinuation symptoms

*Drug interactions due to inhibition of isoenzymes of the cytochrome P450 system.

KEY POINT

Antidepressants treat both mild-severe perimenopausal depressive symptoms and vasomotor symptoms.

over 4 weeks at 75 and 150 mg/day).[32,34] In all of these studies, the effect of the antidepressant on reduction in vasomotor symptoms was independent of any effect on mood. The mechanism by which the serotonin reuptake inhibitors alleviate vasomotor symptoms is unknown, but may be related to the role of serotonin in thermoregulation.[35]

Antidepressant and Estrogen Combination Therapy It is possible that, for some perimenopausal women with depression, the combination of estrogen and an antidepressant might produce a better treatment response than either treatment alone. However, there are few controlled studies of evaluating the efficacy of estrogen therapy in combination with antidepressants in peri-or postmenopausal women. In addition, results of studies of the augmentation effect of estrogen on antidepressant response are mixed. In one retrospective study, estrogen therapy was found to enhance response rates to fluoxetine compared with placebo in depressed women over age 60.[36] However, another retrospective study of fluoxetine in younger depressed menopausal women 45 years of age or older found no differences in efficacy between those taking estrogen with fluoxetine and those on fluoxetine alone.[37] A retrospective study in depressed women over 60 also found little evidence that taking estrogen with an SSRI (sertraline) produced greater improvement in depressive symptoms than the SSRI alone.[38] Recent open trials of adjunctive antidepressant treatment in depressed peri-and postmenopausal women on estrogen therapy suggest that this approach may be useful for those women who continue to experience or develop depression while taking estrogen. In one study, women on estrogen therapy who had major depression were treated with mirtazapine, which enhances central serotonin and norepinephrine activity by antagonizing serotonin types 2 and 3 receptors and presynaptic alpha 2 adrenergic receptors. Remission of the depression was achieved in 14 of 16 subjects (87.5% who received 30–45 mg/day of mirtazapine for 8 weeks.[39] Another study found that adjunctive citalopram 20–60 mg/day for 8 weeks in women who had continued to experience depression after treatment with estrogen resulted in remission of depression in 11 of 12 women (91.6%).[31]

Psychosocial Interventions Multiple psychosocial factors may influence the development of depressive symptoms during perimenopause. Women with a negative attitude toward menopausal or aging may be more likely to report negative mood states.[40] In addition, changes to the body that are associated with aging such as changes in body shape, weight, and wrinkled skin, as well as physical symptoms of perimenopause (e.g., hot flushes) may adversely affect a woman's body image and self-esteem, which could contribute to the development of depressive symptoms.[41] Adverse life events (e.g., death of a significant other, marital conflict) and high levels of reported stress are associated with depressive symptoms during the menopausal transition.[42] Difficulty adjusting to changing roles in the family or at work, unemployment, and lack of social support are also factors that may increase risk of depressive symptoms.[41] Finally, physically inactive women report decreased well-being around menopause.[43]

Psychotherapy is an important treatment modality to address and resolve stresses experienced by many perimenopausal women. Two forms of psychotherapy, cognitive-behavioral and interpersonal psychotherapy, are particularly helpful in the treatment of women with depression. These problem-solving approaches may be more effective for women than less structured, open-ended, psychoanalytically-based therapies.[44] Couples' therapy is useful in addressing interpersonal problems with significant others. Exercise may also help to increase a sense of well-being and reduce depressive and other physical symptoms in perimenopausal women.[45]

Guidelines for the Evaluation and Treatment of Perimenopausal Depression

An important part of the evaluation of women who present with depressive symptoms during perimenopause is an assessment for major depressive disorder and a determination of the severity of the disorder (Fig. 15-1). Self-report questionnaires, such as the Edinburgh Depression Scale,[46] effectively screen for the presence of depressive symptoms, but a mental status examination and a clinical interview that assesses for the DSM-IV criteria are necessary to confirm the diagnosis of major depressive disorder. Of course, a careful assessment of suicidal risk is critical in the evaluation of all patients with depression, and patients at risk for suicide should be referred for hospitalization. Other possible medical or psychiatric causes of depression should be ruled out, including medications (e.g., corticosteroids, antihypertensives, and benzodiazepines), endocrine disorders (particularly thyroid disease), neurologic disorders, cancer, immunologic abnormalities, anemia, infections, metabolic aberrancies, bipolar disorder, and substance use disorders. It is important to obtain a family history of major mood disorders and past psychiatric history, especially prior depressive episodes and response to any treatments. Other factors to consider are the presence of stressors, health problems, lifestyle concerns (e.g., level of physical activity), conflicts in relationships,

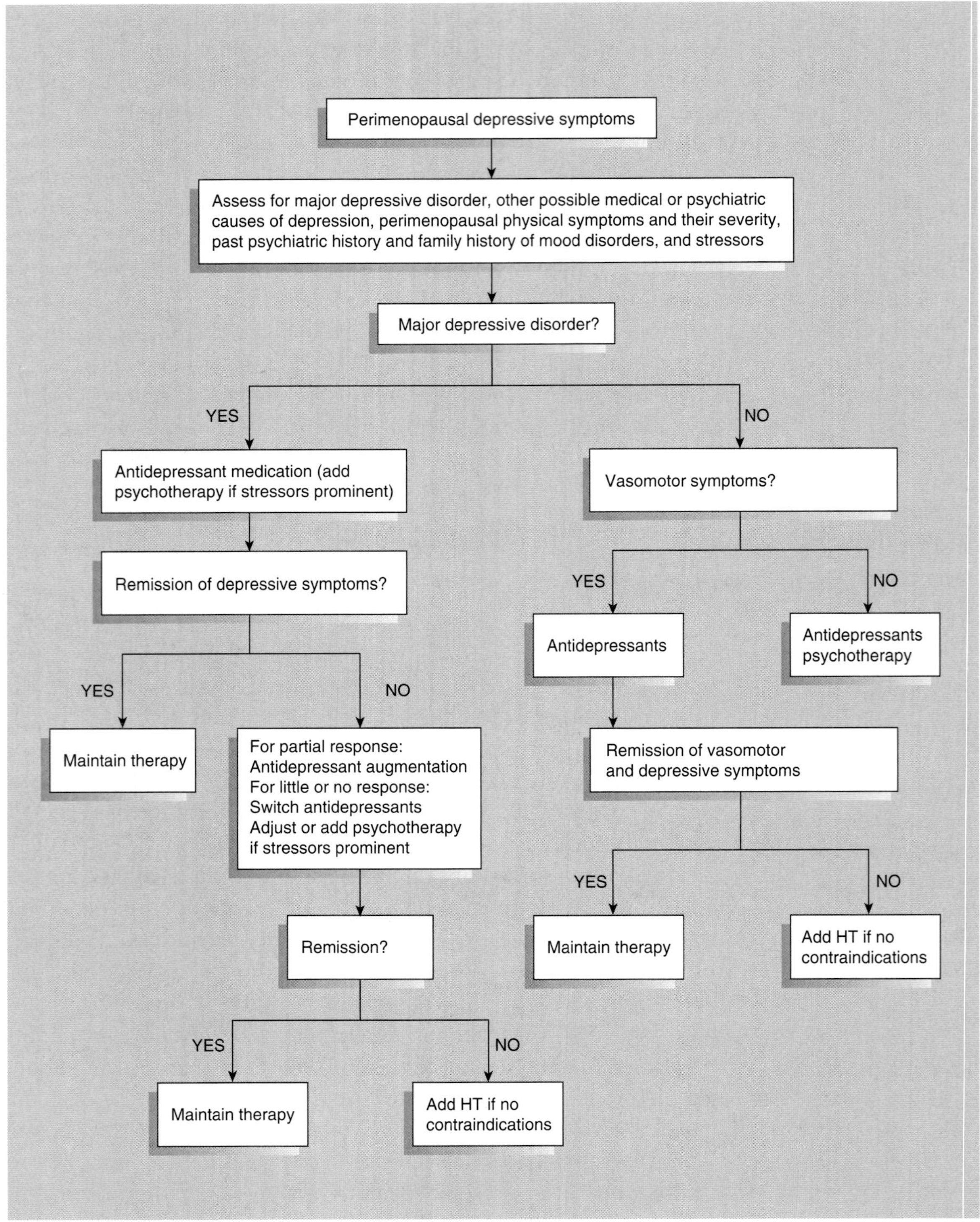

Figure 15-1: Algorithm for the diagnosis and treatment of perimenopausal depression.

losses, changing responsibilities or roles, or negative attitudes about menopause or aging. The evaluation also includes characterization of physical symptoms associated with perimenopause (e.g., vasomotor symptoms) and the degree to which these symptoms disrupt sleep or interfere with daily function.

Treatment strategies are presented in Fig. 15-1. This algorithm assumes that perimenopause has already been confirmed through history of menstrual irregularity, presence of vasomotor symptoms, or measurement of reproductive hormones if necessary (e.g., estradiol and follicle-stimulating hormone). Findings from the Women's Health Initiative Study of the risks associated with HT and the recent evidence of efficacy of several antidepressants in the treatment of vasomotor symptoms suggest that antidepressants, particularly SSRIs, may be the preferred initial approach to treatment of perimenopausal depression ranging in severity from mild subsyndromal depressive symptoms to major depressive disorder with and without vasomotor symptoms. Furthermore, most of the available evidence regarding hormonal treatment of perimenopausal depression is limited to small, short-term studies using estrogen monotherapy in mostly mildly depressed women, making it difficult to determine whether long-term benefits outweigh the potential risks associated with estrogen use.

Women who present with major depressive disorder require treatment with antidepressant medication, but milder depressive symptoms will also likely respond to antidepressants. Psychotherapy can also be considered in women who have prominent stressors that may be contributing to the depressive symptoms. Increasing physical activity may help to alleviate both the mood and physical symptoms associated with perimenopause. If vasomotor symptoms are severe, do not adequately respond to antidepressants, or there are other physical symptoms (e.g., vaginal dryness) that do not typically respond to antidepressants, then HT could be added if there are no contraindications to this treatment. HT could also be added if the depression does not adequately respond to antidepressants alone, however, other strategies should be tried first. These include augmenting with an additional antidepressant or another psychotropic agent (e.g., lithium), switching to another antidepressant, or adding or increasing psychotherapy.

In women with an intact uterus, combination therapy with estrogen and progestogen is usually recommended, but may complicate the management of depression because of progestogen-induced mood disturbances. If women develop cyclic mood symptoms associated with cyclic progestogen regimens, then a switch to continuous HT may be indicated. Higher doses of estrogen or different combination hormone preparations may also be helpful in women who experience mood disturbances while taking HT. The evidence for use of androgens to treat perimenopausal depression is very limited, and androgens are not currently recommended.

Guiding Questions in Approaching a Perimenopausal Patient with Depressive Symptoms

- Has perimenopause been confirmed?
- What is the severity of the depressive symptoms?
- Does she have major depressive disorder?
- Are there other medical or psychiatric causes of her symptoms?
- Has she had prior episodes of depression and responded to antidepressants?
- Does she have prominent vasomotor symptoms?
- Are there contraindications to hormone replacement therapy?

Discussion of Cases

CASE 1

Perimenopausal Depression

The patient is a 48-year-old married homemaker who presents with a 9-month history of irregular menses and hot flushes that occur several times during the day and awaken her in the middle of the night. Over the past month, she has been unable to return to sleep for 1–2 hours after awakening with a hot flush. During this time, she has also been very tired and irritable, and at times, sad and tearful. She is worried about how her increasing "moodiness" is affecting her relationships with her husband and children. She presented with a full, normal range of affect and had no abnormalities on mental examination.

What other information would you gather at this point?

- **Review symptoms of major depressive disorder**
  - **Depressed mood was mild in severity and not present most days**
  - **Mild anhedonia and decreased motivation some days but still able to complete housework and enjoy most activities**

- **Increase in appetite, especially for sweets and a 10-lb weight gain over the past year**
- **Severe middle insomnia**
- **Marked fatigue and feelings of being slowed down**
- **Mild decrease in concentration**
- **No feelings of worthlessness, excessive guilt, or suicide**

- **Ask about psychosocial stressors**
  - **No recent stressors except for concern about impact of irritability on family**
- **Review family history, past psychiatric history, including past antidepressant trials**
  - **Premenstrual dysphoria beginning around age 38**
  - **Mother and sister with history of major depressive disorder**
- **Assess for other medical or psychiatric problems that may be contributing to mood symptoms, including medications**
  - **No other health problems or medications**

What tests, if any, would you recommend?

- **Obtain screening thyroid stimulating hormone**
  - **Normal**
- **Other tests based on suspicion of other medical causes of mood symptoms**
  - **None**

What is your recommendation for initial management?

- **Although the patient does not meet full criteria for major depressive disorder, she has some mood disturbances associated with multiple physical symptoms, including vasomotor symptoms that may respond to antidepressants.**
- **A trial of an SSRI would be the initial approach. Titrate to a therapeutic dose and follow closely**
- **If no response or only partial response, consider adding combination HT, if there are no contraindications to hormone use**

Premenstrual Syndrome and Premenstrual Dysphoric Disorder

EPIDEMIOLOGY

PMS is common and affects about 75% of women with regular menstrual cycles.[47] PMDD, which could be conceptualized as a more severe form of PMS, affects about 3–8% of women with regular menstrual cycles.[47–49] The first, large community-based study of 513 women with prospective diaries and more refined criteria and rigorous assessments demonstrated a 6% prevalence rate of PMDD in women aged 36–44 years.[50]

CLINICAL CHARACTERISTICS AND COURSE

The International Classification of Diseases (ICD-10) defines PMS as any one of the following: mild psychological discomfort, bloating and weight gain, breast tenderness and swelling, swelling of the hands and feet, various aches and pains, poor concentration, sleep disturbance, and change in appetite.[51] In April 2000, the

American College of Obstetricians and Gynecologists (ACOG) published diagnostic and treatment guidelines for PMS.[52] The ACOG criteria require at least one affective (depression, angry outbursts, irritability, anxiety, confusion, social withdrawal) or physical (breast tenderness, abdominal bloating, headaches, swelling of extremities) symptoms during the 5 days before menses in each of the three prior menstrual cycles. The symptoms should be relieved within 4 days of menses, present in absence of medication or drug or alcohol use, and occur reproducibly during two cycles of prospective recording. Finally, the symptoms must cause identifiable dysfunction in social or economic performance. The DSM-IV[9] includes research diagnostic criteria for PMDD in the appendix for criteria sets requiring further study. Establishment of PMDD criteria, albeit provisionally, validates the clinical observation that some women have extremely distressing physical, behavioral, and emotional symptoms premenstrually. The strict criteria requiring evidence of marked premenstrual symptoms that substantially interfere with function also emphasizes that not all women with PMS have a mental disorder. Both the ACOG PMS and DSM-IV criteria require luteal phase timing, prospective symptoms monitoring, and nonattribution to other causes. The main differences are that PMDD requires at least five symptoms, at least one of which must be affective, and marked impairment of psychosocial functioning. The prospective symptoms monitoring is important to help distinguish PMDD from major depressive disorder, in which symptoms persist daily for weeks without a specific relationship to the menstrual cycle.

KEY POINT

The diagnosis of PMDD requires prospective monitoring of mood and physical symptoms.

PMDD can develop at any time from menarche to menopause, but it seems to increase as women get older and most often develops in the late twenties to the mid-thirties.[47–49] PMDD can be confused with symptoms of perimenopause in older women. There is considerable cycle-to-cycle stability in PMDD symptoms and once symptoms begin, they rarely resolve spontaneously. PMDD may worsen over time in some women, and severe premenstrual symptoms are predictive of later development of major depressive disorder.[53] Among the mood symptoms associated with PMDD, tension, anger, and irritability are common, have an adverse effect on relationships, and are often the mood symptoms that bring a woman to treatment. Impairment in relationships and social functioning (most frequently observed at home) are affected more than work efficiency.[54]

RISK FACTORS AND ETIOLOGY

Although PMDD and major depressive disorder are distinct, there is a strong association between PMDD and a previous history of depression.[50,55,56] Between 31% to 70% of women with PMDD report a history of major depression.[57,58] Like major depressive disorder, PMDD is also a familial disorder, but the genetic and environmental risk factors for premenstrual symptoms and lifetime major depression are not closely related.[59] The etiology of PMDD is unknown, but studies indicate that the symptoms occur in the context of normal endocrine function. PMDD may be triggered by a reproductive stimulus in vulnerable women.[60,61] One possible vulnerability trait may be abnormal serotonergic function.[62] Emerging evidence also implicates the gamma-amino butyric acid (GABA) system and the neurosteroid allopregnanolone in the pathophysiology of PMDD.[63] Allopregnanolone, a metabolite of progesterone produced in the brain, has anxiolytic effects (decreased anxiety and tension) probably through its action on the $GABA_A$ receptor.[64] Decreased levels of allopregnanolone are implicated in PMDD, while increased levels could decrease PMDD symptoms.[65] Women with PMDD also appear to have decreased sensitivity of GABA receptors to allopregnanolone during the luteal phase. This deficient GABA neurotransmission could play a role in the development of PMDD symptoms of anxiety, tension, irritability, and sleep symptoms.

What's the Evidence?

TREATMENT

KEY POINT

The serotonergic antidepressants are the first-line treatment for PMDD.

PSYCHOPHARMACOLOGICAL THERAPY The SSRIs are considered by many clinicians to be the first-line treatment for women with PMDD.[66] These medications may improve PMDD symptoms by correcting an underlying vulnerability trait of abnormal central serotonergic function. SSRIs have also been found to increase the production of allopregnanolone by increasing the efficiency of one of the enzymes involved in the synthesis of allopregnanolone from progesterone.[67] This latter mechanism of action could explain the rapid treatment response of PMDD to SSRIs compared with the typically delayed response in major depressive disorder.

Sixty to seventy percent of women with PMDD report significant improvement on serotonergic antidepressants,[68–77] which alleviate the mood and physical symptoms (particularly breast tenderness and bloating) [68–70] as well as the psychosocial dysfunction associated with PMDD.[68,71] Serotonergic antidepressants have shown superiority over predominately noradrenergic antidepressants such as desipramine and maprotiline as well as over bupropion.[72–74] Fluoxetine was the first prescribed medication approved for the treatment of the mood and physical symptoms of PMDD, followed recently by sertraline.

In most studies of antidepressant treatment of PMDD, the medication was given daily throughout the menstrual cycle, but studies have also demonstrated that clomipramine, fluoxetine, sertraline, and citalopram were effective as intermittent treatment during the luteal phase.[76,78–80] Intermittent citalopram was actually more effective than continuous treatment.[76] Advantages of intermittent treatment include decrease in duration of adverse effects and reduced cost.

Other Pharmacological Therapy Other medication approaches to PMDD have been directed at the reproductive endocrine trigger. Ovarian suppression or anovulation appears to reduce the symptoms of PMDD. Leuprolide acetate depot, a gonadotropin-releasing hormone agonist that stops the cyclic release of estrogen and progesterone, reduces symptoms of PMDD in 50–75% of women.[60] Add-back regimens of low doses of estrogen and progestogen may prevent health risk related to the hypoestrogenic state without leading to a recurrence of PMDD.[81] Oophorectomy is an extreme step taken for severe and intractable PMDD. Other hormonal treatments have had mixed results. Exogenous progestogen is ineffective for the treatment of PMDD.[82] Estradiol was effective for PMDD but also suppressed ovulation.[60] Danazol, a synthetic steroid with weak androgenic activity, reduced symptoms of PMDD at low doses (200 mg/day) that did not suppress ovulation.[83] One controlled study using a triphasic contraceptive showed no benefit in PMDD.[84] Notably, concurrent use of oral contraceptives with antidepressants does not alter the efficacy of antidepressants in the treatment of PMDD.[85] Recently, a unique oral contraceptive containing a combination of drospirenone (a spironolactone-like progestin with antiandrogenic and antimineralocorticoid activity) and ethinyl estradiol was found to significantly improve PMDD symptoms of increased appetite, acne, and food cravings, with nonsignificant trends for improvement in mood symptoms.[86]

Other Treatments

Vitamins and Minerals Vitamin B_6 (up to 100 mg/day) may be effective for treating premenstrual symptoms based on a meta-analysis of randomized placebo-controlled trials.[87] However, not all of the studies showed a benefit and they were for PMS, not PMDD. Calcium carbonate 1200 mg/day was found to improve moderate-severe symptoms of PMS by the second or third cycle in 48% on calcium and 30% for placebo.[88] Vitamin E (400 IU d-alpha-tocopherol) was studied in a randomized double-blind trial and found to improve some PMS symptoms.[89] Finally, magnesium pyrrolidone carboxylic acid (360 mg/day) was shown in one study to improve negative affect and arousal in women with PMS.[90]

Diet and Exercise There are no published controlled studies of specific dietary recommendations in PMDD. However, some clinicians suggest limiting intake of alcohol, caffeine, and salt. In a nonrandomized study, 6 months of exercise training was associated with decreased premenstrual symptoms in both sedentary women and marathon trainers.[91] A randomized study found that women with PMS who did aerobic exercise improved in symptoms while those doing nonaerobic exercise did not.[92] However, there are no exercise studies for women with PMDD.

Cognitive-Behavioral Therapy Several studies suggest that cognitive-behavioral therapy may be beneficial as part of the treatment of PMDD, but results of studies have been mixed. Compared with a wait-list control group, women who received 12 weeks of individual cognitive therapy experienced significant improvement in premenstrual psychological and physical symptoms and functioning.[93] Six weeks of group cognitive-behavioral therapy was also superior to group awareness through movement training and a waitlist control.[94] However, 13 weeks of group cognitive-behavioral therapy was equal in efficacy to group information-focused therapy.[95]

Guidelines for the Evaluation and Treatment of Premenstrual Dysphoric Disorder

An important part of the evaluation of a woman who reports premenstrual symptoms is to assess for the presence and severity of both mood and physical symptoms and determine the impact of the symptoms on functioning. The next step is to rule out other medical or psychiatric disorders that may be contributing to the symptoms (Fig. 15-2). Possible medical or psychiatric disorders to consider include endocrine disorders (particularly thyroid disease), neurologic disorders, cancer, immunologic abnormalities, metabolic aberrancies, anemia, perimenopause, major depressive disorder, dysthymia, bipolar disorder, generalized anxiety disorder, and substance use disorders. Other information that is helpful in establishing the diagnosis includes current stressors, and personal and family history of PMS/PMDD, postpartum depression, or major mood disorders. Prospective charting over at least two menstrual cycles by the patient will establish the severity and luteal cyclicity of symptoms, helping to confirm the diagnosis of PMDD.

Treatment strategies are presented in Fig. 15-2. For most women, the preferred initial approach to treatment of PMDD is SSRIs or other serotonergic antidepressants (Table 15-1). The response of PMDD to the SSRIs is often rapid, occurring within days rather than weeks as occurs in the treatment of major depression. To avoid prolonged exposure to side effects of SSRIs, women may elect to use the medication intermittently only during the luteal phase, typically starting 7–14 days before onset of menses or when premenstrual symptoms first appear, and discontinuing the medication at the start of menses. If this regimen does not adequately control symptoms, then continuous use throughout the menstrual cycle is recommended. PMDD may also respond to lower doses of antidepressants than typically used to treat major depression, but the dose should be adjusted to reach a therapeutic level. Because PMDD is a chronic condition, maintenance treatment with SSRIs is recommended. Adjunctive diuretics, over-the-counter analgesics, or prescription strength nonsteroidal anti-inflammatory drugs (NSAIDs) may be helpful for women with body pain, bloating, and water retention. If there is no response to one SSRI, switching to another may be effective. If antidepressants are ineffective and women continue to experience severe,

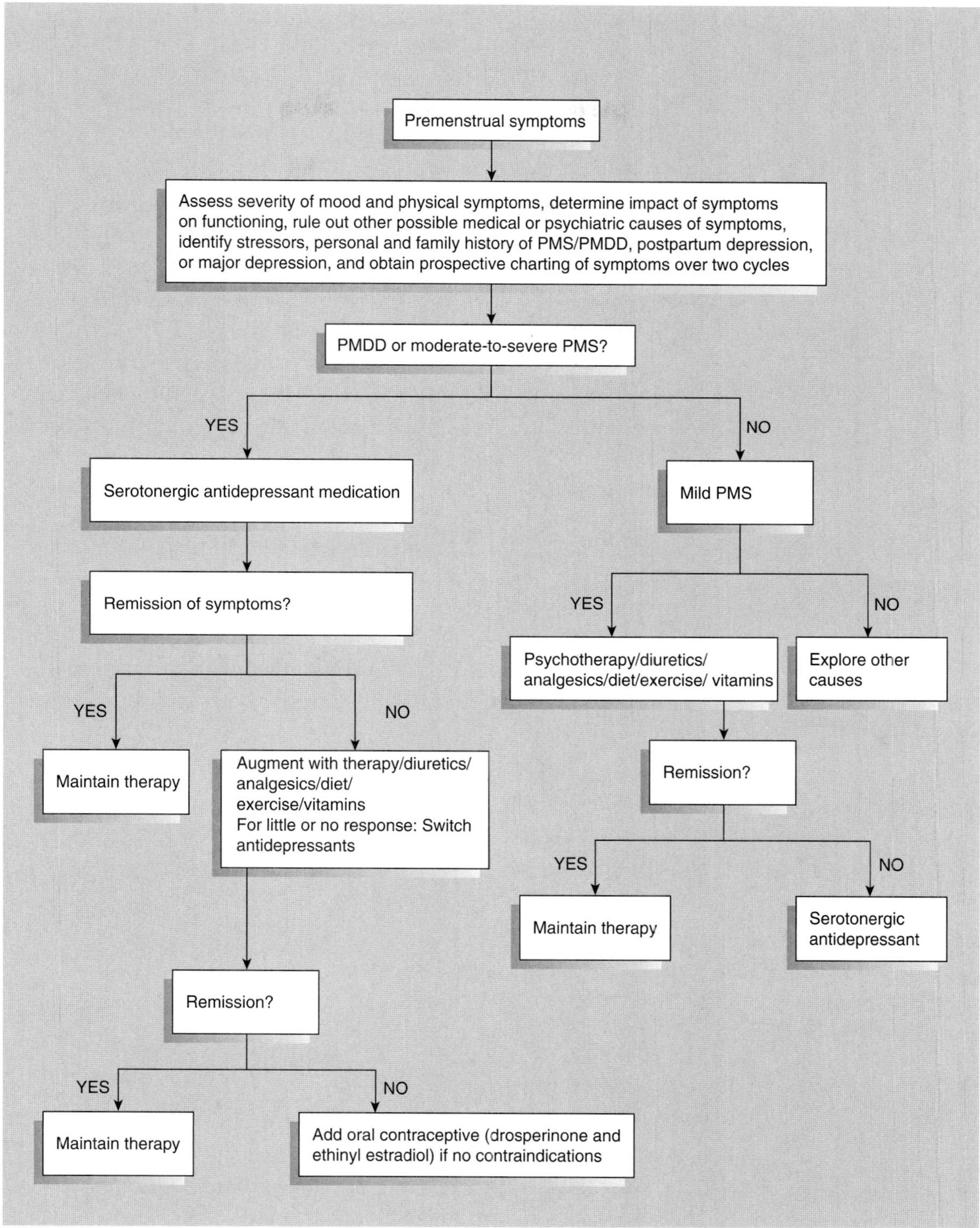

Figure 15-2: Algorithm for the diagnosis and treatment of premenstrual dysphoric disorder.

disruptive PMDD symptoms, then a hormonal approach may be considered. Although oral contraceptives are not usually recommended for PMDD, recent preliminary evidence suggests that a unique oral contraceptive containing a combination of drospirenone (a spironolactone-like progestin with antiandrogenic and antimineralocorticoid activity) and ethinyl estradiol may be helpful in women who do not have contraindications to use of oral contraceptives. This oral contraceptive may be added to the antidepressant if there was a partial response to the antidepressant. Women who do not respond to any of these strategies and continue to have severe symptoms may be candidates for a trial of gonadotropin-releasing hormone agonists such as leuprolide with add-back regimens of estrogen and progestogen. Exercise, cognitive-behavioral therapy, and vitamins (B_6 or calcium) or minerals (magnesium) may be helpful for milder symptoms of PMS or as adjunctive treatment for PMDD.

Guiding Questions in Approaching a Patient with Premenstrual Symptoms

- Are the symptoms cyclical, occurring during the luteal phase and resolving a few days after the onset of menses?
- What is the severity of the mood and physical symptoms?
- Are there other medical or psychiatric causes of her symptoms?
- What is the impact of the symptoms on function at work, school, activities, and relationships?
- Has she had prior episodes of depression and responded to antidepressants?

CASE 2

Premenstrual Dysphoric Disorder

The patient is a 38-year-old woman (G2P2) with regular menstrual cycles who presents with a 12-month history of increasingly severe premenstrual symptoms. She reports feeling extremely irritable beginning about 10 days before the onset of menses. She becomes argumentative with her husband and fears that she will lose control of her anger. She yells more at the children and is concerned about the impact of her behavior on them. She withdraws socially to avoid any conflict with other people. She has difficulty sleeping, is very tired during the day, and has trouble focusing. She is much less efficient at work and sometimes feels completely overwhelmed and unable to get anything done. Her breasts become exquisitely tender, and she has to wear a bra to bed to reduce the uncomfortable sensations. In the morning she notes that her hands are swollen and she feels bloated. All of the symptoms resolve beginning on the second day of her menstrual flow.

What other information would you gather at this point?

- **Assess for other medical or psychiatric problems that may be contributing to symptoms**
  - **No other health problems**
- **Ask her to complete a prospective daily symptom record for 2 months**
  - **The charting indicates that she has many mood and physical symptoms of sufficient severity to meet the criteria for PMDD**
  - **Her symptoms occur only in the luteal phase of the menstrual cycle**
- **Ask about psychosocial stressors**
  - **No recent stressors except for concern about impact of irritability on family**
- **Review family history, past psychiatric history, including past antidepressant trials**
  - **Sister has a history of severe PMS**

What tests, if any, would you recommend?

- **Obtain screening thyroid stimulating hormone**
  - **Normal**
- **Other tests based on suspicion of other medical causes of mood symptoms**
  - **None**

What is your recommendation for initial management?

- **A trial of an SSRI would be the initial approach. Titrate to a therapeutic dose and follow closely. Consider intermittent dosing during luteal phase only**
- **If a partial response, add a diuretic for bloating and water retention, over-the-counter analgesics or prescription NSAIDs for body pain, vitamin (B_6 and calcium), mineral supplementation, or exercise. Limit alcohol, caffeine, and salt**
- **If no response, consider adding oral contraceptive (with drospirenone and ethinyl estradiol), if there are no contraindications to hormone use**

References

1 Burt VK, Altshuler LL, Rasgon N. Depressive symptoms in the perimenopause: prevalence, assessment, and guidelines for treatment. Harv Rev Psychiatry. 1998;6:121–132.

2 Schmidt PJ, Roca CA, Bloch M, et al. The perimenopause and affective disorders. *Semin Reprod Endocrinol.* 1997;15:91–100.

3 Hay AG, Bancroft J, Johnstone EC. Affective symptoms in women attending a menopause clinic. *Br J Psychiatry.* 1994;164:513–516.

4 Soares CN. Depression during the perimenopause. *Arch Gen Psychiatry.* 2001;58:306.

5 Dennerstein L, Lehert P, Guthrie J. The effects of the menopausal transition and biopsychosocial factors on well-being. *Arch Women Ment Health*. 2002;5:15–22.

6 Robinson GE. Psychotic and mood disorders associated with the perimenopausal period. *CNS Drugs*. 2001;15:175–184.

7 Bromberger JT, Meyer PM, Kravitz HM, et al. Psychologic distress and natural menopause: a multiethnic community study. *Am J Public Health*. 2001;91:1435–1442.

8 Joffe H, Hall JE, Soares CN, et al. Vasomotor symptoms are associated with depression in perimenopausal women seeking primary care. *Menopause*. 2002;9:392–398.

9 American Psychiatric Association. *Diagnostic and Statistical Manual for Mental Disorders, Fourth Edition, Text Revision*. Washington, DC: American Psychiatric Association; 2000.

10 Avis NE, Brambilla D, McKinlay SM, et al. A longitudinal analysis of the association between menopause and depression. Results from the Massachusetts Women's Health Study. *Ann Epidemiol*. 1994;4: 214–220.

11 Stewart DE, Boydell K, Derzko C, et al. Psychologic distress during the menopausal years in women attending a menopause clinic. *Int J Psychiatry Med*. 1992;22:213–220.

12 Kessler RC, McGonagle KA, Swartz M, et al. Sex and depression in the National Comorbidity Survey. I: lifetime prevalence, chronicity and recurrence. *J Affect Disord*. 1993;29:85–96.

13 Soares CN, Poitras JR, Prouty J. Effect of reproductive hormones and selective estrogen receptor modulators on mood during menopause. *Drugs Aging*. 2003;20:85–100.

14 Avis NE, Crawford S, Stellato R, et al. Longitudinal study of hormone levels and depression among women transitioning through menopause. *Climacteric*. 2001;4:243–249.

15 Richardson TA, Robinson RD. Menopause and depression: a review of psychologic function and sex steroid neurobiology during the menopause. *Prim Care Update Ob/Gyns*. 2000;7:215–223.

16 Stewart DE, Boydell KM. Psychologic distress during menopause: associations across the reproductive life cycle. *Int J Psychiatry Med*. 1993;23:157–162.

17 Rapkin AJ, Mikacich JA, Moatakef-Imani B, et al. The clinical nature and formal diagnosis of premenstrual, postpartum, and perimenopausal affective disorder. *Curr Psychiatry Rep*. 2002;4: 419–428.

18 Zweifel JE, O'Brien WH. A meta-analysis of the effect of hormone replacement therapy upon depressed mood. *Psychoneuroendocrinology*. 1997;22:189–212.

19 Schmidt PJ, Nieman L, Danaceau MA, et al. Estrogen replacement in perimenopause-related depression: a preliminary report. *Am J Obstet Gynecol.* 2000;183:414–420.

20 Soares CN, Almeida OP, Joffe H, et al. Efficacy of estradiol for the treatment of depressive disorders in perimenopausal women. *Arch Gen Psychiatry.* 2001;58:529–534.

21 Rasgon NL, Altshuler LL, Fairbanks LA, et al. Estrogen replacement therapy in the treatment of major depressive disorder in perimenopausal women. *J Clin Psychiatry.* 2002;63:45–48.

22 Cohen LS, Soares CN, Poitras JR, et al. Short-term use of estradiol for depression in perimenopausal and postmenopausal women: a preliminary report. *Am J Psychiatry.* 2003;160:1519–1522.

23 Grigoriadis S, Kennedy SH. Role of estrogen in the treatment of depression. *Am J Ther.* 2002;9:503–509.

24 Sherwin BB. The impact of different doses of estrogen and progestin on mood and sexual behavior in postmenopausal women. *J Clin Endocrinol Metab.* 1991;72:336–343

25 Rohr UD. The impact of testosterone imbalance on depression and women's health. *Maturitas.* 2002;41(Suppl.):S25–S46.

26 Shifren JL. Androgen deficiency in the oophorectomized woman. *Fertil Steril.* 2002;77(Suppl. 4):60–62

27 Sherwin BB, Gelfand MM. Sex steroids and affect in the surgical menopause: a double-blind, cross-over study. *Psychoneuroendocrinology.* 1985;10:325–335.

28 Shifren JL, Braunstein GD, Simon JA, et al. Transdermal testosterone treatment in women with impaired sexual function after oophorectomy. *N Engl J Med.* 2000;343:682–688.

29 Rossouw JE, Anderson GL, Prentice RL, et al. Risks and benefits of estrogen plus progestin in healthy postmenopausal women: principal results from the Women's Health Initiative randomized controlled trial. *JAMA.* 2002;288:321–333.

30 Kornstein SG, Schatzberg AF, Thase ME, et al. Gender differences in chronic major and double depression. *J Affect Disord.* 2000;60:1–11.

31 Soares CN, Poitras JR, Prouty J, et al. Efficacy of citalopram as a monotherapy or as an adjunctive treatment to estrogen therapy for perimenopausal and postmenopausal women with depression and vasomotor symptoms. *J Clin Psychiatry.* 2003;64:473–479.

32 Loprinzi CL, Kugler JW, Sloan JA, et al. Venlafaxine in management of hot flashes in survivors of breast cancer: a randomised controlled trial. *Lancet.* 2000;356:2059–2063.

33 Stearns V, Isaacs C, Rowland J, et al. A pilot trial assessing the efficacy of paroxetine hydrochloride (Paxil) in controlling hot flashes in breast cancer survivors. *Ann Oncol.* 2000;11:17–22

34 Loprinzi CL, Sloan JA, Perez EA, et al. Phase III evaluation of fluoxetine for treatment of hot flashes. *J Clin Oncol*. 2002;20:1578–1583.

35 Stearns V, Beebe KL, Iyengar M, et al. Paroxetine controlled release in the treatment of menopausal hot flashes. A randomized controlled trial. *JAMA*. 2003;289:2827–2834.

36 Schneider LS, Small GW, Hamilton SH, et al. Estrogen replacement and response to fluoxetine in a multicenter geriatric depression trial. *Am J Geriatr Psychiatry*. 1997;5:97–106.

37 Amsterdam J, Garcia-Espana F, Fawcett J, et al. Fluoxetine efficacy in menopausal women with and without estrogen replacement. *J Affect Disord*. 1999;55:11–17.

38 Schneider LS, Small GW, Clary CM. Estrogen replacement therapy and antidepressant response to sertraline in older depressed women. *Am J Geriatr Psychiatry*. 2001;9:393–399.

39 Joffe H, Groninger H, Soares C, et al. An open trial of mirtazapine in menopausal women with depression unresponsive to estrogen replacement therapy. *J Womens Health*. 2001;10:999–1004.

40 Avis NE, McKinlay SM. A longitudinal analysis of women's attitudes toward the menopause: results from the Massachusetts Women's Health Study. *Maturitas*. 1991;13:65–79.

41 Deeks AA. Psychological aspects of menopause management. *Best Pract Res Clin Endocrinol Metab*. 2003;17:17–31.

42 Kaufert PA, Gilbert P, Tate R. The Manitoba project: a re-examination of the link between menopause and depression. *Maturitas*. 1992;14: 143–155.

43 Bosworth HB, Bastian LA, Kuchibhatla MN, et al. Depressive symptoms, menopausal status, and climacteric symptoms in women at midlife. *Psychosom Med*. 2001;63:603–608.

44 Pajer K. New strategies in the treatment of depression in women. *J Clin Psychiatry*. 1995;56(Suppl. 2):30–37.

45 Slaven L, Lee C. Mood and symptom reporting among middle-aged women: the relationship between menopausal status, hormone replacement therapy, and exercise participation. *Health Psychol*. 1997;16:203–208.

46 Becht MC, Van Erp CF, Teeuwisse TM, et al. Measuring depression in women around menopausal age. Towards a validation of the Edinburgh Depression Scale. *J Affect Disord*. 2001;63:209–213.

47 Rivera-Tovar AD, Frank E. Late luteal phase dysphoric disorder in young women. *Am J Psychiatry*. 1990;147:1634–1636.

48 Johnson SR, McChesney C, Bean JA. Epidemiology of premenstrual symptoms in a nonclinical sample. I. Prevalence, natural history and help-seeking behavior. *J Reprod Med*. 1988;33:340–346.

49 Freeman EW, Rickels K, Schweizer E, et al. Relationships between age and symptom severity among women seeking medical treatment for premenstrual symptoms. *Psychol Med.* 1995;25;309–315.

50 Cohen LS, Soares CN, Otto MW, et al. Prevalence and predictors of premenstrual dysphoric disorder (PMDD) in older premenopausal women. The Harvard Study of Moods and Cycles. *J Affect Disord.* 2002;70:125–132.

51 World Health Organization. *International Statistical Classification of Diseases and Related Health Problems.* 10th rev. Geneva: WHO; 1992.

52 ACOG Practice Bulletin, Number 15, April 2000.

53 Graze KK, Nee J, Endicott J. Premenstrual depression predicts future major depressive disorder. *Acta Psychiatr Scad.* 1990;81:201–205.

54 Yonkers KA, Halbreich U, Freeman E, et al. Symptomatic improvement of premenstrual dysphoric disorder with sertraline treatment. A randomized controlled trial. Sertraline Premenstrual Dysphoric Collaborative Study Group. *JAMA.* 1997;278:983–988.

55 Fava M, Pedrazzi F, Guaraldi GP. Comorbid anxiety and depression among patients with late luteal phase dysphoric disorder. *J Anxiety Disord.* 1992;6:325–335.

56 Bancroft J, Rennie D, Warner P, Vulnerability to perimenopausal mood change: the relevance of a past history of depressive disorder. *Psychosom Med.* 1994;56:225–231.

57 Harrison WM, Endicott J, Nee J, et al. Characteristics of women seeking treatment for premenstrual syndrome. *Psychosomatics.* 1989;30:405–411.

58 Steinberg S. The treatment of late luteal phase dysphoric disorder. *Life Sci.* 1991;49:767–802.

59 Kendler KS, Karkowski LM, Corey LA, et al. Longitudinal population-based twin study of retrospectively reported premenstrual symptoms and lifetime major depression. *Am J Psychiatry.* 1998;155:1234–1240.

60 Roca CA, Schmidt PJ, Bloch M, et al. Implications of endocrine studies of premenstrual syndrome. *Psychiatr Ann.* 1996;26:576–580.

61 Steiner M. Premenstrual syndromes. *Ann Rev Med.* 1997;48:447–455

62 Halbreich U. Reflections on the cause of premenstrual syndrome. *Psychiatr Ann.* 1996;26:581–585.

63 Poromaa IS, Smith S, Gulinello M. GABA receptors, progesterone and premenstrual dysphoric disorder. *Arch Womens Ment Health.* 2003;6:23–41.

64 Paul SM, Purdy RH. Neuroactive steroids. *FASEB J.* 1992;6:2311–2312.

65 Rapkin AJ, Morgan M, Goldman L, et al. Progesterone metabolite allopregnanolone in women with premenstrual syndrome. *Obstet Gynecol.* 1997;90:709–714.

66 Wyatt KM, Dimmock PW, O'Brien PM. Selective serotonin reuptake inhibitors for premenstrual syndrome. *Cochrane Database Syst Rev.* 2002;4:CD001396.

67 Griffin LD, Mellon S. Selective serotonin reuptake inhibitors directly alter activity of neurosteroidogenic enzymes. *Proc Natl Acad Sci USA.* 1999;96:13512–13517.

68 Steiner M, Steinberg S, Stewart D, et al. Fluoxetine in the treatment of premenstrual dysphoria. *N Engl J Med.* 1995;332:1529–1534.

69 Yonkers KA, Halbreich U, Freeman E, et al. Sertraline in the treatment of premenstrual dysphoric disorder. *Psychopharmacol Bull.* 1996;32: 41–46.

70 Steiner M, Romano S, Babcock S. Fluoxetine's efficacy in improving physical symptoms associated with PMDD. *Eur Neuropsychopharmacology.* 1999;9(Suppl. 5):S208.

71 Pearlstein TB, Halbreich U, Batzar ED, et al. Psychosocial functioning in women with premenstrual dysphoric disorder before and after treatment with sertraline or placebo. *J Clin Psychiatry.* 2000;61: 101–109.

72 Eriksson E, Hedberg MA, Andersch B, et al. The serotonin reuptake inhibitor paroxetine is superior to the noradrenaline reuptake inhibitor maprotiline in the treatment of premenstrual syndrome. *Neuropsychopharmacology.* 1995;12:167–176.

73 Freeman EW, Rickels K, Sondheimer SJ, et al. Differential response to antidepressants in women with premenstrual syndrome/premenstrual dysphoric disorder. A randomized controlled trial. *Arch Gen Psychiatry.* 1999;56:932–939.

74 Pearlstein TB, Stone AB, Lund SA, et al. Comparison of fluoxetine, bupropion and placebo in the treatment of premenstrual dysphoric disorder. *J Clin Psychopharmacol.* 1997;17:261–266.

75 Sundblad C, Modigh K, Andersch B, et al. Clomipramine effectively reduces premenstrual irritability and dysphoria: a placebo-controlled trial. *Acta Psychiatr Scand.* 1992;85:39–47.

76 Wikander I, Sundblad C, Andersch B, et al. Citalopram in premenstrual dysphoria: is intermittent treatment during luteal phases more effective than continuous medication throughout the menstrual cycle? *J Clin Psychopharmacol.* 1998;18:390–398.

77 Freeman EW, Rickels K, Yonkers KA, et al. Venlafaxine in the treatment of premenstrual dysphoric disorder. *Obstet Gynecol.* 2001;98:737–744.

78 Sundblad C, Hedberg MA, Eriksson E. Clomipramine administered during the luteal phase reduces the symptoms of premenstrual syndrome: a placebo-controlled trial. *Neuropsychopharmacology.* 1993;9:133–145.

79 Halbreich U, Smoller JW. Intermittent luteal phase sertraline treatment of dysphoric premenstrual syndrome. *J Clin Psychiatry.* 1997;58:399–402.

80 Steiner M, Korzekwa M, Lamont J, et al. Intermittent fluoxetine dosing in the treatment of women with premenstrual dysphoria. *Psychopharmacol Bull.* 1997;33:771–774.

81 Mezrow G, Shoupe D, Spicer D, et al. Depot leuprolide acetate with estrogen and progestin add-back for long-term treatment of premenstrual syndrome. *Fertil Steril.* 1994;62:932–937.

82 Wyatt K, Dimmock P, Jones P, et al. Efficacy of progesterone and progestogens in management of premenstrual syndrome: systematic review. *BMJ.* 2001;323:776–780.

83 Sarno AP, Miller EJ Jr, Lundblad EG. Premenstrual syndrome: beneficial effects of periodic, low-dose danazol. *Obstet Gynecol.* 1987;70: 33–36.

84 Graham CA, Sherwin BB. A prospective treatment study of premenstrual symptoms using a triphasic oral contraceptive. *J Psychosom Res.* 1992;36:257–266.

85 Freeman EW, Rickels K, Sondheimer SJ, et al. Concurrent use of oral contraceptives with antidepressants for premenstrual syndromes. *J Clin Psychopharmacol.* 2001;21:540–542.

86 Freeman EW, Kroll R, Rapkin A, et al. Evaluation of a unique oral contraceptive in the treatment of premenstrual dysphoric disorder. *J Womens Health Gend Based Med.* 2001;10:561–569.

87 Wyatt KM, Dimmock PW, Jones PW, et al. Efficacy of vitamin B-6 in the treatment of premenstrual syndrome: systematic review. *BMJ.* 1999;318:1375–1381.

88 Thys-Jacobs S, Starkey P, Bernstein D, et al. Calcium carbonate and the premenstrual syndrome: effects on premenstrual and menstrual symptoms. Premenstrual Syndrome Study Group. *Am J Obstet Gynecol.* 1998;179:444–452.

89 London RS, Murphy L, Kitlowski KE, et al. Efficacy of alphatocopherol in the treatment of the premenstrual syndrome. *J Reprod Med.* 1987;32:400–404.

90 Facchinetti F, Borella P, Sances G, et al. Oral magnesium successfully relieves premenstrual mood changes. *Obstet Gynecol.* 1991;78:177–181.

91 Prior JC, Vigna Y, Sciarretta D, et al. Conditioning exercise decreases premenstrual symptoms: a prospective, controlled 6-month trial. *Fertil Steril.* 1987;47:402–408.

92 Steege JF, Blumenthal JA. The effects of aerobic exercise on premenstrual symptoms in middle-aged women: a preliminary study. *J Psychosom Res.* 1993;37:127–133.

93 Blake F, Salkovskis P, Gath D, et al. Cognitive therapy for premenstrual syndrome: a controlled trial. *J Psychosom Res.* 1998;45: 307–318.

94 Kirkby RJ. Changes in premenstrual symptoms and irrational thinking following cognitive-behavioral coping skills training. *J Consult Clin Psychol.* 1994;62:1026–1032.

95 Christensen AP, Oei TP. The efficacy of cognitive behaviour therapy in treating premenstrual dysphoric changes. *J Affect Disord.* 1995;33: 57–63.

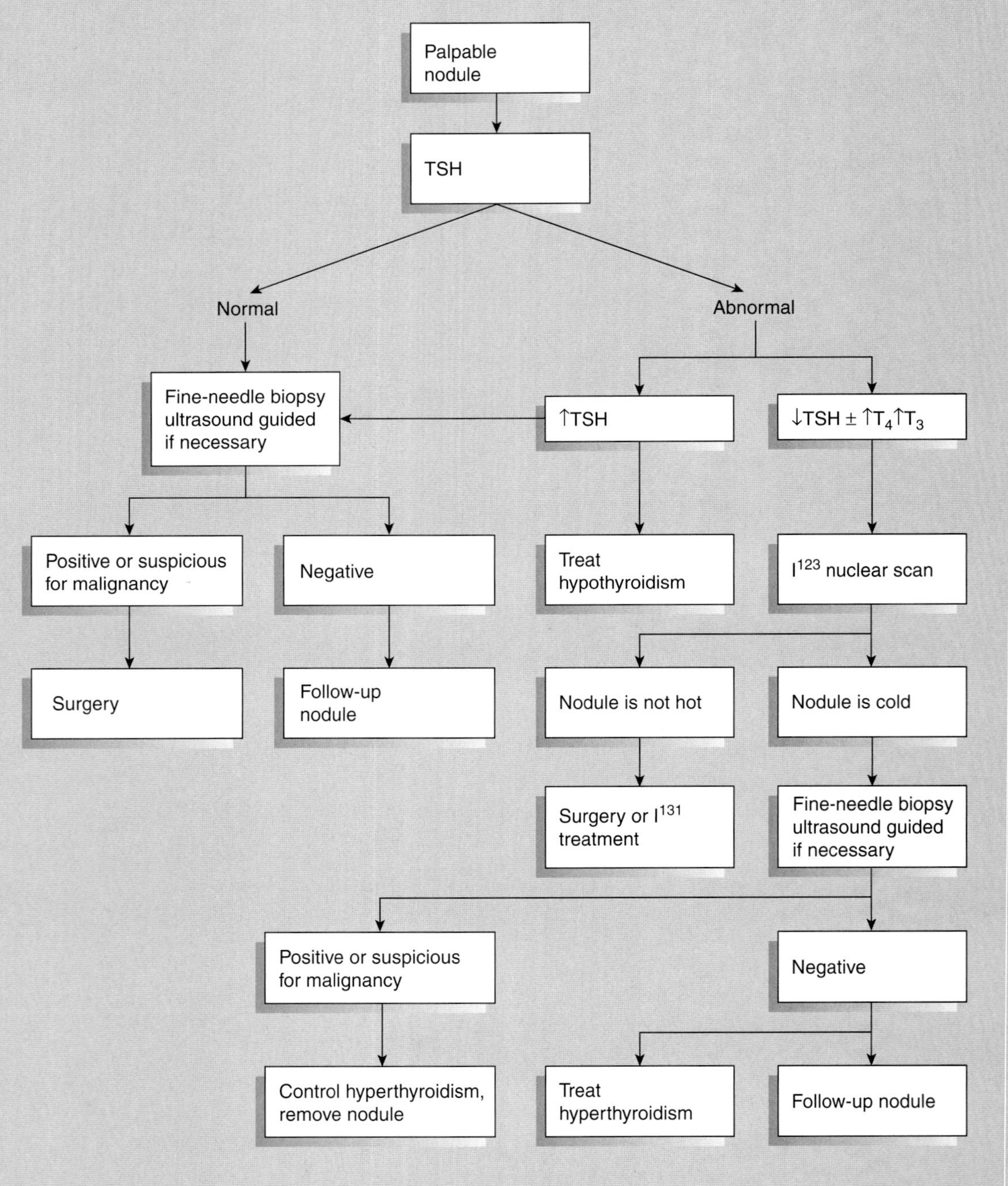

Workup and Management of Thyroid Nodule
Palpable nodule
TSH
Normal
Abnormal
Fine-needle biopsy ultrasound guided if necessary
↑TSH
↓TSH ± ↑T_4↑T_3
Positive or suspicious for malignancy
Negative
Treat hypothyroidism
I^{123} nuclear scan
Surgery
Follow-up nodule
Nodule is not hot
Nodule is cold
Surgery or I^{131} treatment
Fine-needle biopsy ultrasound guided if necessary
Positive or suspicious for malignancy
Negative
Control hyperthyroidism, remove nodule
Treat hyperthyroidism
Follow-up nodule

16 Thyroid Dysfunction

Sona Kashyap
Shahla Nader

KEY POINT

Thyroid disorders are very common in women of peri menopausal age.

In women of perimenopausal age, thyroid disorders are common. Many of these disorders relate to altered immunity. As changes in the hormonal milieu during this phase of life may influence the thyroid hormone concentrations, it is essential to have a basic knowledge of the anatomy and physiology of the thyroid to understand the common thyroid diseases afflicting women in this group. This chapter provides such a synopsis.

Thyroid Anatomy

The normal thyroid gland is the shape of a butterfly. It is firmly attached by fibrous tissue to the anterior and lateral parts of the larynx and trachea. The weight of the thyroid of the normal non-goitrous adult is 10–20 g depending on body size and iodine intake. The width and length of the isthmus average 20 mm, and its thickness is 2–6 mm. The lateral lobes from superior to inferior poles usually measure 4 cm. Their breadth is 15–20 mm, and their thickness is 20–40 mm.

Thyroid Hormone Physiology

SYNTHESIS AND SECRETION

Thyroid hormone production is highly regulated by the hypothalamus through the secretion of TRH, which in turn stimulates the release of TSH from the pituitary. In response to TSH, the thyroid follicle is then stimulated to produce thyroid hormone. The first step involves a Na/I symporter, which binds sodium and iodide and transports them into the cell. The next step is catalyzed

KEY POINT

Thyroid hormone synthesis and secretion involves several coordinated processes in the thyroid follicle, which are stimulated by thyrotropin (thyroid-stimulating hormon [TSH]).

by thyroperoxidase (TPO) and involves the oxidation of iodide and its binding to tyrosyl residues which are part of a large glycoprotein–thyroglobulin. The monoiodotyrosine (MIT) and diiodotyrosine (DIT) residues undergo coupling reaction; this step also mediated by TPO, is one in which either two DIT molecules couple to form T4 or a DIT molecule couples with a MIT molecule and forms T3. Thyroglobulin is stored in the lumen of the follicle as colloid. For secretion, thyroglobulin enters the thyrocytes by pinocytosis and then undergoes hydrolysis liberating the iodoamino acids. Some of the thyroxine (T4) molecules undergo monodeiodination within the gland to form triiodothyronine (T3). The ratio of secretion of T4 and T3 is usually 15:1. DIT and MIT released by hydrolysis are deiodinated by an iodotyrosine dehalogenase and the iodide is reused.

Circulating Thyroid Hormones

Similar to many hormones, both T3 and T4 are protein bound. The main carrier protein is thyroxine-binding globulin (TBG) for T4 and T3. Other binders are transthyretin (TTR), which primarily binds T4 and albumin, which binds both hormones. Only 0.03% of T4 and 0.2% of T3 are unbound. The strong protein binding influences the rate of turnover; the biologic half-life of circulating T4 is about 7 days and of T3 is about 1–3 days. Changes in levels of binding globulin can significantly affect total hormone levels measured (Table 16-1).

KEY POINT

T4 and T3 are both highly protein bound.

Hormone Action

Free thyroid hormones bind to nuclear receptors. T3 has tenfold higher affinity for these receptors than T4, which helps explain the greater biological activity of T3. The major effects of thyroid

Table 16-1. **CAUSES OF ALTERED THYROID HORMONE-BINDING PROTEINS**

Increased Binding	*Decreased Binding*
Pregnancy	Androgens
Estrogen treatment	Glucocorticoids
Oral contraceptives	Salicylates, furosemide, heparin
Hepatitis	L-asparaginase
Tamoxifen, Raloxifene	Nicotinic acid
Mitotane, 5-fluorouracil	Severe illness, nephrotic syndrome
Hereditary	Hereditary

hormones are genomic, stimulating transcription and translation of new proteins. This results in their diverse effects on cellular growth, development, and metabolism.

Hormone Metabolism

The major mechanism is sequential monodeiodination. The first step is deiodination of T4 to produce either T3 or rT3 (reverse T3), which is metabolically inactive. Removal of iodine from the outer ring of T4 results in T3 formation and when iodine is removed from the inner ring, reverse T3 is produced. Most (85%) of the T3 in circulation is derived from monodeiodination of T4 in the periphery. Further deiodination forms diiodothyronines and monoiodothyronines and finally thyronine.

Another pathway is the hepatic uptake, conjugation, and biliary excretion of T4, T3 and its metabolites. This involves the P450 pathway and accounts for 25% of hormone disposal.

Regulation of Thyroid Hormones

Thyroid hormone levels in circulation are determined in two ways. One is regulation of hormone production and secretion by TSH and the other is regulation of extrathyroidal conversion of T4 to T3 by hormonal, nutritional, and stress-related factors.

Thyrotropin-releasing hormone (TRH) is a peptide hormone synthesized and secreted by the hypothalamus. It reaches the pituitary via the portal system to determine the set point of thyroid hormone regulation by TSH.

TSH is a glycoprotein synthesized and secreted by the anterior pituitary. It shares the structure of its alpha subunit with follicle-stimulating hormone (FSH), luteinizing hormone (LH), and human chorionic gonadotropin. (HCG) but has a unique beta subunit.

KEY POINT

TSH stimulates every step in thyroid hormone synthesis and secretion outlined above and induces thyroid gland hyperplasia and hypertrophy.

TSH secretion is controlled by negative feedback. A very small decrease in T4 and T3 levels stimulates the secretion of TSH and very small increments of thyroid hormone levels suppress it. This tight control results in maintenance of thyroid hormone levels within quite narrow limits. Somatostatin, glucocorticoids, and dopamine have inhibitory actions on TSH, whereas TRH stimulates it.[2]

Various factors affecting the enzyme deiodinase influence the peripheral conversion of T4 to T3. Nutritional, hormonal, and other illness-related factors, for example, uncontrolled diabetes and uremia, regulate the activity and mass of this enzyme. Medications like beta-blockers, glucocorticoids, propylthiouracil and iodothyronine analogues also reduce the activity of this enzyme.

Thyroid Testing

SERUM T4 AND T3

Serum total T4 and T3 is measured by radioimmunoassay (RIA), chemiluminometric, or other immunometric assays. These assays measure both the bound and unbound fractions of the hormones. The limitation of these tests is that the results may not be concordant with actual free hormone levels in the body. Alterations in binding proteins (Table 16-1) significantly influence the total hormone levels.[3,4] This is very relevant to women who might be on hormone therapy or birth control pills both of which will increase the level of TBG. In addition, changes in binding proteins might reflect in changes in thyroid hormone requirements in patients with underlying hypothyroidism. For example, thyroid hormone requirements can be higher in hypothyroid patients during pregnancy, oral contraceptives, and on initiation of hormone therapy.

SERUM FREE T4 AND FREE T3

It is the free fraction of the hormones, that is biologically active and binds to nuclear receptors. Many illnesses and drugs affect the binding proteins and may thus affect the levels of total hormones. Accordingly, estimates of free hormones are used to overcome this shortcoming of total hormone measurements.

Various methodologies are used. None of the current assays provide absolutely accurate free hormone levels after accounting for all binding abnormalities. Each methodology has its own normal range.

If free hormone determinations are not available, a free T4 index can be calculated. It is a measurement that uses the value of total T4 and T3 resin uptake. This gives the clinician a better indication of the presence of a binding abnormality. The T3 resin uptake is directly related to the free T4 fraction and inversely related to binding protein. For example, when TBG level is high, as with estrogen use, the total T4 is high, the T3 resin uptake is low, and the free T4 index will be normal.

$$\text{Formula: Free T4 index} = \frac{\text{Total T4} \times \text{T3 resin uptake}}{100}$$

SERUM TSH CONCENTRATION

First-generation assays have a detection limit of 1 mU/L, second-generation assays have a detection limit of 0.1 mU/L, and third generation assays have a limit of 0.01 mU/L. Therefore, the newer third generation assays reliably provide distinguishable levels within patients with hyperthyroidism, hypothyroidism, and euthyroidism.

KEY POINT

The TSH level, using a highly sensitive TSH assay, is the single best test for assessing thyroid function.

When TSH is high, the patient has primary hypothyroidism. When TSH is below the normal range, the patient usually has hyperthyroidism. Exceptions to this rule happen when thyroid dysfunction is secondary to hypothalamic/pituitary disease, secondary to hormone resistance syndromes, or when there is ectopic production of hormones or in the presence of nonthyroidal illnesses.

THYROID ULTRASOUND

Thyroid ultrasonography allows identification of structures as small as 2–3 mm in diameter. It is useful in the following clinical situations—supplements physical examination in evaluating nodular thyroid disease and helps to identify characteristics suggestive of malignancy. In patients with established thyroid malignancy, ultrasound helps in surveillance, localization, and quantification of residual and recurrent disease.

THYROID SCINTISCAN

I-123 and I-131 radioisotopes are employed to image the thyroid gland. Thyroid scanning determines if a given nodule accumulates radioiodine or not. It also gives a two-dimensional scan of functioning thyroid tissue.

Thyroid Disorders

KEY POINT

It is recommended that women be screened with TSH measurements at age 50 and then every 3–5 years.

Thyroid disease is very common and women have a higher prevalence of hypothyroidism, hyperthyroidism, and thyroid nodules as compared to men. The prevalence of hypothyroidism and thyroid nodules increases with age. Autoimmune thyroiditis may also occur in this population. Therefore, it is reasonable to screen women with TSH measurements at age 50 and then every 3–5 years.

HYPOTHYROIDISM

Hypothyroidism results when tissues have inadequate supply of thyroid hormone. It is common especially in women in their mid-fifties with a prevalence of about 10%. Two most common causes are chronic lymphocytic thyroiditis and radioiodine-induced hypothyroidism. Other less common but important causes include subacute thyroiditis, external radiation to neck, drugs, congenital defects, and central hypothyroidism. Hypothyroidism due to iodine deficiency, which is common outside the United States, is rarely seen here (Table 16-2).

Symptoms of hypothyroidism are nonspecific such as cold intolerance, fatigue, weight gain, constipation, depression, dry skin, hair loss, and some menstrual irregularities. With moderate-to-severe disease, physical examination might reveal bradycardia, diastolic hypertension, periorbital swelling, coarse yellow skin, puffy face, and delayed relaxation of deep tendon reflexes. Rare presentations would be congestive heart failure, megacolon, and cardiomegaly. A rare complication is myxedema coma which

Table 16-2. **CAUSES OF HYPOTHYROIDISM**

Cause	*Mechanism*	*Specific Findings*
Chronic lymphocytic thyroiditis (Hashimoto's disease)	Lymphocytic infiltration	TPO Ab, TG Ab Goiter
Iatrogenic destruction of thyroid tissue—radioiodine, thyroidectomy, radiation	Destruction	Positive history
Subacute thyroiditis—viral	Granulomatous inflammation	Pain, fever, malaise, ↑↑ ESR
Acute thyroiditis—infectious	Suppurative infection	Pain, fever
Pituitary lesions (secondary hypothyroidism) surgery, Sheehan's, irradiation, lymphocytic hypophysitis	TSH deficiency	↓↓ TSH and ↓↓ FT4
Hypothalamic lesions (tertiary hypothyroidism)	TRH deficiency	↓↓ TSH and ↓↓ FT4
Drugs—iodides, lithium, IFN-α, thionamides, amiodarone	Destruction/blockage of enzymes	
Congenital	Enzyme defect, aplasia, hypoplasia, maternal I deficiency, TSH receptor defect	
Iodine deficiency	Decreased hormone production	Goiter

Abbreviations: TPO AB, thyroid peroxidase antibody; TG Ab, thyroglobulin antibody; ESR, erythrocyte sedimentation rate; TSH, thyroid-stimulating hormone; FT4, free thyroxine; TRH, thyrotropin-releasing hormone; IFN, interferon.

KEY POINT

In elderly patients, thyroid replacement should begin with low doses with a slow, gradual increase.

is severe hypothyroidism leading to hypothermia, bradycardia, hypoventilation, hypotension, hypoglycemia, and hyponatremia.

An elevated TSH, with a low T4 confirms hypothyroidism. Other laboratory findings are hyponatremia, elevated creatinine phosphokinase (CPK) levels, elevated low-density lipoprotein (LDL) cholesterol, and mild anemia.

Treatment is replacement of thyroxine. Full dose can be used in healthy patients, which is estimated to be approximately 1.6 mcg/kg/day. Elderly patients should be started on low doses and increased gradually in 25 mcg increments every 2–3 months to avoid any exacerbation of cardiac problems. It is essential that patients do not take thyroxine with medications like calcium, iron, sucralfate, and occasionally other medications, which impair absorption significantly. Patients can be monitored by means of TSH testing every 5–6 weeks until the dose is stabilized and then every 6–12 months thereafter. Overreplacement of thyroid hormones increases the risk of bone loss and atrial fibrillation.[5,6]

Hyperthyroidism

Hyperthyroidism results when excessive amounts of thyroid hormone are delivered to responsive tissues. Thyrotoxicosis can result from an overproduction of thyroid hormones or an exaggerated release of preformed hormones from the thyroid gland. The overproduction may be due to increased stimulation by means of thyroid-stimulating immunoglobulins (Graves' disease), autonomous nodules, HCG (choriocarcinoma, molar pregnancy, hyperemesis gravidarum), or TSH (pituitary tumor, TSH resistance). Examples of exaggerated release of preformed hormones include exposure to radiation, inflammation due to an autoimmune/viral phenomenon and trauma. Increased intake of exogenous thyroid hormones in the form of certain weight-loss products or abuse of thyroid hormone preparations can lead to thyrotoxicosis too. It is essential to identify the correct cause, because treatment would depend on the underlying mechanism.

KEY POINT

Graves' disease is the most common form of hyperthyroidism.

In order to delineate the underlying process, one way of classifying causes of thyrotoxicosis is based on 24-hour radioactive iodine uptake (RAIU) (Fig. 16-1). Thyroid–stimulating immunoglobulins and other thyroid antibodies help identify autoimmune thyroid disease.

Antibodies directed against the TSH receptor result in continuous stimulation of the thyroid gland in Graves' disease and autoimmune

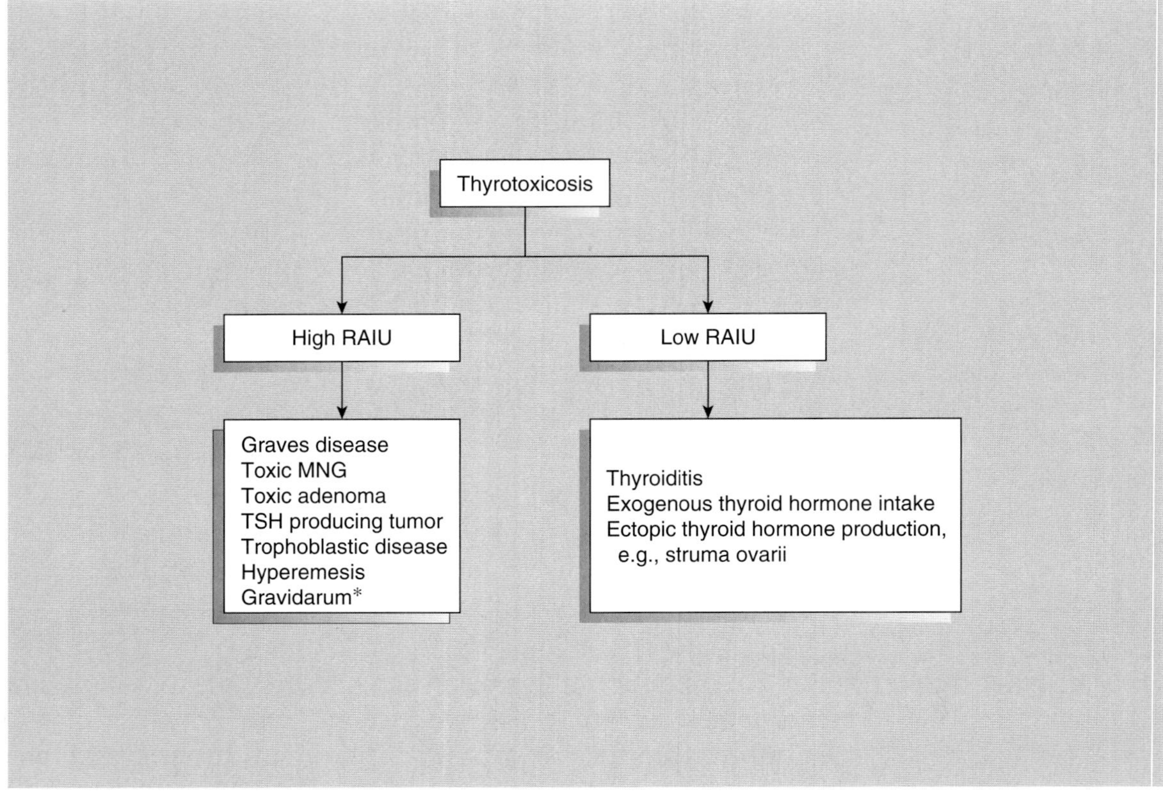

Figure 16-1: Thyrotoxicosis—differential diagnosis of high and low iodine uptake states. RAIU: radioactive iodine uptake; MNG: multinodular goiter; TSH: thyroid-stimulating hormone. *RAIU is not recommended in pregnancy.

disorder. It is more common in women of childbearing age. In addition to a diffuse goiter, patients can have extrathyroidal manifestations, which include ophthalmopathy (20–25%), pretibial myxedema (5%), and thyroid acropachy, which is clubbing and osteoarthropathy of phalanges of fingers and toes.

Toxic multinodular goiter (Plummer's disease) arises in the setting of longstanding multinodular goiter in which certain nodules develop autonomy. It is usually seen in women in their fifties. Exposure to iodine may also trigger hyperthyroidism in this setting.

KEY POINT

Thyroiditis may have a transient hyperthyroid phase in about 33% of the patients.

Toxic adenomas have excessive constitutive activation of the thyroid tissue and frequently produce overt hyperthyroidism when larger than 3–3.5 cm.

Thyroiditis can be acute, subacute, or silent/postpartum thyroiditis. There is an initial phase of thyrotoxicosis with the release of stored hormones, followed by hypothyroidism, which eventually resolves and euthyroidism is restored. About 8% of women develop postpartum thyroiditis and these women have a high rate of progression (20%) to hypothyroidism.

Other rare causes of hyperthyroidism are ectopic thyroid hormone production, e.g., struma ovarii or increased HCG production, e.g., choriocarcinoma, pituitary-specific thyroid hormone resistance and TSH-producing tumors.

Symptoms of hyperthyroidism include heat intolerance, fatigue, weight loss, nausea, diarrhea, palpitations, anxiety, insomnia, shakiness, and menses with lighter flow. Elderly patients may present with lack of typical adrenergic features. They may have apathy, weight loss, and cardiac decompensation—termed as apathetic hyperthyroidism.[7]

Signs include tachycardia, tremors, warm moist skin, hyperreflexia, thyroid bruit (Graves' disease), and eye signs such as lid lag, stare, and proptosis in Graves' disease.

Treatment alternatives for hyperthyroidism are radioactive iodine, antithyroid drugs, and surgery. These treat the underlying overproduction of thyroid hormones and beta-blockers may be used to treat the hyperadrenergic symptoms. The choice of treatment depends on the underlying disease process and patient response.[8]

Antithyroid drugs (methimazole and propylthiouracil) are up to 90% successful in achieving euthyroidism in Graves' disease. The initiation dose is 30–60 mg/day for methimazole and 150–600 mg/day for propylthiouracil. Maintenance doses are 50–70% lower.[9] Long-term remission rate in Graves' disease is only 30% after 12–18 months of treatment. Antithyroid drugs are not effective in patients with low RAIU states such as thyroiditis. In patients with toxic adenomas and toxic multinodular goiters, antithyroid drugs are unlikely to cause long-term remission and are used temporarily to reduce overproduction prior to treatment that is more definitive. The significant side effects of antithyroid drugs are agranulocytosis (<0.5%), hepatotoxicity (necrotic hepatitis with propylthiouracil and cholestatic jaundice with methimazole), and rashes (3–5%). Propylthiouracil is the preferred agent in younger patients of reproductive age as methimazole has been reported to cause aplasia cutis and possible other embryopathy in exposed fetuses.

I-131 treatment is a more definitive treatment. It emits destructive beta particles over a period of several months. It is about 90% effective in rendering the patient euthyroid over 6 months. Younger patients should be advised to avoid pregnancy for at least 6 months after treatment. This modality is used for patients with Graves' disease, toxic adenomas, and toxic multinodular goiters.

Surgery is reserved for patients intolerant of medications, when I-131 is contraindicated and in patients with suspicious cold nodules or for extremely large goiters. Patients should be euthyroid before surgery.

Thyroid Nodules

The presence of thyroid nodules is a very common finding that might first be noticed by the patient, the physician, or by an imaging procedure done for a different reason. Approximately 5–7% of these nodules eventually turn out to be malignant.

KEY POINT

Evaluation of a thyroid nodule requires screening for hyperthyroidism, a thyroid scan, and a fine needle biopsy.

The risk of malignancy is increased if age is over 45 years and there is history of exposure to radiation at a young age. Clinical features that suggest malignancy are rapid growth of the mass, a hard tumor, obstructive symptoms, cervical lymphadenopathy, and vocal cord paralysis. Ultrasonogrophic features suggestive of malignancy are microcalcifications, irregular borders, and central blood flow.

The first step in evaluating a thyroid nodule is to do thyroid function tests to exclude hyperthyroidism. Evidence of hyperthyroidism warrants a thyroid scan. In all other cases, fine needle aspiration biopsy (FNAB) would be a reasonable initial diagnostic test. Ultrasound guided FNAB is done when palpation guided FNAB is technically difficult.

FNAB is about 95% accurate in its diagnosis when performed by experienced physicians. The results are reported as benign, indeterminate/suspicious, or malignant when sufficient specimen is collected. The nodules reported as indeterminate or suspicious can be either follicular or Hurthle cell cancers or adenomas. The presence of capsular or vascular invasion indicates malignancy and this cannot be determined by FNAB. Thus, surgery is recommended for indeterminate/suspicious lesions.[10]

Thyroid Cancer

Malignancies arising from follicular cells are classified as papillary, follicular, or anaplastic thyroid cancer based on the microscopic appearance, and they occur in this order of frequency. Medullary thyroid cancer arises from C cells.

Differentiated thyroid cancer (papillary and follicular) usually presents as a painless thyroid nodule and the peak incidence is in fourth-fifth decade of life. Rarely these cancers may present with obstructive symptoms or with difficulty speaking.

Therapy of differentiated thyroid cancer is surgical removal of the primary tumor followed by radioablation by radioactive iodine (I-131). Lifelong suppression of TSH with exogenous thyroid hormone subsequently reduces the risk of recurrence. It is important to be aware of this in patients with a history of thyroid cancers that are on thyroid hormone as the aim is to have their TSH levels suppressed below the normal levels. Whole-body scans, thyroglobulin levels, and radiological studies are used to monitor these patients for recurrent or residual disease. The 10-year mortality is 5–10% and is slightly worse in follicular cancers as compared to papillary cancers.

Anaplastic thyroid carcinoma is more aggressive and usually presents with symptoms related to aggressive local growth—dysphagia, dyspnea, hoarseness, and pain. It accounts for 1–10% of thyroid carcinomas. Surgery along with external beam radiation or chemotherapy has been used but average survival is 6–10 months.

Medullary thyroid cancers (MCT) arise from parafollicular cells (C cells), and account for 2–10% of all thyroid carcinomas. These cells produce calcitonin, which modulates release of calcium from skeletal stores. It occurs in sporadic and hereditary forms, presenting in the fourth-fifth decade of life. The hereditary form occurs within kindreds as a component of MEN (multiple endocrine neoplasia) 2A, as a component of MEN 2B, or as familial MCT. In addition to the symptoms of aggressive local growth, these tumors secrete a wide range of peptides, which result in multiple extrathyroidal symptoms. Surgery is the main modality of treatment. External beam radiotherapy and chemotherapy have been used but do not have any clear survival benefit.

Nonthyroidal Illnesses

Patients with nonthyroidal illnesses frequently have abnormal thyroid function tests. It is not known whether these changes are an adaptation to the severe illness or a part of the illness itself. The usual findings are that of a low serum T3 and T4 and a low TSH. However, TSH can also be normal or even slightly elevated.

Undetectable TSH levels are not a common finding in nonthyroidal illness and should alert the physician to the presence of hyperthyroidism. Hence, thyroid function should be interpreted very cautiously under these circumstances. Distinguishing nonthyroidal illness from early mild thyroid dysfunction can be difficult and requires complementary testing such as thyroid antibody studies, repeat assays, and looking for associated autoimmune diseases.

One of the mechanisms of low T3 is hypothesized to be high endogenous cortisol levels, high free fatty acid levels, cytokines, and certain drugs like amiodarone or propranolol that reduce 5′-monodeiodinase activity. This enzyme is responsible for T4 conversion to T3 and causes deiodination of rT3 to diiodothyronines. Hence, rT3 accumulates in such circumstances. The other proposed mechanism for the observed changes in hormone levels is reduced binding and reduced concentrations of the thyroid hormone-binding proteins.[11,12] Another hypothesis is the inhibition of hypothalamic-pituitary-thyroid axis in states of stress.

Currently, there is no evidence of benefit with respect to mortality or morbidity to support replacement of thyroid hormones in patients with nonthyroidal illness with low T3 and T4. It is advised that thyroid function tests be repeated on recovery.

Discussion of Cases

CASE 1

A 52-year-old postmenopausal woman presents for evaluation of menopausal hormonal treatment. She has had hysterectomy with bilateral salpingo-oophorectomy for fibroids and has been symptomatically menopausal for 3 years. She gives a history of irregular heartbeat. On examination, her vital signs are within normal limits. Head and neck examination reveals a 20–25 g thyroid with no palpable nodules. Rest of the examination including cardiac, respiratory, abdomen is benign.

On investigation, the patient is mildly anemic—normocytic normochromic. Chemistries, liver profile, and lipid panel are within normal ranges. A TSH is checked and it is 9.8 mIU/L.

The patient has hypothyroidism. Hypothyroidism is a common diagnosis in women in this age group and may present insidiously with nonspecific symptoms. It is advisable to maintain a low threshold to check TSH levels in postmenopausal women.

No further tests are needed before initiating treatment. Patient is initiated on levothyroxine replacement at a dose of 50 mcg daily. Six weeks later, repeat tests showed TSH of 3.8 mIU/L (0.04–5.5), which is within normal range. The patient is symptomatically better. She feels more energetic. She is continued on her current dose of levothyroxine and she should be monitored by means of checking TSH levels every 6 months.

CASE 2

A 58-year-old postmenopausal female complains of unintentional 16 lb weight loss. Appetite is normal. Review of symptoms is otherwise negative. She has a history of osteoporosis and poliomyelitis affecting her right leg. Her current medications include Fosamax.

On examination, her pulse is 90–100/minute and regular. Head and neck examination reveals a 30 g goiter, which is diffuse. Eye examination is normal. Rest of the head and neck examination is normal. Cardiac examination reveals tachycardia. Chest and abdomen examination is normal. Extremities reveal smooth warm skin. Reflexes are brisk and no tremors are noted on outstretched hands.

Investigations reveal a TSH of 0.01 mIU/L (0.04–5.5), free T4 of 2.5 ng/dL (0.8–1.8 ng/dL), and total T3 of 353 ng/dL (60–181 ng/dL). A RAIU and scan reveals homogenous uptake, 13.5% at 4 hours and 12.4% at 24 hours.

Repeat laboratory investigations continue to show a suppressed TSH of 0.01 mIU/L (0.04–5.5).

The history, physical examination, and investigations are consistent with a diagnosis of hyperthyroidism. Because her thyroid gland is diffusely enlarged without nodules, her thyrotoxicosis is most likely secondary to Graves' disease (see Table 16-3). While the RAIU is not elevated, the fact that it is *not* suppressed lends further support to our diagnosis of Graves' disease rather than thyroiditis. The patient is initiated on methimazole, which blocks thyroid hormone synthesis and the plan is to treat her with radioactive iodine to ablate her thyroid during a follow-up visit.

Table 16-3. **EVALUATION OF THYROTOXICOSIS**

	GRAVES'	*TOXIC MNG*	*TOXIC ADENOMA*	*FACTITIOUS*	*THYROIDITIS*
TSH	↓↓	↓↓	↓↓	↓↓	↓↓
T4/T3	↑↑	↑↑	↑↑	↑↑	↑↑
RAIU	↑↑	↑↑	↑↑	↓↓	↓↓
Others	TSI/thyroid scan*	Thyroid scan†	Thyroid scan‡	Thyroglobulin, thyroid scan§	Thyroid scan, TPO, anti-TG Ab¶

Abbreviations: TSH, thyroid-stimulating hormone; T4, thyroxine; T3, triiodothyronine; RAIU, radioactive iodine uptake; TSI, thyroid-stimulating immunoglobulin; TPO, thyroid peroxidase antibody; anti-TG Ab, anti thyroglobulin antibody; MNG, multinodular goiter.

*TSI high and diffuse enlargement on scan.

†Patchy areas of increased iodine uptake.

‡Uptake of iodine increased in adenoma only.

§Low thyroglobulin and decreased iodine intake.

¶Decreased iodine uptake and positive TPO and anti-TG Ab.

References

1 Larsen PR, Davies TF, Hay ID. The thyroid gland. Williams Textbook of Endocrinology; 1998:389–515.

2 Scanlon MF, Toft AD, Braverman LE, et al. Regulation of TSH secretion. *Werner and Ingbar's The Thyroid: A fundamental and Clinical Text*. 7th ed. 1996:220–240.

3 Gorman CA. Thyroid function testing: a new era. *Mayo Clin Proc.* 1988;63:1026–1027.

4 Klee GG, Hay ID. Biochemical thyroid function testing. *Mayo Clin Proc.* 1994;69:469–470.

5 Sawin CT, Geller A, Wolf PA, et al. Low serum thyrotropin concentration as a risk factor for atrial fibrillation in older persons. *N Engl J Med.* 1994;331:1249–1252.

6 Faber J, Galloe AM. Changes in bone mass during prolonged subclinical hyperthyroidism due to L-thyroxine treatment: a meta analysis. *Eur J Endocrinol.* 1994;130:350–356.

7 Trivalle C, Doucet J, Chassagne P, et al. Differences in the signs and symptoms of hyperthyroidism in older and younger patients. *J A Geriatric Soc.* 1996;44(1):50–53.

8 Solomon B, Glinoer D, Lagasse R, et al. Current trends in the management of Graves' Disease. *J Clin Endocrinol Metab.* 1990;70: 1518–1524.

9 Cooper DS. Antithyroid drugs. *N Engl J Med.* 1984;22:311(21): 1353–1362.

10 Mazzaferri EL. Management of a solitary thyroid nodule. *N Engl J Med.* 1993;328:553–559.

11 Utiger RD. Altered thyroid function in nonthyroidal illness and surgery. To treat of not to treat? *N Engl J Med.* 1995;333:1562.

12 McIver B, Gorman CA. Euthyroid sick syndrome: an overview. *Thyroid.* 1997;7:125–132.

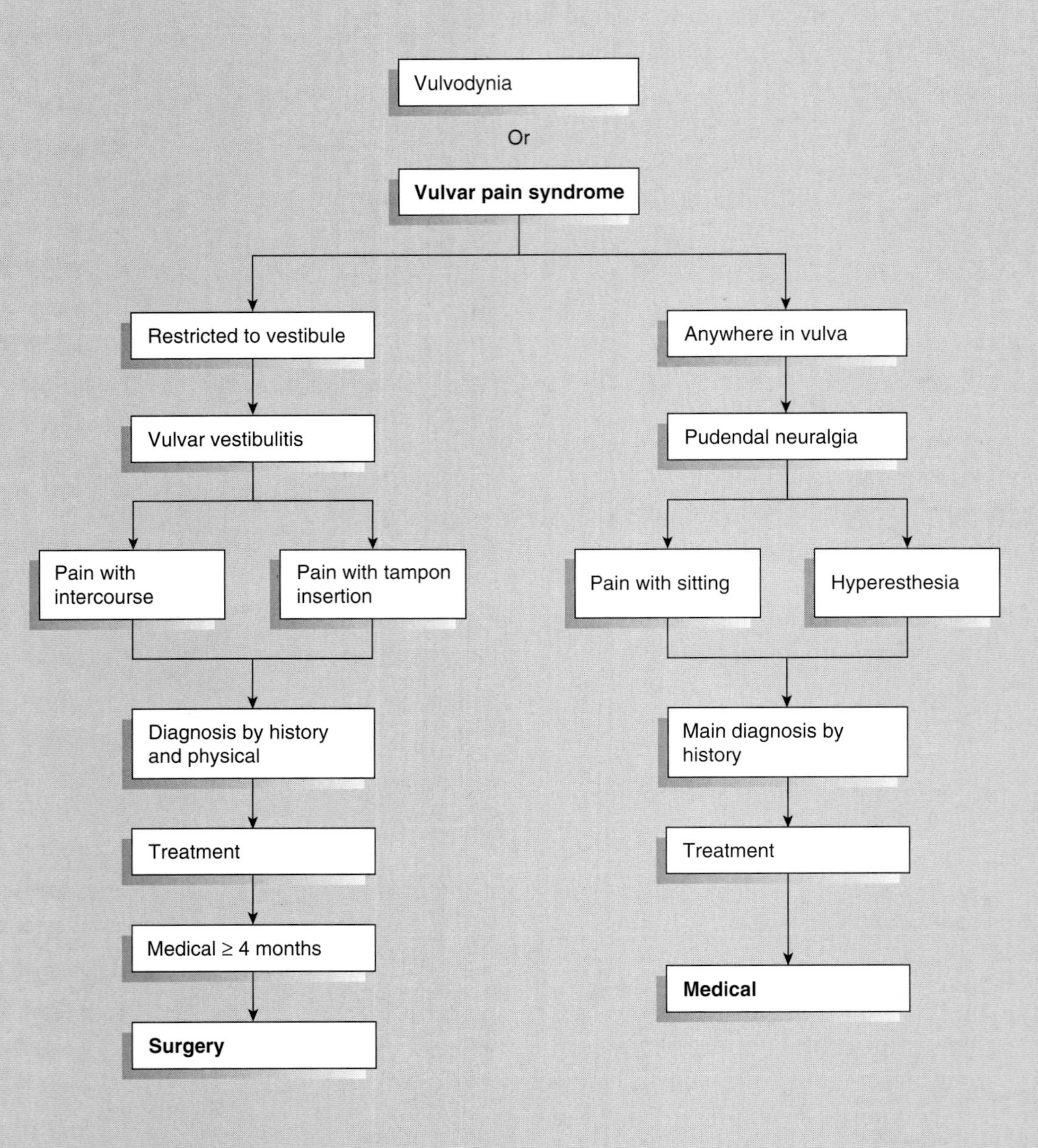

Vulvodynia
Or
Vulvar pain syndrome
Restricted to vestibule
Anywhere in vulva
Vulvar vestibulitis
Pudendal neuralgia
Pain with intercourse
Pain with tampon insertion
Pain with sitting
Hyperesthesia
Diagnosis by history and physical
Main diagnosis by history
Treatment
Treatment
Medical ≥ 4 months
Medical
Surgery

17 Vulvodynia

Michael S. Baggish

Introduction

KEY POINT

The vulvodynia group of disorders should be referred to as vulvar pain syndromes.

The term *vulvodynia* was adopted at the Seventh Congress for the International Society for the Study of Vulvar Disease (ISSVD) in 1983 and subsequently published in the Journal of Reproductive Medicine (1984).[1] The term means pain and refers nonspecifically to the vulva. Rather than using a pseudo-Greek, circuitous derivative, a more logical approach could refer to the disorder(s) as *vulvar pain syndromes*.

The foregoing naming event was preceded by two investigations and two subsequent reports. Fortuitously, the author of this chapter had first hand knowledge of these data. At a course sponsored by SUNY Syracuse in the Bahamas in early 1983, both Ed Friedrich and Don Woodruff were invited speakers. They discussed their recent research relating to a nebulous but real pain syndrome associated with severe burning pain during intercourse. Papers were published later in 1983 about the pain syndrome and its surgical treatment.[2,3] Friedrich, between 1983 and 1986, gathered 86 patients and anatomically defined specific pain related to touch or attempted vaginal entry. He called the problem vulvar vestibulitis syndrome.[4] Historically, descriptions of vulvar hyperesthesia and contact burning discomfort can be documented in the literature over a span of 100 years. In 1889, Skene described hyperesthesia of the vulva in his *Treatise on the Disease of Women*.[5] TG Thomas and PF Munde also described a syndrome of excessive vulvar sensitivity in their *Practical Treatise on Diseases of Women* (1891).[6]

In Charles West's *Diseases of Women* (1861), a condition called *prurigo* is described. He describes the condition: "it is sometimes an unpleasant sense of creeping, or formication, at other times a feeling of smarting, while in other cases the positive itching is so distressing as to be almost unbearable. ...the very rubbing of the parts both aggravates the patient's condition, and also helps to produce and to keep up a state of morbid sexual excitement which in some of these cases constitutes by no means the least of her suffering."[7]

In 1928, after an interval of >40 years, the condition resurfaced in the gynecology literature.[8] Kelly observed a condition associated with vestibular red spots which made sexual intercourse impossible. He described "exquisitely sensitive deep-red spots in the mucosa of the hymenal ring as a fruitful source of dyspareunia."

Several sporadic but pertinent articles appeared in the literature over the next five decades. In 1942, Hunt described the minor vestibular glands[9]; in 1948, Dickinson defined the architecture of the female vestibule.[10] In 1976, Pelisse and Hewitt reported 30 women with erythematous vulvitis.[11] In 1988, Pyka et al. described the histopathology of vulvar vestibulitis syndrome.[12]

Nomenclature

KEY POINT

The two main disorders of the vulvar pain syndrome are vulvar vestibulitis syndrome and pudendal neuralgia.

The nomenclature for vulvar pain syndromes is unnecessarily confusing. The two main idiopathic disorders are (1) vulvar vestibulitis syndrome and (2) pudendal neuralgia.

Vulvar vestibulitis syndrome is characterized by pruritus (early), burning pain especially with provocative acts, e.g., tampon insertion, sexual intercourse, and gynecological examination. The pain or discomfort is limited to the anatomic boundaries of the vestibule. The condition is associated with vestibular erythema and vascular ectasia (Table 17-1).

Table 17-1. **NONEFFICACIOUS MEDICAL THERAPY**

Topical steroids
- Cortisone preparations, estrogen creams, testosterone proportionate in petroleum have no therapeutic benefit or logical usage in the treatment of vulvar vestibulitis syndrome

Antiviral therapy
- Vulvar vestibulitis syndrome is not causally related to HSV, HPV, HIV, or any other viruses. The use of antiviral drugs, e.g., Interferon, lacks justification. These drugs are expensive and have significant side effects

5-Fluorouracil cream
- Trichloracetic acid, Aldura, and Condylox are inappropriate and contraindicated for vulvar vestibulitis syndrome

Pudendal neuralgia is a condition of hyperesthesia. Pain occurs anywhere in the vulvar, periclitoral, perianal tissues. The pain occurs with no specific provocation. Wearing of undergarments may precipitate discomfort. Sitting always aggravates the pain or initiates it. No erythema or other visible vulvar abnormalities are seen.

Etiology

No known etiology exists for pudendal neuralgia or vulvar vestibulitis syndrome. Several hypotheses have emerged including general decreased pain tolerance, psychologic desire to avoid intercourse, and psychiatric disorders. Clearly, the causes of the vulvar pain syndromes are not rooted in mental disorders. Obviously, people who have unexplained chronic pain, which interferes with basic and physiologic life functions may become depressed after months or years of incorrect diagnosis. Similarly, individuals who have chronic pain at one site are more sensitive to painful stimuli at other locations. Likewise, stress aggravates pain. It is important to accept the mostly pure physical aspects of the pain associated with vestibulitis and pudendal neuralgia.

Other hypothetical etiologies include infections (fungal, bacterial, viral). No published data conclusively supports the notion(s) that vulvar pain syndrome is caused by a specific bacterial or fungal organism. Additionally, the notion that fungal antibodies produce an autoimmune condition creating pain is speculative.

KEY POINT

No known etiology exists for vulvar pain syndromes.

Positive cultures for fungus, Chlamydia, aerobic bacteria, Mycoplasma and Ureaplasma in vestibulitis patients compared to nonafflicted gynecology patients are equivalent. There are no increased numbers compared to the general gynecologic patients of sexual abuse, glucose intolerance, drug therapy, or allergies.

Certain facts suggest that the mucous glands of the vestibule are dysfunctional in vulvar vestibulitis syndrome.[13] Consistently, the erythema, ectasia, light touch pain, and severe pressure pain are located around the Bartholin's duct and gland. The vestibule is mostly red in the tissues around the Bartholin's duct opening in vestibulitis patients. The pain resulting from light pressure over the underlying Bartholin's gland is seen with 100% consistency in women with vulvar vestibulitis. Although pain may be elicited at the posterior fourchette and over the paraurethral glands, its frequency is two-thirds to three-fourth less than that observed over the Bartholin's glands.

KEY POINT

Onset of vestibulitis most commonly occurs following a surgical operation, childbirth, honeymoon, or a new sex partner.

Historically, the beginning symptoms of vestibulitis most commonly follow a surgical operation, childbirth, honeymoon, or a new sex partner. The former two may be associated with chemical scrubbing of the vestibular tissues, e.g., Iodine prep solution, and chlorhexidine. The initiation of pain with a honeymoon may well relate to direct trauma to the gland and duct orifice because of a tight introitus as well as with poor lubrication. The dynamics of the new sex partner may be the sudden increase in frequency of sexual activity associated with the new relationship.

Anatomically, the Bartholin's gland is intimately related to the lower portion of the bulbocavernosus muscle, which is likewise intimately applied to the levator ani muscle. The gland cannot be physically separated from the muscle. If the Bartholin's gland is to be excised then a segment of the bulbocavernosus muscle must accompany the gland.

KEY POINT

Pathology of vestibular skin will demonstrate chronic inflammation in almost all cases.

The pathology sections of removed vestibule skin demonstrate chronic inflammation in all (100%) cases. This is *not* a normal finding. The pathology of removed Bartholin's glands shows chronic inflammation in 85–90% of the sections. Fungal stains have been uniformly negative and bacterial cultures are uniformly negative.

In summation, although the exact etiology of vulvar vestibulitis is unknown, the focus of the disorder is the Bartholin's gland and secondarily the inflamed vestibular skin. The role played by topical medicinal agents, such as topical antifungals, surgical preparatory agents (iodine, alcohol, chlorhexidine), chlorhexidine- based lubricants, or 5-Fluorouracil cream is substantial in the initiation of the chronic inflammation and dysfunction of the Bartholin's gland, Bartholin's duct, and the surrounding vestibular tissue (Table 17-1).

Anatomy

The vestibule occupies the area external to the vagina and urethra between the labia minora. Opening into the vestibule are the urethra meatus, vagina, Skene's Ducts, paraurethral ducts, Bartholin's ducts, and minor vestibular gland ducts. The lateral boundaries of the vestibule are marked by Hart's line on the inner aspect of the labia minora. The medial margins are the hymenal ring or the hymenal remnants. The anterior margin stops just below the clitoral frenula. The posterior margin is the junction between the fossa navicularis and posterior commissure.[13] Compared to the tissues of the labia majora, labia minora, and perineum, the vestibular skin is pinker because the keratinized layer of the stratified squamous epithelium is thin. Beneath the epithelium, no skin appendages are evident. Mucous glands are however present. Typically, minor vestibular glands and Bartholin's glands consist of acini lined by mucous secreting columnar cells. The Bartholin's duct consists of a transitional cell and mucous cell epithelial lining.[14,15]

Epidemiology

Since vestibulitis and pudendal neuralgia are not reportable diseases, no accurate data exists relative to the number of women afflicted with these disorders. Goetsch found that 78 out of 210 gynecologic patients seen in a routine practice had light, cotton tip touch sensitivity and 31 patients were overtly diagnostic for vulvar vestibulitis syndrome.[16] Of 400 patients with vulvar pain syndrome seen at the Center for Advanced Gynecology at Good Samaritan Hospital in Cincinnati, 40% had symptoms of pain for >2 years.

The age range for women with vulvar pain syndrome ranges from 18 to 75 years. The mean age was 38 years. The mean age for vestibulitis is 31 years, whereas the mean age for women with pudendal neuralgia is 45 years. Out of 400 cases seen by the author, only 1 patient was African American, 2 patients were Asiatic, the rest were Caucasian.

Symptoms

Evolution

The evolution of symptoms between vestibulitis and pudendal neuralgia is different. Vulvar vestibulitis syndrome's initiating events can be fixed relative to a specific date or time. In contrast, pudendal neuralgia begins insidiously. Although tolerable, discomfort can be dealt with on a short-term basis; the constant day-after-day burning and hyperesthesia eventually brings the patient to her gynecologist's attention. Both disorders may present with varying degrees of severity. Passage of time does not necessarily equate with ameliorating symptomatology. No factual data are available relative to quantifying spontaneous cures. Dyspareunia and apareunia are associated with both vulvar vestibulitis and pudendal neuralgia but are definitely more notable and severe with the former. Anxiety, frustration, and depression are the later sequelae of chronic pain. Numerous trips to doctor's offices; inevitable misdiagnoses by general practitioners, gynecologists, dermatologists, psychiatrists; myriads of useless topical and systemic drugs together with spousal suspicions as well as pressure to resolve the issue are the ingredients which conjure up a cauldron of despair and hopelessness for the unfortunate woman with vulvar pain syndrome.

Many patients obtain information via the Internet. Patient support groups as well as chat rooms may or may not provide accurate information. As with most open forums, zealots will dominate a palate of skewed remedies emphasizing natural, herbal, holistic monikers. Most of these are not harmful but typically useless. Occasionally, however, these largely unregulated agents produce toxicity and actually make the afflicted woman's condition worse.

History

A natural history obtained in the words of the patient is the most valuable piece of information obtainable. The physician can, after obtaining the patient's history, ask focused questions. Data pinpointing the early aspects of the disorder are very helpful in the differential diagnosis. Was the patient asymptomatic prior to a hysterectomy or a delivery? When, if ever, was intercourse not associated with pain?

Early vestibulitis is principally associated with vestibular pruritus. Most patients believe they have a yeast infection. Most gynecologists do not culture prior to treating a woman for vaginitis. Inevitably, the patient is told that she has a yeast infection and receives a topical agent, e.g., miconazole or terconazole vaginal cream. When her symptoms persist, she is treated with a systemic antifungal drug, e.g., fluconazole. When this does not relieve symptoms, a microscopic examination is performed revealing white cells in the saline preparation and she and her husband are treated with another antimicrobial agent, e.g., metronidazole. This cycle continues over and over again. The pruritus then assumes a less prominent role as irritation becomes the dominant feature of the disorder. Patients try over-the-counter agents, e.g., miconazole or cortisone cream, which usually provide temporary relief. This can be explained by the cream providing a covering barrier effect rather than a root therapeutic action. Relentlessly, the irritation becomes worse with each sexual encounter. Burning pain supercedes the irritation with each attempt at intercourse for the woman with vulvar vestibulitis. The act itself results in burning pain and the burning usually continues several hours post intercourse. A cold douche or dousing in a tub of warm water provides temporary relief. When pressed to describe the discomfort encountered during intercourse, women provide the following adjectives: raw, swollen, dry. A typical description analyzes the sensation as akin to rubbing the tissues with sandpaper. Urination produces a distinct burning sensation when the urine contacts the inflamed vestibular skin. Showering and cleansing with soap similarly produces a burning sensation. The pain associated with vestibulitis is typically *not* constant, but waxes and wanes throughout the menstrual cycle. It tends to be at its lowest ebb during menstruation. It is at its acme premenstrually and early in the follicular phase. If there is no provocation there is little pain, i.e., if no sex occurs then there is no pain. At some point, the discomfort and pain reach a degree of severity such that the patient prefers to avoid intercourse altogether. This situation may have adverse effects on the relationship and further distress the woman.

KEY POINT

Pudendal neuralgia is characterized by burning or shooting pain in the vulvar area.

Pudendal neuralgia is characterized by burning or shooting pain. A component of pruritus is unusual. A key question to ask the patient is what activities worsen the pain. Sitting, particularly for extended periods, such as during long car or plane rides, produces exacerbation of pain. Bicycle or horseback riding creates similar aggravation of pain symptoms. As the disorder worsens, even light contact with clothing apparel creates discomfort. At some point, patients prefer to clothe themselves with dresses and avoid wearing underpants whenever feasible. At night, sheets and bedclothes add to vulvar discomfort. Desperate patients may spend a better part of their day sitting on icepacks or lying in a tub of cool water. Soap definitely aggravates the problem for many women.

Unproven remedies have included testosterone ointment and 5-fluoruracil. These approaches are not recommended and could aggravate this condition

It is important to avoid implying that the condition is a figment of the patient's imagination, a conscious desire to avoid sex, or a primary psychiatric disorder.

Finally, although the superficial discomfort of an inflamed vestibule or a hyperesthetic vulva may be masked by a topical local anesthesia, e.g., 2% viscous Xylocaine, that maneuver which provides short-term relief simply masks symptoms, doing nothing to eliminate the disorder. The potential harm relates to the creation of systemic allergy to the medication.

Signs

EXAMINATION

KEY POINT

The area of pain sensitivity should be systematically mapped using a Q-tip method during a colposcopic examination.

The author prefers to perform the vulvar examination with the aid of magnification. The ideal instrument to accomplish a thorough vulvar examination is the colposcope. Although my equipment is elaborate and equipped with a television camera (for the benefit of the patient) attached via beam splitter, simpler equipment will suffice. During the examination, a small cotton-tipped applicator is utilized to manipulate the tissues. It is useful to gently draw the cotton across the patient's inner thigh skin and ask her whether this causes any discomfort. Typically, the answer to that question is no. Next, light pressure is placed on the inner thigh skin with the same applicator. Again, the patient is questioned whether this causes pain. Again, she answers no. These simple techniques instill confidence to the already anxious patient and reinforce the fact that you will not unnecessarily cause her discomfort. Further, I show the patient the cotton-tipped applicator to reassure her that it is not a pain-producing device. After systematically examining the labia, clitoris, perineum, and perianal skin and gently drawing the cotton tip over the tissues, the patient is questioned regarding discomfort. Next, the labia minora are parted exposing the vestibule. If vestibulitis exists, redness is seen around the Bartholin's duct opening. This structure is easily seen as a pin-sized hole adjacent to the hymenal ring. It is specifically located lateral to the lower third of the hymenal ring. In severe cases, the entire vestibule will show a red color. Stretching of the brittle, inflamed tissue will often create a fissure usually in the area of the posterior fourchette. As the cotton-tipped applicator is drawn across the red tissue, the patient exclaims that this hurts or will physically draw back on the examining table. The same applicator next is pushed onto the tissue just lateral and slightly below the duct opening in the exact manner that light pressure was applied to the thigh. This again creates point discomfort and withdrawal. The procedure is repeated for both right and left sides. The stimulation of the gland to secrete mucous will produce even greater erythema and will be clearly visualized while viewing under colposcopic magnification. The patient will comprehend that the burning discomfort she had experienced during intercourse was exactly recreated in the examining room. The entire vestibule should be systematically mapped inclusive of the paraurethral and urethral glands. Higher power colposcopic examination will usually reveal vascular ectasia. The latter will appear as large punctuate terminal vessels around the Bartholin's duct orifice within the vestibular epithelium. Next, the applicator is carefully placed into the vagina and gently drawn across the vaginal epithelium taking care not to place any friction on the hymen. Pressure is placed on the vagina with the device. No pain is elicited. The erythema and relative pain is scored utilizing a digital scale (1–10). A 10/10 is scored for extreme erythema and physical withdrawal produced by the pain.

A Pederson speculum is shown to the patient and then gently inserted into the vagina under colposcopic vision (no lubrication). The speculum is gently opened and the vagina and cervix are examined. Cultures are routinely obtained and plated for fungus, aerobes, Chlamydia, Gonorrhea, Mycoplasma/Ureaplasma. Mucous and debris are swabbed out utilizing a large cotton-tipped applicator (soaked in 4% acetic acid) (scopette) and the entire cervix and vagina again are examined colposcopically. The examination is completed with a bimanual examination and rectovaginal examination utilizing an Astroglide lubricated gloved hand. The findings above have described the physical appearance of vulvar vestibulitis syndrome.

In the case of pudendal neuralgia, the vulva and vestibule will appear absolutely normal. Light Q-tip touch to the labia, clitoral hood, and perineum may create pain. Light touch in the vestibule and vagina will not elicit any pain. If the examiner pushes his or her index finger into the tissue of the lowest most portion of the labia majora just medial to the ischial tuberosity, pain will be elicited in women afflicted with neuralgia. This maneuver will not cause discomfort in women with vestibulitis unless hymenal traction occurs. Furthermore, vaginal examination will not produce pain unless pressure is applied through the vaginal wall at the level of the ischial spine.

Differential Diagnosis

KEY POINT

Differentiation between vestibulitis and neuralgia is important because the treatment approaches for each disorder are very different.

The major differential diagnosis that must be made in vulvar pain syndrome focuses upon differentiation between vestibulitis and neuralgia since the ultimate treatment programs are very different. Other vulvar disorders including infections can coexist with either of these entities but the astute gynecologist should easily be able to diagnose other pain-producing conditions. Erosive lichen planus produces vestibular ulceration and creates pain that precludes intercourse, tampon insertion. Cleansing and wiping the vestibule is also painful. In this condition, the lack of epithelial covering and/or thinning of the epithelium are diagnostic. A biopsy will confirm the diagnosis. In the case of vulvar vestibulitis syndrome, a biopsy is not diagnostic or for that matter useful. Additionally, vaginal and buccal involvement are common with lichen planus.

Behcet's disease affects the vestibule and medial aspects of the *labia minora*. Behcet's characteristically produces a large, necrotic, painful ulcer and is also associated with lesions in the mouth.

Acute vulvitis secondary to bacterial or fungal infection produces vestibular symptoms characteristic of vulvar vestibulitis syndrome. Acute vulvitis is more diffuse with respect to inflammation. A positive culture will corroborate the diagnosis and specific antibiotic or antifungal treatment rapidly resolves the problem.

Any chemical reaction or burn can produce vestibulitis and mimic vulvar vestibulitis syndrome. The history will help in the differential diagnosis relative to cause and effect. These chemical injuries or hypersensitivity reactions are acute in onset and do not follow the evolutionary pathophysiology described earlier. The injury improves with time; however, this type of problem can be an instigator of vulvar vestibulitis syndrome. Several cases of bona fide vulvar vestibulitis syndrome have followed exposure to bromides in hot tubs, antifungal topicals instilled in the vagina, latex and spermicide allergies, 5-fluourouracil vaginal infusions, and bizarre caustic douching (e.g. bleach).

Much has been written relative to herpes simplex virus (HSV) infections and human papilloma virus (HPV) infections as instigators of both vulvar vestibulitis syndrome and pudendal neuralgia. HPV even in its most florid presentations is not a pain-producing entity. HPV DNA typing does not show vulvar pain syndrome patients to have a greater degree of infectivity than the general gynecologic population. Biopsies of the vestibular epithelium do not show any greater pathology characteristic of HPV than the general gynecologic population. Therefore, HPV is not an instigator of vulvar pain syndrome although it can occasionally coexist. Herpes simplex virus infections of the vulva and vestibule create ulcers which have a characteristic appearance.[17–20] Culture will prove the presence of the virus particularly when vesicles are aspirated. Biopsy shows multinucleate giant cells with large viral inclusions. Neutralizing antibody studies will show specific increased titers of immunoglobulin G (IgG) and immunoglobulin M (IgM) to HSV I and/or II. HSV infections are not difficult to differentiate from the physical or historical findings associated with vulvar pain syndrome. There is no evidence to support HSV or HPV is a cause of chronic vulvar pain.

Diagnosis

The diagnosis is based on precise historical data and careful physical assessment. The correct diagnosis is not difficult. Finally, observation while undergoing conservative (medical) therapy is the watchword even if uncertainty is not an issue. Clearly, precipitous surgical intervention in the mistaken belief that the vulvar pain syndrome is due to vestibulitis when in fact the data point to neuralgia is an error. Continuous and frequent follow-up with history and examination will over time differentiate vestibulitis from neuralgia. Referral to a subspecialty clinic or to a gynecologist specializing in vulvar disorders is always useful for the general gynecologist to confirm the correctness of the diagnosis.

Treatment

Medical

The basis for medical therapy at the Vulvar-Vaginal Disorders Clinic at Good Samaritan Hospital, Cincinnati, Ohio is to utilize those reported techniques which will cause the patient no harm, i.e., will not worsen the condition and which have reported some reasonable efficacy.

Vulvar Vestibulitis Syndrome The initial advice given to all new patients specifies that no topical drugs are to be placed onto the vulva or into the vagina and that no intercourse be attempted for at least 6 weeks.

Based on the work of Glazer et al., all patients are referred to our physical therapist for biofeedback.[21] Pre- and posttreatment levator ani testing is performed. Tricyclic antidepressive drugs, e.g., nortriptyline (25 mg daily), amitriptyline (20 mg daily), are effective as pain-modulating formulations. Alternatively, gabapentin 300 mg tid or qid may be prescribed. The major side effect of these drugs is drowsiness particularly during the early morning hours.

Although the role of oxalates in the genesis of vulvar vestibulitis is doubtful and the data regarding the mechanism of its effects on the disorder are sparse, we will at least offer the patient a low oxalate diet the first 6 weeks and will prescribe calcium citrate 400 gm tid.[22–24]

Additionally, a patient is given a squirt bottle and a 500 mL bottle of sterile water and is instructed to irrigate the vestibule after urination and prior to wiping. Any patient who has a positive culture relative to the work-up is treated with specific systemic medication for the diagnosed infection.

Following an interval of 6 weeks, the patient returns for subjective and objective assessment. The regimen remains the same for the next 6 weeks with the addition of trying to have intercourse once per week utilizing the liberal application of Astroglide or other suitable substitute lubricant.

If no appreciable response to the conservative therapeutic program is witnessed during the 12-16-week period of time, then surgical options are discussed with the patient and her family. Our philosophy is to support and continue the medical treatment for however long the patient wishes to pursue it. Unfortunately, only 15–20% of women with vulvar vestibulitis syndrome will respond, i.e., elimination of pain and pain-free, pleasurable intercourse.

Pudendal Neuralgia In contrast to vulvar vestibulitis, this disorder should be managed by conservative, nonsurgical methods. A specific regimen is prescribed which includes the following:

- Minimizing sitting time: Patients are advised against long periods in the sitting position. They are advised to recline on a couch at home in preference to sitting.
- A biofeedback program is prescribed via our physical therapist.

- Systemic antidepressive drugs are prescribed according to the following schema: amitriptyline 20 mg hs or gabapentin 300 mg tid or qid.
- If the patient does not experience significant relief within 6 weeks then she is begun on serial dexamethasone injections into the pudendal nerve area, 2 mg dexamethasone each side at monthly intervals. Patients may report a transient increase in pain at the injection site due to the carrier vehicle.

At the Vulvar-Vaginal Disorders Clinic, >85% of all patients will respond by significant pain reduction or elimination of pain utilizing this regimen.

SURGICAL

Surgery is reserved for those individuals who have not responded to medical management of vulvar vestibulitis syndrome[25] (Table 17-2). Surgery is not indicated for pudendal neuralgia. The operation we perform is based on the role played by a dysfunctional Bartholin's duct and gland. The glands are radically excised together with the vestibular skin. The vaginal margin is undermined and advanced to cover the deficit and forms the new introitus.[26]

- Preparation: It is preferred to meet in the office setting well in advance of surgical date with the patient and her spouse or significant other. The details of the surgical procedure are fully disclosed. I prefer to make a simple drawing to illustrate what tissues will be removed and how they will be repaired. The patient should be told about untoward effects of the surgery, which include pain and pain management. Possible complications and their frequency should

Table 17-2. **INDICATIONS FOR SURGERY RELATIVE TO TREATMENT FOR VULVAR VESTIBULITIS SYNDROME**

Minimum trial of medical therapy for 4 months
Continuing disabling pain after the medical trial
Objective demonstration of continuing erythema and pain at ≥8/10 level
Subjective and objective findings limited to vestibule
Absence of concurrent bacterial or fungal infection as demonstrated by culture
Patient's desire to undergo surgery after suitable informed consent
No medical contraindication to surgery

be discussed. The latter should include in the short-term excessive bleeding (uncommon), wound infection (uncommon), vaginal pullback, that is, vaginal separation from the vestibule and perineal sutured margins (low), nausea and vomiting (common), swelling (common), ecchymosis (common), and rectal injury (rare). The most troublesome long-term complications which must be clearly delineated are lack of natural introital lubrication and surgically induced pudendal neuralgia. Finally, I give the patient a reprint of an article detailing the surgery, which shows pictures and illustrations as well as statistical data relative to the surgery. Finally, the prospective surgical candidate is provided with a list of former patients who have completed surgery and who have volunteered to speak directly with preoperative women in order to relay their experiences. Patients who require medical or surgical consultation are referred. Consultation recommendations are discussed with the patient and implemented. In some cases, preoperative psychiatric consultation is obtained.

I discuss with patients who are in the childbearing years details regarding future pregnancy and fertility. Vulvar vestibulitis syndrome has no effect on the ability of a patient to conceive and to carry a pregnancy. I recommend that the patient who has undergone therapeutic surgery for vestibulitis not deliver vaginally because of the risk of scar formation after episiotomy or perineal tearing. A cesarean section is a better alternative for them.

- Surgical Technique: The surgery is performed in the lithotomy position. The anatomy of the Bartholin's gland, bulbocavernosus muscle, bulb of the vestibule, and vagina has been adequately detailed elsewhere (Fig. 17-1).[14,15] To gain exposure, the labia are sutured to the skin of the groin. Vasopressin solution 1:100 is injected beneath the vestibular skin. Utilizing a superpulsed CO_2 laser coupled via a micromanipulator to an operating microscope, a linear cut approximately 2 cm long is made just lateral to the hymenal ring and carried down through Colles' fascia (Fig. 17-2A and B). Utilizing Tenotomy scissors, the inner aspect of the vagina is dissected away from the bulbocavernosus muscle to a depth of 2-3 cm (Fig. 17-3). A double gloved finger is placed in the rectum to accurately determine its relationship to the area of dissection. Next,

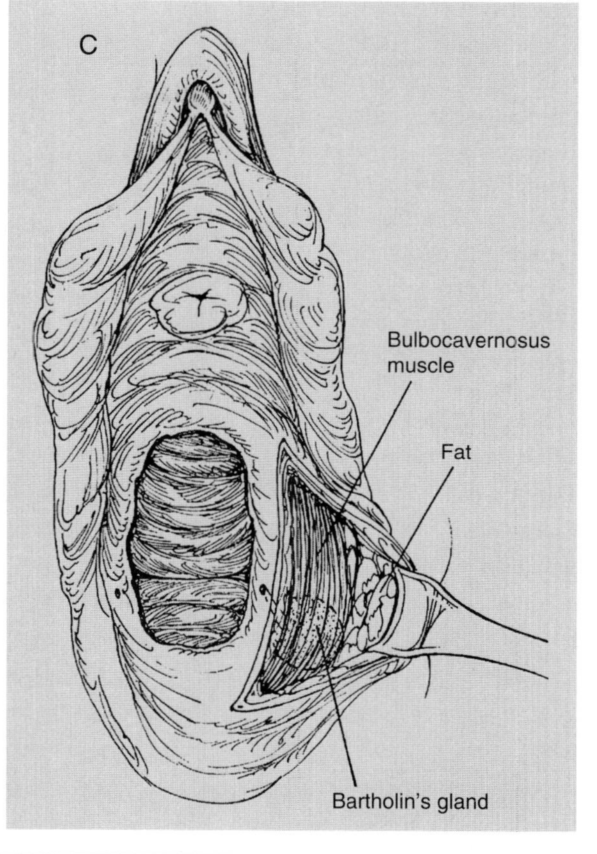

Figure 17-1: Schematic drawing of vulvar vestibule anatomy showing the relationships of Bartholin's gland to the bulbocavernosus muscle and vagina. (*Source*: Baggish MS, Karram M. *Atlas of Pelvic Anatomy and Gynecologic Surgery*. Philadelphia, PA: W.B. Saunders; 2001.)

Colles' fascia is opened at the lateral margin of the muscle. The bulbocavernosus muscle is now isolated and exposed (Fig. 17-4). The fascia overlying the levator ani (perineal membrane) located between the bulbo and ischiocavernosus muscles is identified. The bulbocavernosus muscle is clamped with a mosquito clamp at the lowest extent of the incision and at the junction of the middle and lower one-third of the muscle (Fig. 17-5A). The muscle is cut with Tenotomy scissors (Fig. 17-5B). Several further clamps are placed more deeply and cut. The Bartholin's gland is identified on the undersurface of the muscle (Fig. 17-6). The gland's blood supply is isolated and clamped. The segment of muscle and gland are removed (Fig. 17-7). The duct is attached to the removed gland. The deep defect created by removal of muscle and gland is closed with 3-0 Vicryl. If the bulb of the vestibule is

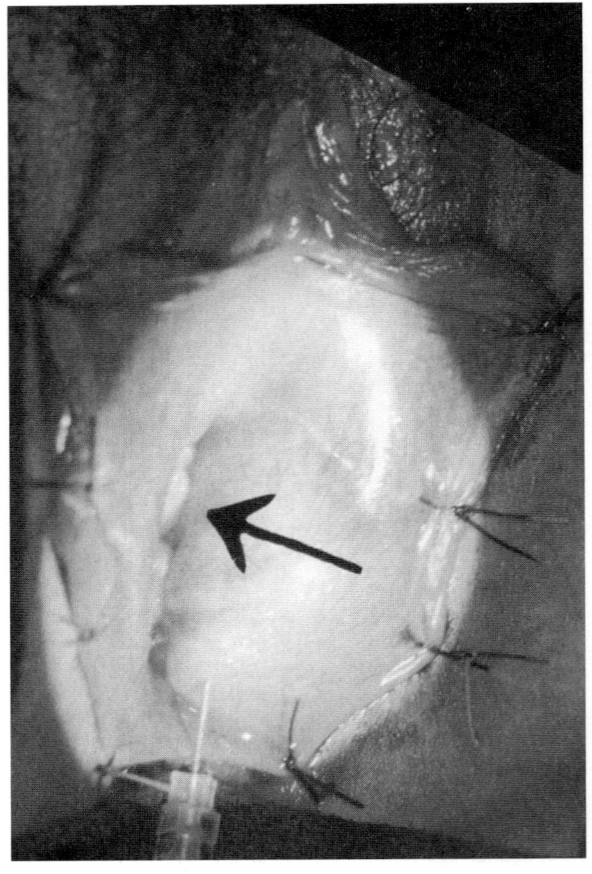

Figure 17-2: (A) A solution of vasopressin 1:100 is injected into the vestibule adjacent to the vaginal introitus (arrow points to vaginal opening). (B) A relatively bloodless incision is made with a superpulsed CO_2 laser beam. The laser micromanipulator is coupled to the operating microscope. Beam diameter is 1.0 mm. (*Source*: Baggish MS, Karram M. *Atlas Of Pelvic Anatomy And Gynecologic Surgery*. Philadelphia, PA: W.B. Saunders; 2001.)

opened during the dissection, it will bleed and the sinus-like, cavernosus structure must then be sutured with 4-0 or 5-0 vicryl; it should not be clamped. The hymen with a 1 cm margin of vagina is excised. The remainder of the vestibule is excised to Hart's line (Fig. 17-8A and B). All excised tissue is sent in separate containers to the pathology laboratory (Fig. 17-9A and B). The vagina is undermined and advanced with use of Steven's scissors. The margins of the vagina are sutured to the residual margins of the labium minus and the perineum. The operation is carried out identically on the opposite side (Fig. 17-10).

At the terminus of the procedure, the wound is thoroughly irrigated with 0.9% sodium chloride solution. The wound is dried. The urethra is catheterized and the bladder emptied.

Figure 17-2: (*Cont.*)

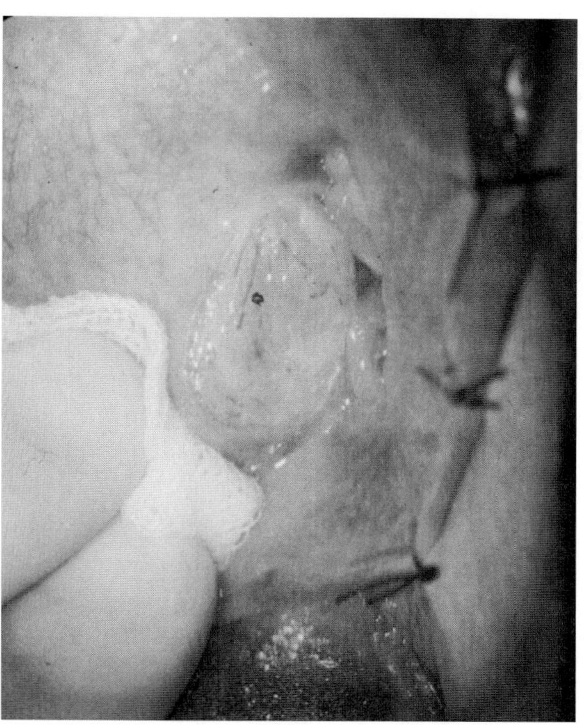

Silvadene cream is applied to the wound and the patient is placed in the supine position and transferred to a stretcher.

- Postoperative Management: The patient is given a prescription for a stool softener, Silvadene cream, Instant Ocean, Toradol 10 gm tid for 3-4 days, Codeine with Tylenol or Aspirin to take after the Toradol expires. I place all patients on Cipro 500 mg bid. All patients are seen in the office within 1 week of discharge and are followed every 1-2 weeks thereafter. At 4 weeks postop, the patients are fitted with a small vaginal form which is inserted twice daily for 10 minutes. A medium form is fitted 2 weeks later. Finally, a large form is given to the patient at 8 weeks postoperatively. The step to intercourse is very easy after utilizing the large form for 2 weeks.

The data (Table 17-3) for pain-free intercourse following surgery is very good, i.e., 95%. Follow-up has ranged from 1 to 9 years. All patients are instructed to use Astroglide or a

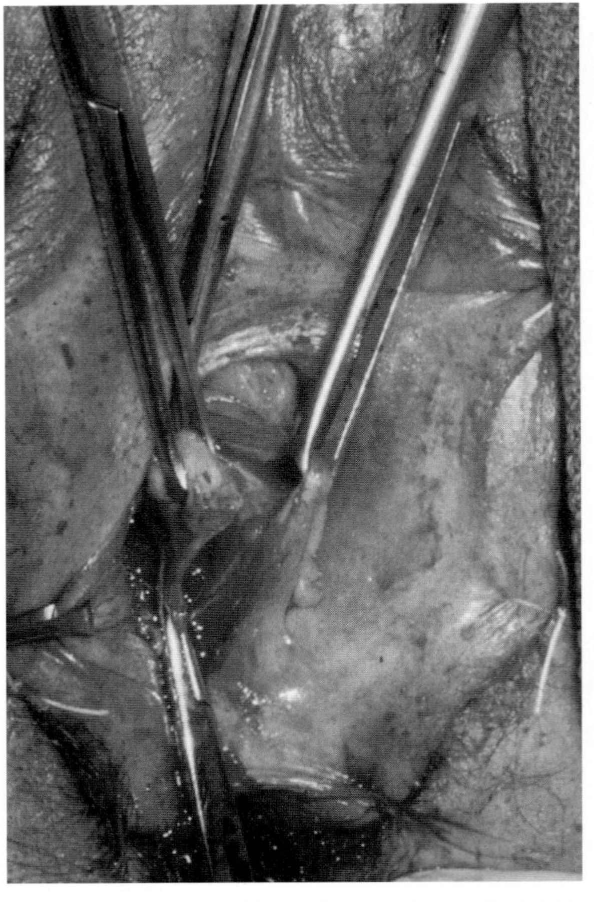

Figure 17-3: A space is sharply dissected between the inner wall of the vagina and the bulbocavernosus muscle, levator ani muscle. (*Source*: Baggish MS, Karram M. *Atlas of Pelvic Anatomy and Gynecologic Surgery*. Philadelphia, PA: W.B. Saunders; 2001.)

suitable substitute with intercourse. None of our patients has had difficulty with sexual response or pregnancy following this type of surgery.

Fifteen percent of patients will have pudendal neuralgia located at the lowest most portion of the labium majus. The pain is described as a sticking discomfort made worse by sitting but not aggravated by intercourse. This pain responds to conservative treatment in >90% of patients.

- Alternative Surgical Procedures: Other vestibular operative procedures have been described but all of them have shortcomings when compared to Bartholin's gland excision. One must bear in mind that Bartholin's gland excision requires greater surgical skill and a detailed knowledge of perineal

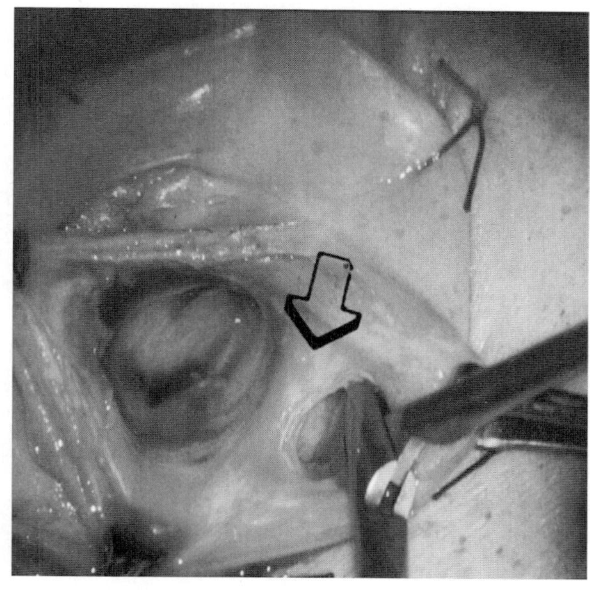

Figure 17-4: Laterally, a second space is developed in order to clearly define and isolate the bulbocavernosus muscle and the Bartholin's gland which clings to the inner (deep) surface of the muscle. This colpophotograph shows the muscle between the inner (arrow) and lateral (outer) anatomical space. (*Source*: Baggish MS, Karram M. *Atlas of Pelvic Anatomy and Gynecologic Surgery*. Philadelphia, PA: W.B. Saunders; 2001.)

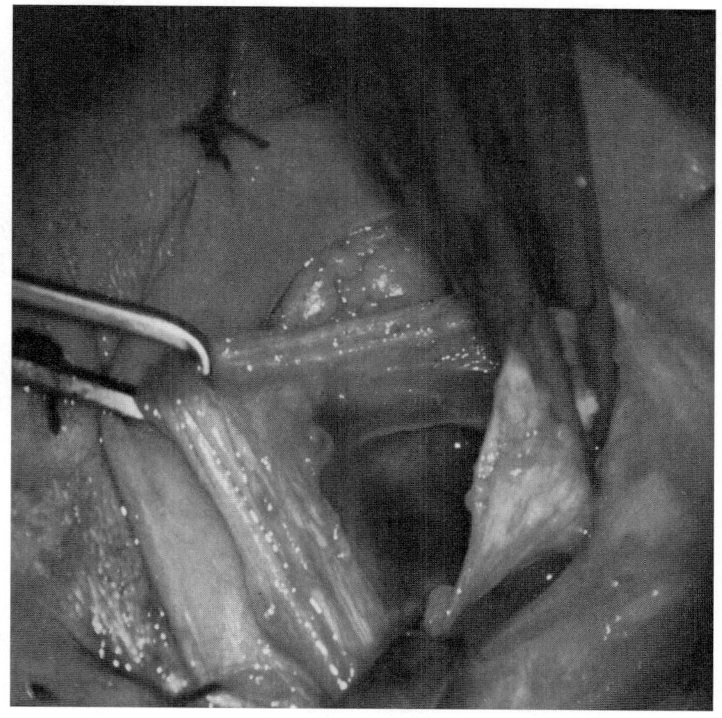

Figure 17-5: (A) Mosquito clamps are placed on the bulbocavernosus muscle preparatory to cutting it. (B) The muscle is cut anteriorly via Steven's scissors. (C) The relationship of the vagina to the operative field is demonstrated by placing traction on the Allis clamp which is attached to the lower vaginal lateral wall. (*Source*: Baggish MS, Karram M. *Atlas of Pelvic Anatomy and Gynecologic Surgery*. Philadelphia, PA: W.B. Saunders; 2001.)

Figure 17-5: (*Cont.*)

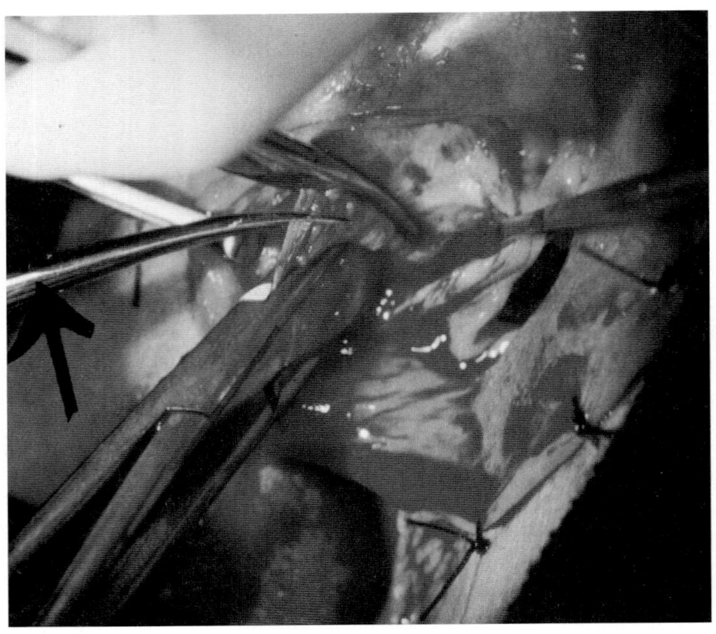

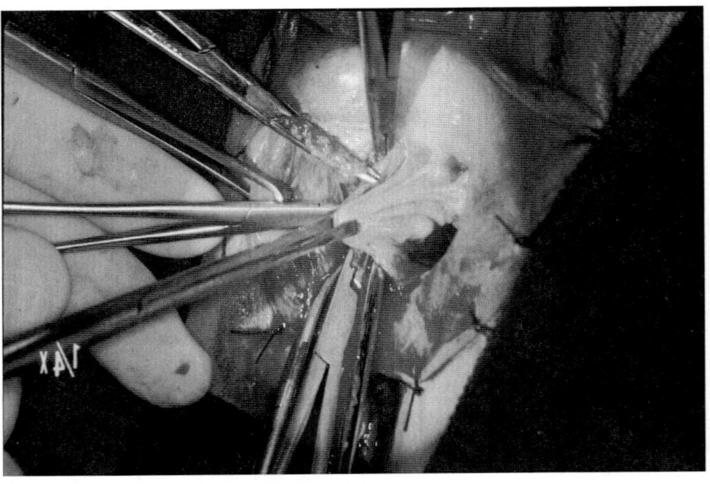

anatomy. Clearly, not every gynecologic surgeon is capable of performing this operation. Therefore, it is quite understandable that the majority of individuals who focus on the treatment of Vulvar Pain Disorders perform only the simplest operations.

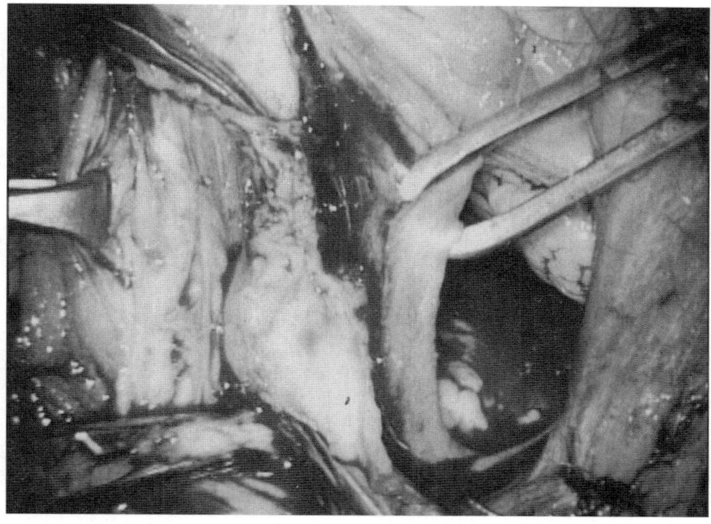

Figure 17-6: The muscle and gland are attached only by small tissue strips which are about to be cut (at upper and lower mosquito clamps). The Allis clamp on the left is attached to the vagina. (*Source*: Baggish MS, Karram M. *Atlas of Pelvic Anatomy and Gynecologic Surgery.* Philadelphia, PA: W.B. Saunders; 2001.)

The surgery recommended by Woodruff and Parmley in 1983 and which most gynecologists have continued to perform without much modification is basically a vestibulectomy with excision of the hymen and a half cm margin of lower vagina. The incision extends to the perineum and terminates

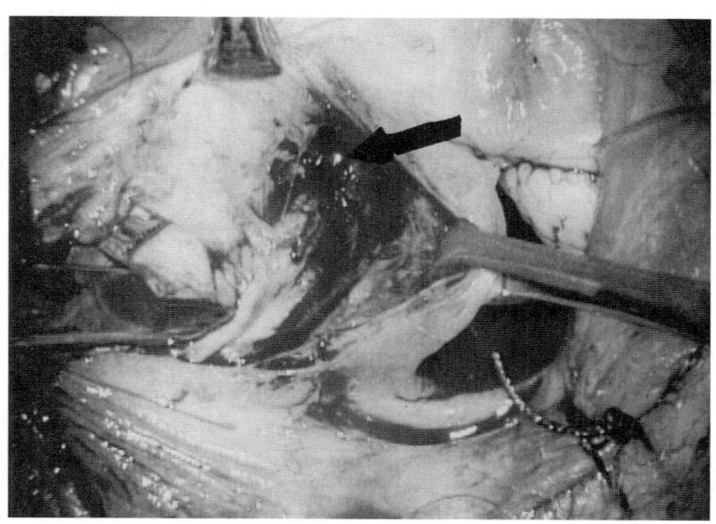

Figure 17-7: The gland has been removed. Note the defect once occupied by the left Bartholin's gland (arrow). (*Source*: Baggish MS, Karram M. *Atlas of Pelvic Anatomy and Gynecologic Surgery.* Philadelphia, PA: W.B. Saunders; 2001.)

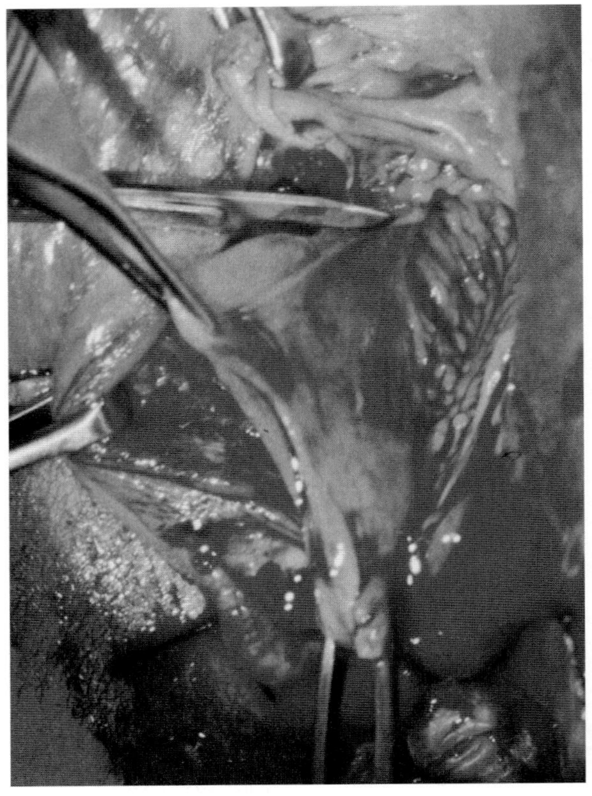

Figure 17-8: (A) The lower vagina (Adson forceps) with the hymenal ring is cut away. (B) The remaining vestibule is cut away to the margin of Hart's line on the labium minus. (*Source*: Baggish MS, Karram M. *Atlas of Pelvic Anatomy and Gynecologic Surgery*. Philadelphia, PA: W.B. Saunders; 2001.)

by advancing the vagina to cover the denuded area. The deficiencies of this operation center about leaving the Bartholin's gland behind and at the same time destroying the duct. One of the root causative factors of the disorder is not treated. Postoperatively patients continue to demonstrate pressure sensitivity and although "improved" are not cured.

Simply excising the vestibular skin including the orifice of the duct is less effective than the Woodruff-Parmley operation. The biggest advantage of the former, which is favored by dermatologists, is its simplicity.

Summation

Vulvar pain syndrome appears to be an emerging cause of disability to a significant number of women in the United States and elsewhere. The symptoms which it creates may account for >15% of all visits to gynecology offices each year. Vulvar

Figure 17-8: (*Cont.*)

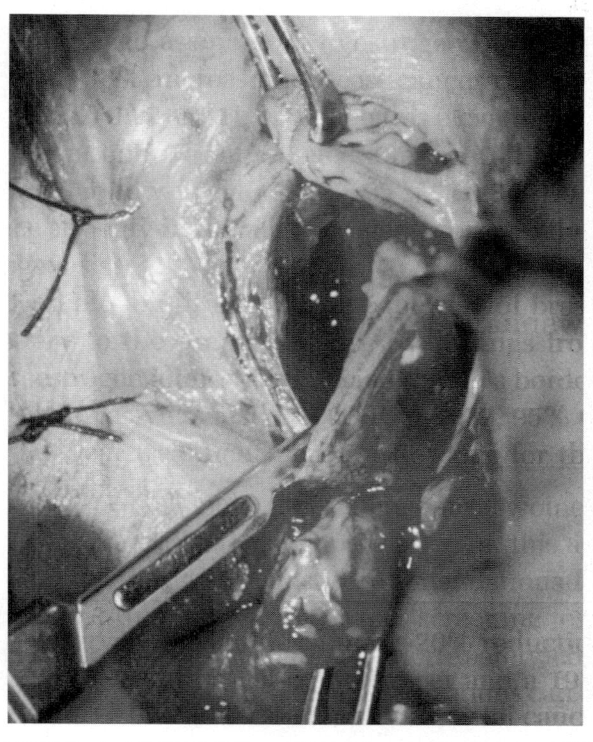

Figure 17-9: (A) Section of the excised Bartholin's gland. This is a true mucous secreting gland. (B) Section of vestibule showing a significant inflammatory infiltration. (*Source*: Baggish MS, Karram M. *Atlas of Pelvic Anatomy and Gynecologic Surgery.* Philadelphia, PA: W.B. Saunders; 2001.)

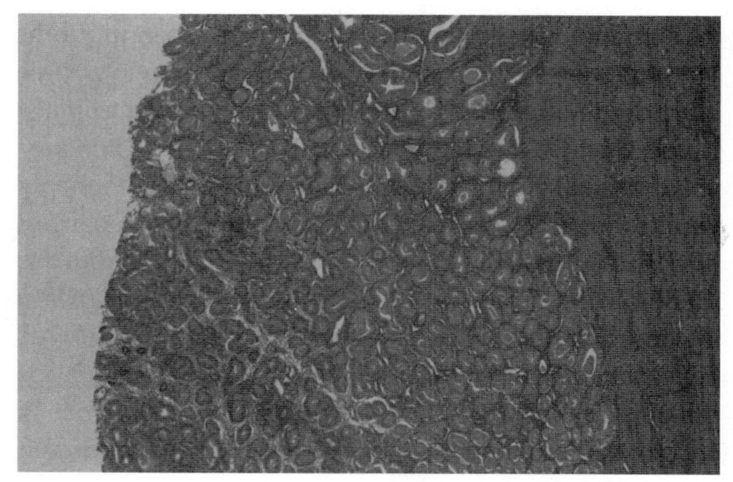

Figure 17-9: (*Cont.*)

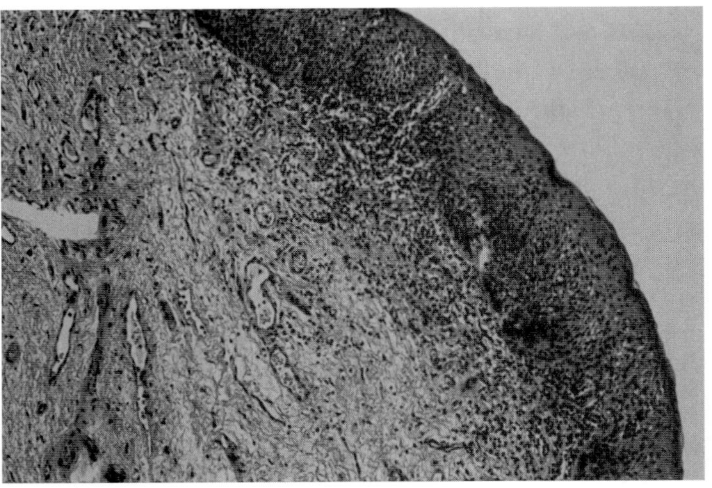

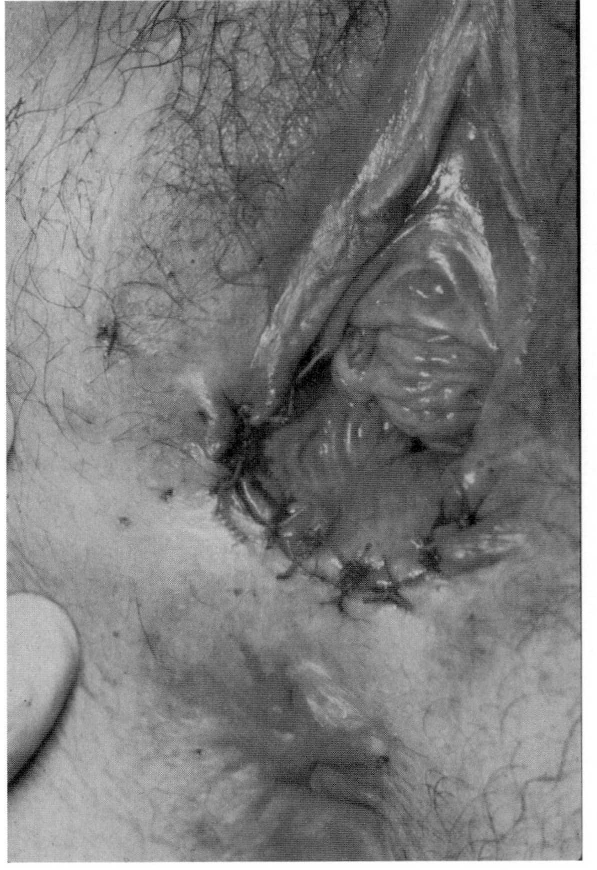

Figure 17-10: Completed surgery showing the advanced vagina attached directly to the labia and perineum, i.e., total absence of a vestibule. (*Source*: Baggish MS, Karram M. *Atlas of Pelvic Anatomy and Gynecologic Surgery.* Philadelphia, PA: W.B. Saunders; 2001.)

Table 17-3. **RESULTS OF RADICAL BILATERAL BARTHOLIN'S GLAND EXCISION, VESTIBULAR EXCISION, VAGINAL ADVANCEMENT SURGERY (N = 72)***

Follow-Up	*N*	*No Pain*	*Pudendal Neuralgia*
Intercourse			
>1 year	4	3	1
>1–2 years	30	36	4
>2 years	38	39	4
Total	72	63	9

*1994–1999.

vestibulitis syndrome is more prevalent than pudendal neuralgia with a proportion of 10 vestibulitis cases versus one case of pudendal neuralgia.

Unwieldy classification systems have retarded the diagnostic process because of confusion. The tendency to attribute pruritus to infection without objective diagnosis further adds to the plague of errors delaying the timely detection of vulvar pain syndrome. A recent obstacle to simplification of diagnosis is the attempt to subdivide vulvar vestibulitis into primary and secondary categories for no clear reason. The justification is lacking for a more complex classification.

Interpretation of therapeutic results is confused by adding the category of "improved" outcomes. As with classification, simplicity will provide the shortest route to the lowest common denominator. The elimination of pain is the bottom line, which determines the success or failure of any treatment most objectively. I find it difficult to interpret the word improvement in a clinical sense since a placebo effect alone may be responsible for the "improvement."

In the most basic terms, a great step forward will occur when gynecologists and other health care professionals recognize that vulvar pain syndrome exists and that it can be successfully treated.

Guiding Questions

- How long has the problem been present?
- Was the patient symptomatic prior to delivery or hysterectomy?
- Was intercourse always painful?

- Is there a history of vaginal infection(s)?
- Is there a history of allergies?

What's the Evidence?

Although vestibulectomy has been viewed as an aggressive treatment approach for vulvar vestibulitis, it is becoming a frequently recommended procedure with over 20 respective studies that have reviewed its efficacy. Two other treatment approaches for *pain syndromes* have also been studied for vulvar vestibulitis. These include surface electromyographic biofeedback, a technique that has been used for chronic headaches and has been adapted for dyspareunia.[27] Another approach is cognitive behavioral therapy. These two latter approaches were evaluated for efficacy in vulvar vestibulitis against surgery in the only prospective randomized clinical trial for treatment of vestibulitis.[28] In this trial, 78 women with well-characterized long-standing vestibulitis of 4-5 years duration were randomized to cognitive-behavioral therapy, surface electromyographic feedback, and vestibulectomy. Women had assessments of pain (McGill Pain Questionnaire), sexual function (Derogatis Sexual Functioning Inventory), and psychological adjustments (Brief Symptom Inventory) at baseline, after 12 weeks of treatment, and at 6-month follow-up. Based on the intent to treat analysis, all three treatments appeared to reduce vestibular pain. However, vestibulectomy was significantly more successful than the other two nonsurgical treatments. Additionally, vestibulectomy had greater pain reduction (mean 52.5% [range 46.8–70%]), than the other two methods. These gains were maintained at the 6-month follow-up. It must be pointed out that the surgical technique described by the author is more extensive than the vestibulectomy procedure in this randomized trial.

Further Reading

Table 17-4 provides general vulvar skin care recommendations for the patient. Other sources of helpful information include the following:

- National Vulvodynia Association *www.nva.org* or 301-299-0775.
- International Society for the Study of Vulvovaginal Disease *www.issvd.org* or 704-814-9493

Table 17-4. **SELF-HELP TIPS FOR VULVAR SKIN CARE***

While you are seeking effective treatment for vulvar pain, here are some coping measures to relieve symptoms and prevent further irritation. Even when your symptoms are under control, these guidelines are recommended as a preventive strategy.

Clothing and laundry

Wear all-white cotton underwear and loose-fitting pants or skirts
Do not wear panty hose (wear thigh high or knee-high hose instead)
Remove wet bathing suits and exercise clothing promptly
Use dermatologically-approved detergent such as Purex or Clear
Double-rinse underwear and any other clothing that comes into contact with the vulva
Do not use fabric softener on undergarments

Hygiene

Use soft, white, unscented toilet paper
Use lukewarm or cool sitz baths to relieve burning and irritation
Avoid getting shampoo on the vulvar area
Do not use bubble bath, feminine hygiene products, or any perfumed creams or soaps
Wash the vulva with cool to lukewarm water only
Urinate before the bladder is full and rinse the vulva with water after urination
Prevent constipation by (a) adding fiber to your diet (if necessary, use a psyllium product such as Metamucil) and (b) drinking at least eight glasses of water daily
Use 100% cotton menstrual pads and tampons

Sexual intercourse

Use a lubricant that is water soluble, e.g., Astroglide, KY Warming Liquid, and so forth
Ask your physician for a prescription for a topical anesthetic, e.g., Lidocaine gel 5%
(This may sting for the first 3–5 minutes after application.)
Apply ice or a frozen blue gel pack (lunch box size) wrapped in a towel to relieve burning after intercourse
Urinate (to prevent infection) and rinse vulva with cool water after sexual intercourse

Physical activities

Avoid exercises that put direct pressure on the vulva such as bicycle riding and horseback riding
Limit intense exercises that create a lot of friction in the vulvar area (try lower intensity exercises such as walking)
Use a frozen gel pack wrapped in a towel to relieve symptoms after exercise
Enroll in an exercise class such as yoga to learn stretching and relaxation exercise
Do not swim in highly chlorinated pools and avoid the use of hot tubs

Everyday living

Use a foam rubber donut for long periods of sitting
If you must sit all day at work, try to intersperse periods of standing (e.g., rearrange your office so that you can stand while you speak on the phone)
Learn some relaxation techniques to do during the day. (*The Relaxation and Stress Reduction Workbook* by Davis, Eshelman, and McKay or *The Chronic Pain Control Workbook* by Catalano and Hardin are recommended.)

*From the National Vulvodynia Association. Note: The National Vulvodynia Association is an educational, nonprofit organization founded to disseminate information on vulvodynia. The NVA does not engage in the practice of medicine. It is not a medical authority, nor does it claim to have medical knowledge. In all cases, the NVA recommends that you consult your own health-care provider regarding any course of treatment or medication.

- Books
  - The V Book: A Doctor's Guide to Complete Vulvovaginal Heath by Elizabeth Steward, M.D. and Paula Spencer.
  - The Vulvodynia Survival Guide: How to Overcome Painful Vaginal Symptoms and Enjoy and Active Lifestyle by Howard Glazer, M.D. and Gae Rodke, M.D.
- Internet
  - *www.nva.org*
  - *www:vulvarhealth.org*
  - *www.vulvodynia.com*

References

1 Young AW. Burning Vulvar Syndrome: Report of the ISSVD. *J Reprod Med.* 1984;29:457.

2 Friedrich EG Jr. The vulvar vestibule. *J Reprod Med.* 1983;11: 773–774.

3 Woodruff JD, Parmley TH. Infection of the minor vestibular glands. *Obstet Gynecol.* 1983;62:609–612.

4 Friedrich EG Jr. Vulvar vestibulitis syndrome. *J Reprod Med.*, 1987;32:110–114.

5 Skene AJC. *Treatise on the Disease of Women.* New York: Appleton and Co.; 1989.

6 Thomas TG, Munde PF. *A Practical Treatise on the Disease of Women.* Philadelphia, PA: Lea Brothers and Co.; 1891.

7 West C. *Diseases of Women.* Philadelphia, PA: Blanchard and Lea; 1861.

8 Kelly HA. *Gynecology.* New York: Appleton and Co.; 1928.

9 Hunt I. *Disease of the Vulva.* St. Louis, MO: The CV Mosby Co.; 1948.

10 Dickinson RL. *Human Sex Anatomy.* 2nd ed. Baltimore, MD: Williams & Wilkins, 1949.

11 Pelisse M, Hewitt J. Erythematous vulvitis en plague. In: *Proceedings of the Third Congress of the International Society for the Study of Vulvar Disease.* 1976:35–37.

12 Pyka RE, Wilkinson EJ, Friedrich EG Jr, et al. The histopathology of vulvar vestibulitis syndrome. *Int J of Gynecol Pathol.* 1988;7:249–257.

13 Baggish MS, Miklos JR. Vulvar pain syndrome: a review. *Obstet Gynecol Surv.* 1995;50:618–627.

14 Baggish MS. *Colposcopy of the Cervix, Vagina, and Vulva.* Philadelphia, PA: Mosby; 2003.

15 Baggish MS, Karram MM. *Atlas of Pelvic Anatomy and Gynecologic Surgery*. Philadelphia, PA: W.B. Saunders; 2001.

16 Goetsch MF. Vulvar vestibulitis: prevalence and historic features in a general gynecologic practice population. *Am J Obstet Gynecol*. 1991;164:1609–1616.

17 Gentile G, Formelli G, Pelusi G, et al. Is vestibular micropapillomatosis associated with human papilloma virus infection? *Eur J Gynaecol Oncol*. 1997;18:523–525.

18 Marks TA, Shroyer KR, Markham NE, et al. A clinical histologic and DNA study of vulvodynia and its association with human papilloma virus. *J Soc Gynecol Investig*. 1995;1:57–63.

19 Prayson RA, Stoler MH, Hart WR. Vulvar vestibulitis: a histopathologic study of 36 cases including human papilloma virus in situ hybridization analysis. *Am J Surg Pathol*. 1995;19:154–160.

20 Bergeron C, Moyal-Barracco M, Pelisse M, et al. Vulvar vestibulitis: lack of evidence for a human papilloma virus etiology. *J Reprod Med*. 1994;39:936–938.

21 Glazer HI, Jantos M, Hartman EH, et al. Electromyographic comparisons of the pelvic floor in women with dysesthetic vulvodynia and asymptomatic women. *J Reprod Med*. 1998;43:959–962.

22 Solomons CC, Melmed MH, Heitler SM. Calcium citrate for vulvar vestibulitis. *J Reprod Med*. 1991;36:879–882.

23 Melmed MH. A low oxalate diet and calcium citrate are effective treatments for vulvar pain syndrome. *J Gynecol Surg*. 1996;12: 217–222.

24 Baggish MS, Sze EHM, Johnson R. Urinary oxalate excretion and its role in vulvar pain syndrome. *Am J Obstet Gynecol*. 1997;177: 507–511.

25 Marinoff SC, Turner MLC. Vulvar vestibulitis syndrome: an overview. *Am J Obstet Gynecol*. 1991;165:1228–1233.

26 Baggish MS. Surgery for vulvar vestibulitis syndrome: operative techniques in gynecologic surgery. 2000;5:48–58.

27 Glazer HI, Rodke G, Swencionis C, et al.. The treatment of vulvar vestibulitis syndrome by electromyographic biofeedback of pelvic floor musculature. *J Reprod Med*. 1995;40:283–290.

28 Bergeron S, Binik YM, Khalife S, et al. A randomized comparison of group cognitive-behavioral therapy, surface electromyographic biofeedback, and vestibulectomy in the treatment of dyspareunia resulting from vulvar vestibulitis. *Pain*. 2001;91:297–306.

HORMONE THERAPIES

18 Sexual Dysfunction and Androgen Replacement Therapy

Elizabeth A. Wise
Carol J. Mack
James A. Simon

Background

Women today are living longer, healthier lives and as life expectancy has increased so has the interest in female sexuality among middle-aged and older women. Low libido, inability to achieve orgasm, and decreased pleasure in sexual activities are common complaints. The National Health and Social Life Survey found that 43% of women in the United States experience sexual dysfunction.[1] However, the importance of sexuality in the later years is not a unique issue to women in the United States. In fact, sexual dysfunctions affect older women of all ages worldwide.[2] As the concept of female androgen insufficiency has been recognized as a valid clinical condition, more research has been devoted to the diagnosis and treatment of women with sexual complaints. Interestingly, the focus of these investigations has centered on women in their postmenopausal years despite the fact that perimenopausal women also suffer many of these same concerns.

In fact, women in this survey who were presumed to be perimenopausal had a greater frequency of sexual complaints than women ages 50–59. Additionally, measurement of serum androgen levels shows that the androgen hormones decline with increasing age during the reproductive years, but they decrease very little or not at all during the first few years following menopause.

KEY POINT

Low sexual desire was the most common complaint in women with sexual dysfunction.

With 22% of women in the United States complaining of low sexual desire, clinicians are faced with the issue of deciding which patients should be evaluated for androgen insufficiency as a cause of the problem. Low sexual desire, often used synonymously with low libido or low sexual interest and motivation, was the most common sexual complaint of women surveyed.[1] Female sexual function is complex and multifactorial. Besides the issue of androgens, other important causes of low libido include depression, anxiety, fatigue (physical and psychological), relationship conflicts, prior sexual abuse, lack of privacy, medications and the diseases they treat, as well as body image While these conditions can affect many aspects of sexual function, the reduction in desire and its relationship to androgens for women in the perimenopausal period will be the primary focus of this chapter.

Evaluation of Low Libido

It is important to remember that the patient seeing her clinician for a sexual function problem often assumes that she has a hormone or anatomic problem. If she thought her loss of sexual interest was due to depression, anxiety, or a psychological disorder she would have gone to a mental health professional instead. This is not a trivial issue since meeting the patient's expectations is very important in establishing a therapeutic alliance with her against the problem. Even though most patients with a sexual dysfunction do not have pure testosterone deficiency, many of them do not recognize that the relationship with their partner may be an issue or that their current life circumstances may be stressful.

In the initial interview, where evaluation for causative factors takes place, it is important to validate the patient's concerns about sexual function by explaining that there can be a variety of causes for the problem and by assuring her that many women experience similar problems. It is also important that the practitioner keep an open mind to the possibility that what appears obvious in the original interview may only be the tip of the iceberg and that other factors may come to light later. One possibility could be testosterone deficiency. The time of onset for low libido is an important factor. A lifelong history of low libido should be referred to a mental health professional. On the other hand, problems with a very specific onset in time may be related to a specific event (social, psychological, or hormonal) worthy of further exploration.

Any history of psychiatric problems, particularly those related to reproductive factors are particularly important. For example, a history of depression, poor adjustment to sexual development, anorexia nervosa or bulimia, depression associated with menarche, or oral contraceptives (OCPs), postpartum blues or depression, anxiety or depression during infertility treatment or, as is the issue here, during the perimenopause or menopause are very important. Investigation of possible sexual abuse or incest is advisable in all such patients. If there is a suggestion of a mood, relationship, or psychological problem preceding the loss of sexual desire, referral to a mental health professional is warranted. Failure to refer such a patient is not in the patient's best interest nor is it cost-effective. Because most antidepressants (i.e., the selective serotonin reuptake inhibitors and selective norepinephrine reuptake inhibitors) have sexual side effects of their own (i.e., delayed and/or absent orgasm) use of these agents in this setting should be reserved for a mental health professional working with a skilled and experienced psychiatrist familiar with the sexual consequences of these medications.

The physical examination should be undertaken with care. It is common for women to project their lack of sexual interest on some ill-defined problem with their genitals. For example, the patient may feel that her vagina is too big, too small, too dry, too painful, and so forth. While some patients may actually have a very small vagina, severe atrophy causing strictures or labial agglutination, these cases are very uncommon. A wide, gaping introitus can reduce sensation and sexual pleasure, but this condition seldom affects sexual interest directly. Likewise, pain syndromes such as vestibulitis and vulvodynia are very real and need to be evaluated by a trained professional, but they seldom lead to a lack of interest. Typically, pain leads to avoidance of intercourse because of pain, not lack of interest. Some women find a way to avoid the painful areas with manual or oral clitoral stimulation but most continue to have difficulty with intercourse. The same can be said for deep pain or cervical motion tenderness found during bimanual examination. These findings may be indicative of pelvic inflammatory disease, endometriosis, pelvic adhesions, and so forth, but only indirectly reduce libido.

KEY POINT

Androgen insufficiency should be evaluated when the physical examination is normal.

If the woman is menopausal, the physical examination may demonstrate vulvar or vaginal dryness and/or frank atrophy. A diagnosis of atrophy is unlikely in the perimenopausal women who is still cycling. If she is making enough estrogen to menstruate, there is sufficient estrogen to prevent vagina atrophy. If vaginal dryness or atrophy is present without specific signs of vestibulitis, vulvodynia, or infection, then adequate estrogenizing of the vagina is relatively straightforward, using one of the available local estrogen creams, suppositories, or tablets. At present, it is unclear if systemic estrogen therapy has an impact on central nervous system sexual responses.

Finally, and only if all of the above evaluations are negative, should one conclude that the patient may have testosterone insufficiency. There are at least two reasons for this approach. The first and most important is the well-established fact that the measurement of free or bioavailable testosterone in postmenopausal women is confounded by poor reliability and the imprecision of the commonly available assays. Using total testosterone as suggested in Fig. 18-1 is marginally better, but is also less accurate in women who are menopausal. In patients who are much younger, the assays perform better because the hormone levels are higher, since most of the commercially available assays are designed to measure male testosterone levels. Because the levels fluctuate throughout the cycle, a standardized approach is helpful. This accounts for the suggestion to measure free and total testosterone in menstruating women between cycle days 7 and 10. This time frame avoids the early menstrual cycle when most women have very low free and total testosterone concentrations. Sampling at this point also avoids the preovulatory peak in testosterone except in those women with very short perimenopausal cycles. By choosing an arbitrary definition of normal as the upper two-thirds of the normal premenopausal range, clinicians can avoid overtreating and undertreating. Dehydroepiandrosterone (DHEA) sulfate levels should also be determined in conjunction with testosterone.

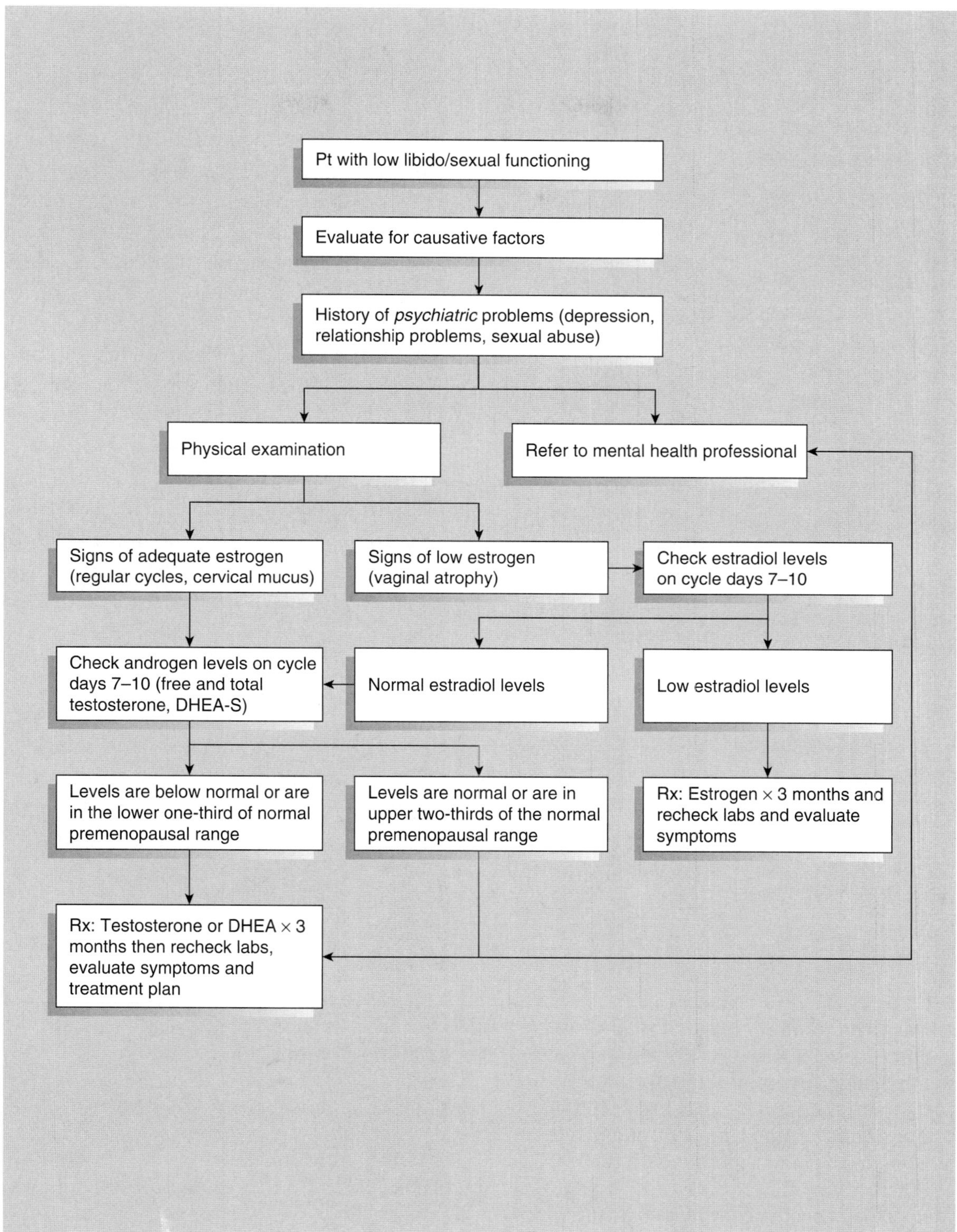
Pt with low libido/sexual functioning
Evaluate for causative factors
History of *psychiatric* problems (depression, relationship problems, sexual abuse)
Physical examination
Refer to mental health professional
Signs of adequate estrogen (regular cycles, cervical mucus)
Signs of low estrogen (vaginal atrophy)
Check estradiol levels on cycle days 7–10
Check androgen levels on cycle days 7–10 (free and total testosterone, DHEA-S)
Normal estradiol levels
Low estradiol levels
Levels are below normal or are in the lower one-third of normal premenopausal range
Levels are normal or are in upper two-thirds of the normal premenopausal range
Rx: Estrogen × 3 months and recheck labs and evaluate symptoms
Rx: Testosterone or DHEA × 3 months then recheck labs, evaluate symptoms and treatment plan

Figure 18-1

DHEA sulfate provides an integrated measure of adrenal androgen production.

Currently, Food and Drug Administration (FDA)-approved treatment options do not exist. For the patient with a low testosterone or very low DHEA one can opt for a trial of empiric therapy using intramuscular or topical testosterone or DHEA. DHEA serves as a precursor drug to deliver systemic testosterone and estradiol. The wide commercial availability of DHEA is offset by the poor reliability of the formulation and absorption. Typical doses are 25–75 mg per day for 1–3 months followed by reevaluation of both symptoms and blood levels (Fig. 18-1). Remember, DHEA in this setting is having an effect through delivery of estradiol and testosterone, not via DHEA per se. Intramuscular testosterone is also available as testosterone enanthate, cypionate, or propionate. Typical doses are 1 mg/kg ideal body weight to 1 mg/kg actual body weight via a once-a-month intramuscular injection. New delivery systems including intranasal, transdermal patches, gels, and emulsions as well as oral testosterone and methyltestosterone are in development. If these approaches fail to provide relief to the patient, referral to an experienced mental health professional is in order.

Perimenopausal Women At Risk of Sexual Dysfunction

The is little scientific information on women during the perimenopausal period because the focus has been primarily on postmenopausal women. However, we might consider how to clinically apply the recommendations of the Princeton Consensus[3] (Table 18-1) to this population.

Table 18-1. **FEMALE ANDROGEN INSUFFICIENCY PRINCETON CONSENSUS STATEMENT, JUNE 2001**

Clinical symptoms
Diminished sense of well-being, dysphoric mood, and/or blunted motivation
Persistent, unexplained fatigue
Sexual function changes, including decreased libido, sexual receptivity, and pleasure
Other potential signs and symptoms
Bone loss, decreased muscle strength, and changes in cognition/memory
As the most common presenting symptoms are nonspecific, symptoms alone are not sufficient for the diagnosis of androgen insufficiency

It is relatively common for women to complain of decreased sexual desire during the perimenopause.[4] A biological explanation for this phenomenon in perimenopausal women who maintain functional ovulatory cycles is difficult since the levels of testosterone do not fall appreciably during the perimenopausal transition. Levels of both testosterone (primarily from the ovary) and the adrenal androgens (DHEA and androstenedione) will decrease from early adulthood to about 50% of their peak adult values by the time of menopause.[5] Libido, sexual functioning, and frequency of sexual activities diminish in concert with the decline in estradiol levels during the menopausal transition.[6] A possible explanation of an androgen-based mechanism for a reduction in sexual interest during the perimenopause has been proposed by Mushayandebvu et al.[7] These investigators found that older but still ovulatory women had a blunting of the periovulatory rise in both testosterone and androstenedione compared to younger women. Since the periovulatory phase of the menstrual cycle is one of the times when women may initiate or are more receptive to sexual activity, these hormonal changes could provide one explanation for the perimenopausal change in sexual behavior in those individuals presenting with the symptom of decreased sexual desire. Recently, Gracia and colleagues suggested that a pronounced fluctuation in total testosterone concentrations over time was associated with a decrease in libido.[8]

Other common comorbidities can cause decreased sexual desire during the perimenopausal transition. While an exhaustive review of this issue goes beyond the scope of this chapter, some discussion is relevant. Any illness or therapy which lowers androgen production could result in a reduction in sexual interest. Examples include any illness treated with chronic corticosteroid therapy since these agents directly suppress adrenal androgen secretion. High corticosteroid doses also reduce ovarian estrogen and androgen production. These compounds are commonly used in asthma, rheumatoid arthritis, and other inflammatory diseases. Hyperthyroidism or excessive thyroid hormone replacement can decrease libido by increasing sex hormone-binding globulin (SHBG) and thereby decreasing free or bioavailable testosterone.

OCPs in premenopausal and perimenopausal women as well as hormone therapy (HT) in postmenopausal women, also reduce androgen bioavailability by increasing SHBG. While the

KEY POINT

Use of contraceptive steroids will decrease androgen bioavailability.

new transdermal combination contraceptive patches (e.g., Ortho Pharmaceutical, Inc.; Evra) and vaginal combination contraceptive rings (e.g., Organon, Inc.; NuvaRing) might be presumed to have a different impact on liver-dependent globulins (i.e., SHBG and CBG), this has not been demonstrated.[9] The impact of these newer contraceptive therapies on androgen bioavailability and action is similar to the standard dose (i.e., 35 mcg) OCPs. Unfortunately, the impact of contraceptive steroids on androgen bioavailability in perimenopausal women is seldom considered prior to initiating such treatments and sexual dysfunction can result.

Clinical Symptoms

One of the more common concerns mentioned by perimenopausal women seeking assistance from the gynecologist is a decrease in sexual interest. A nonjudgmental atmosphere facilitates discussion of this topic. Whether lower libido is a physiologic or pathophysiologic change is clearly subject to interpretation. However, when a decrease in sexual desire causes distress in the woman or initiates or aggravates conflict for a couple, some intervention appears warranted. Obviously, all such complaints are not related to androgens. In fact, documenting androgen deficiency in perimenopausal women is difficult. Many other causes are likely to be operative in this setting. These include the empty nest syndrome, financial problems related to higher education of children, and aging and disabled parents or grandparents to name just a few. All of these issues can put an added strain on the relationship that can lead to reduced interest in sexual activity.

Although a decrease in sexual desire or receptivity to one's partner is the most common presenting complaint, other sexual symptoms including a reduction in pleasure, a decrease in the intensity of orgasm, and/or reduced sensitivity of the clitoris and surrounding labia minora can accompany decreased desire or present as the primary symptom. In addition, symptoms related to a sense of a decrease in quality of life, a diminished sense of well-being, a dysphoric mood, and/or blunted motivation may be primary complaints or may simply accompany a reduction in desire. Persistent and unexplained fatigue without other symptoms of depression can be a reliable clinical symptom of androgen deficiency.

Other potential signs or symptoms which may become apparent are a reduction in bone density, decreased muscle strength, and nonspecific changes in cognition and memory, especially changes related

KEY POINT

There are no clear symptoms associated with androgen deficiency.

to visual spatial function and math problem solving. Examples might be an altered proficiency in parallel parking (visual-spatial dysfunction), or ability to do simple mathematical problems both from the standpoint of accuracy and of speed (math problem solving). Unfortunately, these symptoms are nonspecific and can be characteristic of depression, sleep disturbance, chronic fatigue syndrome, and underlying malignancy. Therefore, these symptoms alone are not sufficient for the diagnosis of androgen insufficiency.

Given that many presenting symptoms are not specific to androgen insufficiency, diagnostic tests that include measurement of androgen levels would be helpful in the assessment of the androgen deficiency condition. Unfortunately, most commercial laboratories will not be helpful as standard commercially available clinical assays are notoriously unreliable for measuring lower testosterone levels found in women, particularly perimenopausal and postmenopausal women. In addition to problems with the assay method (sensitivity), accurate measurement depends on when the blood sample is drawn. Drawing blood samples before menstrual cycle day 7[7] commonly leads to erroneously low total or free testosterone levels giving practitioners the unfortunate assessment that the patient is, in fact, androgen deficient. Testosterone levels drawn between menstrual cycle days 7 and 10 are ideal if the serum is assayed in a reference assay (often not available clinically). Testosterone levels drawn after day 10 the midcycle events in perimenopausal women with short cycles often can be lower than expected. As a general recommendation, serum samples for testosterone or free testosterone should *not* be used to determine the adequacy of androgens in perimenopausal or postmenopausal women unless specialized reference assays are being utilized.[10–12] However, current testosterone assays are perfectly adequate to assess excess androgen, or tumor levels of androgen(s) in women. There is a need for the development of readily available assays that currently measure the low levels of testosterone found in peri- and postmenopausal women.

Androgen Supplementation in Perimenopausal Women with Low Sexual Desire

Only recently has the importance of androgen therapy in women been investigated in a systematic fashion. These investigations have focused on postmenopausal women and in particular surgically postmenopausal women. This latter group is more hormonally homogenous than naturally menopausal women, and more likely to be clinically symptomatic. These investigations have shown that androgen replacement therapy in postmenopausal women does improve sexual function and other aspects of behavior. These studies demonstrate that testosterone replacement can improve arousability, sexual desire and fantasy, frequency of sexual activity and orgasm, and satisfaction and pleasure from sexual activity. Furthermore, Davis et al. assert that testosterone therapy enhances quality of life. Low libido, generalized fatigue, and an overall decreased sense of well-being may also be improved.[13]

To extend the existing research on androgen replacement to women in their premenopausal and perimenopausal years, Goldstat et al. conducted a study that evaluated the efficacy of transdermal testosterone therapy on women.[14] Thirty-four premenopausal women with low libido participated in the study, which lasted 28 weeks. From start to finish, 31 women provided complete data for the study. These women were between the ages of 30 and 45 and had reported diminished sexuality on the Sabbatsberg Sexual Self-Rating Scale, a sexual assessment scale specifically validated in this population. These women were also found to have early morning serum total testosterone levels of less than 2.2 nmol/L, which is considered the low-normal range for reproductive-age women. These authors excluded women who had relationship problems, dyspareunia, depression, high testosterone levels, and various other medical problems. In a placebo-controlled, crossover design, the participants treated themselves during two double-blind 12-week treatment periods, which were separated by a single-blind 4-week washout period. During the 12-week periods, some of the women applied 10 mg of testosterone cream to the thigh on a daily basis, while other women applied identical-appearing placebo cream. During the washout period, all women administered the placebo cream. At each visit, serum total testosterone, SHBG, and estradiol (E_2) concentrations were measured. These levels were measured between days 7 and 28 of the menstrual cycle because testosterone typically rises to a higher level and remains relatively constant throughout the mid to late follicular phase and the luteal phase.

The Psychological General Well-Being Index (PGWB) was employed to evaluate the overall general well-being of the women.

This 22-item multiple-choice questionnaire assesses anxiety, depressed mood, self-confidence, general health, well-being, and vitality. Furthermore, the Beck Depression Inventory measured depressed mood. The Sabbatsberg Sexual Self-Rating Scale evaluated the following elements of sexuality: sexual interest, sexual activity, satisfaction with sexual life, experience of sexual pleasure, sexual fantasy, orgasm capacity, and sexual relevancy.

During the testosterone cream treatment phase, serum total testosterone levels increased as anticipated. The mean serum total testosterone showed an increase of 1.54 nmol/L, starting from a baseline that was within the lower one-third of the normal female reproductive range. For the placebo participants, the serum total testosterone increased 0.22 nmol/L (a nonsignificant change). The Free Androgen Index (FAI), a ratio of total testosterone to SHBG, increased by 3.6 with testosterone, and by 0.4 with placebo. Serum E_2 levels did not change in either group.

The results of the PGWB and Sabbatsberg Sexual Self-Rating Scale indicated a significant improvement in general well-being, mood, and sexual function. The PGWB and the Sabbatsberg Scale showed improvements of 12.9 and 15.7 units, respectively. Testosterone showed beneficial effects on all subscale scores of the PGWB. Results from the Beck Depression Inventory were not significantly changed, yet testosterone treatment significantly improved scores on the PGWB and on the sexual self-rating scores (Sabbatsberg) relative to placebo. Furthermore, 46% of the women exhibited a 50% or higher increase in their total sexual self-rating score with testosterone treatment, compared to 19% of the women administering placebo treatment.

Numbers aside, how can one interpret these results? According to the authors of the above study, the effects of testosterone therapy on healthy premenopausal women are "substantial and clinically meaningful improvements in psychological and sexual well-being." Moreover, the mean total serum testosterone level of the women at baseline was in the low-normal female range when measured in the morning and outside the menstrual phase. Due to the testosterone treatment, the mood of the women was restored to general well-being average levels exhibited by the general population, based on the results of the PGWB. The average composite score, as applied to the general population in the National Health and Nutrition Examination Survey (NHANES) sample, was 80.3. The results of the Beck Depression Inventory were just outside the limit of statistical significance; however, the authors of the study see potential in the magnitude of improvement in mood with testosterone treatment. Perhaps most impressive, the results of the Sabbatsberg Sexual Self-Rating Scale showed a large improvement *and* carried over after no treatment during the 4-week washout period. The authors reported, "Not only did the mean sexual score increase from being in the lowest quartile for premenopausal women to the median for such women, but nearly half of the women had a 50% improvement in their individual sexual function score." In addition to these benefits of testosterone cream, none of the participants developed virilizing features during the short period of treatment. The cream was reported as otherwise well tolerated by the women. As a result of the transdermal application of the cream, total testosterone levels were raised to the high-normal range, and values for the FAI crossed the upper limit of normal. Although limited in its size and large amount of missing data (high dropout rate), these authors should be commended for their contribution to research as one of the first trials to evaluate the efficacy of testosterone therapy in premenopausal women.

Other studies have proven the efficacy of testosterone therapy on women in their mid to late reproductive years as well. Adrian Tuiten et al.[15] led a small study on the time course of effects of testosterone administration on sexual arousal in women. The authors examined whether a single dose of testosterone given to sexually functional women increased vaginal blood flow and subjective sexual arousal by exposing the women to erotic visual stimuli. Eight healthy premenopausal Caucasian women participants were tested within 10 days of the end of their menstrual cycle. The women were not taking any medication, and they were all heterosexuals who had engaged in sexual intercourse during the past year. Five of the women had a steady relationship, and the other three had multiple partners.

The study was a double-blind, randomly assigned, placebo-controlled crossover design. The authors exposed the women to six consecutive erotic film segments depicting heterosexual intercourse. The first excerpt (a 5-minute neutral film followed by a 5-minute hard core pronography videotape) was shown immediately before using a rapidly absorbed sublingual troche of placebo or testosterone 0.5 mg.

The second excerpt was shown 15 minutes afterward. The last four segments were shown at $1^1/_2$ hour intervals thereafter. Psychophysiologic and subjective evaluation of sexual functioning was conducted after exposure to the videos. Blood sampling was taken after 15 minutes and then after 105 minutes. These samples were then analyzed for total testosterone and SHBG.

In order to determine vaginal blood flow, vaginal pulse amplitude (VPA) was measured by vaginal photoplethysmograph. Variations in the amplitude of the signal indicate variation in vaginal vasocongestion. The VPA was recorded continuously during the experimental sessions, and its output corrected for changes in heartbeat. Peak-to-trough amplitude of the waves were calculated per pulse and then averaged over 5 minutes. This calculation counted as one data point for each baseline trial (VPA: BA), and one data point for each erotic trail (VPA: ET). Using these values, the authors were able to calculate the relative increase, percent-wise, in vasocongestion during the erotic condition, as compared to the neutral condition. In addition to the VPA calculations, self-report ratings of sexual functioning were noted after each session. The ratings were based on subjective experiences, regarding *bodily arousal*, *genital sensations*, and *sexual lust*.

The results of the study indicated that testosterone treatment does indeed increase vaginal responsiveness in a time-dependent fashion. Fifteen minutes following testosterone therapy, total testosterone levels increased tenfold or more in some cases. Within 90 minutes, however, testosterone returned to baseline levels. SHBG levels did not change between and on test days. Results from the Wilcoxon test indicated a difference in effect of testosterone compared to placebo treatment on the variation of VPA over time. There was a time-course effect of testosterone treatment on genital arousal of approximately 3–$4^1/_2$ hours suggesting that testosterone induced the increased readiness and activity of the responsive network in the brain in about 3–$4^1/_2$ hours. This time-delayed effect may reflect the role of brain mechanisms in regulating female sexual behavior.

The authors also concluded that there is a strong correlation between an increase in genital arousal and the occurrence of genital sensation and sexual lust. The study showed that changes in genital sensations and sexual lust in the testosterone treatment condition were correlated with testosterone concentrations albeit in a temporally delayed fashion suggesting that pharmacodynamic changes could have influenced the neurophysiological outcomes (genital sensation and sexual lust). While these results are promising, the authors of the study concede that a larger sample would extend their findings.

An important confounding variable in all studies of naturally-occurring androgens (i.e., testosterone, androstenedione, DHEA, and DHEA-S) in the treatment of sexual dysfunction is their potential to be converted to estrogens or to increase the bioavailability of estrogens. It has been shown that estrogen levels are strongly associated with sexual function in women[6] and that estradiol can improve depression symptoms in perimenopausal and postmenopausal women.[16] In a 4-week study of estrogen therapy on depression in perimenopausal women, remission of depression was noted in 8 of the 20 women who completed the study. Six of these women, who were taking 100 mcg of transdermal estradiol a day, were perimenopausal. Although some perimenopausal women with depression clearly benefited from short-term use of estrogen therapy, it would be wise to further investigate the role of such treatment in a larger more robust cohort. Nevertheless, because androgens can be easily aromatized to estrogens (i.e., testosterone→estradiol, androstenedione→estrone), clinicians must be careful not to assume that the ultimate effect of the androgen treatment is mediated through the androgen receptor. In addition, since both oral androgens and transdermal androgens in adequate doses commonly reduce the circulating levels of SHBG, these treatments may increase both free estradiol and free androgen.

Another study of perimenopausal and postmenopausal women taking androgen supplements also reported improved sexual behavior.[17] Thirty-eight women, who had androgen deficiency as a result of hypopituitarism and were between the ages of 25 and 65 years, received treatments of oral DHEA. These women took between 20 and 30 mg daily, based on their age, for a 6-month study. The administration of DHEA increased the serum levels of DHEA-S to normal age-related ranges. In women taking the 30-mg dose, androstenedione and T levels increased by 50%. Furthermore, the women's partners reported improved sexual relations, as compared to the placebo group. Eighty-four percent of the women reported androgenic effects on skin and hair growth. In contrast, a different study on the effect of DHEA supplementation to perimenopausal women did not exhibit any benefits.[18] In this randomized double-blind placebo-controlled study, 60 perimenopausal women were assigned to take either 50 mg of oral DHEA or a placebo tablet on a daily basis for 3 months. These women had heretofore complained of altered mood and well-being. There were no statistically significant differences in the participant's baseline hormone levels, including DHEA levels. After DHEA treatment, the serum androgen levels of the women greatly increased, as compared to those women in the placebo group. However, the women receiving DHEA supplementation did not report any greater improvements in their perimenopausal symptoms, mood, dysphoria, libido, cognition, memory, or well-being than the women in the placebo group.

Androgen therapy should be considered for women who are perimenopausal or premenopausal and who exhibit symptoms of androgen insufficiency syndrome or low free testosterone levels when measured in a reference laboratory. Androgens can be administered orally, by injection, or transdermally (Table 18-2). The transdermal treatment seems to give the best balance between achieving

Table 18-2. **ANDROGEN THERAPY FOR WOMEN: TYPES OF ANDROGENS**

Intramuscular
Testosterone propionate
Testosterone cypionate
Testosterone enanthate
Subcutaneous
Testosterone propionate pellets
Sublingual
Testosterone in propylene glycol
Oral
Methyltestosterone
Transdermal*
Testosterone
Gel*
Testosterone
Tibolone†

*In development

†Not FDA approved in USA

stable testosterone concentrations, and having minimal lipid and hepatic effects. Adverse effects and potential risks of androgen replacement therapy include acne, hirsutism, virilization, fluid retention, polycythemia, hepatic injury, sleep apnea, aggressive behavior, and a lowering of the high-density lipoprotein level.[19] The patient should be monitored for these effects. Additionally, one study suggested that *Andro* prohormones might increase a person's risk for developing pancreatic cancers.[20]

What's the Evidence

Although a decline in sexual desire has been observed during perimenopause, levels of testosterone and DHEA sulfate do not abruptly change. Therefore, it is difficult to determine whether these observed changes are due to menopause, aging, or a combination of the two factors.[4] Assessment of lower testosterone levels in the perimenopausal and menopausal woman is more difficult because of the lack of sufficiently precise and sensitive commercial assays for testosterone. If androgen deficiency is identified, treatment with testosterone or DHEA preparations can be considered. At the present time, no FDA-approved products are available and clinicians must rely on compounded pharmaceutical preparations. Any patient started on androgen therapy should be carefully monitored for response to therapy, androgenic side effects, and lipoprotein changes.

Conclusion

The importance of androgens in health and disease is emerging only now. Androgen actions at the cellular level are mediated by direct binding of the androgenic hormone to the androgen receptor or by conversion to other active androgens or estrogens. The primary source of estrogen in postmenopausal women comes from the aromatization of circulating adrenal androgen in the peripheral fat tissue.[7]

There is a growing body of evidence demonstrating the positive effects of estrogen-androgen therapy after menopause with regard to sexual desire, mood, cognitive functioning, and overall well-being.[2,6,8] In addition, androgens have been shown to have direct bone-stimulating effects in postmenopausal women,[21] although this use of androgens remains controversial. These potential beneficial effects must be understood to be preliminary and must be viewed against a backdrop of the complexities of the androgen production, metabolism, and interaction with estrogen and estrogen-induced binding globulins. Our current knowledge of the biological effects of androgens in women is very superficial, particularly the effects on the central nervous system. This void in our knowledge offers opportunity for further investigation.

Discussion of Cases

Case 1

AP is a 45-year-old married woman with a history of hypothyroidism. She experienced multiple episodes of irregular vaginal bleeding requiring D&C and hysteroscopy. She began OCPs to control her vaginal bleeding. AP was previously diagnosed with hypothyroidism, the result of a thyroid nodule, which is being suppressed with higher doses of levothyroxine. She is currently euthyroid by all biochemical tests. Since the initiation of her OCPs, she finds that she has extraordinarily low sexual desire, a dramatic change. Her family physician suggests that this is normal, perhaps secondary to the demands of AP's career and taking care of her ill mother. AP's physician suggests that she cut down on her work hours, hire a caregiver at home for her mother, and that "in time" AP's sexual desire will likely return. Six additional months ensue without significant improvement in AP's sexual desire, despite a significant reduction in her work hours, an increase in the amount of help she has at home, and by her own admission an extremely supportive and patient spouse. AP presents to the reproductive endocrinologist seeking further evaluation, thinking that her low sexual desire could be related to her hormones.

Physical evaluation reveals an otherwise healthy female in no acute distress with normal appearing external genitalia, without evidence of vaginal atrophy or vulvar tenderness, and a history of regular although "light" nonpainful withdrawal bleeding episodes on OCPs.

Laboratory tests document normal thyroid function and very low free testosterone, largely due to very high SHBG concentrations. AP's total testosterone is, in fact, in the upper normal range.

AP admits that she is willing to try almost anything in order to regain her sexual desire, and is determined to go off her OCPs, having already discussed this possibility with her husband who will use condoms.

Within 6 weeks of discontinuing her OCPs, AP calls the office to make another appointment. She returns at that time, noting that there is a marked increase in her desire. Her reproductive endocrinologist states that he is not certain that her change in libido is related to the discontinuation of her OCPs, since this has transpired very quickly, and determines to repeat her total and free testosterone levels. Total testosterone levels are again within the normal range; SHBG has returned to the mid to lower range and free testosterone is now at the mid to upper portion of the normal range.

Discussion

AP had a number of potential reasons for low libido. Her gynecologist was correct in assuming a large component of her low desire to be related to the stresses of career and being a caregiver for her ill mother. This scenario is very common and such everyday stresses and lack of sleep commonly reduce one's desire. AP also had several potential endocrinological causes for her low desire. Her use of levothyroxine and OCPs both of which can dramatically increase SHBG are also potential causes of her reduced desire. Contraception using vaginal rings and patches, while originally thought to avoid the SHBG increases seen with OCPs by avoiding the liver *first-pass* effect has been found to increase SHBG also. Discontinuing the OCPs in favor of a barrier form of contraception can obviate this issue. In the future, testosterone replacement therapies approved for women may allow "replacement" in situations like this. Although, this case was "managed" by measuring the total and free testosterone levels, this approach is not required since an understanding of the biology in this circumstance allow for clinical management strategies.

CASE 2

KS is a 46-year-old Caucasian female who has had an otherwise normal, healthy sex life with her husband of 20 years. She has recently been diagnosed with rheumatoid arthritis, and has begun a course of steroids to suppress the disease. Her rheumatologist anticipates her use of prednisone (30 mg daily) will last 3–6 months, depending upon her joint symptoms, after which time he anticipates initiating a *disease modifying agent* in an effort to reduce or discontinue her corticosteroid therapy, and to maintain her inflammatory disease at a manageable level. A baseline bone density test (dual energy x-ray absorptiometry [DXA]) is found to be normal. Her inflammatory markers are all elevated and she has been utilizing her prednisone for approximately 6 weeks. As she was due for her routine gynecological examination, she came to the office and had an unremarkable gynecologic physical and pelvic examination, with the exception that she complained of a dramatic and profound decline in her interest in sex particularly since starting on her prednisone. Upon further discussion, her cycles were found to be somewhat irregular, although this had been the case many times in the past without any associated psychosexual symptomatology. Her relationship with her husband of many years seems to be solid, although she does comment that her sleep pattern has been disturbed by both her joint stiffness and pain, as well as by her use of corticosteroids.

Laboratory assessment demonstrated normal gonadotropins and low-normal estradiol. However, the adrenal androgens, DHEAS, androstenedione and the ovarian androgens, total testosterone and free testosterone, were all extremely low for a woman of her age.

The rheumatologist was consulted regarding the possibility of using OCPs to regulate her menstrual cycles and to provide adequate estrogen in an effort to reduce bone loss during the time of maximal corticosteroid therapies. He had no objection. OCPs were initiated. In addition, a compounded preparation of 2%

testosterone in lightweight petrolatum was prescribed for local application to the clitoris and labia minora. A small amount of the testosterone preparation was applied three times weekly and the patient returned for a repeat of her lab tests after 4 weeks of therapy. At that time, total testosterone levels were in the upper limit of normal for a premenopausal woman, SHBG concentrations were likewise elevated, and free testosterone was within the normal range (high). The patient noted a marked increase in clitoral and nipple sensitivity, as well as a return of her normal sexual desire and adequate functioning despite her joint stiffness.

Discussion

Rheumatologic disorders whether treated or not are sometimes associated with a reduction in sexual desire. Whether the incidence is higher than with other chronic conditions remains to be determined. With glucocorticoid treatment, the resulting adrenal and ovarian androgen suppression contributes to altered sexual desire. Although serum levels of both total and free testosterone can be confirmatory, they are not required for the diagnosis or empiric treatment with testosterone. In this case, locally applied testosterone while very effective in increasing clitoral sensitivity, is also absorbed systemically and results in better libido as well as nipple sensitivity. It is important in such cases that adequate estrogen is present since all available studies to date have been done in an adequate estrogenic milieu. However, estrogen or OCP treatment is not acceptable in all rheumatological disorders. Collaboration with the rheumatologist is required for the successful management of these cases. It would be prudent to monitor lipid levels in women who are maintained on long-term testosterone therapy.

References

1 Laumann EO, Paik A, Rosen RC. Sexual dysfunction in the United States: Prevalence and predictors. *JAMA.* 1999;281:537–544.

2 Nicolosi A, Laumann EO, Glasser DB, et al., and Global Study of Sexual Attitudes and Behaviors Investigators' Group. Sexual behavior and sexual dysfunctions after age 40: the global study of sexual attitudes and behaviors. *Urology.* 2004;64:991–997.

3 Bachmann G, Bancroft J, Braunstein G, et al. Female Androgen Insufficiency: The Princeton Consensus Statement On Definition, Classification And Assessment. *Fertil Steril.* 2002;77(4):660–665.

4 Dennerstein L, Dudly E, Burger H. Are changes in sexual functioning during midlife due to aging or menopause? *Fertil Steril.* 2001;76:456–460.

5 Longcope C. Adrenal and gonadal androgen secretion in normal females. *Clin Endocrinol Metab.* 1986;15(2):213–228.

6 Dennerstein L, Randolph J, Taffee J, et al. Hormones, mood, sexuality, and the menopausal transition. *Fertil Steril.* 2002;77:(Suppl. 4): S42–S48.

7 Mushayandebvu T, Castracane VD, Gimpel T, et al.. Evidence for diminished midcycle ovarian androgen production in older reproductive aged women. *Fertil Steril.* 1996;65:721–723.

8 Gracia CR, Sammel MD, Freeman EW, et al. Predictors of decreased libido in women during the late reproductive years. *Menopause.* 2004;11:144–150.

9 Timmer CJ, Mulders MT. Pharmacokinetics of etonogestrel and ethinylestradiol released from a combined contraceptive vaginal ring. *Clin Pharmacokinet.* 2000;39:233–242.

10 Judd HL, Yen SS. Serum androstenedione and testosterone levels during the menstrual cycle. *J Clin Endocrinol Metab.* 1973;36:475–481.

11 Vierhapper H, Nowotny P, Waldhausl W. Determination of testosterone production rates in men and women using stable isotope dilution and mass spectrometry. *J Clin Endocrinol Metab.* 1997;82: 1492–1496.

12 Simon J, Houston V. *Restore Yourself: A Women's Guide to Reviving Her Sexual Desire and Passion for Life.* New York: Berkley Books; 2001:147–149.

13 Davis SR, McCloud P, Strauss BJ, et al. Testosterone enhances estradiol's effects on postmenopausal bone density and sexuality. *Maturitas.* 1995;21:227–236.

14 Goldstat R, Briganti E, Tran J, et al. Transdermal testosterone therapy improves well-being, mood, and sexual function in premenopausal women. *Menopause.* 2003;10:390–398.

15 Tuiten A, Van Honky J, Koppeschaar H, et al. Time course of effects of testosterone administration on sexual arousal in women. *Arch Gen Psychiatry.* 2000;57:149–153.

16 Cohen LS, Soares CN, Poitras JR. Short-term use of estradiol for depression in perimenopausal and postmenopausal women: a preliminary report. *Am J Psychiatry.* 2003;160:1519–1522.

17 Johannsson G, Burman P, Wiren L, et al. Low dose dehydroepiandrosterone affects behavior in hypopituitary androgen-deficient women: a placebo-controlled trial. *J Clin Endocrinol Metab.* 2002;87:2046–2052.

18 Barnhart KT, Freeman E, Grisso JA, et al. The effect of dehydroepiandrosterone supplementation to symptomatic perimenopausal women on serum endocrine profiles, lipid parameters, and health-related quality of life. *J Clin Endocrinol Metab.* 1999;84:3896–3902.

19 Braunstein GD. Androgen insufficiency in women: summary of critical issues. *Fertil Steril.* 2002;77:S98.

20 Broeder CE. Oral andro-related prohormone supplementation: do the potential risks outweigh the benefits? *Can J Appl Physiol.* 2003;28: 102–116.

21 Raisz LG, Wiita B, Artis A, et al. Comparison of the effects of estrogen alone and estrogen plus androgen on biochemical markers of bone formation and resorption in postmenopausal women. *J Clin Endocrinol Metab.* 1996;81:37–43

19 Postmenopausal Hormone Therapy: Observational Studies to Clinical Trials

Shari S. Bassuk
JoAnn E. Manson

One of the most complex health-care decisions facing women is whether or not to use postmenopausal hormone therapy (HT). Once prescribed primarily to relieve hot flushes and other menopausal symptoms, HT has been promoted as a strategy to forestall various disorders that accelerate after menopause, including coronary heart disease (CHD), cognitive decline, and osteoporosis. In 2001, an estimated 42% of postmenopausal women in the United States used HT.[1] This widespread use was unwarranted, given the paucity of conclusive data from randomized clinical trials on the health consequences of such therapy. Indeed, the recent publication of trial findings indicating unexpected adverse effects on clinical cardiovascular outcomes has led to a steady decline in HT use. Relative to January-June 2002, U.S. prescriptions in January-June 2003 declined by 33% for Premarin, the most widely used estrogen, and by 66% for Prempro, the most widely used estrogen-progestin combination.[1]

Although observational studies suggest that HT prevents a number of chronic diseases, the apparent benefits may result at

KEY POINT

Data from the large-scale WHI trial do not indicate a favorable balance of benefits and risks associated with estrogen-progestin or estrogen-only therapy when used for chronic disease prevention in postmenopausal women aged 50–79 years.

least in part from differences between women who opt to take postmenopausal hormones and women who do not. Those choosing HT tend to be healthier, have greater access to medical care, are more compliant with prescribed treatments, and maintain more health-promoting lifestyles, all of which may influence risk of CHD and other outcomes. Clinical trials, which minimize the problem of confounding by these factors by randomly assigning subjects to treatment groups, have not consistently confirmed the benefits found in observational studies—most notably, the finding that HT appears to protect against the development of CHD. Because CHD is a major cause of morbidity and mortality in postmenopausal women, consideration of potential coronary effects is important in evaluating the balance of benefits and risks of HT. Indeed, the hormone components of the Women's Health Initiative (WHI), a large prevention trial in healthy postmenopausal women aged 50–79 years, were stopped early as a result of such considerations. The estrogen-progestin arm, which enrolled more than 16,000 women with an intact uterus at baseline, was terminated after 5.2 years because of an overall unfavorable risk-benefit ratio associated with the hormone combination.[2] The estrogen-only arm, which enrolled more than 10,000 women with hysterectomy, was terminated after 6.8 years because of an excess risk of stroke that was not offset by a reduced risk of CHD in the hormone group.[3] Whether administration of hormones to younger women when they first reach menopause would confer the same balance of benefits and risks was not addressed by this trial, however.

Although many women rely on their health-care providers for a definitive answer to the question of whether to use postmenopausal hormones, balancing the benefits and risks for an individual patient can challenge even experienced clinicians. This chapter, which summarizes evidence from observational studies and clinical trials on the risks and benefits of HT, along with the following chapter on the "when and how" of HT prescribing, provides guidance to physicians and others who may be perplexed by this rapidly evolving clinical area. Table 19-1 gives an overview of empirical findings reviewed in this chapter, and Table 19-2 summarizes considerations in the application of study results to clinical practice.

Table 19-1. **POSTMENOPAUSAL HT AND DISEASE OUTCOMES: RESULTS FROM THE WOMEN'S HEALTH INITIATIVE (WHI), HEART AND ESTROGEN/PROGESTIN REPLACEMENT STUDY (HERS), AND OBSERVATIONAL STUDIES**

	WHI		*HERS*[a]		*Observational Studies*	
	Estrogen-Progestin	*Estrogen Alone*	*Randomized Treatment*	*Randomized Treatment and Observational Follow-Up*	*Estrogen-Progestin*	*Estrogen Alone*
	Relative Risk (95% confidence interval)[b]					
CHD	1.24 (1.00–1.54)[16]	0.91 (0.75–1.12)[3]	0.99 (0.80–1.22)[9]	0.99 (0.84–1.17)[9]	0.64 (0.49–0.85)[5]	0.55 (0.45–0.68)[5]
Stroke	1.31 (1.02–1.68)[27]	1.39 (1.10–1.77)[3]	1.23 (0.89–1.70)[28]	Not available[c]	1.45 (1.10–1.92)[5]	1.18 (0.95–1.46)[5]
VTE	2.11 (1.58–2.82)[2]	1.33 (0.99–1.79)[3]	2.66 (1.41–5.04)[32,35]	2.08 (1.28–3.40)[35]	2.1 (1.2–3.8)[31d,e]	
Endometrial cancer	0.81 (0.48–1.36)[36]	Not applicable	0.39 (0.08–2.02)[35]	0.25 (0.05–1.18)[35]	0.8 (0.6–1.2)[34]	4.1 (2.9–5.7)[34f]
Breast cancer	1.26 (1.00–1.59)[2]	0.77 (0.59–1.01)[3]	1.38 (0.82–2.31)[35]	1.27 (0.84–1.94)[35]	1.35 (1.21–1.49)[37d,g]	
Colorectal cancer	0.63 (0.43–0.92)[48]	1.08 (0.75–1.55)[3]	0.69 (0.32–1.49)[35h]	0.81 (0.46–1.45)[35h]	0.66 (0.59–0.74)[45d]	
Gallbladder disease	Not available	Not available	1.39 (1.00–1.93)[35]	1.48 (1.12–1.95)[35]	2.1 (1.9–2.4)[49d]	
Dementia	2.05 (1.21–3.48)[62]	1.49 (0.83–2.66)[61]	Not assessed	Not assessed	0.66 (0.53–0.82)[53d,i]	
Hip fracture	0.67 (0.47–0.96)[76]	0.61 (0.41–0.91)[3]	1.16 (0.55–2.44)[35,75]	1.61 (0.98–2.66)[35]	0.75 (0.68–0.84)[71d]	

[a] In HERS, the randomized treatment period lasted 4.1 years. Participants were then followed for an additional 2.7 years, with open-label treatment at the discretion of participants' personal physicians.

[b] Relative risks are for assignment to HT vs. assignment to placebo in the WHI and HERS trials, and, except where indicated, for current use vs. never use of HT in the observational studies. Confidence intervals are nominal.

[c] Stroke alone was not reported. For the combined end point of stroke and transient ischemic attack, the relative risks (and associated 95% confidence intervals) after the randomized treatment period and after the additional observational follow-up were 1.09 (0.84–1.43) and 1.09 (0.88–1.35), respectively.[9]

[d] Estimate is for use of any hormones.

[e] Estimate is for pulmonary embolism only.

[f] Estimate is for recent (within past 1 year) vs. never use.

[g] Estimate is for 5 or more years of current hormone use.

[h] Estimate is for colon cancer only.

[i] There is significant heterogeneity in results across individual observational studies.

Table 19-2. CONSIDERATIONS IN THE APPLICATION OF STUDY RESULTS TO CLINICAL PRACTICE

Observational Study	Randomized Clinical Trial
Methodology	**Methodology**
Participants engage in their usual health behaviors and medical practices while researchers observe them over time, often for years or decades, to determine whether these behaviors are associated with the risk of developing a given outcome—either a disease or clinical biomarker	Participants are randomly assigned to active agent or placebo. In a double-blind design, neither participants nor investigators know participants' treatment assignment. An independent Data and Safety Monitoring Board (DSMB) periodically reviews the data to determine the effect of treatment on a defined outcome (disease or clinical biomarker). If a clear benefit or harm emerges before the scheduled end of the trial, the DSMB recommends early termination
Strengths	**Strengths**
Investigates "real-world" exposures and medical practices	In a large-enough sample, randomized treatment assignment is an effective way to control confounding. On average, both known confounders and unknown or unmeasured confounders will be distributed equally among the active agent and placebo groups.
Permits examination of diverse exposures (e.g., various HT regimens) in a single study	Double blinding ensures that expectations of a benefit or harm do not bias participants' responses or investigators' analysis and interpretation of the data
Permits examination of harmful exposures (e.g., smoking) that cannot ethically be studied in a randomized trial	
Less expensive to conduct and less onerous to participants than a randomized trial, thus facilitating long-term follow-up to detect late effects	
Weaknesses	**Weaknesses**
Confounding (healthy-user bias, compliance bias): Investigators must identify and measure differences between participants that could influence observed exposure-disease associations and then use statistical modeling to control for such differences	Participants may not reflect typical users of the agent under investigation, limiting the generalizability of findings. In HT trials, participants were older, were further away from menopause, had fewer menopause symptoms, and had higher BMI than HT users in observational studies.
Incomplete capture of early clinical events due to discontinuous monitoring of exposures	Subgroup analyses to identify subsets of patients who experience greater benefit or harm from the agent under investigation must be interpreted with caution, as such analyses tend to be post hoc and are susceptible to confounding. In addition, analyses limited to good compliers can be misleading.
Cautious application of findings to clinical practice; findings require replication in randomized clinical trials	Trials usually focus on one or two specific regimens; thus, whether differences in HT formulation, dose, or route of administration affect outcomes is unclear
	Expensive; recruitment can be difficult; trials that provide information about long-term effects are scarce

Coronary Heart Disease

KEY POINT

Neither primary nor secondary prevention of CVD should be viewed as an expected benefit of HT, and the possibility of an early increase in risk of coronary events should be considered.

Until recently, much of the enthusiasm for postmenopausal HT had been due to its putative cardioprotective effects. During the past three decades, dozens of observational studies have, in the aggregate, suggested that women who take estrogen are 35 to 50% less likely to develop CHD than women who do not take estrogen.[4] This inverse association has been observed in both primary and secondary prevention settings. The 20-year Nurses' Health Study (NHS) is the largest prospective investigation of HT and risk of developing CHD. Among 70,533 postmenopausal participants with no history of cardiovascular disease (CVD), current use of HT, as compared with never use, was associated with a relative risk (RR) of a major coronary event of 0.61 (95% confidence interval [CI] 0.52–0.71), after adjustment for age, body mass index (BMI), diabetes, hypertension, high cholesterol, age at menopause, smoking, and parental history of premature heart disease.[5] A protective effect has also been found among women with established CHD. Among the 2489 postmenopausal NHS participants with previous myocardial infarction (MI) or documented atherosclerosis, the RR for recurrent coronary events associated with current HT use, as compared with never use, was 0.65 (95% CI 0.45–0.95).[6]

That HT reduces cardiovascular events is biologically plausible. In randomized trials, exogenous estrogen lowers plasma low-density lipoprotein (LDL) cholesterol levels by 10–14% and raises high-density lipoprotein (HDL) cholesterol levels by 7–8%, changes known to be associated with a reduced risk of CHD.[7] Oral administration of estrogen has also been shown to reduce levels of lipoprotein(a), inhibit oxidation of LDL cholesterol, improve endothelial vascular function, and reverse postmenopausal increases in fibrinogen and plasminogen-activator inhibitor type 1—changes that should lower CHD risk.[7] At the same time, however, estrogen has potentially detrimental effects on other biomarkers of cardiovascular risk; it boosts triglyceride levels; promotes coagulation through increases in factor VII, prothrombin fragments 1 and 2, and fibrinopeptide A; and raises levels of the inflammatory marker C-reactive protein.[7] Estrogen therapy also increases the production and activity of matrix metalloproteinases, degradative enzymes important in the destabilization and rupture of plaque.[7]

As shown in Table 19-3, randomized trials of estrogen or combined estrogen-progestin in women with preexisting CHD have not

Table 19-3. RANDOMIZED CLINICAL TRIALS OF POSTMENOPAUSAL HT AND CHD

Trial Name	Study Population	Age Range (Mean), Years	Treatment	Mean Duration, Years	Results
Secondary Prevention (i.e., among women with preexisting CHD)					
Heart and Estrogen/Progestin Replacement Study (HERS)[8,9]	2763 women with documented CHD	44–79(66.7)	0.625 mg oral CEE and 2.5 mg MPA daily, or placebo	4.1*	CHD events (nonfatal MI, CHD death): Overall: RR = 0.99 (95% CI 0.80–1.22) Year 1: RR = 1.52 (95% CI 1.01–2.29) Year 2: RR = 1.00 (95% CI 0.67–1.49) Year 3: RR = 0.87 (95% CI 0.55–1.37) Year 4/5: RR = 0.67 (95% CI 0.43–1.04)
Estrogen Replacement and Atherosclerosis (ERA)[10] Trial	309 women with angiographically verified CHD	42–80 (65.8)	0.625 mg oral CEE daily, or 0.625 mg oral CEE and 2.5 mg MPA daily, or placebo	3.2	No significant differences in progression of stenosis No significant differences in CHD events (nonfatal MI, CHD death) overall or during year 1
Papworth Hormone-Replacement Therapy Atherosclerosis Study[11]	255 women with documented CHD	≥55 (67)	Transdermal 17-β estradiol alone or with cyclic norethisterone, or placebo	2.5	CHD events (MI, hospitalization for unstable angina, cardiac death): RR = 1.29 (95% CI 0.84–1.95)
Women's Angiographic Vitamin and Estrogen (WAVE)[12] Trial	423 women with at least one 15–75% coronary stenosis	range not provided (65)	0.625 mg oral CEE with or without 2.5 mg MPA daily, or placebo	2.8	Slightly greater progression of stenosis with HT than with placebo CVD events (MI, stroke) or death: RR = 1.9 (95% CI 0.97–3.6)
Estrogen in the Prevention of Reinfarction Trial (ESPRIT)[13]	1017 women with prior MI	50–69 (62)	2 mg oral estradiol valerate, or placebo	2	CHD evens (nonfatal MI, cardiac death): RR = 0.99 (95% CI 0.70–1.41)

Primary Prevention (i.e., among women at usual risk of CHD)					
Overview of 22 HT trials[17]	4124 women	Not provided	HT (various regimens) vs. placebo or other therapy	<3	Cardiovascular events: RR = 1.39 (95% CI 0.48–3.95)
Women's Health Initiative (WHI): Estrogen-progestin arm[2,16]	16,608 women at usual risk of CVD	50–79 (63)	0.625 mg oral CEE and 2.5 mg MPA daily, or placebo	5.6	CHD events (nonfatal MI, CHD death): Overall: RR = 1.24 (95% CI 1.00–1.54) Year 1: RR = 1.81 (95% CI 1.09–3.01) Year 2: RR = 1.34 (95% CI 0.82–2.18) Year 3: RR = 1.27 (95% CI 0.64–2.50) Year 4: RR = 1.25 (95% CI 0.74–2.12) Year 5: RR = 1.45 (95% CI 0.81–2.59) Year ≥ 6: RR = 0.70 (95% CI 0.42–1.14)
Women's Health Initiative (WHI): Estrogen-only arm[3]	10,739 women at usual risk of CVD	50–79 (63)	0.625 mg oral CEE or placebo	6.8	CHD events (nonfatal MI, CHD death): Overall: RR = 0.91 (95% CI 0.75–1.12) Year 1: RR = 1.16 Year 2: RR = 1.20 Year 3: RR = 0.89 Year 4: RR = 0.79 Year 5: RR = 1.28 Year 6: RR = 1.24 Year ≥7: RR = 0.42 (p for trend = 0.02)

Abbreviations: CEE: conjugated equine estrogen; CI: confidence interval; CVD: cardiovascular disease; MI: myocardial infarction; MPA: medroxyprogesterone acetate, RR: relative risk.

* An additional 2.7 year of observational follow-up yielded an overall RR of 0.99 (0.84–1.17) and a RR in years 6 and 7 of 1.00 (0.77–1.29).[9]

confirmed the benefits reported in observational studies.[8–15] In the Heart and Estrogen/progestin Replacement Study (HERS), a seminal secondary prevention trial designed to test the efficacy and safety of HT (0.625 mg of oral conjugated equine estrogen plus 2.5 mg of medroxyprogesterone acetate per day) in relation to clinical cardiovascular outcomes, the 4.1-year incidence of coronary mortality and nonfatal MI among 2763 women with documented CHD was similar in the active treatment and placebo groups.[8] A 50% increase in risk of CHD events was noted during the first year of the study among women assigned to active treatment, although this elevation was offset by a decreased risk in years 4 and 5. An additional 2.7 years of observational follow-up, with open-label treatment at the discretion of participants' personal physicians, did not alter these findings.[9] This temporal pattern could result from an acceleration of the rate of events in susceptible women, leaving a lower-risk group for continued follow-up. It is also possible that progestins may have adverse cardiovascular effects and may mitigate beneficial effects of estrogen. However, in the placebo-controlled Estrogen Replacement and Atherosclerosis (ERA) trial, neither estrogen alone nor estrogen in combination with progestin (i.e., oral conjugated equine estrogen alone or with medroxyprogesterone acetate) affected the angiographically determined progression of coronary atherosclerosis.[10] The Papworth Hormone-Replacement Therapy Atherosclerosis Study,[11] which evaluated transdermal estradiol alone or with norethindrone, and the Women's Angiographic Vitamin and Estrogen (WAVE) trial,[12] which evaluated oral conjugated equine estrogen alone or with medroxyprogesterone acetate, also showed no cardiovascular benefit of the regimens studied. Indeed, the Papworth trial was terminated ahead of schedule because of an early increase in cardiovascular events in the active treatment group. In the Estrogen in the Prevention of Reinfarction Trial (ESPRIT), estradiol valerate (2 mg/day) did not reduce the risk of subsequent cardiac events in women with a history of MI.[13] Thus, on the basis of data from randomized trials, postmenopausal HT has not proven effective for the secondary prevention of CHD.

Primary prevention trials also indicate an early increase in cardiovascular risk and absence of cardioprotection with postmenopausal HT. In the WHI, women assigned to 5.6 years of estrogen-progestin therapy were 24% more likely to develop CHD than those assigned to placebo.[16] The increased risk was most evident during the first year of randomized treatment and was augmented among women with higher LDL cholesterol levels at baseline.[16] Women assigned to 6.8 years of estrogen-only therapy also experienced no reduction in CHD risk as compared with those assigned to placebo; RRs were slightly elevated during early follow-up and diminished over time.[3] Similar results were found in an aggregate analysis of 22 mostly short-term trials examining other outcomes of HT.[17]

Methodologic and biologic explanations for the discrepancy between the CHD results from observational studies and those from clinical trials have been proposed.[18,19] Methodologic explanations often focus on the well-recognized potential for confounding in observational studies. Women who choose HT tend to be healthier and to adhere more frequently to other types of health-promoting behaviors than women who choose not to take postmenopausal hormones. These *healthy-user* and *compliance* biases may lead to an underestimate of the true coronary risk associated with HT. Statistical methods can adjust for such effects, but only to the extent that confounders are known and accurately measured. Residual confounding due to unknown or imperfectly measured covariates is a threat to the validity of inferences drawn from observational data. Yet the concordance between findings from trials and observational studies for other outcomes, especially stroke, which have similar lifestyle determinants as CHD, argues against confounding as the major reason for the discrepancy in findings for CHD.

Another methodologic shortcoming of many observational studies is their inability to capture early clinical events that occur soon after initiation of HT. In prospective studies with long-term follow-up, information on HT use is generally updated only at infrequent intervals, if at all. Thus, clinical events that develop shortly after HT is begun may be incorrectly classified as having taken place in a nonuser or during a "nonusing" interval, which would lead to attenuated risk estimates. This misclassification may be particularly salient for CHD outcomes, because, in both HERS and WHI, HT-associated increases in CHD risk were most pronounced soon after randomization to treatment, whereas delayed or persistently elevated risks were seen for most of the other outcomes of interest, including stroke, venous thromboembolism (VTE), and breast cancer.

These temporal trends in HERS and WHI prompted closer attention to timing of exposure in recent analyses of observational data. Among NHS participants with prior coronary disease, there was a strong trend of decreasing risk of recurrent CHD events with increasing duration of HT use. Among women using hormones for less than 1 year, 1–1.9 years, and 2 or more years, as compared with never users, the RRs of recurrent events were 1.25 (95% CI 0.78–2.00), 0.55 (95% CI 0.13–2.27), and 0.38 (95% CI 0.22–0.66), respectively (*P* for trend = 0.002).[6] On the other hand, the opposite trend was observed among NHS participants without prior coronary disease. In this group, the protective effect decreased as duration of use increased, with RRs for durations of less than 1 year, 1–1.9 years, 2–4.9 years, 5–9.9 years, and 10 years or more of 0.40, 0.41, 0.53, 0.58, and 0.74, respectively.[5] However, the impact of HT in the first few months of use could not be assessed, because participants reported current use or nonuse of HT only at 2-year intervals and were classified as users or nonusers for the duration of a given interval. In the Group Health Cooperative Study, a 3.5-year follow-up of 981 postmenopausal women with prior MI, information on hormone use was continually updated from a computerized pharmacy database, allowing a more precise estimate of exposure timing than was possible in the Nurses' cohort[20] or other observational studies. Although this study found no overall association between current HT use and risk of recurrent coronary events (RR = 0.96, 95% CI 0.62–1.50), there was an apparent doubling of risk of CHD events in the first 60 days following initiation of HT (RR = 2.16, 95% CI 0.94–4.95). However, ongoing hormone use lasting more than 1 year was associated with reduced coronary risk (RR = 0.76, 95% CI 0.42–1.36).

Biologic explanations may also account in part for differences in results from observational studies and randomized clinical trials. For example, whereas the hormone regimen most often tested in clinical trials has been a daily estrogen-progestin combination, the majority of women studied in observational settings have used estrogen-only formulations. Nevertheless, in the NHS, one of the few cohorts in which the number of combination-therapy users was large enough to allow subgroup analyses, combination therapy appeared to be nearly as protective as unopposed estrogen against first CHD events. Compared with nonusers of

HT, users of oral conjugated estrogen alone had a RR of CHD of 0.55 (95% CI 0.45–0.68), and users of estrogen plus progestin had a RR of 0.64 (95% CI 0.49–0.85).[5] Among women with preexisting CVD, there were also no clear differences in the coronary effect of estrogen alone versus estrogen combined with progestin.[6] Most women taking combination hormones reported cyclic (10–14 days/month) rather than continuous progestin use, however. Whether differences in HT formulations, or in doses or routes of administration, can account for conflicting observational and randomized findings remains uncertain.

Differing clinical characteristics of observational and randomized study populations may also influence the relationship between HT use and coronary outcomes. One striking difference between participants in observational studies and those in clinical trials is that of body weight. Whereas the mean BMI among HT users without prior CVD in the NHS was 26.1 kg/m^2, the mean BMIs among women in the estrogen-progestin and estrogen-only arms of the WHI were 28.5 and 30.1 kg/m^2, respectively. BMI is strongly and positively correlated with endogenous estrogen levels in postmenopausal women. Because leaner women have lower levels of endogenous estrogen than their heavier counterparts, they may be more likely to have vasomotor symptoms, to opt for HT to relieve these symptoms, and to benefit uniquely from such use. Indeed, in a 12-year observational follow-up of nearly 300,000 postmenopausal women with no history of CVD or cancer (the American Cancer Society's Cancer Prevention Study II [CPS II]), the inverse association between estrogen therapy and CHD mortality was strongest in lean women; for BMIs of less than 22, 22–25, 25 to less than 30, and 30 kg/m^2 or more, the RRs were 0.49, 0.72, 0.77, and 1.45, respectively (P for interaction = 0.02).[21] In the WHI, however, this pattern was not observed. Indeed, in the estrogen-progestin arm, there was a weak trend in the opposite direction; among women with BMIs of less than 25, 25 to less than 30, and 30 or more kg/m^2, the RRs of CHD associated with HT were 1.38, 1.23, and 1.16, respectively.[16] On the other hand, the harmful coronary effects of estrogen plus progestin seemed more prominent among participants without hot flushes at baseline. Among 50–59-year-old women, assignment to HT doubled the risk of CHD in those without hot flushes (RR = 1.98), but was unrelated to CHD risk in those with hot flushes (RR = 0.95).[16] However, statistical power to detect an interaction was low, and the apparent effect modification largely disappeared when the classification of vasomotor status was widened to include night sweats. At the time of chapter preparation, detailed analyses of the estrogen-only arm of the WHI were not available.

A woman's age, time since menopause, and underlying stage of atherosclerosis may additionally modify the influence of exogenous hormones on CHD risk. Women taking postmenopausal hormones in observational studies tend to initiate therapy at the onset of menopause, whereas clinical trial participants are typically randomized to hormones years after menstruation has ceased. Menopause occurs, on average, at age 51 in U.S. women. The baseline ages of participants in the NHS ranged from 30 to 55 years, and about 80% of cohort members who chose to use HT did so within 2 years of menopause. In contrast, the mean baseline ages of WHI and HERS participants were 63 and 67 years, respectively; thus, the majority of these women had been postmenopausal for many years at the time of enrollment. It is likely that these older women, on average, had more extensive subclinical atherosclerosis than did their younger counterparts. It has been suggested that the prothrombotic effect of estrogens manifests itself predominantly among women with subclinical lesions who initiate HT well after the menopausal transition, whereas women with less arterial damage who start HT early in menopause may derive cardiovascular benefit. Nonhuman primate data support this hypothesis. Conjugated estrogen had no effect on the extent of coronary artery plaque in cynomolgus monkeys assigned to estrogen alone or to estrogen combined with medroxyprogesterone acetate starting 2 years (about 6 human years) after oophorectomy and well after the establishment of atherosclerosis. On the other hand, administration of exogenous hormones immediately after oophorectomy, during the early stages of atherosclerosis, reduced the extent of plaque by 50%.[22] Subgroup analyses of WHI data provide mixed support for the idea that these variables influence the HT-CHD association. The risk of developing CHD associated with estrogen-only therapy sharply increased with age; among participants aged 50–59, 60–69 years, and 70–79 years; RRs were 0.56 (95% CI 0.30–1.03), 0.92 (95% CI 0.69–1.23), and 1.04 (95% CI 0.75–1.44), respectively.[3] Although this pattern was not observed in the estrogen-progestin arm (the corresponding RRs were 1.27, 1.05, and 1.44), the RRs associated with this regimen steadily increased with years since menopause (for <10, 10–19, and ≥20 years; RRs were 0.89, 1.22, and 1.71, respectively).[16]

However, in neither the estrogen-only nor the estrogen-progestin arm did the presence of preexisting CHD appreciably modify the relationship between HT and new coronary events. The RRs associated with estrogen alone were 0.91 (95% CI 0.73–1.14) in women without prior CHD and 1.02 (95% CI 0.63–1.71) among women with prior CHD. For estrogen plus progestin, the corresponding RRs were 1.23 (95% CI 0.97–1.55) and 1.44 (95% CI 0.77–2.70).

Further research on clinical characteristics, including biochemical and genetic markers that predict increases or decreases in coronary risk associated with exogenous hormone use is needed. Some data suggest that women with elevated serum lipoprotein(a) levels[23] or specific polymorphisms in the estrogen receptor gene[24] might benefit, whereas those with hypertension and a prothrombin mutation might be at particularly high risk.[25]

Stroke

Observational studies of HT and stroke have yielded inconsistent results. In a 20-year follow-up of 70,533 postmenopausal NHS participants without prior CVD, there was little association between HT and total stroke incidence or mortality.[5] The RR of incident stroke was 1.13 (95% CI 0.94–1.35) for current use of any duration and 1.32 (95% CI 0.76–2.32) for current use of less than 1 year (but see the above caveat regarding measurement of exposure duration), as compared with never use, after adjustment for vascular risk factors. Upon closer examination, however, current hormone use appeared to increase the risk of ischemic stroke (RR = 1.26, 95% CI 1.00–1.61) but not hemorrhagic stroke (RR = 0.93, 95% CI 0.64–1.34). In addition, although there was little association between current use of unopposed oral conjugated estrogen and total stroke (RR = 1.18, 95% CI 0.95–1.46), a significantly elevated stroke risk among women taking estrogen plus progestin was noted (RR = 1.45, 95% CI 1.10–1.92). Moreover, risk of stroke increased with increasing dose of oral conjugated estrogen; for doses of 0.3, 0.625, and 1.25 mg/day or more, the RRs were 0.54 (95% CI 0.28–1.06), 1.35 (95% CI 1.08–1.68), and 1.63 (95% CI 1.18–2.26), respectively. On the other hand, in a large case-control study at Group Health Cooperative, a health-maintenance organization with detailed computer records of hormone use, current use of estrogen with or without progestin was not related to risk of either ischemic or hemorrhagic stroke.[26]

However, risk of both stroke types doubled during the first 6 months of HT use (ischemic stroke: RR = 2.16 [95% CI 1.04–4.49]; hemorrhagic stroke: RR = 2.20 [95% CI 0.83–5.81]), and ischemic stroke risk also increased with estrogen dose (*P* for trend = 0.03).

In the WHI, women assigned to 5.6 years of estrogen-progestin were 31% more likely to develop stroke than those assigned to placebo (RR = 1.31, 95% CI 1.02–1.68), although there was no difference between treatment groups with respect to stroke mortality.[27] Unlike the pattern for CHD, where the risk was highest in the year following initiation of HT, the excess stroke risk emerged during the second year and remained elevated throughout the randomized treatment period. Similar findings were observed for estrogen alone; assignment to 6.8 years of the hormone was associated with a significant increase in the risk of total stroke (RR = 1.39, 95% CI 1.10–1.77) but not fatal stroke[3]; the increase persisted for the duration of randomized follow-up. For estrogen plus progestin, the increased risk was found for ischemic stroke (RR = 1.44, 95% CI 1.09–1.90) but not hemorrhagic stroke (RR = 0.82, 95% CI 0.43–1.56).[27] Parallel analyses of stroke subtypes are not yet available for estrogen alone.

Two trials in women at high risk of stroke have evaluated the effect of HT on this outcome. In HERS, a secondary CHD prevention trial, estrogen-progestin therapy was not significantly associated with risk of stroke (RR = 1.23, 95% CI 0.89–1.70) or a combined end point of stroke and transient ischemic attack (RR = 1.09, 95% CI 0.84–1.43).[28] When stroke subtypes were examined, no significant findings emerged for ischemic or hemorrhagic stroke, or for nonfatal or fatal stroke. Unlike the HT-CHD association, the relationship between HT and incident cerebrovascular events did not vary over the course of the trial. The results were unchanged after an additional 2.7 years of observational follow-up.[9]

The Women's Estrogen for Stroke Trial (WEST) enrolled 664 women with a history of ischemic stroke or transient ischemic attack. Participants assigned to 17-beta-estradiol (1 mg/day) were much more likely to experience a fatal stroke (RR = 2.9, 95% CI 0.9–9.0) than were those assigned to placebo, a finding that was particularly pronounced for fatal ischemic stroke (RR = 4.4, 95% CI 0.9–20.2). Although estradiol therapy was unrelated to the incidence of nonfatal stroke, the nonfatal strokes that occurred in the estradiol group were associated with slightly worse functional deficits than were those in the placebo group.[29] Post hoc analysis indicated a sharp increase in total stroke incidence during the first 6 months of HT use (RR = 2.3, 95% CI 1.1–5.0), but the association did not persist for the duration of the 2.8-year trial.

Venous Thromboembolism

In the WHI, randomized assignment to estrogen-progestin therapy was associated with a twofold increased risk of VTE (RR = 2.11, 95% CI 1.58–2.82),[2] and randomized assignment to estrogen alone was associated with a 33% increase in risk (RR = 1.33, 95% CI 0.99–1.79).[3] A meta-analysis of 12 previous studies – eight case-control, one cohort, and three trials – found that current estrogen use doubled VTE risk (RR = 2.14; 95% CI 1.64–2.81).[30] In the NHS, which was the sole cohort study included in the meta-analysis, the RR of pulmonary embolism was 2.1 (95% CI 1.2–3.8).[31] RRs of VTE were higher in the three trials: 2.66 (95% CI 1.41–5.04) in HERS,[32] 3.70 (95% CI 0.45–30.44) in ERA,[10] and 5.10 (95% CI 0.30–86.66) in the Postmenopausal Estrogen/Progestin Interventions (PEPI) trial,[33] a 3-year study of 875 healthy women randomly assigned to HT or placebo in which change in cardiovascular risk profile—rather than CVD itself—was the primary end point.

Endometrial Cancer

A combined analysis of 30 observational studies found a tripling of risk of endometrial cancer among short-term (1–5 years) users of unopposed estrogen (RR = 2.8, 95% CI 2.3–3.5) and a nearly tenfold elevation in risk among users for 10 or more years (RR = 9.5, 95% CI 7.4–12.3).[34] These findings are supported by results from the PEPI trial, in which 24% of women assigned to unopposed estrogen for 3 years developed atypical endometrial hyperplasia, a premalignant lesion, compared with only 1% of women assigned to placebo.[33] Use of a progestin, which opposes the effects of estrogen on the endometrium, eliminates these risks.[34] Neither HERS[35] nor the WHI[2,36] reported an increase in the risk of endometrial cancer when a daily combined regimen was used.

Breast Cancer

An increased risk of breast cancer has been found among current or recent estrogen users in observational studies; this risk is directly related to duration of use. In a meta-analysis

KEY POINT

Recent data from both observational studies and clinical trials suggest that estrogen-progestin therapy may increase risk of breast cancer more rapidly than previously believed.

of 51 case-control and cohort studies (80% of HT use involved estrogen-only preparations), short-term use (<5 years) of postmenopausal HT did not appreciably elevate breast cancer incidence, whereas long-term use (≥ 5 years) was associated with a 35% increase in risk (RR = 1.35, 95% CI 1.21-1.49).[37] In contrast to findings for endometrial cancer, combined estrogen-progestin preparations appear to increase breast cancer risk more than estrogen alone.[37–43] For example, the Million Woman Study recently examined the relationship between HT and breast cancer incidence among 829,000 postmenopausal participants.[43] During 2.6 years of follow-up, current use of unopposed estrogen increased the incidence of invasive breast cancers by almost one third (RR = 1.30, 95% CI 1.21–1.40), and current use of estrogen plus progestin doubled the risk (RR = 2.00, 95% CI 1.88–2.12). These risks steadily rose with increasing duration of use; for current estrogen-only use of less than 1, 1–4, 5–9, and 10 or more years' duration, RRs were 0.81, 1.25, 1.32, and 1.37, respectively. The corresponding estimates for estrogen plus progestin were 1.45, 1.74, 2.17, and 2.31. For conjugated equine estrogen and medroxyprogesterone (i.e., the combination regimen tested in WHI and HERS), the RRs were 1.62 (95% CI 1.34–1.96) for current use of less than 5 years' duration and 2.42 (95% CI 2.08–2.81) for current use of 5 or more years. In the NHS, for each year of use among current HT users, the risk of breast cancer rose by 9% for combination therapy and by 3.3% for estrogen alone.[39]

Randomized trial data confirm that estrogen plus progestin raises breast cancer risk. In the WHI, women assigned to estrogen plus progestin for an average of 5.6 years were 24% more likely to develop invasive breast cancer ($P = 0.003$) or total (i.e., invasive and *in situ*) breast cancer ($p < 0.001$) than women assigned to placebo, with the increased risk evident by the third year of the trial.[44] Invasive breast cancers diagnosed in women allocated to HT were larger (1.7 vs. 1.5 cm, $P = 0.04$), were more likely to be node positive (26% vs. 16%, $p = 0.03$), and were more likely to have spread (25% vs. 16%, $p = 0.04$) than those diagnosed in women allocated to placebo. In addition, the percentage of women with abnormal mammograms was higher in the HT group than in the placebo group (32% vs. 21%, $p < 0.001$). These results suggest that estrogen-progestin therapy induces the development of breast cancer relatively rapidly and at the same time delays detection, perhaps by increasing breast tissue density. In HERS, randomized assignment to estrogen plus progestin was predictive of a 38% increase in breast cancer risk over 4.1 years (RR = 1.38, 95% CI 0.82–1.31). Although this elevation was not statistically significant and was attenuated after an additional 2.7 years of observational follow-up (RR = 1.27, 95% CI 0.84–1.94), the totality of evidence strongly implicates estrogen-progestin therapy in breast carcinogenesis.

In the WHI, estrogen alone did not increase the risk of breast cancer. Indeed, contrary to the preponderance of findings from observational studies, estrogen alone was associated with a borderline reduction in risk of invasive breast cancer (RR = 0.77, 95% CI 0.59–1.01) over the 6.8-year treatment period.[3] Reasons for this unexpected finding are unclear.

Colorectal Cancer

A meta-analysis of 18 observational studies found a 20% reduction (RR = 0.80, 95% CI 0.74–0.86) in risk of colon cancer and a 19% reduction (RR = 0.81, 95% CI 0.72–0.92) in the risk of rectal cancer among postmenopausal women who had ever taken HT compared with those who had never used HT.[45] Much of the apparent reduction in colorectal cancer was limited to current hormone users (RR = 0.66, 95% CI 0.59–0.74), but among such users, longer duration of use did not afford greater protection (duration of use <5 years, RR = 0.61 [95% CI 0.48–0.79]; duration of use ≥ 5 years, RR = 0.67 [95% CI 0.56–0.79]). Because most participants in observational studies used unopposed estrogen, there were insufficient data for a separate analysis of combination regimens.

The two largest prospective investigations included in the meta-analysis were the CPS II and NHS. In the CPS II, a 7-year follow-up of 422,000 postmenopausal women without cancer at baseline, ever versus never use of HT was associated with a 29% reduction in colon cancer mortality (RR = 0.71, 95% CI 0.61–0.83) and rectal cancer mortality (RR = 0.71, 95% CI 0.49–1.04).[46] In the NHS, a 14-year follow-up of 59,000 postmenopausal women without a history of cancer, current use of HT was associated with a decreased risk of colorectal cancer (RR = 0.65, 95% CI 0.50–0.83), after adjustment for potential confounders.[47] The association remained strong even after exclusion of women who had had a screening sigmoidoscopy

(RR = 0.64, 95% CI 0.49–0.82), suggesting that the apparent protection is not due to better screening among HT users. The association between HT and colorectal adenomas, which tend to arise 10–15 years before cancer develops, was also examined. As compared with never users, current users of HT were at decreased risk of large adenoma (>1 cm) (RR = 0.74, 95% CI 0.55–0.99), but there was no association between HT and small adenoma.

In the WHI, women assigned to 6.8 years of estrogen-only therapy did not have a reduced risk of colorectal cancer compared with women assigned to placebo (RR = 1.08, 95% CI 0.75–1.55), although subgroup analyses suggest a beneficial effect among the youngest participants (women aged 50 to 59 years: RR = 0.59, 95% CI 0.25–1.41).[3] On the other hand, women assigned to 5.6 years of estrogen-progestin therapy rather than placebo experienced a large and significant risk reduction (RR = 0.61, 95% CI 0.42–0.87),[48] but the proportion of cancers diagnosed at an advanced stage was unexpectedly higher in the hormone group than in the placebo group. In HERS, assignment to estrogen plus progestin for 4.1 years appeared to protect against the development of colon cancer (RR = 0.69, 95% CI 0.32–1.49), although the association was attenuated after an additional 2.7 years of observational follow-up (RR = 0.81, 95% CI 0.46–1.45).[35]

Biologic data support a possible protective effect of HT on colorectal cancer.[45] Administration of estrogen decreases the secondary production of bile acids, compounds that are believed to initiate or promote malignant change in the colonic epithelium. In addition, the estrogen receptor gene may directly promote development of colonic tumors. Finally, estrogen decreases serum levels of insulin-like growth factor 1, a mitogen that may be associated with colorectal cancer.

Gallbladder Disease

Several large observational studies report a 2- to 3-fold increased risk of gallstones or cholecystectomy among postmenopausal women taking estrogen.[49,50] For example, the NHS found that, as compared with never users, current hormone users had a RR of 2.1 (95% CI 1.9–2.4) for cholecystectomy.[49] This risk increased with increasing duration of use (RR = 2.6 [95% CI 2.0–3.1] for ≥10 years of use) and higher doses of estrogen (RR = 2.4 [95% CI 2.0–2.9] for doses ≥1.25 mg/day). In HERS, women randomized to 4.1 years of estrogen-progestin therapy had a 39% greater risk of biliary tract surgery than those assigned to placebo (RR = 1.39, 95% CI 1.00–1.93),[51] a risk that climbed to 48% after 2.7 additional years of observational follow-up (RR = 1.48, 95% CI 1.12–1.95).[35] At the time of chapter preparation, WHI findings with respect to gallbladder outcomes had not yet been reported.

Cognitive Decline and Dementia

KEY POINT

Data from clinical trials suggest that HT does not prevent the onset of dementia or the progression of cognitive decline.

Meta-analyses of observational studies, most of which utilized a retrospective case-control design, suggest that postmenopausal hormone use is associated with a 30% to 45% decreased risk of Alzheimer's disease (AD), but there is significant heterogeneity in results across individual studies.[52–54] In the recent prospective Cache County Study, which followed 1889 postmenopausal women (mean age, 74.5 years) for 3 years, ever users of HT were less likely than never users to develop AD (RR = 0.59, 95% CI 0.36–0.96).[55] Upon closer examination, however, nearly all of the HT-related risk reduction occurred among former users (RR = 0.33, 95% CI 0.15–0.65). In fact, current users appeared to be at elevated risk of AD unless they had been using HT for more than 10 years. The RRs associated with current HT use of less than 3, 3–10, and more than 10 years' duration were 2.41 (95% CI 0.70–6.34), 2.12 (95% CI 0.83–4.71), and 0.55 (95% CI 0.21–1.23), respectively. A similar pattern of results was observed in a cohort of 9651 women aged 65 years and older without dementia at baseline who were followed for 4–6 years as part of the Study of Osteoporotic Fractures; women who had initiated HT at menopause experienced less cognitive decline than women who had never used HT, but women who started HT later in life did not.[56] It has been suggested that women must initiate HT in early menopause and before the onset of subclinical neuropathologic changes in the brain to derive cognitive benefit. Indeed, several small trials suggest that estrogen therapy is ineffective at slowing cognitive decline in women with established AD.[57–59]

Findings from HERS and WHI suggest an adverse effect of estrogen-progestin therapy on cognitive outcomes. In HERS, 1063 women (mean age, 67 years) with coronary disease completed a battery of standardized cognitive tests after an average treatment interval of 4.2 years.[60] The hormone and placebo groups differed only on a test of verbal fluency, and the difference favored the placebo group. Cognitive function was not assessed at baseline.

The WHI Memory Study followed WHI participants aged 65 years and older without probable dementia at enrollment, including 4532 women in the estrogen-progestin arm and 2947 women in the estrogen-only arm.[61] In analyses that pooled the data across both arms, assignment to active treatment was associated with a 76% increase in the risk of probable dementia (RR = 1.76, 1.19–2.60) and a 25% increase in the risk of mild cognitive impairment (RR = 1.25, 95% CI 0.97–1.89).[61] (In treatment-specific analyses, estrogen-progestin therapy was associated with a doubling of the risk of probable dementia [RR = 2.05, 95% CI 1.21–3.48] but was unrelated to the development of mild cognitive impairment [RR = 1.07, 95% CI 0.74–1.55].[62] Estrogen-only therapy was associated with a trend toward increased risks of both probable dementia [RR = 1.49, 95% CI 0.83–2.66] and mild cognitive impairment [RR = 1.34, 95% CI 0.95–1.89].[61]) AD, which has an insidious onset and a slowly progressive course, was the most common dementia classification, accounting for 52% of the cases in the pooled data. The relatively short follow-up interval during which probable cases were diagnosed suggests that some participants had already experienced cognitive decline at enrollment, and that HT did not initiate the underlying dementia but rather accelerated its progression or manifestation. Nevertheless, when women with low baseline cognitive scores were excluded from analysis, an elevated risk for probable dementia in the hormone group remained (pooled RR = 2.19, 95% CI 1.25–3.84).[61]

Given the significant increase in stroke incidence associated with HT in the larger WHI study population, it is possible that vascular dementia, which tends to have a more abrupt onset than AD, is the outcome responsible for the WHI dementia findings. Although vascular dementia was less often diagnosed than AD in the WHI, standard diagnostic methods favor the latter over the former when both are present. However, the HT-associated elevation in risk of probable dementia was present even among women without previous or incident stroke. Nevertheless, it remains possible that undetected cerebrovascular events could account for the increased dementia risk in the hormone group.

Quality of Life

Compelling evidence, including data from randomized trials such as PEPI,[63] HERS,[64] and the WHI,[65] indicates that estrogen therapy (with or without a progestin) is highly effective for controlling vasomotor, sleep, and some vulvovaginal symptoms.[66,67] However, the impact of HT on other quality-of-life outcomes is less certain. In the WHI, women assigned to estrogen plus progestin experienced no significant improvement in vitality, mental health, depressive symptoms, or sexual satisfaction as compared with those assigned to placebo.[65] In HERS, amelioration of mental health and depressive symptoms in participants assigned to HT was confined to those with vasomotor complaints at baseline.[68] Indeed, women without such complaints experienced HT-associated declines in energy and physical function, perhaps as a result of an increased rate of cardiovascular events. Clinical trials do not indicate a benefit of HT with respect to urinary incontinence.[66,69]

Osteoporosis

By reducing bone turnover and resorption rates, estrogen slows the aging-related bone loss experienced by most postmenopausal women. More than 50 randomized trials have demonstrated that postmenopausal estrogen therapy, with or without a progestin, rapidly increases bone mineral density at the spine by 4–6% and at the hip by 2–3%, and maintains those increases over at least 3 years of treatment.[70] Discontinuation of estrogen therapy leads to a rapid diminution of protection.

The reduction in fracture risk associated with HT use exceeds that expected based on increases in bone density alone. Data from observational studies indicate a 50% lower risk of vertebral fracture and a 25–35% lower risk of hip, wrist, and other peripheral fractures among current estrogen users; addition of a progestin does not appear to modify this benefit.[71–73] In the Study of Osteoporotic Fractures, which followed a population-based cohort of 8816 white women aged 65 years and older at baseline, the adjusted 10-year probability of nonvertebral fracture among current estrogen users who had taken the hormone without interruption since the onset of menopause was 19.6%, similar to that among current users who had not used menopausal hormones continuously (22.4%), but significantly lower than that among past users (29.6%) and never users (30.9%).[73] Probabilities of vertebral fracture over 3.7 years of follow-up were 2.5% among current users who had taken estrogen continuously since menopause and 4.0% among never users. A meta-analysis of 22 randomized trials found that use of HT for 1 year or more significantly reduced the risk of hip and wrist fractures (RR = 0.60, 95% CI 0.40–0.91) and total nonvertebral fracture (RR = 0.73, 95% CI 0.56–0.94); the protective effect was most marked in study populations who were, on average, in early menopause.[74] However, the questionable quality of some of the trials renders these summary statistics less than persuasive. Moreover, the observed effect modification by age was based primarily on the results of only one trial in women who were, on average, well into their menopausal years—HERS, which contributed 80% of the older participants and 80% of the fractures in this age group. In this trial, 5 years of HT (0.625-mg conjugate equine estrogen plus 2.5-mg medroxyprogesterone acetate daily) among a population unselected for osteoporosis was not associated with a reduced fracture risk after 4.1 years of randomized therapy[75] or after an additional 2.7 years of nonrandomized treatment.[35] On the other hand, in the WHI, the same regimen in a similarly unselected population was associated with 33% fewer hip (RR = 0.67, 95% CI 0.47–0.96) and 24% fewer total (RR = 0.76; 95% CI 0.69–0.83) fractures.[76] For estrogen alone, the RRs for hip and total fracture were 0.61 (95% CI 0.41–0.91) and 0.70 (95% CI 0.63–0.79), respectively.[3] These RRs did not significantly differ across age groups. Large randomized trials evaluating the effectiveness of HT in reducing fracture risk in women with osteopenia or osteoporosis are lacking.

Other Disorders

On the basis of limited observational and randomized trial data, it has been hypothesized that HT increases the risk of ovarian cancer,[36,77,78] certain collagen vascular diseases (rheumatoid arthritis and systemic lupus erythematosus),[79–81] and asthma,[82] and reduces the risk of type 2 diabetes mellitus.[83] These hypotheses require confirmation in additional clinical trials.

What's the Evidence?

In summary, although HT ameliorates menopausal symptoms and prevents osteoporotic fractures and possibly colorectal cancer, such benefits may be offset by heightened risks of CHD, stroke, VTE, breast cancer, gallbladder disease, and cognitive dysfunction.

Neither primary nor secondary prevention of CVD should be viewed as an expected benefit of HT, and the possibility of an early increase in risk of vascular events should be considered. The WHI findings suggest that among 10,000 postmenopausal women taking estrogen plus progestin each year, there would be six fewer colorectal cancers and five fewer hip fractures, but also seven more coronary events, eight more strokes, eight more pulmonary emboli, and eight more invasive breast cancers. Overall, the net effect would be 19 additional adverse events per 10,000 women per year.[2] Additionally, there would be 23 excess cases of dementia.[62] Even among women at high risk of osteoporotic fracture, the benefits do not appear to outweigh the risks associated with estrogen-progestin use.[76] Parallel analyses of the estrogen-only data of the WHI also show no evidence of a favorable balance of benefits and risks for such therapy when used for chronic disease prevention among postmenopausal women as a whole.[3] More detailed examinations, including subgroup analyses, of these data are ongoing.

Clinical Guidelines

The publication of results from HERS, WHI, and other trials has led to revisions of clinical guidelines for postmenopausal hormone use. The U.S. Preventive Services Task Force (USPSTF)[84] and the Canadian Task Force on Preventive Health Care[85] recommend against the routine use of estrogen with or without progestin for the prevention of chronic conditions; these are *grade D* recommendations, indicating at least fair evidence that treatment is not effective or that risks outweigh benefits. The U.S. Food and Drug Administration (FDA) has approved new labels for estrogen and estrogen-progestin preparations that warn against the use of these products for CVD protection.[86,87] The labels for estrogen-progestin products additionally highlight the increased risks of MI, stroke, thromboembolic events, and breast cancer found in the WHI. The American Heart Association,[88] the North American Menopause Society,[89,90] and the American College of Obstetricians and Gynecologists[91] also recommend that HT not be used for primary or secondary prevention of CVD.

HT is currently approved by the FDA for the treatment of menopausal symptoms and the prevention of osteoporosis. Physicians should counsel their postmenopausal patients to have realistic expectations about the benefits and risks of HT as well as an appreciation of existing uncertainties in clinical knowledge. Physicians should also emphasize alternative approaches to control menopausal symptoms and prevention of chronic disease, including lifestyle choices such as smoking abstention, adequate physical activity, and a healthy diet. An expanding array of pharmacologic options—including antidepressants, clonidine, or phytoestrogens for vasomotor symptoms; bisphosphonates or selective estrogen receptor modulators for osteoporosis; and lipid-lowering or antihypertensive agents for CVD—should also reduce reliance on HT.[15]

Discussion of Cases

Case 1

Hypothetical study: A new study on postmenopausal hormones is reported. It involves the use of a transdermal estrogen given to 835 women ages 45–55 years who have had a hysterectomy. The investigators report that after 3 years of use, the participants did not have a significant increase in cardiovascular problems, thromboembolism, breast cancer, or dementia. Bone density remained stable, but there were too few fractures to comment on fracture efficacy. The product reduced hot flushes and was well tolerated.

What questions should the clinician be asking after reading this report?

Among the questions that should be asked are the following: Was this study an observational study or a clinical trial? If a trial, was treatment randomly allocated, and was a double-blind design used? What are the characteristics of the study population? Do participants have a low or high baseline risk of developing the outcomes of interest? Is this a study of primary or secondary prevention—e.g., do participants have documented atherosclerotic disease? osteopenia? Do participants have characteristics that might make them more likely to derive benefit or experience harm from HT than other women? Do they have severe menopausal symptoms? How many years from menopause were they at study entry? Are the study participants similar enough to the patients in my clinical practice to permit generalization of study findings to the women that I treat?

Does this study provide evidence that transdermal estrogen is safer than oral estrogen?

This is a small study. One would expect few clinical events of interest in this young, perimenopausal sample during the 3 years of the study. Thus, there will be much statistical uncertainty associated with the RR estimates, and the 95% CI surrounding the risk estimates will be wide. That is, although no clear harm was seen, the study's findings are likely to be consistent with protective, neutral, or harmful effects. Moreover, the trial was not long enough to observe a potential increase in risk of breast cancer. This study does not provide compelling evidence that transdermal estrogen is safer than oral estrogen.

How do these data compare to data from the WHI or observational studies?

The WHI is not examining transdermal estrogen. Because transdermal preparations are less commonly prescribed than oral ones, many observational studies have insufficient data on transdermal estrogen use to permit a separate analysis of such use. Thus, the results of this study are not directly comparable to findings from the WHI or most existing observational studies.

Should oral estrogen users be switched to this product?

Higher levels of endogenous estrogen in women may be partly responsible for their lower age-specific CHD rates as compared with men. Such estrogen enters the bloodstream directly, without initially being metabolized by the liver. Because transdermal administration allows exogenous hormones to enter the bloodstream without early hepatic processing, it has been hypothesized that estrogen patches may be safer than pills in terms of thromboembolic and cardiovascular sequelae. However, data from large clinical trials in a variety of patient populations are needed to draw definitive conclusions about the relative efficacy and safety of oral and transdermal estrogen. On the basis of findings from one small study, oral estrogen users should not be switched to this transdermal product.

References

1 Hersh AL, Stefanick ML, Stafford RS. National use of postmenopausal hormone therapy: annual trends and response to recent evidence. *JAMA*. 2004;291:47–53.

2 Writing Group for the Women's Health Initiative Investigators. Risks and benefits of estrogen plus progestin in healthy postmenopausal women: principal results from the Women's Health Initiative randomized controlled trial. *JAMA*. 2002;288:321–333.

3 The Women's Health Initiative Steering Committee. Effects of conjugated equine estrogen in postmenopausal women with hysterectomy: the Women's Health Initiative randomized controlled trial. *JAMA*. 2004;291:1701–1712.

4 Grodstein F, Stampfer M. The epidemiology of postmenopausal hormone therapy and cardiovascular disease. In: Goldhaber SZ, Ridker PM, eds. *Thrombosis and Thromboembolism*. New York: Marcel Dekker; 2002:67–78.

5 Grodstein F, Manson JE, Colditz GA, et al. A prospective, observational study of postmenopausal hormone therapy and primary prevention of cardiovascular disease. *Ann Intern Med*. 2000;133:933–941.

6 Grodstein F, Manson JE, Stampfer MJ. Postmenopausal hormone use and secondary prevention of coronary events in the Nurses'

Health Study. A prospective, observational study. *Ann Intern Med.* 2001;135:1–8.

7 Chae CU, Manson JE. Postmenopausal hormone therapy. In: Manson JE, Buring JE, Ridker PM, Gaziano JM, eds. *Clinical Trials in Heart Disease.* Philadelphia, PA: W.B. Saunders; 2004:349–363.

8 Hulley S, Grady D, Bush T, et al. Randomized trial of estrogen plus progestin for secondary prevention of coronary heart disease in postmenopausal women. Heart and Estrogen/progestin Replacement Study (HERS) Research Group. *JAMA.* 1998;280:605–613.

9 Grady D, Herrington D, Bittner V, et al. Cardiovascular disease outcomes during 6.8 years of hormone therapy: Heart and Estrogen/progestin Replacement Study follow-up (HERS II). *JAMA.* 2002;288:49–57.

10 Herrington DM, Reboussin DM, Brosnihan KB, et al. Effects of estrogen replacement on the progression of coronary-artery atherosclerosis. *N Engl J Med.* 2000;343:522–529.

11 Clarke SC, Kelleher J, Lloyd-Jones H, et al. A study of hormone replacement therapy in postmenopausal women with ischaemic heart disease: the Papworth HRT atherosclerosis study. *BJOG.* 2002;109:1056–1062.

12 Waters DD, Alderman EL, Hsia J, et al. Effects of hormone replacement therapy and antioxidant vitamin supplements on coronary atherosclerosis in postmenopausal women: a randomized controlled trial. *JAMA.* 2002;288:2432–2440.

13 ESPRIT team. Oestrogen therapy for prevention of reinfarction in postmenopausal women: a randomised placebo controlled trial. *Lancet.* 2002;360:2001–2008.

14 Manson JE, Martin KA. Clinical practice. Postmenopausal hormone-replacement therapy. *N Engl J Med.* 2001;345:34–40.

15 Manson JE, Bassuk SS. The perimenopause transition and postmenopausal hormone therapy. In: Kasper DL, Braunwald E, Fauci AS, Hauser SL, Longo DL, Jameson JL, eds. *Harrison's Principles of Internal Medicine.* 16th ed. New York: McGraw-Hill; 2004: pp. 2209–2213.

16 Manson JE, Hsia J, Johnson KC, et al. Estrogen plus progestin and the risk of coronary heart disease. *N Engl J Med.* 2003;349:523–534.

17 Hemminki E, McPherson K. Impact of postmenopausal hormone therapy on cardiovascular events and cancer: pooled data from clinical trials. *BMJ.* 1997;315:149–153.

18 Grodstein F, Clarkson TB, Manson JE. Understanding the divergent data on postmenopausal hormone therapy. *N Engl J Med.* 2003;348: 645–650.

19 Michels KB, Manson JE. Postmenopausal hormone therapy: a reversal of fortune. *Circulation.* 2003;107:1830–1833.

20 Heckbert SR, Kaplan RC, Weiss NS, et al. Risk of recurrent coronary events in relation to use and recent initiation of postmenopausal hormone therapy. *Arch Intern Med.* 2001;161:1709–1713.

21 Rodriguez C, Calle EE, Patel AV, et al. Effect of body mass on the association between estrogen replacement therapy and mortality among elderly US women. *Am J Epidemiol.* 2001;153:145–152.

22 Mikkola TS, Clarkson TB. Estrogen replacement therapy, atherosclerosis, and vascular function. *Cardiovasc Res.* 2002;53: 605–619.

23 Shlipak MG, Simon JA, Vittinghoff E, et al. Estrogen and progestin, lipoprotein(a), and the risk of recurrent coronary heart disease events after menopause. *JAMA.* 2000;283:1845–1852.

24 Herrington DM, Howard TD, Hawkins GA, et al. Estrogen-receptor polymorphisms and effects of estrogen replacement on high-density lipoprotein cholesterol in women with coronary disease. *N Engl J Med.* 2002;346:967–974.

25 Psaty BM, Smith NL, Lemaitre RN, et al. Hormone replacement therapy, prothrombotic mutations, and the risk of incident nonfatal myocardial infarction in postmenopausal women. *JAMA.* 2001;285: 906–913.

26 Lemaitre RN, Heckbert SR, Psaty BM, et al. Hormone replacement therapy and associated risk of stroke in postmenopausal women. *Arch Intern Med.* 2002;162:1954–1960.

27 Wassertheil-Smoller S, Hendrix SL, Limacher M, et al. Effect of estrogen plus progestin on stroke in postmenopausal women: the Women's Health Initiative: a randomized trial. *JAMA.* 2003;289:2673–2684.

28 Simon JA, Hsia J, Cauley JA, et al. Postmenopausal hormone therapy and risk of stroke: The Heart and Estrogen-progestin Replacement Study (HERS). *Circulation.* 2001;103:638–642.

29 Viscoli CM, Brass LM, Kernan WN, et al. A clinical trial of estrogen-replacement therapy after ischemic stroke. *N Engl J Med.* 2001;345: 1243–1249.

30 Miller J, Chan BK, Nelson HD. Postmenopausal estrogen replacement and risk for venous thromboembolism: a systematic review and meta-analysis for the U.S. Preventive Services Task Force. *Ann Intern Med.* 2002;136:680–690.

31 Grodstein F, Stampfer MJ, Goldhaber SZ, et al. Prospective study of exogenous hormones and risk of pulmonary embolism in women. *Lancet.* 1996;348:983–987.

32 Grady D, Wenger NK, Herrington D, et al. Postmenopausal hormone therapy increases risk for venous thromboembolic disease. The Heart and Estrogen/progestin Replacement Study. *Ann Intern Med.* 2000; 132:689–696.

33 Writing Group for the PEPI Trial. Effects of estrogen or estrogen/progestin regimens on heart disease risk factors in postmenopausal women. The Postmenopausal Estrogen/Progestin Interventions (PEPI) Trial. *JAMA.* 1995;273:199–208.

34 Grady D, Gebretsadik T, Kerlikowske K, et al. Hormone replacement therapy and endometrial cancer risk: a meta-analysis. *Obstet Gynecol.* 1995;85:304–313.

35 Hulley S, Furberg C, Barrett-Connor E, et al. Noncardiovascular disease outcomes during 6.8 years of hormone therapy: Heart and Estrogen/progestin Replacement Study follow-up (HERS II). *JAMA.* 2002;288:58–66.

36 Anderson GL, Judd HL, Kaunitz AM, et al. Effects of estrogen plus progestin on gynecologic cancers and associated diagnostic procedures: the Women's Health Initiative randomized trial. *JAMA.* 2003;290:1739–1748.

37 Collaborative Group on Hormonal Factors in Breast Cancer. Breast cancer and hormone replacement therapy: collaborative reanalysis of data from 51 epidemiological studies of 52,705 women with breast cancer and 108,411 women without breast cancer. *Lancet.* 1997;350: 1047–1059.

38 Persson I, Weiderpass E, Bergkvist L, et al. Risks of breast and endometrial cancer after estrogen and estrogen-progestin replacement. *Cancer Causes Control.* 1999;10:253–260.

39 Colditz GA, Rosner B, for the Nurses' Health Study Research Group. Use of estrogen plus progestin is associated with greater increase in breast cancer risk than estrogen alone. *Am J Epidemiol.* 1998; 147(Suppl.):64S.

40 Schairer C, Lubin J, Troisi R, et al. Menopausal estrogen and estrogen-progestin replacement therapy and breast cancer risk. *JAMA.* 2000;283:485–491.

41 Porch JV, Lee IM, Cook NR, et al. Estrogen-progestin replacement therapy and breast cancer risk: the Women's Health Study (United States). *Cancer Causes Control.* 2002;13:847–854.

42 Li CI, Malone KE, Porter PL, et al. Relationship between long durations and different regimens of hormone therapy and risk of breast cancer. *JAMA.* 2003;289:3254–3263.

43 Million Women Study Collaborators. Breast cancer and hormone-replacement therapy in the Million Women Study. *Lancet.* 2003;362: 419–427.

44 Chlebowski RT, Hendrix SL, Langer RD, et al. Influence of estrogen plus progestin on breast cancer and mammography in healthy postmenopausal women: the Women's Health Initiative Randomized Trial. *JAMA.* 2003;289:3243–3253.

45 Grodstein F, Newcomb PA, Stampfer MJ. Postmenopausal hormone therapy and the risk of colorectal cancer: a review and meta-analysis. *Am J Med.* 1999;106:574–582.

46 Calle EE, Miracle-McMahill HL, Thun MJ, et al. Estrogen replacement therapy and risk of fatal colon cancer in a prospective cohort of postmenopausal women. *J Natl Cancer Inst.* 1995;87:517–523.

47 Grodstein F, Martinez ME, Platz EA, et al. Postmenopausal hormone use and risk for colorectal cancer and adenoma. *Ann Intern Med.* 1998;128:705–712.

48 Chlebowski RT, Wactawski-Wende J, Ritenbaugh C, et al. Estrogen plus progestin and colorectal cancer in postmenopausal women. *N Engl J Med.* 2004;350:991–1004.

49 Grodstein F, Colditz GA, Stampfer MJ. Postmenopausal hormone use and cholecystectomy in a large prospective study. *Obstet Gynecol.* 1994;83:5–11.

50 Mamdani MM, Tu K, van Walraven C, et al. Postmenopausal estrogen replacement therapy and increased rates of cholecystectomy and appendectomy. *CMAJ.* 2000;162:1421–1424.

51 Simon JA, Hunninghake DB, Agarwal SK, et al. Effect of estrogen plus progestin on risk for biliary tract surgery in postmenopausal women with coronary artery disease. The Heart and Estrogen/progestin Replacement Study. *Ann Intern Med.* 2001;135:493–501.

52 Hogervorst E, Williams J, Budge M, et al. The nature of the effect of female gonadal hormone replacement therapy on cognitive function in post-menopausal women: a meta-analysis. *Neuroscience.* 2000; 101:485–512.

53 LeBlanc ES, Janowsky J, Chan BK, et al. Hormone replacement therapy and cognition: systematic review and meta-analysis. *JAMA.* 2001;285:1489–1499.

54 Nelson HD, Humphrey LL, Nygren P, et al. Postmenopausal hormone replacement therapy: scientific review. *JAMA.* 2002;288: 872–881.

55 Zandi PP, Carlson MC, Plassman BL, et al. Hormone replacement therapy and incidence of Alzheimer disease in older women: the Cache County Study. *JAMA.* 2002;288:2123–2129.

56 Matthews K, Cauley J, Yaffe K, et al. Estrogen replacement therapy and cognitive decline in older community women. *J Am Geriatr Soc.* 1999;47:518–523.

57 Henderson VW, Paganini-Hill A, Miller BL, et al. Estrogen for Alzheimer's disease in women: randomized, double-blind, placebo-controlled trial. *Neurology.* 2000;54:295–301.

58 Mulnard RA, Cotman CW, Kawas C, et al. Estrogen replacement therapy for treatment of mild to moderate Alzheimer disease: a randomized controlled trial. Alzheimer's Disease Cooperative Study. *JAMA.* 2000;283:1007–1015.

59 Wang PN, Liao SQ, Liu RS, et al. Effects of estrogen on cognition, mood, and cerebral blood flow in AD: a controlled study. *Neurology.* 2000;54:2061–2066.

60 Grady D, Yaffe K, Kristof M, et al. Effect of postmenopausal hormone therapy on cognitive function: the Heart and Estrogen/progestin Replacement Study. *Am J Med.* 2002;113:543–548.

61 Shumaker SA, Legault C, Kuller L, et al. Conjugated equine estrogens and incidence of probable dementia and mild cognitive impairment in postmenopausal women: Women's Health Initiative Memory Study. *JAMA.* 2004;291:2947–2958.

62 Shumaker SA, Legault C, Thal L, et al. Estrogen plus progestin and the incidence of dementia and mild cognitive impairment in postmenopausal women: the Women's Health Initiative Memory Study: a randomized controlled trial. *JAMA.* 2003;289:2651–2662.

63 Greendale GA, Reboussin BA, Hogan P, et al. Symptom relief and side effects of postmenopausal hormones: results from the Postmenopausal Estrogen/Progestin Interventions Trial. *Obstet Gynecol.* 1998;92: 982–988.

64 Barnabei VM, Grady D, Stovall DW, et al. Menopausal symptoms in older women and the effects of treatment with hormone therapy. *Obstet Gynecol.* 2002;100:1209–1218.

65 Hays J, Ockene JK, Brunner RL, et al. Effects of estrogen plus progestin on health-related quality of life. *N Engl J Med.* 2003;348: 1839–1854.

66 Barrett-Connor E, Hendrix S, Ettinger B. Best Clinical Practices: Chapter 13 from the International Position Paper on Women's Health and Menopause: A Comprehensive Approach: National Heart Lung and Blood Institute, National Institutes of Health Office of Research on Women's Health, Giovanni Lorenzini Medical Science Foundation; 2002:5–32.

67 MacLennan A, Lester S, Moore V. Oral estrogen replacement therapy versus placebo for hot flushes: a systematic review. *Climacteric.* 2001;4:58–74.

68 Hlatky MA, Boothroyd D, Vittinghoff E, et al. Quality-of-life and depressive symptoms in postmenopausal women after receiving hormone therapy: results from the Heart and Estrogen/Progestin Replacement Study (HERS) trial. *JAMA.* 2002;287:591–597.

69 Grady D, Brown JS, Vittinghoff E, et al. Postmenopausal hormones and incontinence: the Heart and Estrogen/progestin Replacement Study. *Obstet Gynecol.* 2001;97:116–120.

70 North American Menopause Society. Management of postmenopausal osteoporosis: position statement of the North American Menopause Society. *Menopause.* 2002;9:84–101.

71 Grady D, Rubin SM, Petitti DB, et al. Hormone therapy to prevent disease and prolong life in postmenopausal women. *Ann Intern Med.* 1992;117:1016–1037.

72 Barrett-Connor E. Hormone replacement therapy. *BMJ.* 1998;317: 457–61.

73 Nelson HD, Rizzo J, Harris E, et al. Osteoporosis and fractures in postmenopausal women using estrogen. *Arch Intern Med.* 2002;162: 2278–2284.

74 Torgerson DJ, Bell-Syer SE. Hormone replacement therapy and prevention of nonvertebral fractures: a meta-analysis of randomized trials. *JAMA.* 2001;285:2891–2897.

75 Cauley JA, Black DM, Barrett-Connor E, et al. Effects of hormone replacement therapy on clinical fractures and height loss: The Heart and Estrogen/progestin Replacement Study (HERS). *Am J Med.* 2001;110:442–450.

76 Cauley JA, Robbins J, Chen Z, et al. Effects of estrogen plus progestin on risk of fracture and bone mineral density: the Women's Health Initiative randomized trial. *JAMA.* 2003;290:1729–1738.

77 Lacey JV Jr, Mink PJ, Lubin JH, et al. Menopausal hormone replacement therapy and risk of ovarian cancer. *JAMA.* 2002;288:334–341.

78 Rodriguez C, Patel AV, Calle EE, et al. Estrogen replacement therapy and ovarian cancer mortality in a large prospective study of US women. *JAMA.* 2001;285:1460–1465.

79 Sanchez-Guerrero J, Liang MH, Karlson EW, et al. Postmenopausal estrogen therapy and the risk for developing systemic lupus erythematosus. *Ann Intern Med.* 1995;122:430–433.

80 Meier CR, Sturkenboom MC, Cohen AS, et al. Postmenopausal estrogen replacement therapy and the risk of developing systemic lupus erythematosus or discoid lupus. *J Rheumatol.* 1998;25:1515–1519.

81 Barrett-Connor E. Postmenopausal estrogen therapy and selected (less-often-considered) disease outcomes. *Menopause.* 1999;6:14–20.

82 Troisi RJ, Speizer FE, Willett WC, et al. Menopause, postmenopausal estrogen preparations, and the risk of adult-onset asthma. A prospective cohort study. *Am J Respir Crit Care Med.* 1995;152:1183–1188.

83 Kanaya AM, Herrington D, Vittinghoff E, et al. Glycemic effects of postmenopausal hormone therapy: the Heart and Estrogen/progestin Replacement Study. A randomized, double-blind, placebo-controlled trial. *Ann Intern Med.* 2003;138:1–9.

84 US Preventive Services Task Force. Hormone therapy for the prevention of chronic conditions in postmenopausal women: recommendations from the U.S. Preventive Services Task Force. *Ann Intern Med.* 2005;142:855–860.

85 Wathen CN, Feig DS, Feightner JW, et al. Hormone replacement therapy for the primary prevention of chronic diseases: recommendation statement from the Canadian Task Force on Preventive Health Care. CMAJ 2004;170:1535–1537.

86 U.S. Food and Drug Administration. FDA Approves New Labels for Estrogen and Estrogen with Progestin Therapies for Postmenopausal

Women Following Review of Women's Health Initiative Data. Available at http://www.fda.gov/cder/drug/infopage/estrogens_progestins/default.htm Accessed July 8, 2004.

87 U.S. Food and Drug Administration. FDA plans to evaluate results of Women's Health Initiative study for estrogen-alone therapy. FDA Talk Paper, March 2, 2004. Available at http://www.fda.gov/bbs/topics/ANSWERS/2004/ANS01281.html Accessed July 8, 2004.

88 American Heart Association. Postmenopausal hormone therapy and cardiovascular disease in women. Available at http://americanheart.org/presenter.jhtml?identifier=4536. Accessed July 8, 2004.

89 North American Menopause Society. NAMS Hormone Therapy Position Statement, Sept 2003. Available at www.menopause.org. Accessed July 8, 2004.

90 North American Menopause Society. The North American Menopause Society responds to published results from the estrogen-only arm of the Women's Health Initiative study. Press release, April 14, 2004. Available at http://www.menopause.org/NR/rdonlyres/BA830BD3-018F-4806-BC83-2EAA0002CE53/0/PR04_0414JAMAETarmWHINew.pdf. Accessed July 8, 2004.

91 American College of Obstetricians and Gynecologists. *Guidelines for Women's Health Care*. Washington, DC: American College of Obstetricians and Gynecologists;2002:130–133, 171–176, 314–318.

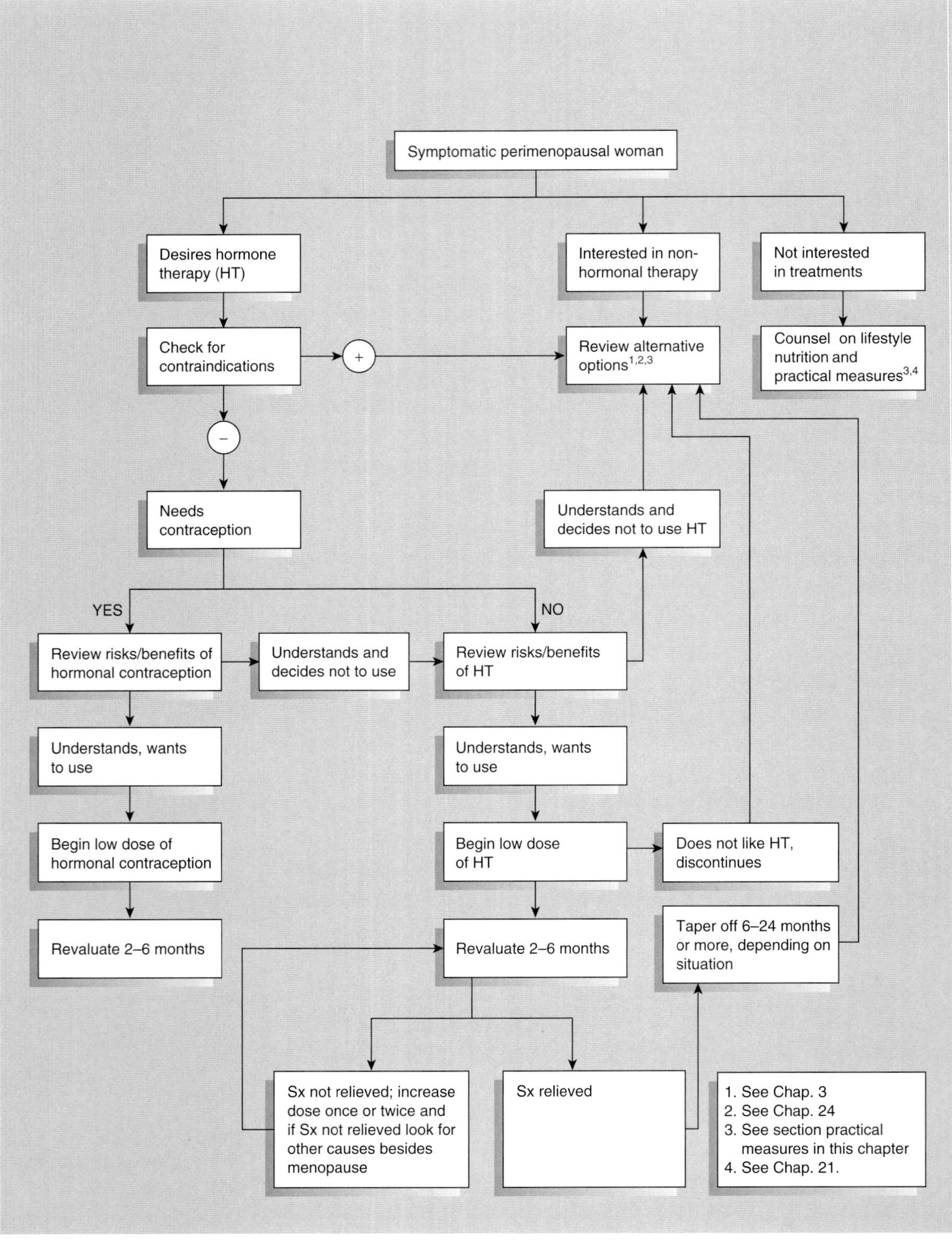

Symptomatic perimenopausal woman
Desires hormone therapy (HT)
Interested in non-hormonal therapy
Not interested in treatments
Check for contraindications
+
Review alternative options[1,2,3]
Counsel on lifestyle nutrition and practical measures[3,4]
−
Needs contraception
Understands and decides not to use HT
YES
NO
Review risks/benefits of hormonal contraception
Understands and decides not to use
Review risks/benefits of HT
Understands, wants to use
Understands, wants to use
Begin low dose of hormonal contraception
Begin low dose of HT
Does not like HT, discontinues
Revaluate 2–6 months
Revaluate 2–6 months
Taper off 6–24 months or more, depending on situation
Sx not relieved; increase dose once or twice and if Sx not relieved look for other causes besides menopause
Sx relieved
1. See Chap. 3
2. See Chap. 24
3. See section practical measures in this chapter
4. See Chap. 21.

20 Hormone Therapy: When and How?

Margery L. S. Gass

Historical Perspective

KEY POINT

HT has been used with varying levels of enthusiasm over the past 100 years.

The concept of hormone therapy (HT) has been discussed in medical circles for more than a century. The Landau Clinic in Berlin began using ovarian extracts as early as 1896. Hormone preparations with the biological activity of estrogen obtained from organs and from animal urinary sources were available to practitioners in the early 1900s.[1]

The synthesis in 1938 of diethylstilbestrol (DES), a nonsteroidal estrogen, and the introduction to the market of natural conjugated equine estrogens in 1942, provided highly effective female HT that could be made available on a widespread basis. The intervening history of HT has been a saga of dramatic upward and downward swings in popularity. In the 1980s and 1990s there was a steady growth in the number of postmenopausal HT prescriptions (Fig. 20-1).

KEY POINT

Observational data suggested that HT would have a wide range of health benefits for postmenopausal women.

A few randomized controlled trials along with observational data from many sources led clinicians to believe that HT would be good preventive therapy for many health problems associated with aging: cardiovascular disease (CVD) (see Chaps. 14 and 19), osteoporosis (see Chap. 23), decline in cognitive function (see Chap. 4), dementia, ostoarthritis, macular degeneration, tooth loss, pelvic relaxation, and urinary tract infection.[2–7] It was in this atmosphere of optimism regarding the presumed benefits of HT that the large randomized controlled trial known as the Women's Health Initiative (WHI) was conceptualized in 1991.

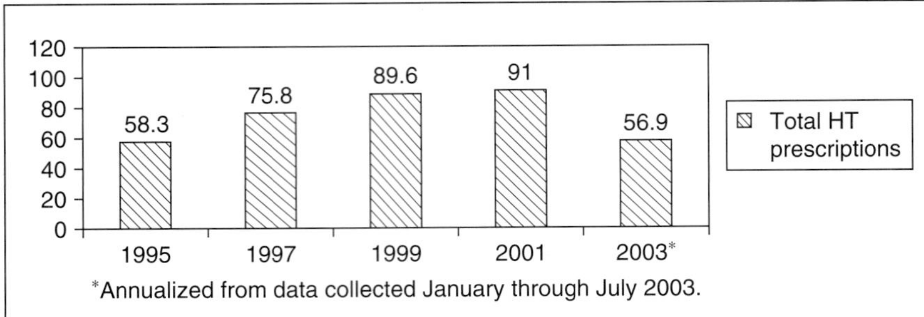

Figure 20-1: Number of hormone therapy prescriptions in millions. (Adapted from Hersh AL, Stefanick ML, Stafford. RS. National use of postmenopausal hormone therapy. *JAMA*. 2004;291:47–53.)

The Women's Health Initiative

The greatest impact on HT use in recent years (Fig. 20-1) resulted from the publication of results from the WHI in 2002.[8] The objective of the WHI was to evaluate the effectiveness of three different interventions in reducing some of the common chronic conditions associated with aging such as CVD, osteoporosis, and breast and colorectal cancer. The interventions were (1) HT, (2) low-fat diet, and (3) calcium plus vitamin D supplementation.

During the approximate 10-year course of the WHI, other randomized controlled hormone trials were completed. The Postmenopausal Estrogen/Progestin Interventions (PEPI) study reported that estrogen plus progestogen had a favorable effect on the lipid profile.[9] The Heart and Estrogen/progestin Replacement study (HERS) and HERS II publications concerning the effect of HT on preexisting CVD indicated that there was no apparent benefit of estrogen plus progestogen on secondary prevention of CVD.[10,11]

Although designed to run until 2005, the estrogen plus progestin intervention of the WHI study was stopped in July 2002 because the data and safety monitoring board noted an increased risk of invasive breast cancer. Additionally, there was lack of evidence for a cardiovascular benefit, as well as lack of overall benefit in the global risk index. The estrogen-alone arm (30% smaller in number) was allowed to continue until March 2004 when the National Institutes of Health requested that the women in the estrogen-alone arm stop their study drug because of an elevated risk of stroke and no evidence of a cardiovascular benefit. The remaining low fat diet arm and calcium-vitamin D arm of the study were stopped in 2005 as scheduled. A 5-year extension of the study was approved to follow the entire WHI cohort until 2010.

The principal results of the estrogen plus progestin arm of the WHI as reported in 2002 indicated a small increase in the risks of invasive breast cancer, coronary heart disease, stroke, deep vein thrombosis, and pulmonary embolus. There was a small reduction in the risks of colorectal cancer and osteoporotic fractures.[8] On the basis of these findings, the authors concluded that estrogen plus progestin should not be used for the primary prevention of chronic diseases.

KEY POINT

THE WHI has quantified risks and benefits of HT.

Principal results from the estrogen arm of the WHI were similar to those of the estrogen plus progestin arm of the study with regard to a decreased risk of fracture and an increased risk of stroke and deep vein thrombosis. Estrogen use, however, showed no statistically significant difference when compared to placebo treatment with regard to CHD, breast or colorectal cancer.[12]

In response to the WHI findings, major medical organizations have recommended limiting the use of HT primarily to the treatment of menopausal symptoms using the lowest effective dose for the shortest amount of time.[13–16]

WHI *and Clinical* Practice

KEY POINT

The challenge for clinicians lies in extrapolating findings from a disease prevention study conducted with older women to a setting involving younger, symptomatic women.

The challenge for clinicians lies in translating the findings from the preventive care setting used in the WHI to the treatment setting that involves a symptomatic menopausal patient. The principal reason women initiate HT at menopausal is to alleviate troublesome menopausal symptoms. Treatment of menopausal symptoms was not a primary focus of the WHI design. The efficacy of HT for treating menopausal symptoms was already well established through randomized controlled trials. The WHI was designed to determine if HT should be offered to the majority of postmenopausal women as a preventive care measure to keep women healthier as they age.

Incorporating the WHI preventive care findings into the setting of treating menopausal symptoms requires the clinician to extrapolate the data to the individual patient's situation. That task is best accomplished by starting with the woman's chief complaint: What concerns the patient? Is she symptomatic? Is she requesting treatment? If she is not symptomatic, it is unlikely she should consider HT (see Discussion of Cases). The asymptomatic menopausal woman would be best served by a discussion of healthy lifestyle.

KEY POINT

An estimated 10–15% of women experience severe symptoms at menopause.

For some women, perimenopause and menopause come and go smoothly with no disruption of their everyday life (15–20% of women do not have hot flushes). However, not all women experience an easy exit from their reproductive years. The clinical significance of perimenopause lies in the disruption of a menstrual pattern and quality of life that had become familiar to a woman during the preceding several decades. Significant changes in menstrual frequency, the amount and duration of menstrual blood flow, dysmenorrhea, mastalgia, duration of premenstrual-type syndrome, migraine exacerbation, hot flushes, and sleep disruption can all be part of the perimenopause experience. The intensity of the symptoms varies from nonexistent to disabling. An estimated 10–15% of women experience severe symptoms at menopause.[17] The duration of the symptoms is also variable and cannot be predicted accurately. Perimenopause, as currently defined, encompasses the most symptomatic years of the entire process.

With the arrival of the final menstrual cycle, hot flushes, night sweats (hot flushes occurring at night), and vaginal dryness become more pronounced. This particular constellation of symptoms extends beyond the time frame of the earlier changes. The severity of the symptoms as well as the woman's personal response to them will both play a role in determining the need for intervention.

KEY POINT

Women often have a preconceived preference regarding treatment of their menopausal symptoms.

The symptomatic menopausal woman has often made a decision about therapy prior to her office visit. She may indicate that her symptoms are manageable. In that scenario, the healthy lifestyle discussion applies, as well as a discussion of practical measures for reducing symptoms (see Practical Measures). The woman who does want treatment may already know whether she prefers HT, nonhormonal prescription therapy, or nonprescription alternative therapies. The role of the clinician at this juncture is to review the reasons behind her choice and to ascertain that the woman has the most recent and the most accurate information on these options (see Chaps. 3 and 24).

For the woman interested in HT, the first step is to determine if she has any contraindications to using hormones. Commonly accepted contraindications include history of venous thrombosis, breast cancer, uncontrolled hypertension, active liver disease, and a recent addition to the list, CVD. Relative contraindications include history of endometriosis, leiomyomata, and hypertriglyceridemia. Hypertension and lipid abnormalities corrected by treatment would not necessarily constitute a contraindication. In general, doses of HT are thought to be low enough that they will not stimulate endometriosis or leiomyomata. Close monitoring of the patient's condition is advisable in these circumstances.

Discussion of Risks and Benefits of HT

Once a woman has been cleared of contraindications, it is important to discuss the current understanding of the risks and benefits associated with hormone use. Generalizing findings from research studies is an imperfect process, but it remains the best option for evidence-based medicine. A summary of the risks and benefits of continuous combined estrogen plus progestin therapy can be seen in Fig. 20-2. The figure illustrates several ways to discuss risks with patients. They can be discussed as the increase or decrease in the number of cases per 10,000 women per year. The original WHI

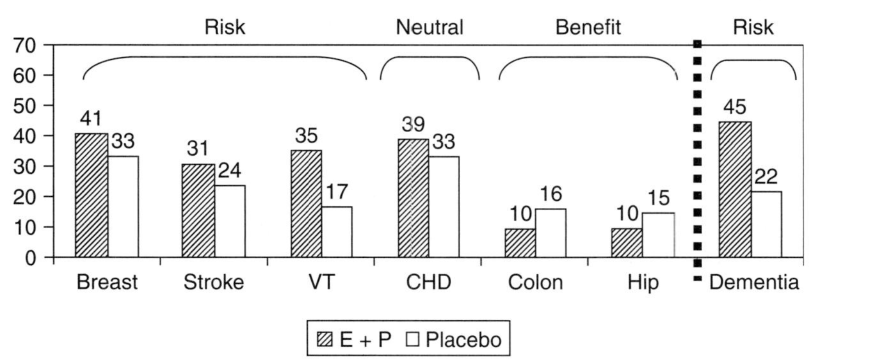

Figure 20-2: Number of adverse events per 10,000 women per year. E + P, estrogen plus progestin; breast, invasive breast cancer; VT, venous thrombosis; CHD, coronary heart disease; colon, colon cancer; hip, hip fracture; dementia, probable dementia over age 65. See references 23, 21, 20, 22, 8, and 18.

report in 2002 indicated there would be 19 excess adverse events per 10,000 women per year or approximately 2 per 1000 women using estrogen plus progestin per year.[8] The figure of 2 per 1000 per year may be more meaningful to many women. The 2002 report presented figures based on the entire estrogen plus progestin cohort of women aged 50–79 at baseline. It did not include the risk of cognitive decline and the twofold increased risk of dementia in the older half of the cohort that were published later.[18,19]

One option in applying WHI findings to symptomatic menopausal women is to use the data from the 50–59-year-old cohort of the study. Some of the hazard ratios for the various outcomes changed across age groups in the WHI; however, the background incidence of the risks under consideration is notably lower in younger women (Table 20-1).

The majority of outcomes studied in the WHI are medical conditions that increase in prevalence with age. Thus, even if hazard ratios are similar across age groups producing a similar *relative* increase in cases, the *absolute* number of cases will be smaller in the younger age range. Given the average age of menopause is 51, it is reasonable to use the absolute number of cases from the youngest cohort of WHI participants for the discussion of HT risks with perimenopausal patients. Table 20-2 reveals that there

Table 20-1. **INCIDENCE OF VARIOUS CONDITIONS BY AGE GROUP AMONG PLACEBO USERS ENROLLED THE EPT OR ET TRIALS IN THE WOMEN'S HEALTH INITIATIVE**

Age Range at Baseline	*Venous Thrombosis*		*Stroke*		*Coronary Heart Disease*		*Invasive Breast Cancer*	
	EPT*	ET†	EPT‡	ET†	EPT§	ET†	EPT¶	ET†
50–59	0.08	0.13	0.10	0.16	0.17	0.24	0.26	0.29
60–69	0.19	0.23	0.23	0.30	0.34	0.59	0.36	0.36
70–79	0.27	0.28	0.48	0.57	0.55	0.84	0.41	0.34

Abbreviations: EPT, combined estrogen and progestogen therapy; ET, estrogen therapy.

*See Ref. 20.

†See Ref. 12.

‡See Ref. 21

§See Ref. 22

¶See Ref. 23

Table 20-2. **HAZARD RATIOS AND ANNUALIZED RATES OF ADVERSE EVENTS FOR ESTROGEN PLUS PROGESTIN USERS AND ESTROGEN ALONE USERS AGES 50-59 IN THE WOMEN'S HEALTH INITIATIVE.**

	Venous Thrombosis		*Stroke*		*Coronary Heart Disease*		*Invasive Breast Cancer*	
	EPT*	**ET†**	**EPT‡**	**ET†**	**EPT§**	**ET†**	**EPT¶**	**ET†**
Hazard ratio	2.27	1.22	1.46	1.08	1.27	0.56	1.20	0.72
95% CI	1.19–4.33	0.62–2.42	0.77–2.79	0.57–2.04	NA	0.30–1.03	0.80–1.82	0.43–1.21
Annualized % in placebo group	0.08	0.13	0.10	0.16	0.17	0.24	0.26	0.29
Number in placebo group per 10,000	8	13	10	16	17	24	26	29
Number in hormone group per 10,000	19	15	14	16	22	14	31.2	21
Excess (decrease) number per 10,000	11	2	4	0	5	(10)	5.2	(8)

*See Ref. 20.

†See Ref. 12.

‡ See Ref. 21

§See Ref. 22

¶See Ref. 23

is less than 1 excess adverse event per 1000 women per year in each chronic disease category except EPT thrombosis.

For the woman without uterus who is considering using estrogen alone, the risks appear to be fewer (Fig. 20-3). The only significantly elevated risks associated with use of estrogen were stroke (HR 1.39) and deep vein thrombosis (HR 1.47).[12] It is important to point out that the cohort of women in the estrogen arm and the cohort of women in the estrogen-progestin arm had different baseline characteristics. All of the women in the estrogen arm had undergone hysterectomy and 40% had undergone bilateral salpingo-oophorectomy. As a group they weighed more, had higher blood pressure, higher cholesterol, and more cases of diabetes mellitus. They had less income, less education, and were less active. There was a higher representation of other ethnic groups in the estrogen arm. The placebo users in the estrogen arm had higher rates of stroke, venous thrombosis, and cardiovascular events than the estrogen-progestin group (Table 20-1).

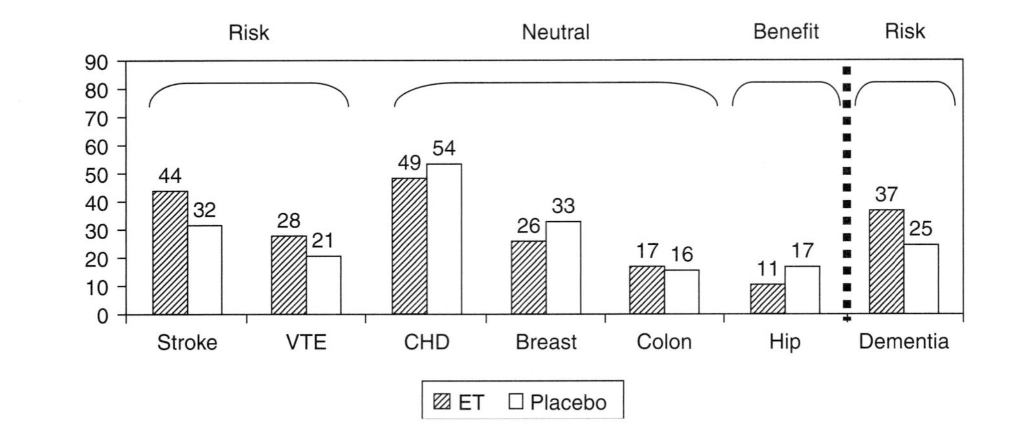

Figure 20-3: Number of adverse events per 10,000 women on estrogen therapy per year. ET, conjugated equine estrogens; VTE, venous thromboembolism; CHD, coronary heart disease; breast, invasive breast cancer; colon, colon cancer; hip, hip fracture; dementia, probable dementia over age 65. See references 12 and 24.

The dementia study, known as the Women's Health Initiative Memory Study or WHIMS, was designed as an ancillary study to the WHI. Only women 65 and older were enrolled because dementia is more common in the older age group. Neither EPT nor ET reduced the incidence of dementia, and the combined analysis produced a statistically significant hazard ratio of 1.76 for dementia with use of either ET or EPT.[18,24] The fact that the occurrence of dementia is rare in women in their early fifties should be reassuring to the perimenopausal woman concerned about dementia yet interested in HT. Nonetheless, the increase in dementia among HT users 65 and older should be mentioned to women considering HT, even though it is not possible to tell them with the current data precisely how that risk applies to women at age 50.

A thorough review of risks and benefits of HT will provide the basis for an informed decision on the part of the patient. If a patient decides against HT at that point, alternative treatments, a healthy lifestyle, and practical measures can be addressed (see Chaps. 3 and 24). It is important to reevaluate and review therapeutic indications at each visit.

KEY POINT

For those on HT, it is important to reevaluate and review therapeutic indications at each visit.

If the patient would like to proceed with HT, it is helpful to know if she prefers oral or alternative modes of drug delivery. The oral route has potential advantages such as familiarity and convenience. It appears to have more pronounced lipid effect than other routes through lowering total cholesterol and low-density lipoproteins while raising high-density lipoproteins. Negative effects include increases in triglycerides and C-reactive protein. The precise clinical risk associated with these last two effects is not known. Cases of pancreatitis secondary to hypertriglyceridemia associated with HT use have been reported.[25] The process of gastrointestinal absorption and hepatic metabolism generally requires a higher dose of hormones resulting in stimulation of hepatic protein production. For example, oral hormones often increase angiotensin and sex hormone binding globulin.[26]

Advantages to the transdermal delivery of HT include avoidance of first-pass hepatic effect by delivery of drug to the blood vessels without first undergoing metabolism in the liver. Often a smaller dose can be used that results in less effect on the lipid profile and other hepatic processes. Some women have skin sensitivity to the transdermal patches; some are simply averse to the concept of wearing their medication visibly on their skin. Newer lotion and gel products as well as vaginal rings eliminate these drawbacks. Whether estradiol increases the risks or benefits compared to other forms of estrogen is not clear. One case-control study indicated there was less risk of thrombosis with transdermal estrogen.[27]

In the case of progestogens, the difference in effect does appear to be related to the type of progestogen. Medroxyprogesterone acetate (MPA) offsets the beneficial lipid effects of conjugated equine estrogens to a greater degree than does micronized progesterone.[9] The progestins derived from 19-nortestosterone have more androgenic effects compared to progesterone and MPA. They also tend to offset the lipid benefits of oral estrogen, although they may have a more beneficial effect on bone density.[28]

Whether any of the various combinations of estrogens and progestrogens have a substantially different risk benefit profile from that found with the continuous combined regimen of conjugated equine estrogens and MPA used in the WHI remains to be seen. The Food and Drug Administration has taken the position that in the absence of data to the contrary, all hormone combinations and regimens should be assumed to carry similar risks and benefits.

This statement would also apply to compounded hormones and the so-called bioidentical hormones (see Chap. 24).

The risk/benefit profile for estrogen alone is less clear. While the Million Women Study[29] and a large meta-analysis[30] both suggest that estrogen does increase the risk of breast cancer, it may do so at a lower and slower rate than estrogen and progestin combined. Because of the lesser risk associated with estrogen alone, women without a uterus are advised not to use a progestogen. The WHI estrogen arm found a decreased risk of breast cancer after a mean of 6.8 years of estrogen use that was not statistically significant.[12]

KEY POINT

Lower doses of HT are recommended.

In view of recent findings, initial treatment should begin with the lowest dose available for any particular product and titrated upward as needed to alleviate symptoms. Hot flushes can be expected to improve over 4 weeks. The following doses of various estrogens have been considered standard in recent years: conjugated or esterified estrogens 0.625 mg, oral estradiol 1 mg, and transdermal estradiol 0.05 mg. Low dose refers to a dose lower than these examples.

The woman with a uterus must also decide between cyclic or continuous progestogen therapies. The principal advantage of continuous therapy is the probability of eliminating all uterine bleeding. The likelihood of no bleeding on continuous therapy increases with the duration of continuous therapy and the length of time since menopause. The woman who is perimenopausal may find a more predictable bleeding pattern using the cyclic method of 12–14 days of progestogen per month until the withdrawal bleeding diminishes. At that point switching to continuous combined therapy is more likely to eliminate all bleeding.

While hot flushes typically diminish in intensity and frequency over time even without HT, symptoms of vaginal atrophy may persist or worsen. If the practical measures discussed in the next section do not suffice, small doses of topical estrogen can be applied directly to the vagina. Estrogen creams for vaginal use have been available for many years. More recently, a vaginal ring and vaginal tablets have been added to the list of options. These low dose options have been demonstrated to provide local benefit without substantially raising serum estradiol levels. The product information sheets indicate endometrial safety at 1 year. Whether the intermittent addition of a progestin is advisable for longer use has not been established. Some clinicians utilize an annual or biannual progestin challenge test consisting of 12–14 days of progestogen. Withdrawal bleeding would suggest the local estrogen is stimulating the endometrium.

The needs of the patient can determine the reevaluation process. An appointment by 3 months provides an opportunity to discuss concerns and adjust therapy as necessary. Patients can be given the option to call in with a message as to how they are doing if they prefer not to miss work for another appointment.

Since no consensus exist at present regarding specific duration of treatment for menopausal symptoms and since recommendations may vary for combined estrogen and progestin versus estrogen alone, the clinician and patient must decide when an attempt at discontinuation would be appropriate. The patient should be advised that she could experience a recurrence of menopausal symptoms whenever she discontinues hormones. One study found that 26% of women who tried to stop HT after the 2002 WHI report requested to resume therapy.[31] Within WHI only 4% of women resumed HT. There is a widespread misconception among patients that menopausal symptoms are strictly a menopause-related phenomenon rather than a phenomenon related to any drop in estrogen, be it endogenous or exogenous. Whether a slow tapering of hormones will minimize menopausal symptoms associated with discontinuation is not known. Patient preference is important in this setting.

Practical Measures

KEY POINT

Practical measures and lifestyle changes suffice for many women.

Few practical measures for hot flushes have undergone the rigorous evaluation of a large, randomized, controlled trial. However, most of the measures are inexpensive and have few to no side effects. As such there is little reason not to try them before initiating prescription therapy. Traditional advice includes dressing in layers so that clothing adjustments can be made according to the environment, wearing clothing open at the neck, and choosing fabrics that ventilate. It may also be helpful to avoid sitting or working under bright lights. At night, keeping a cool environment may mean not using comforters, electric blankets, and heated waterbeds. Other triggers for hot flushes could include alcoholic beverages, spicy foods, and stress. The chapter on hot flushes provides information on other techniques that may provide relief of hot flushes (see Chap. 3).

The other main category of menopausal symptoms is vaginal atrophy. For some symptomatic women a vaginal moisturizer may be sufficient. Others may need a lubricant in order to make intercourse comfortable. In the absence of HT, it is all the more important to continue sexual intercourse, if that is an option. This advice presumes the woman wants to preserve the capacity to have intercourse. Without intercourse and without HT, the introitus can constrict considerably making it extremely difficult to resume intercourse later. If tightness has already occurred, graduated vaginal dilators can be used by the woman to reach the point where she no longer experiences discomfort with intercourse. Local estrogen treatment may be required in conjunction with vaginal dilators. Vaginal tightness and vaginal dryness are two different causes of dyspareunia, and it is important to differentiate the two, as the treatments are different. Estrogen, however, can facilitate improvement in both conditions.

Future Options

The majority of women experience perimenopause with symptoms that are manageable. Others find the experience quite disruptive and seek treatment. More research is needed to find safer options for these symptomatic women. Data are needed on parenteral estrogen, lower doses of estrogen, as well as alternative progestrogen regimens such as vaginal or intrauterine delivery systems. New selective estrogen receptor modulators and drugs such as tibolone that have tissue selectivity may provide additional options. Of critical importance is a better understanding of the mechanisms underlying the adverse effects of HT. Being able to identify subpopulations at risk for thrombosis, early cardiac events, breast cancer, and dementia could markedly improve the safety of HT use. For now, the prudent use of HT would consist of a short-term use of the lowest dose of hormones that provides symptom relief.

Conclusion

Lifestyle changes and practical measures should be the first approach to perimenopausal symptoms, but low-dose, short-term

HT will remain an important choice for many women. Discussions informing and updating women on the known risks and benefits will facilitate informed decision-making on this important issue during perimenopause.

Discussion of cases

Questions often arise about the possible use of HT in special circumstances. There are many situations in which an ideal solution does not exist and/or data are incomplete for the particular situation. Nonstandard cases are described below with possible management options that will need to be modified when more data become available.

Case 1

A 41-year-old gravida 3, para 3, with a last menstrual period 6 months ago, complains of disruptive hot flushes, poor sleep, and irritability. She has read about results from the WHI and is reluctant to use HT. She seeks advice from her clinician.

What is the patient's main concern?

She is concerned about experiencing one of the side effects reported in the WHI.

At this point it would be important to explain that we do not know if the findings from the WHI can be directly applied to women under age 50 since the study enrolled women age 50–79, average age 63. The percent increase in risk in the WHI is very small and represents an increase above the usual occurrence of a particular event in a certain age group. For a woman in her forties, the risks of heart attack, stroke, thrombosis, and breast cancer are quite small. Thus, the absolute risk for this patient would be very low. The risk may be altered further by the fact that the comparison group would be women her own age, most of whom would still be producing their own estrogen, unlike the WHI, where the control group has extremely low levels of estrogen. In the absence of contraindications, using the lowest dose of HT that alleviates her symptoms and reevaluating her situation each year appears appropriate. Theoretically, further decrease in risks may accrue through use of parenteral estrogen.

Case 2

A 62-year-old gravida 2, para 2, Caucasian female presents for an annual visit with no complaints. She has been using HT since menopause. For the past 5 years she has been on a continuous combined oral regimen, and she believes it is keeping her healthy and youthful. She is pleased to know she is getting bone protection and perhaps other preventive care benefits as well.

How might a clinician approach this patient given the current research findings?

The patient should be made aware that the background rate of CVD, stroke, and thrombosis increases with age, so that her absolute risk of experiencing one of these side effects may be increasing. In particular, she is nearing the age where Alzeheimer's disease begins

to occur, and the WHI reported an increased risk of dementia in women who participated in the study. Only women who were 65 and older were allowed to enroll in that ancillary study. Not known at this time is whether an older woman who has used HT since menopause could be at lower risk since she has survived earlier use of HT with no adverse events. For example, the elevated hazard ratio for venous thrombosis with EPT use declined with years from randomization in the WHI from 4.01 in year 1 to 1.04 in year 6 suggesting that susceptible women were gradually eliminated from the HT user pool as they had thrombotic events leaving the less susceptible women to continue HT.[20]

Recommendation?

Taper off HT: Adverse events have been identified with HT use and randomized controlled trial data fail to show a predominating benefit. If the patient is opposed to discontinuation, recommend a lower HT dose and be sure that she is aware of and willing to accept the known risks.

What are her alternatives?

Other drugs, calcium, vitamin D, and lifestyle measures are available for prevention of osteoporosis (see Chap. 23). Skin moisturizers and sunscreen can help to preserve skin appearance. Exercise and good nutrition have numerous benefits. Vaginal atrophy can be addressed with the practical measures above or low-dose topical estrogen.

Case 3

A 54-year-old woman has severe osteopenia, a strong family history of osteoporosis and no secondary causes of her condition. She experienced side effects with available osteoporosis treatments that were unacceptable to her. She was happy on HT in the past and wants to resume it. Several options exist. This woman might do well on low-dose HT but she would need to understand the risks of long-term HT. Alternatively, she might be followed with bone density measurements and conscientious attention to calcium and vitamin D plus exercise. Parenteral bisphosphonates are available and alternative selective estrogen receptor modulators may be available in the near future.

Case 4

A 53-year-old breast cancer survivor reports that severe vaginal atrophy has seriously affected her quality of life and her sexual relationship. She understands the risks of HT including the possible recurrence of cancer and is willing to take those risks. If practical measures and alternative therapies have all failed, this patient may benefit from a short course of low-dose vaginal estrogen and possible vaginal dilator until sexual activity is comfortable. At that point, discontinuing HT while maintaining regular sexual activity with lubricants should suffice. The patient should be advised that a trial investigating the use of HT in breast cancer survivors was discontinued because of an increased recurrence of breast cancer in the HT group.[32]

Guiding Questions

- Is the woman interested in HT for menopausal symptoms?
- Does she have contraindications to HT?
- Is she aware that symptoms are generally transient?
- Is she aware that symptoms may recur upon discontinuing HT later?
- Is she aware of alternative approaches to managing symptoms?
- Is she adequately informed about the risks and benefits of HT?
- What would be the lowest dose of HT likely to alleviate her symptoms?

What's the Evidence?

Randomized controlled trial evidence does not support the long-term use of HT for prevention of chronic disease in healthy post-menopausal women. Estrogen alone appears to have fewer risks and benefits than combined estrogen and progestin. Consensus is that use of HT at the lowest effective dose to treat menopausal symptoms for a limited amount of time is acceptable because absolute risks are small for women in the perimenopausal age group.

References

1 Sevringhaus E. *Endocrine Therapy.* Chicago, IL: Year Book Publishers, Inc.; 1938.

2 Zandi PP, Carlson MC, Plassman BL, et al. Hormone replacement therapy and incidence of Alzheimer disease in older women: the Cache County Study. *Journal of the American Medical Association.* 2002;288(17):2133–2139.

3 Nevitt M, Cummings S, Lane N, et al. Association of estrogen replacement therapy with osteoarthritis of the hip in elderly white women. Study of Osteoporotic Fractures Research Group. *Arch Intern Med.* 1996;156:2073–2080.

4 Smith W, Mitchell P, Wang JJ. Gender, oestrogen, hormone replacement and age-relate macular degeneration: results from the Blue Mountains Eye Study. *Aust N Z J Opphthalmol.* May 25 (Suppl. 1): S13–S15.

5 Grodstein F, Colditz G, Stampfer M. Postmenopausal hormone use and tooth loss: a prospective study. *J Am Dent Assoc.* 1996;127: 370–377.

6 Wall LL. Medical management of pelvic relaxation. *Curr Opin Obstet Gynecol.* Aug 1993;5(4):440–445.

7 Raz R, Stamm W. A controlled trial of intravaginal estriol in postmenopausal women with recurrent urinary tract infections. *N Engl J Med.* 1993;329:753–756.

8 Writing Group for the Women's Health Initiative Investigators. Risks and benefits of estrogen plus progestin in healthy postmenopausal women: principal results from the Women's Health Initiative randomized controlled trial. *JAMA.* 2002;288:321–333.

9 Effects of estrogen or estrogen/progestin regimens on heart disease risk factors in postmenopausal women. *JAMA.* 1995;273:199–208.

10 Hulley S, Grady D, Bush T, et al. Randomized trial of estrogen plus progestin for secondary prevention of coronary heart disease in postmenopausal women. *JAMA.* 1998;280:605–613.

11 Grady D, Herrington D, Bittner V, et al. Cardiovascular disease outcomes during 6.8 years of hormone therapy. *JAMA.* 2002;288:49–57.

12 The Women's Health Initiative Steering Committee. Effects of conjugated equine estrogen in postmenopausal women with hysterectomy. *JAMA* 2004;291:1701–1712.

13 ACOG News Release. *ACOG Statement on the NIH Announcement to Halt Estrogen-Only Arm of the WHI Study.* March 2, 2004. communications@acog.org Accessed June 20, 2004. Members only.

14 Recommendations for estrogen and progestogen use in peri- and postmenopausal women: October 2004 position statement of The North American Menopause Society. *Menopause.* 2004;11:589–600.

15 USPSTF. Postmenopausal hormone replacement therapy for the primary prevention of chronic conditions. *Ann Intern Med.* 2002;137:834–839.

16 RCPE. Consensus Conference on Hormone Replacement Therapy, October 2003. Final Consensus Statement. Royal College of Physicians of Edinburgh. *http://www.rcpe.ac.uk/esd/consensus/hrt_03.html.* Accessed 04-01-04.

17 Kronenberg F. Hot flashes: epidemiology and physiology. *Ann NY Acad Sci.* 1990;592:52–86.

18 Shumaker SA, Legault C, Rapp SR, et al. Estrogen plus progestin and the incidence of dementia and mild cognitive impairment in postmenopausal women. *JAMA.* 2003;289:2651–2662.

19 Rapp SR, Espeland MA, Shumaker SA, et al. Effect of estrogen plus progestin on global cognitive function in postmenopausal women. The Women's Health Initiative Memory Study. A Randomized controlled trial. *JAMA.* 2003;289:2663–2672.

20 Cushman M, Kuller LH, Prentice R, et al. Estrogen plus progestin and risk of venous thrombosis. *JAMA.* 2004;292:1573–1580.

21 Wassertheil-Smoller S, Hendrix S, Limacher M, et al. Effect of estrogen plus progestin on stroke in postmenopausal women. *JAMA.* 2003;289:2673–2684.

22 Manson J, Hsia J, Johnson K, et al. Estrogen plus progestin and the risk of coronary heart disease. *N Engl J Med.* 2003;349:523–534.

23 Chlebowski R, Hendrix S, Langer R, et al. Influence of estrogen plus progestin on breast cancer and mammography in healthy postmenopausal women. *JAMA.* 2003:289:3243–3253.

24 Shumaker SA, Legault C, Kuller L, et al. Conjugated equine estrogens and incidence of probable dementia and mild cognitive impairment in postmenopausal women. *JAMA.* 2004;291:2947–2058.

25 Glueck C, Scheel D, et al. Estrogen induced pancreatitis in patients with previously covert familiar type V hyperlipoproteinemia. *Metabolism.* 1972;21:657–666.

26 Chetkowski R MD, Steingold KA. Biologic effects of transdermal estradiol. *N Engl J Med.* 1986;314:1615–1620.

27 Scarabin PY, Oger E, Plu-Bureau G. Differential association of oral and transdermal oestrogen-replacement therapy with venous thromboembolism risk. *Lancet.* 2003;362:428–432.

28 McClung M, et al. *Changes in BMD Lumbar Spine (L1–L4) with E2 Alone and Combined with NETA.* San Francisco, CA: ASBMR; 1998.

29 Million Women Study Collaborators. Breast cancer and hormone-replacement therapy in the Million Women Study. *Lancet.* 2003;362: 419–427.

30 Collaborative Group on Hormonal Factors in Breast Cancer. Breast cancer and hormone replacement therapy: collaborative reanalysis of data from 51 epidemiological studies of 52,705 women with breast cancer and 108,411 women without breast cancer. *Lancet.* 1997;350: 1047–1059.

31 Grady D, Ettinger B, Tosteson AN, et al. Predictors of difficulty when discontinuing postmenopausal hormone therapy. *Obstet Gynecol.* 2003;102:1233–1239.

32 Holmberg L, Anderson H, for the HABIT steering and data monitoring committees. HABITS trial looking at use of HT in breast cancer survivors terminated early due to safety concerns. *Lancet.* 2004;363: 453–455.

PREVENTIVE HEALTH STRATEGIES

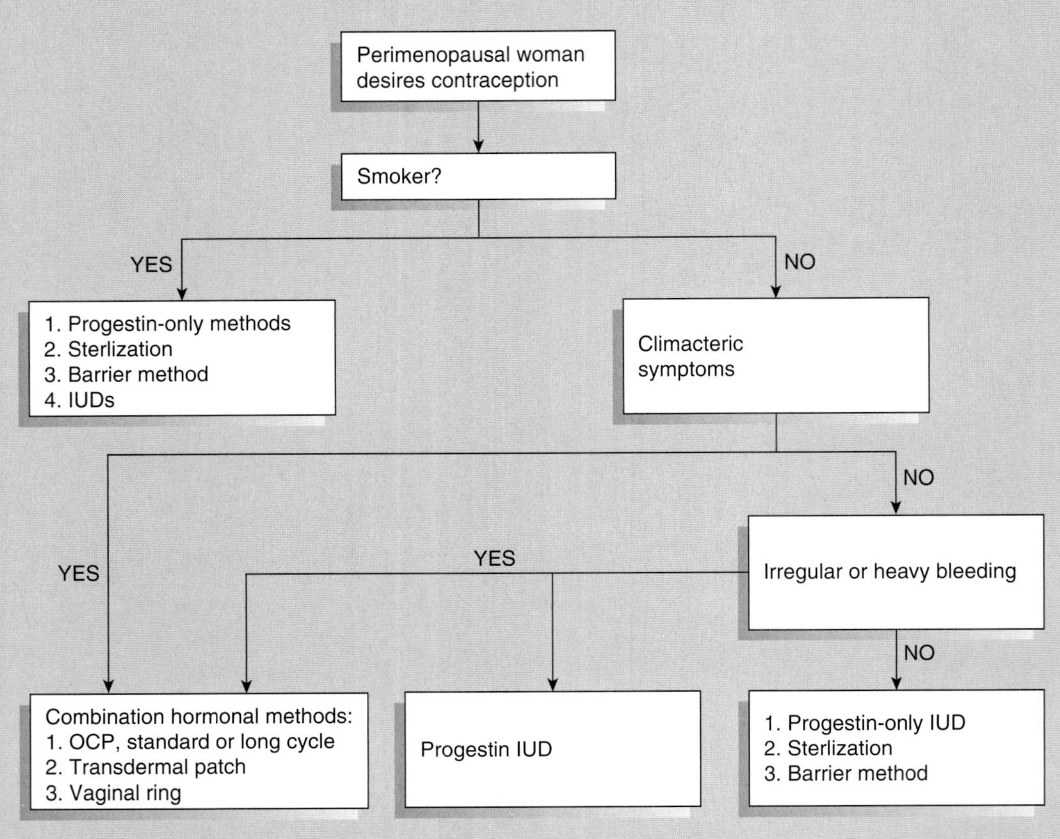

Perimenopausal woman desires contraception
Smoker?
YES
NO
1. Progestin-only methods
2. Sterlization
3. Barrier method
4. IUDs
Climacteric symptoms
NO
YES
YES
Irregular or heavy bleeding
NO
Combination hormonal methods:
1. OCP, standard or long cycle
2. Transdermal patch
3. Vaginal ring
Progestin IUD
1. Progestin-only IUD
2. Sterlization
3. Barrier method

21 Contraception

Paul A. Robb
Daniel B. Williams

Guiding Questions

- Does the couple desire future fertility?
- How devastating would a contraceptive failure be?
- Is the woman having irregular or heavy cycles?
- Is the woman having any hypoestrogenic symptoms?
- Does the woman have risk factors for osteoporosis in addition to age?

What's the Evidence

Though somewhat ironic, women seeking pregnancy in perimenopause period often have difficulty conceiving, while those not seeking to add to their families remain at risk for pregnancy. Indeed some 80% of women ages 40–44 are able to conceive.[1] Often, for women in this age group, an unplanned pregnancy is also an unwanted pregnancy. This leads to an abortion rate as high as 35% among pregnant women over the age of 40, and an even higher rate for women over the age of 45, making this the highest rate of any group except for preteens.[2] The types of contraceptive options available for women in advanced reproductive ages are the same as those in younger aged groups. Due to declining fertility, the efficacy of contraceptive methods is likely enhanced in this age group. In general, women of this age are more compliant; however, an awareness of decreased fertility could possibly make women less compliant. While no form of contraception is necessarily contraindicated on the basis of age alone some contraceptive choices may have added benefits for this age group. Options include sterilization, barrier methods, intrauterine devices (IUDs), and hormonal methods. Many new options have recently become available, especially in the last group.

Sterilization

KEY POINT

Sterilization remains very popular but offers no other benefits beyond contraception.

Female sterilization, despite lack of noncontraceptive benefits, is the most common method of contraception used by perimenopausal women in the United States.[3]

The rate of sterilization is higher in the United States compared with other countries, perhaps because in the United States insurance often covers the sterilization procedure and often does not cover reversible contraceptive methods. The failure rate is very low but is method dependant with a range from 0.75% to 3.65%.[4] It also requires outpatient surgery with its attendant surgical and anesthetic risks. This is in contrast to male sterilization with vasectomy, which requires only an outpatient procedure under local anesthesia. Although there are reports of menstrual irregularities following female sterilization, most studies would suggest that there is no change in menstrual function.[5] The problem of sterilization regret, which can be significant in a younger population, is usually minimal in this age group.

Barrier Methods

These methods have typical efficacy rates around 85% and may be even more effective in the older age group due to declining fertility. One must consider the consequences of a contraceptive failure for this age group when counseling about these relatively less effective methods. Side effects are rare and the method is totally patient controlled. Diaphragm use requires fitting by a physician. The condom has the added benefit of protection from sexually transmitted infections. However, these methods have no cycle control benefit.

Natural Methods

While natural methods can be used, changes in the menstrual cycle in the perimenopause make these methods unreliable. Again, the consequences of contraceptive failure are often very high making these methods less than desirable for most women.

Intrauterine Devices

KEY POINT

The levonorgestrel IUD offers protection from dysfunctional bleeding and hyperplasia in addition to very effective long-term contraception.

IUDs offer very effective, long-term protection from pregnancy with efficacy rates above 99% that often make them very attractive for women in their late reproductive years. The copper-containing IUDs are effective for 10 years, while the levonorgestrel system is effective for 5 years. Either of these may serve a woman well during her perimenopausal years. The risks of IUDs include the risk of infection within 20 days of insertion,[6] perforation at the time of insertion, and the risk of an ectopic pregnancy should a contraceptive failure occur. The copper-containing devices may have the disadvantage of increased menstrual cramping and bleeding which may add to the disordered menstruation already present in many perimenopausal women. Nonsteroidal anti-inflammatory agents may alleviate these effects. The levonorgestrel system bridges the gap between IUDs and hormonal methods by combining a progestin with an IUD system. It may have the added benefit of preventing uterine bleeding and hyperplasia that can result from the unopposed estrogen in the anovulatory cycles that are common at this time in woman's life.

A recent 3-year follow-up study showed that 77% of women were very satisfied with the levonorgestrel system.[7]

Hormonal Methods

PROGESTIN ONLY

Injectable depot medroxyprogesterone acetate (DMPA) has been available for many years as an intramuscular injection every 3 months. It has very good efficacy with little opportunity for compliance failure. The common side effects are weight gain, bloating, acne, headache, mood changes, and a delayed return to fertility. There are several additional concerns for the perimenopausal woman. The use of DMPA has been shown to cause a decrease in bone mineral density.[8] There is evidence that these losses are recovered within 12–24 months of stopping DMPA.[9] For the perimenopausal women, however, if DMPA is used up to the time of menopause, it is possible that any decreases in bone mineral density would not be fully recovered, since recovery of bone mass is thought to depend on return of the DMPA suppressed estrogen levels to a normal premenopausal state. In the perimenopausal setting, use of DMPA may cause the usual menopausal bone loss to occur earlier. This method can also induce a hypoestrogenic state that could exacerbate any hypoestrogenic symptoms of hot flushes and night sweats that are common in the perimenopause period. There is also an unpredictably long delay in the return of fertility following DMPA use making it a less desirable choice for those over 35 years of age who are contemplating future pregnancies. Finally, DMPA often causes menstrual irregularity prior to causing amenorrhea that may worsen the irregularity already present in the perimenopausal period. The new single-rod levonorgestrel implant and other progestin-only forms of contraception are also not likely to be the best choice of a contraceptive for a woman in the perimenopause due to their inherent problems of irregular bleeding. On the other hand, progestin- only contraception may help correct the relative progesterone deficiency experienced by some women. The progestin-only pill may be used in older women who smoke[10] but as with injectable forms, menstrual irregularity may become a problem.

Combination Estrogen/Progestin Methods

Oral

There is a decrease in oral contraceptive (OCP) use with age that is likely due the widespread belief that the use of OCPs incurs a greater health risk in women after the age of 35. Earlier studies had suggested an increased cardiovascular risk, but once confounding factors such as smoking were removed, the risk disappeared.[11] The OCP is therefore no longer recommended to women over the age of 35 who continue to smoke. Newer pills are of a lower dose compared to the pills in the earlier studies and may have lower risk, although a small risk of venous thrombosis remains. For the perimenopausal woman all the usual benefits of the pill apply, such as a reduction in ovarian and endometrial cancer, anemia, pelvic infection, ovarian cysts, benign breast disease, and dysmenorrhea. In addition, combination OCPs offer a number of advantages that apply particularly to women in the perimenopause. The pill is associated with a reduction in climacteric symptoms such as vasomotor symptoms,[12] a reduction in the incidence of dysfunctional bleeding,[13] and preservation of bone mineral density.[14] For the perimenopausal woman with climactic symptoms, the long-cycle (84 days)OCP might be particularly helpful in relieving symptoms. It needs to be mentioned that the recent data from

KEY POINT

Combination estrogen/progestin methods offer added benefits particularly applicable to the perimenopausal women including reduced vasomotor symptoms, reduced dysfunctional bleeding, and preservation of bone mass.

the Women's Health Initiative (WHI)[15] study does not necessarily apply to the perimenopausal patient population as it included only postmenopausal women with a mean age of 63 who given hormone replacement therapy. However, an increase in relative risk for heart disease, breast cancer, stroke, and venous thrombotic events was also seen in the women ages 50–54, who were using continuous combined estrogen and progestin. Even though the relative risk was similar across all age groups in the WHI, the absolute risk would be lower in younger women because the background rate of events is lower.

Low-dose OCPs provide an excellent low-risk option for the older woman toward the end of her reproductive years.

TRANSVAGINAL

The monthly vaginal ring is another nonoral method that contains ethinyl estradiol and etonogestrel (active metabolite of desogestrel). It releases 15 μg of ethinyl estradiol daily and 120 μg of etonogestrel daily. Its efficacy compared favorably with OCPs.[16] Clinically, there appears to be less breakthrough bleeding with the vaginal ring compared to other hormonal contraceptive methods.[17] The approved regimen involves inserting the ring for 3 weeks and then removing it for 1 week before inserting a new ring. Following removal, return to ovulation can be expected in several weeks.[18] The ring may cause an increase in vaginal secretions due to a mechanical effect.[19] The ring may not be appropriate for women with significant prolapse and the same contraindications that apply to OCPs apply to the ring.

TRANSDERMAL

The weekly patch is another modality to administer contraceptive hormones. The patch contains ethinyl estradiol (20 μg daily) and norelgestromin (150 μg daily; an active metabolite of norgestimate). The contraceptive efficacy compares with that of OCPs. The approved regimen is to apply one patch weekly for 3 weeks followed by a patch-free week before starting a new cycle. Should the patch detach (occurrence of about 1%), it should be replaced immediately. The patch can be placed on the abdomen, buttocks, upper torso (avoid the breasts), or the upper outer arm. Again, the same precautions that apply to other combination hormonal contraceptive methods apply to the patch, and the same benefits can be expected. There are reports that the contraceptive efficacy may be reduced in women weighing more than 90 kg.[20] A study comparing the patch to an OCP (Triphasil) showed an increase in breast tenderness in the patch group in the first two cycles.[21] The hepatic *first-pass effect* is avoided with this parenteral source. There have been recent reports of a slight increase in thrombotic risk in contraceptive patch users.

When to Discontinue Hormonal Contraception?

One question that often arises with the perimenopausal women on contraceptive doses of hormones is when to stop them and consider hormone therapy (HT) for menopausal symptoms. One easy way is to obtain an follicle-stimulating hormone (FSH) level at the end of the hormone-free week (day 6 or 7) and to stop contraceptives when the FSH is above 20 IU/L. Some women may not show an increase in FSH after 1 week,[22] but it is not a problem to simply retest in 1 year or the hormone-free period can be extended to 2 weeks with retesting of FSH and estradiol at that time (a back-up method of contraception is required in this instance). Castracane et al.[22] concluded that after 2 weeks off hormones either a rise in FSH or no change in basal estradiol levels was strong evidence that it was safe to discontinue contraceptives. A woman could then consider switching to HT if she were symptomatic and desiring HT. Nonhormonal methods of contraception have the advantage of not obscuring a woman's natural menopause.

What's the Evidence?

The nonsmoking woman in perimenopause has the same contraceptive choices as younger women. The natural decline in fertility likely increases the efficacy of all modalities. Sterilization remains a popular choice but offers no additional contraceptive benefits and involves a surgical procedure. Barrier methods have a higher failure rate, which need to be factored into the decision process. Hormonal choices offer additional benefits and few risks in the healthy woman. The progestin in the levonorgestrel IUD may offer improvement in patients with dysfunctional bleeding as well as prevention of endometrial hyperplasia. In other forms, progestin-only methods may exacerbate irregular bleeding patterns inherent in this age group and DMPA may result in bone loss at a time when it cannot be fully recovered. Choices that involve the use of estrogens may be advantageous in that they are likely to have a positive effect on some of the particular symptoms that the perimenopausal woman may encounter. Estrogens will reduce vasomotor symptoms, protect against bone loss, and regulate the menstrual cycle so that dysfunctional uterine bleeding may be reduced. The estrogen content in OCPs has been decreasing which may serve to minimize side effects. Newer delivery systems for combined contraceptive methods including depot injections, vaginal rings, and patches have extended choices for women, and by not using intestinal absorption they avoid a first-pass effect on liver metabolism.

Women in their older reproductive years still face the significant issue of unwanted pregnancy. Women in this age group have numerous options for contraception that are similar to their younger counterparts. It is imperative for these patients to receive proper counseling to allow them to select the method that is optimal for them.

Discussion of Cases

Case 1

Mrs. W is a 46-year-old woman in a monogamous 23-year relationship with three children and desires contraception. She has no desire to add to her family in the future. She and her husband have been using condoms but she is worried about the higher failure rate with condoms, especially since she does not think they could cope with another child. She had tried OCPs in the past but did not like having to take a pill every day. Usually her menses occur every 30–32 days but she occasionally misses a cycle or two with a subsequent heavy period. She is a healthy individual with no medical problems at this time.

On examination, she has a normal-sized anteverted uterus. Because of the irregular bleeding, an endometrial biopsy is performed in the office. It reveals proliferative endometrium, negative for hyperplasia or malignancy. After a discussion of contraceptive methods, she decides to try the levonorgestrel-containing IUD. It is inserted 5 days after her next menstrual period. She notes some spotting in the first 2 months but this resolves and her periods actually cease. She is doing well and plans to continue with the device until she turns 51 years of age.

References

1 Schmidt-Sarosi C. Infertility in the older woman. *Clin Obstet Gynecol.* 1998;41:940–950.

2 Henshaw SK. Unintended pregnancy in the United States. *Fam Plann Perspect.* 1998;30:24–29.

3 Williams JK. Contraceptive needs of the perimnopausal woman. *Obstet Gynecol Clin North Am.* 2002;29:575–588.

4 Peterson HB, Xia Z, Hughes JM, et al. The risk of pregnancy after tubal sterilization: findings from the US Collaborate Review of sterilization. *Am J Obstet Gynecol.* 1996;174:1161–1170.

5 Peterson HB, Jeng G, Folger SG, et al. The risk of menstrual abnormalities after tubal sterilization: findings from the US Collaborative Review of Sterilization. *N Engl J Med.* 2000;343L:1681–1687.

6 Farley TMM. Intrauterine device and pelvic inflammatory disease: an international perspective. *Lancet.* 1992;339:785–788.

7 Baldaszti E, Beate WP, Löschke. Acceptability of the long-term contraceptive levonorgestrel-releasing intrauterine system (Mirena®): a 3-year follow-up study. *Contraception.* 2003;67:87–91.

8 Ott SM, Scholes D, LaCroix AZ, et al. A prospective controlled study on the bone biochemical markers in women. *J Clin Endocrinol Metab.* 2001;86:179–185.

9 Cundy T, Cornish X, Evans MC, et al. Recovery of bone density in women who stop using medroxyprogesterone acetate. *BMJ.* 1993;308: 247–248.

10 Medical Eligibility Criteria for Contraceptive Use Third edition—2004. *htt://www.who.int/reproductive-health/publications/mec*, accessed 10-02-05.

11 Croft P, Hannaford PC. Risk factors for acute myocardial infarction in women: evidence from the Royal College of General Practitioners' oral contraceptive study. *Br Med J.* 1989;298:165–168.

12 Shargil AA. Hormone replacement therapy in perimenopausal women with a triphasic contraceptive compound: a three-year prospective study. *Int J Fertil.* 1985;30(1):15, 18–28.

13 Davis A, Godwin A, Lippman J, et al. Triphasic norgestimate-ethinyl estradiol for treating dysfunctional uterine bleeding. *Obstet Gynecol.* 2000;96(6):913–920.

14 Gambacciani M, Spinetti A, Cappagli B, et al. Hormone replacement therapy in perimenopausal women with a low dose or contraceptive preparation: effects on bone mineral density and metabolism. *Maturitas.* 1994;19(2):125–131.

15 Rossouw J, Anderson G, Prentice R. Risks and benefits of estrogen plus progestin in healthy postmenopausal women: principal results from the Women's Health Initiative randomized controlled trial. *JAMA.* 2002;288:321–333.

16 Dieben TO, Roumen FJ, Apter D. Efficacy, cycle control, and user acceptability of a novel combined contraceptive vaginal ring. *Obstet Gynecol.* 2002;100:585–593.

17 Roumen FJ, Apter D, Mulders TM, et al. Efficacy, tolerability and acceptability of a novel contraceptive vaginal ring releasing releasing etonogestrel and ethinyl estradiol. *Hum Reprod.* 2001;16:469–475.

18 Mulders TM, Dieben TO, Bennik HJ. Ovarian function with a novel combined contraceptive vaginal ring. *Hum Reprod.* 2002;75:2594–2599.

19 Roumen F, Dieben T, Assendorp R, et al. The clinical acceptability of a non-medicated vaginal ring. *Contraception.* 1990; 42(2):201–207.

20 Ortho-McNeil Pharmaceutical Inc., Ortho Evra (norelgestromin/ethinyl estradiol transdermal system) package insert. Raritan, NJ; 2001.

21 Audet MC, Moreau M, Koltun WD, et al. ORTHO EVRA/EVRA 004 Study Group. Evaluation of contraceptive efficacy and cycle control of a transdermal contraceptive patch vs an oral contraceptive: a randomized controlled trial. *JAMA.* 2001;285(18):2347–2354.

22 Castracane VD, Gimpel T, Goldzieher JW. When is it safe to switch from oral contraceptives to hormonal replacement therapy? *Contraception.* 1995;52(6):371–376.

22 Cancer Screening and Prevention

Elizabeth V. Brandewie

Screening Tests

Cancer is the leading cause of death among perimenopausal women; therefore, it is crucial that physicians caring for women, in this age group, be well informed regarding the latest recommendations for cancer screening.[1] An ideal time to discuss cancer screening tests with a patient is during her annual examination. Unfortunately, conflicting recommendations from various national organizations can be confusing and can impair a physician's likelihood for implementing cancer screening. This chapter focuses on national recommendations for cancer screening in perimenopausal women; specifically, screening for breast, colon, cervical, uterine, and ovarian cancer. In addition, new screening techniques are also highlighted.

National agencies have adhered to specific principles regarding screening tests prior to making their recommendations. These include the following.[2]

Guiding Principles for Screening Tests

The disease to be screened must represent a significant health burden to society.

- The disease should have a detectable, preclinical phase, defined as the mean sojourn time.
- Early treatment of the patient should improve morbidity and mortality from the disease, thus justifying the cost of the screening test.
- The screening test should have good sensitivity and specificity.
- The screening test should be safe and well tolerated by the patient.

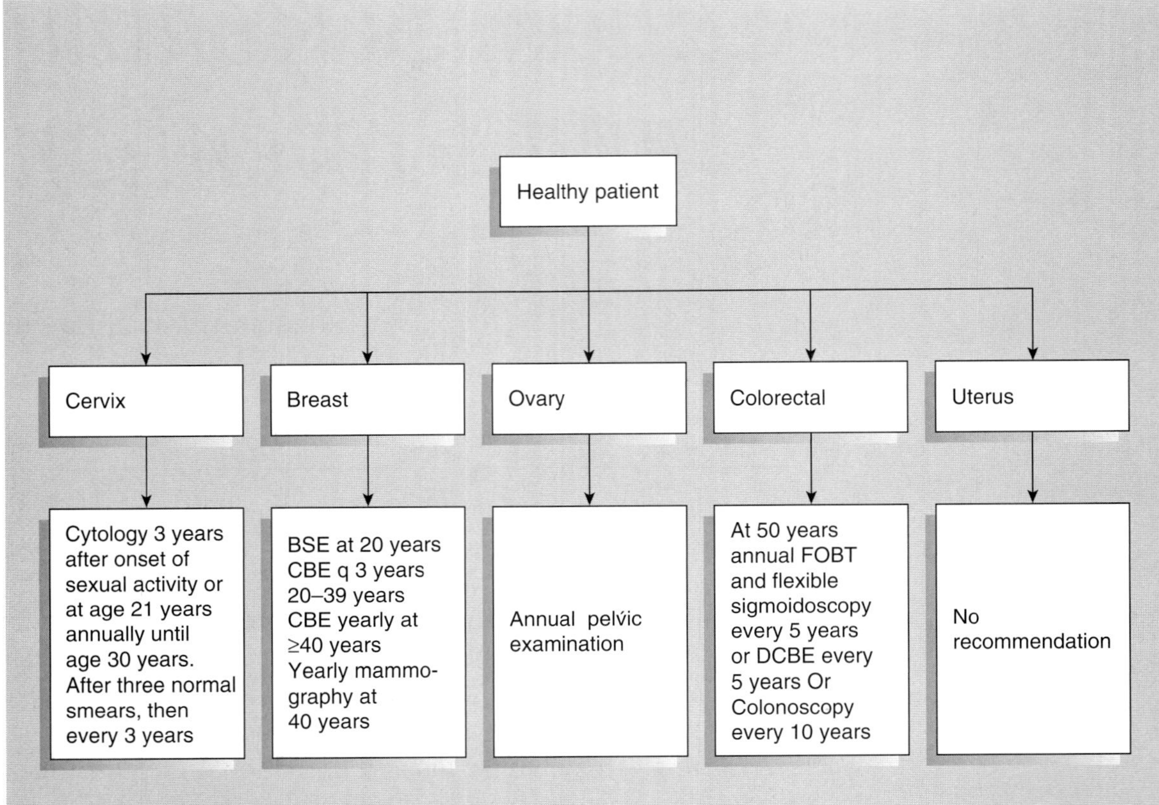

American Cancer Society Screening guidelines.

BSE, breast self-examination
CBE, clinical breast examination
FOBT, fecal occult blood test
DCBE, dual contrast barium enema

Obviously, if the screening test, or the follow-up test it provokes, is very uncomfortable to the patient, it will be difficult to implement such screening. Also, the disease must be prevalent enough to justify the expense of screening large populations of patients. The screening test should have good specificity to accurately identify those patients with preclinical disease, thereby preventing a large number of patients from having invasive diagnostic procedures unnecessarily. Finally, the disease itself must have a preclinical stage that the screening test targets with the intention of either obtaining a cure, or dramatically reducing morbidity and mortality.

Breast Cancer Screening

Breast cancer is the most common cancer in women, excluding skin cancers. It is the number one cause of cancer death in women aged 20–59. In the year 2003, it was estimated that there will be 39,800 deaths from this disease.[3] Certainly breast cancer meets the "burden of disease" criterion for cancer screening. Multiple studies on breast cancer screening demonstrate that a detectable preclinical stage exists.

KEY POINT

Early Detection of breast cancer will reduce overall mortality associated with breast cancer.

Early detection reduces tumor size and lymph node status, both of which are predictors of breast cancer mortality. Specifically, the Swedish Two-County Trial noted an 88%, 16-year survival for tumors less than or equal to 5 mm versus a 69%, 16-year survival for tumors greater than 1 cm.[4] The latest recommendations regarding screening mammography, breast self-examination (BSE), and clinical breast examination (CBE) from the American Cancer Society (ACS, 2003), United States Preventive Services Task Force (USPSTF, 2002), and American College of Obstetricians and Gynecologists (ACOG, 2003) are reviewed. In addition, other screening tests including magnetic resonance imaging (MRI), ultrasound, and ductal lavage are discussed.

Mammography

In average-risk women, the ACS recommends yearly screening mammography commencing at age 40.[5] On the other hand, the USPSTF advises screening mammography for women of average risk age 40 and older every 1–2 years.[6] ACOG takes the middle ground and recommends mammography every 1–2 years for average-risk women aged 40–49, and annual mammography starting at age 50.[7] These recommendations are based on analyses of at least eight randomized control trials of screening mammography in women aged 40–74 which demonstrate approximately a 20–30% reduction in mortality from breast cancer with screening mammography.[8] Unfortunately, the studies differed regarding screening interval, use of other screening tests like CBE, and proportion of women in the 40–50 age range. The ACS identifies the decreased sojourn time of breast cancer in women aged 40–49 versus older women as further evidence to support annual screening commencing at age 40. In a study of women aged 40–49, diagnosed with invasive breast cancer, 32.1% were diagnosed by mammography and 67.9% had a palpable mass. Of the patients with a palpable mass, 41.5% had nodal metastases versus 6.3% of patients diagnosed by mammography.[9]

Concerns regarding annual screening mammography in perimenopausal women have been raised. Approximately 40% of breast cancers diagnosed by mammography are ductal carcinoma in situ (DCIS).[10] The natural history of DCIS is unknown, and the majority of women with DCIS have a surgical procedure performed. Evidence strongly suggests that DCIS is a precursor to invasive cancer; however, Smith argues that DCIS should not be considered a "cost" of screening mammography.[2] The sensitivity of one-time screening mammography has been estimated to be 71–96% with a specificity of 94–97%. The positive predictive value of an abnormal diagnostic mammogram, requiring biopsy, ranges from 12% to 78%.[8] Over a 10-year period, 23% of women in one community setting were noted to have an abnormal mammogram requiring a repeat mammogram or a biopsy.[11] Lastly, mammography involves a radiation exposure. Feig and Hendrick estimated that annual mammography of 100,000 women, beginning at age 40, would induce no more than eight deaths per 100,000 from breast cancer.[12]

Clinical Breast Examination

KEY POINT

The sensitivity for detection of breast cancer by the clinical breast examination is low.

The ACS recommends CBE for average-risk women, starting in their twenties, as a part of general health examinations, preferably every 3 years. By age 40, a yearly CBE is recommended.[5] The ACOG also endorses the CBE.[7] On the other hand, the USPSTF concludes that there is insufficient evidence to recommend for, or against CBE for breast cancer screening.[6] While the sensitivity of CBE is low, Oestreicher noted 5.7% of breast cancers were diagnosed by CBE alone.[13] In addition, the ACS suggests that the CBE is an important opportunity to discuss breast symptoms, genetic factors, and new screening technologies.

Breast Self-Examination

The ACS states that average-risk women, beginning in their twenties, should be informed of the benefits and limitations of BSE, and that it is acceptable for women to choose not to do BSE.[5] The ACS recommendations are supported by the ACOG .[7] The USPSTF states that there is insufficient evidence to recommend for or against BSE.[6] Both recommendations followed the final report from the randomized control trial based in Shanghai. This trial failed to show a decreased breast cancer mortality rate with BSE instruction. It also noted an increase in the benign biopsy rate.[14] The ACS maintains that as a significant percentage of breast cancers are first noted incidentally by the patient, there may be some benefit for women to have increased awareness of their breasts' anatomy.

KEY POINT

A randomized control trial of BSE failed to demonstrate a reduction in breast cancer mortality.

New Technologies

Digital Mammography Digital mammography (DM) refers to the use of digital detectors to obtain an x-ray generated image of the breast. This is compared to standard screen-film mammography (SFM) in which a phosphor screen serves as the detector subsequently generating a permanent film image. Both techniques involve similar radiation doses. Lewin performed a prospective study of 4945 patients who underwent both SFM and DM. He noted no significant difference in the cancer detection rate, however, there were significantly fewer recalls with DM.[15] DM allows for *postacquisition image processing*. Thus, the radiologist can alter the brightness of the image, virtually eliminating the problem of possible under- or overexposure.[16] In addition, the digital images can be easily accessed and stored. Finally, DM can be employed in conjunction with computer-aided detection (CAD) as discussed below.

KEY POINT

In one study, computer-aided analysis of DM images resulted in an increase in the number of cancers detected.

Computer-Aided Detection CAD refers to the use of computers to review digitized mammograms, in order to detect and prompt mammography signs of cancer. This technology is used as an adjunct to interpretation by a radiologist. Ideally, the radiologist reviews the image prior to CAD, and then repeats this review after considering prompts produced by the computer. Thus, this technology is not intended to replace the radiologist, but rather its purpose is to help avoid the false negatives associated with mammography.[16]

In a prospective study of 12,860 patients undergoing screening mammography, Freer noted that CAD resulted in a 19.5% increase in the number of cancers detected without an unacceptable increase in recall rate.[17] Also, Warren Burhenne reviewed 286 cancers that were noted on re-review of previous films. CAD could have reduced the false-negative rate of 21% by 77%.[18] However, it is very important to consider CAD as an adjunct to review by a radiologist as CAD detected 100% of malignancy microcalcifications versus 67% of malignant masses.[18] In summary, CAD is a promising new technique; although, its cost effectiveness is yet to be evaluated.

Breast Ultrasound Ultrasound of the breast is primarily utilized as adjunct to screening mammography to aid in the distinction between benign and malignant breast lesions.[19] Bilateral-whole breast sonography (BWBS) has been studied as a screening test mostly in women with radiologically dense breasts. BWBS is limited by the technical abilities of the sonographer. If a lesion is not noted during the examination, it will not be noted by a radiologist reviewing a hard copy of the study. In addition, ultrasound cannot completely replace mammography as a screening test because of ultrasound's inability to demonstrate microcalcifications.[19] However, Kolb studied 3626 patients with dense breasts noted on mammogram. BWBS increased cancer detection by 17%. In order to detect these additional 11 out of 41 tumors, fine needle aspiration biopsy (FNAB) or surgical biopsy was performed on 123 patients.[20] Gordon reviewed 1575 solid masses detected by ultrasound that were nonpalpable and occult on mammogram. Breast cancer was detected in 44 cases (2.8%) after 279 patients underwent FNAB.[21]

KEY POINT

Ultrasound is a complementary test to mammography and may be effective in radiologic dense breasts. Ultrasound has a decreased overall sensitivity for breast cancer detection relative to mammography.

In summary, ultrasound can detect breast cancer that is occult on mammogram particularly in patients with dense breasts. At this point, it is a complimentary test to mammogram as it has an overall sensitivity less than mammography. However, in premenopausal patients with dense breasts, particularly patients at high risk of developing breast cancer, ultrasound can be used as an adjunct to mammography for screening.

Magnetic Resonance Imaging of the Breast MRI of the breast has a sensitivity that approaches 100% and a specificity of 90%

in high-risk populations.[22] Given the high cost of this test along with its high specificity, it has mostly been evaluated in high-risk populations. MR imaging involves scanning each breast before and after administration of an intravenous contrast agent, gadolinium. Warner studied 196 women aged 26–59 years with either proven breast cancer associated gene 1 or 2 (BRCA-1), or (BRCA-2) mutations, or a strong family history of breast, or ovarian cancer who underwent mammography, ultrasound, MR imaging, and CBE on a single day. Six invasive cancers were detected by MR imaging, and only two of these cases were detected on mammography. Overall, 23 women were required to have a breast biopsy in order to diagnose those six cases.[22]

KEY POINT

MR imaging of the breast may be of value in high-risk patients.

MR imaging quality is not influenced by breast density, and thus may become the ideal screening test for those premenopausal patients at high risk of breast cancer. Often, these patients have breasts that are too dense for a quality mammogram. In addition, data suggest that patients genetically predisposed to develop premenopausal breast cancer may have breasts that are more sensitive to the effects of radiation.[23] MR imaging of the breast is not as sensitive for the detection of DCIS; although this lesion is less common in high-risk patients as compared to patients of average risk.[24] At this point, MR imaging of the breast, as a screening test, remains investigational.

KEY POINT

Ductal lavage should be viewed as a tool for surveillance of patients at increased risk of developing breast cancer.

Ductal Lavage Atypical ductal hyperplasia is a known risk factor for the development of breast carcinoma. In 2001, Dooley reported the use of a new technique, ductal lavage, to obtain a sampling of breast intraductal cells.[25] This study enrolled 507 women with increased risk of developing breast cancer—prior personal history of breast cancer, 5-year Gail model risk of greater than or equal to 1.7%, or BRCA-1 or BRCA-2 carrier. These patients underwent nipple aspiration, followed by ductal lavage of the ducts that produced nipple aspirate. All patients had a negative CBE and mammogram within the past year. Ductal lavage involves the cannulation of breast ducts followed by the infusion and collection of saline. Ductal lavage detected abnormal intraductal breast cells in 24% of patients versus nipple aspiration which detected atypical cells in 6% of patients.[25] Currently, there are no data on the sensitivity or specificity of ductal lavage for the detection of breast cancer. Thus, this technique is not considered a screening test for breast cancer. Rather, ductal lavage may be a test which can aid in the decision between surveillance mode or surgery for risk-reduction therapy in patients at increased risk of developing breast cancer.[25]

Patients at Increased Risk of Breast Cancer

KEY POINT

BRCA-1 and BRCA-2 mutations involve tumor suppressor genes that are inherited in an autosomal dominant manner. Carriers of BRCA-1 or BRCA-2 have a lifetime risk of breast cancer that range from 50% to 85% and an increased risk for ovarian cancer of up to 44%.

The identification of the Breast Cancer-Associated Gene 1 and 2 (BRCA-1 and BRCA-2) mutations in 1994 and 1995, respectively, has greatly improved our understanding of genetic predisposition for developing breast cancer.[26,27] Both genes are considered tumor suppressor genes involved in assessing DNA damage and/or repair. They are inherited in an autosomal dominant fashion. Ford presented data from the Breast Cancer Linkage Consortium which noted that in families with at least four cases of breast cancer disease was linked to BRCA-1 in 52% and BRCA-2 in 32%.[28] In addition, approximately 10% of patients under age 35, with breast cancer, carry one of these genes.[29] There are reports of hundreds of mutations in these genes, and most are unique to families. Two founder mutations are identified which mainly occur in patients of Ashkenazi Jewish heritage. It is estimated that the lifetime risk of breast cancer in carriers of BRCA-1, or BRCA-2 mutations is about 50–85% with 60% of these cancers occurring prior to menopause.[30]

The ACS lists the following as risk factors for carrying BRCA-1 or BRCA-2[31]:

- Two or more relatives with breast or ovarian cancer
- Breast cancer occurring before age 50 in an affected relative
- Relatives with both breast and ovarian cancer
- One or more relatives with two cancers (breast and ovarian cancer or two independent breast cancers)
- Male relatives with breast cancer
- A family history of breast or ovarian cancer and Ashkenazi Jewish heritage

Many models have been developed to estimate a woman's risk of developing breast cancer. The Gail model was developed prior to the identification of BRCA-1.[32] This model focuses mostly on reproductive risk factors and first-degree relatives with disease. The Claus model includes both first and second degree relatives with disease.[33] A more recent model, BRCAPRO, estimates a woman's risk of carrying a BRCA mutation.[34] The American

Society of Clinical Oncology recommends genetic testing for women with a risk of 10% or greater for carrying these mutations.[35] Unfortunately, as most mutations are unique to families, genetic testing is of more value if the index case of breast cancer is still living and willing to undergo genetic testing.

In 1997, the Cancer Genetics Consortium issued recommendations for screening patients with a known BRCA-1 or BRCA-2 mutations.[23] These recommendations are for patients at very high risk of developing breast cancer, and can only be extended to patients with predicted risk that is similar to the mutation carriers. BSE is recommended starting at age 18, and CBE is recommended either annually or semiannually starting at age 25–35. Annual mammography is recommended starting at age 25–35 years, taking into account the adequacy of the first study. As discussed above, ultrasound may be a useful adjunct to mammography in these patients. MR imaging of the breast may be an alternative but is still investigational.

Colorectal Cancer Screening

KEY POINT

Adenomatous polyps can be a precursor stage for colon cancer.

Colorectal cancer is another ideal disease for screening. It is the third most common cause of cancer death in women.[1] A person at age 50 has a 5% lifetime risk of developing colorectal cancer.[36] In addition, there is an identifiable preclinical stage, as 80% of colorectal cancers arise from adenomatous polyps.[37] About 20–25% of people at age 50 have colon polyps, and 10% of adenomatous polyps greater than 1 cm become malignant within 10 years.[38] The National Polyp Study demonstrated that identifying and removing adenomatous polyps reduced the incidence of colon cancer.[39] In addition to colon polyps, a family history of colon cancer in two or more first-degree relatives with colon cancer can help to identify higher risk individuals (see Table 22-1).

KEY POINT

The digital rectal examination is not considered a screening test for colorectal cancer.

Multiple screening tests are available to screen for colon cancer. These include fecal occult blood testing (FOBT), flexible sigmoidoscopy, FOBT and flexible sigmoidoscopy, double contrast barium enema (DCBE), and colonoscopy. These are addressed individually further. In addition, newer techniques including computed tomographic colonoscopy (CTC) or *virtual colonoscopy*, fecal DNA testing, and fecal immunologic tests are discussed. The digital rectal examination is no longer considered a screening test

Table 22-1. HIGHER RISK INDIVIDUALS

Higher Risk Individuals	
Familial Risk Category	*Screening Recommendation*
Two or more first-degree relatives with colon cancer, or a single first-degree relative with colon cancer or adenomatous polyps diagnosed at an age <60 years	Colonoscopy every 5 years, beginning at age 40 years or 10 years younger than the earliest diagnosis in the family, whichever comes first
First-degree relative affected with colorectal cancer or an adenomatous polyp at age ≥60 years, or two second-degree relatives affected with colorectal cancer	Same as average risk but starting at age 40 years
One second-degree or any third-degree relative with colorectal cancer	Same as average risk

Source: U.S. Multisociety Task Force on Colorectal Cancer guidelines.

for colorectal cancer. Recommendations from the U.S. Multisociety Task Force on Colorectal Cancer, the USPSTF, and the ACS are discussed. These recommendations are for *average-risk* individuals: no first-degree relatives with colon cancer or adenomatous polyps before age 60, no medical condition predisposing to colorectal cancer like inflammatory bowel disease, and no personal history of colorectal cancer or adenomatous polyps.

Fecal Occult Blood Testing

The U.S. Multisociety Task Force on Colorectal Cancer, the USPSTF, and the ACS all recommend yearly FOBT starting at age 50.[40–42] The guaiac tests are the most commonly used, and include brand names such as Hemoccult II and Hemoccult II SENSA (Beckman Coulter, Inc., Fullerton, CA). The test consists of three cards impregnated with guaiac. When treated with a developer containing hydrogen peroxidase, the cards give a color-coded result based on the presence or absence of peroxidase-like activity of the heme in the stool.[43] These tests typically require abstaining from red meat for 3 days and nonsteroidal anti-inflammatory drugs (NSAIDs) for 1 week before the testing. All societies recommend performing the FOBT on spontaneously passed stools. Three large randomized controlled trials have demonstrated decreased mortality from colorectal cancer with the use of FOBT.[44–46] There is one study that showed a comparable positive predictive value with FOBT performed at the time of a digital rectal examination; however, there are no data on sensitivity or specificity.[47] In addition, the three-sample protocol was developed based on the concept that colonic polyps bleed intermittently. All positive results should be followed up with colonoscopy.

KEY POINT

FOBT should be performed beginning at age 50. All positive fecal occult blood tests should be followed by a colonoscopy.

There are new immunochemical tests such as the !nSure FOBT, Hemeselect (SmithKline Diagnostics, San Jose, CA), and Flexsure OBT (SmithKline Diagnostics, San Jose, CA).[43] These detect the intact globin portion of human hemoglobin. This negates the need for dietary restriction; since hemoglobin does not survive passage through the upper gastrointestinal tract, this test is specific for bleeding from the colon and rectum.[43] !nSure FOBT was approved by the Food and Drug Administration (FDA) in 2001, and has demonstrated a sensitivity for colorectal cancer of 87% in a group of individuals at risk for colorectal cancer.[48] Unfortunately, this test requires the sample to be sent to the laboratory where the test is performed. The ACS has endorsed the immunochemical tests as acceptable alternatives to traditional guaiac-based tests.

Flexible Sigmoidoscopy

Flexible sigmoidoscopy ideally examines the distal one-third of the colon. The ACS, the U.S. Multisociety Task Force on Colorectal Cancer, and the USPSTF recommend flexible sigmoidoscopy in addition to the annual FOBT every 5 years for patients ages 50 and older.[40–42] Several case-control trials have demonstrated reduced mortality from colorectal cancer with screening sigmoidoscopy. Analysis of findings from colonoscopies on 2885 veterans suggested that a flexible sigmoidoscopy, followed by colonoscopy, if a polyp were found, would have identified 70–80% of patients with advanced proximal neoplasia. The decision to perform colonoscopy if polyps are found on sigmoidoscopy is complex and should be based on polyp size and histology.

Dual-Contrast Barium Enema

Dual-contrast barium enema (DCBE) is recommended as an alternative screening test for colorectal cancer by the ACS and the U.S. Multisociety Task Force on Colorectal Cancer with a frequency of every 5 years for patients ages 50 and older.[40,42] DCBE has several limitations. It has been shown to detect only 48% of adenomas greater than 1 cm compared to colonoscopy.[49] It also requires a bowel preparation. In addition, Dachman acknowledges that fewer radiologists are adequately trained to interpret the films.[50] This test is now performed less frequently.

Colonoscopy

KEY POINT

Colonoscopy appears to be the more sensitive technique for colon cancer screening.

Colonoscopy is recommended as a possible colon cancer screening test by the ACS and the U.S. Multisociety Task Force on Colorectal Cancer with a frequency of every 10 years for patients ages 50 and older.[40,42] Although it is more expensive, and involves slightly more risk to the patient, colonoscopy is more thorough than sigmoidoscopy as two studies demonstrated that approximately 50% of advanced proximal neoplasms had no distal colonic neoplasms.[51,52] Also, there is a trend of increased proportion of proximal neoplasia with increasing age and male gender. No test is perfect, however, as one study demonstrated: colonoscopy missed 6% of polyps greater than 1 cm.[53]

New Technology

Computed Tomographic Colonoscopy or Virtual Colonoscopy CTC or *virtual colonoscopy* uses a combination display technique combining both two- and three-dimensional CT images to screen for colon cancer. Studies have demonstrated sensitivities of up to 94% for polyps greater than 1 cm in high-risk individuals.[54] This test requires a bowel preparation along with distention of the colon with either room air or carbon dioxide gas. If a polyp is noted, colonoscopy is then required to biopsy the polyp. Another application of this test is to evaluate the proximal colon in patients with an incomplete colonoscopy.

Fecal DNA Testing Testing for altered genetic material in stool is a new screening technique. One study demonstrated a sensitivity of 71% for colorectal cancer in high-risk individuals.[43] More research is needed, but if this test proves to be reliable, it has the advantage of being noninvasive.

Cervical Cancer Screening

Papanicolaou Smear

Since the introduction of the Papanicolaou (Pap) smear, the rate of death from cervical cancer in the United States has decreased approximately 80%.[55] Cervical cancer is a prevalent disease, with approximately 12,200 cases estimated for 2003, and it has a detectable preclinical phase. Thus, cervical cancer is an ideal disease for regular screening. In addition, the 5-year survival for localized disease is 92% versus 32% for patients with regional spread.[55] With new information regarding the method of Pap smear collection, the optimal screening intervals, and the association of human papilloma virus (HPV) with cervical cancer, the ACS, USPSTF, and ACOG have recently released new guidelines for cervical cancer screening.

KEY POINT

Annual cervical cytological screening is recommended for women <30 years and every 3 years in those with three consecutive negative screenings.

In 2003, the ACS guidelines for cervical cancer screening recommend a Pap smear approximately 3 years after first intercourse or by age 21. Pap smears are then recommended every year with conventional Pap smear or every 2 years with liquid-based collection. At age 30, after three consecutive, negative Pap smears that are satisfactory for evaluation, screening should continue at intervals of every 2–3 years.[42] The ACOG recommendations published in 2003 agree with the ACS recommendations regarding the age of first pap smear.[56] However, ACOG recommends annual Pap smears for patients under age 30, not distinguishing between method of collection. In addition, ACOG extends the screening interval for women aged 30 and over to every 3 years with the previous negative history as above. Automatic HPV testing for women aged 30 and over is also considered "appropriate" as studies have demonstrated that women in this age group with both a negative Pap test and negative high-risk HPV testing were at very low risk of developing moderate or severe dysplasia over the next 3–5 years. The USPSTF also agrees upon the age at which to initiate Pap smears. It then recommends Pap smears at least every 3 years.[57] The recent change in screening guidelines regarding sexually active women under age 21 is based on evidence that HPV infection in these individuals is often transient and also that cervical cancer in this age group is rare.[58]

KEY POINT

After a complete hysterectomy (with removal of the cervix), cervical cytological screening should no longer be needed.

Of course there are exceptions to these extended screening intervals. Both the ACS and ACOG agree that women with a history of HIV, history of exposure to diethylstilbestrol, or women who are immunocompromised should be screened more frequently. ACOG recommends that women with HIV have two Pap smears in the first year after diagnosis and then annually. Also, women treated in the past for high-grade squamous intraepithelial lesions should continue annual screening.[42,56] All three organizations agree that after a complete hysterectomy for benign indications, Pap smears should no longer be performed. ACOG refers to a study of 9610 Pap tests performed after complete

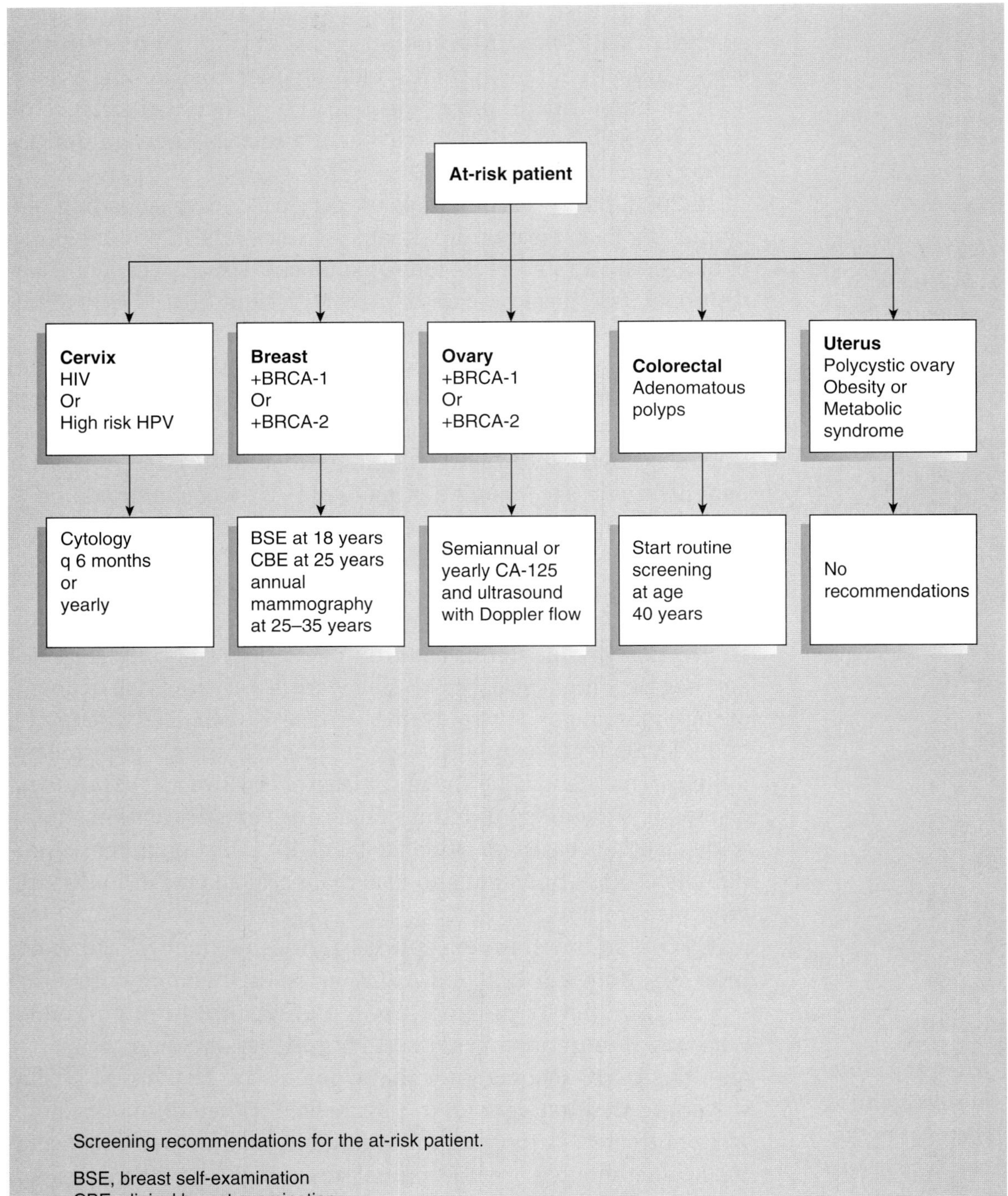

Screening recommendations for the at-risk patient.

BSE, breast self-examination
CBE, clinical breast examination
FOBT, fecal occult blood test
DCBE, dual contrast barium enema

hysterectomies for benign indications that identified zero cases of vaginal intraepithelial neoplasia grade 3 or cancer.[59] Women who had high-grade intraepithelial lesions of the cervix prior to hysterectomy should continue to be screened postoperatively for several years until three negative vaginal smears are documented. ACOG acknowledges that if the hysterectomy pathology and prior screening history cannot be confirmed, these posthysterectomy guidelines may have to be altered.[56]

New Technology

These guidelines allude to two more recently developed screening technologies: liquid-based collection and high-risk HPV typing. The impetus for developing new technologies is partially based on recent analyses estimating the sensitivity of a single Pap smear for a threshold of moderate dysplasia to be 58%.[60] Also, it is has been estimated that 25% of cervical cancers were not detected earlier secondary to errors in cervical sampling technique and interpretations of the findings.[61] In 1996, the FDA approved the ThinPrep liquid-based collection system. With this system, the Pap smear sampling device is rinsed in a vial containing a buffered alcohol preservative solution. The cells are then transferred to a slide for evaluation. Studies have noted increased detection of cervical dysplasia with ThinPrep compared to conventional Pap smears, although there is little data on specificity.[62] Another benefit of the ThinPrep collection system is the ability to perform high-risk HPV testing on the cells remaining in solution. HPV triage of Pap smears reported as atypical squamous cells of undetermined significance (ASCUS) was noted in the ASCUS/low-grade squamous intraepithelial lesion (LSIL) Triage Study (ALTS) to have excellent sensitivity (96.3%) in the detection of severe dysplasia.[63] Now more recent data indicates that HPV testing performed in conjunction with even normal cervical cytology improves sensitivity.[64]

In summary, cervical cancer is an ideal disease for a screening test. The Pap smear has been successful in significantly reducing mortality from cervical cancer in the United States. Now, efforts must focus on providing screening to all women in an attempt to decrease the percent of women diagnosed with cervical cancer who had not received screening within 5 years prior to diagnosis. Also, new technologies are aimed at reducing the number of women with cervical cancer who fell victim to a false-negative screening test.

Ovarian Cancer Screening

KEY POINT

The inability to identify the preclinical phase of ovarian cancer has made establishing an effective screening modality difficult.

Ovarian cancer represents the fifth most common cancer in women and is responsible for 14,300 cancer deaths each year.[1] Thus, it is responsible for more cancer deaths in women than cervical cancer and uterine cancer combined. A woman's lifetime risk is approximately 1 in 60. The median age of diagnosis is 59, and the 5-year survival is 52%.[55] Unfortunately, 75% of women initially present with advanced disease. Women who present with disease confined to the ovaries have a much-improved survival. Therefore, it would be very beneficial to develop an ideal screening test for ovarian cancer. Both the lack of specificity of the screening tests along with the unknown preclinical lesion of ovarian cancer has hindered the adoption of ovarian cancer screening (see Chap. 12).

ULTRASONOGRAPHY AND CA-125

The two main screening tests currently being evaluated in large trials are transvaginal ultrasonography and serum CA-125. Base et al. in 1984 first reported the identification of a glycoprotein, CA-125, that was elevated 10–12 months prior to the development of a stage III ovarian carcinoma.[65] Unfortunately, only 50% of stage I ovarian cancers have an elevated CA-125, and other diseases have been associated with an elevated CA-125 also.[66] In the only randomized controlled trial published to date on multimodal ovarian cancer screening, Jacobs et al. evaluated sequential screening with CA-125 followed by transvaginal ultrasound in cases of an elevated CA-125 (>30 U/mL) for postmenopausal women aged 45 and older.[67] He reported a positive predictive value of 20.7%, and a statistically significant increased ovarian cancer survival in the screened group. In the University of Kentucky Ovarian Cancer Screening Project, transvaginal ultrasonography, with an abnormal screen defined by ovarian volume and patient age, achieved a sensitivity of 81%, and a positive predictive value of 9.4%. More than 50% of the ovarian cancers were stage I. Overall, 180 surgeries were performed in order to diagnose the 17 cases of ovarian cancer.[68]

Two major randomized trials are underway to evaluate the use of serum CA-125 and transvaginal ultrasonography to screen for ovarian cancer in postmenopausal women. The United Kingdom

KEY POINT

Screening tests should not be done in patients at average risk for ovarian cancer.

trial of ovarian cancer screening (UKTOCS) is a randomized trial that commenced in 2001 involving 200,000 postmenopausal women aged 50–74 years randomized to either no screen, multimodal screen as described above, or transvaginal ultrasonography. The PLCO study, Prostate, Lung, Colon, and Ovarian cancer screening study sponsored by the National Institutes of Health (NIH), involves 74,000 women aged 60–74 randomized to annual CA-125 and transvaginal ultrasonography versus routine medical care. Both studies are powered to detect decreases in ovarian cancer mortality; however, results will not be available for several years.[69]

Patients at Increased Risk for Ovarian Cancer

Currently, the ACS and the USPSTF do not support a screening test for patients at average risk of ovarian cancer. A case for ovarian cancer screening can be made for those patients with increased risk of developing the disease based on family history. Approximately 5–10% of ovarian cancer cases are familial, and the BRCA-1 and BRCA-2 genes are responsible for most of these cases.[70,71] In addition, it was originally estimated that BRCA-1 carriers had a cumulative risk of ovarian cancer by age 70 of 44%, however, more recent data suggest that this was an overestimation.[28] Also, BRCA-2 carriers have a lower risk of ovarian cancer than BRCA-1 carriers. In 1997, the Cancer Genetics Studies Consortium recommended that female carriers of the BRCA-1 mutation and possibly the BRCA-2 mutation undergo annual or semiannual transvaginal ultrasonography with the addition of color flow Doppler and serum CA-125 testing commencing at age 25–35.[23] Prophylactic oophorectomy in these patients is also an option and the reader is referred to the Cancer Genetics Studies Consortium statement for further discussion.

KEY POINT

Women with BRCA-1 or BRCA-2 mutations should consider screening with transvaginal ultrasound using color flow Doppler and CA-125 annually or semiannually.

Finally, new molecular markers including both proteins and genetic material are currently under investigation including lysophosphatidic acid, mesothelin, and HE4.[69] It is hoped that the use of multiple markers will have improved sensitivity and specificity in ovarian cancer screening. (see Chap. 12)

Uterine Cancer

Uterine cancer is the most common gynecological cancer in women in the United States. It ranks as the fourth most common cancer diagnosed in women after breast, lung, and colon cancer.[1] Unfortunately, it still lacks a routine mass-screening tool. Most uterine cancers originate from the endometrium. The ACS concluded in its Guidelines for the Early Detection of Cancer that there was insufficient evidence to recommend screening for endometrial cancer for women with average or increased risk.[3] In concordance, the ACOG acknowledges that total population screening for endometrial cancer and its precursors is neither cost effective nor warranted.[72] Fortunately, 97% of uterine cancers involve the endometrium and hence announce themselves by abnormal vaginal bleeding. This prompts further investigation leading to the diagnosis. Seventy-five percent of women with endometrial cancers are postmenopausal, placing age as an important risk factor for the disease. Other risk factors include obesity, diabetes mellitus, hypertension, unopposed estrogen intake or anovulation, tamoxifen intake, and familial and genetic factors.[73] Both the ACS and the ACOG recommend that at the onset of menopause, women should be informed about risks and symptoms of endometrial cancer. Also, women are strongly encouraged to report any unexplained bleeding or spotting to their physicians.

What's the Evidence

- The sensitivity of one-time screening mammography has been estimated to be 71–96% with a specificity of 94–97%. The positive predictive value of an abnormal diagnostic mammogram, requiring biopsy, ranges from 12% to78%.[8]

  Analyses of at least eight randomized control trials of screening mammography in women aged 40–74 demonstrate approximately a 20–30% reduction in mortality from breast cancer with screening mammography.[8]
- For high-risk women with BRCA-1 or BRCA-2 mutations, the Cancer Genetics Consortium issued the following recommendations.[23] BSE is recommended starting at age 18, and CBE is recommended either annually or semiannually starting at ages 25–35. Annual mammography is recommended starting at ages 25–35 years, taking into account the adequacy of the first study.

- Three large randomized controlled trials have demonstrated decreased mortality from colorectal cancer with the use of FOBT.[44–46]
- The ThinPrep cervical cytologic screening has demonstrated an increased detection of cervical dysplasia compared to conventional Pap smears, although there is little data on specificity.[62] HPV screening of Pap smears reported as ASCUS was noted in the ALTS to have excellent sensitivity (96.3%) in the detection of severe dysplasia.[63]

Discussion of Case

CASE

A 47-year-old female presents for evaluation and treatment of vasomotor symptoms. She is of Ashkenazi heritage. In review of her family history, she has two maternal aunts with breast cancer and her mother died of ovarian cancer at age 48 years. She is an only child. The patient should consider which of the following tests:

- BRCA-1/ BRCA-2
- Cervical cytology screening
- Mammography
- Rectal examination
- Transvaginal ultrasound with Doppler flow
- CA-125 levels

Discussion

This woman meets the criteria as having risk factors for carrying BRCA-1 or BRCA-2 mutations because of a family history of breast and ovarian cancer and her Ashkenazi Jewish heritage. She should be counseled to the availability of BRCA testing and its potential implications if she is BRCA positive. Both genes encode for tumor suppressors and are involved in cellular surveillance for DNA damage and repair. Estimates for lifetime breast cancer risks for carriers of BRCA-1 or -2 mutations range from 50 to 85% with the majority of these cancers occurring prior to menopause. If the clinician is uncomfortable in providing key information, the patient should be referred to a genetics counseling center or a cancer center that offers genetic counseling services. If this patient is BRCA-1 or -2 positive, she should have mammography performed annually and a CBE annually or semiannually. MR imaging may be helpful in patients with dense breast tissue. If testing is negative but the patient is a BRCA carrier, hormone therapy for vasomotor symptoms should be considered with caution.

These women are also at increased risk for ovarian cancer with a lifetime risk of up to 44%. The Cancer Genetics Studies Consortium has recommended that these women be screened with annual CA-125 levels and transvaginal ultrasonography with Doppler flow of the ovaries annually or semiannually. Screening for colon and cervical cancers should follow routine guidelines.

References

1 Jemal A, Murray T, Samuels A, et al. Cancer statistics, 2003. *CA Cancer J Clin.* 2003;53:5–26.

2 Smith R. Screening fundamentals. *J Natl Cancer Inst Monogr.* 1997; 22:15–19.

3 Smith RA, Cokkinides V, Eyre HJ. American Cancer Society guidelines for the early detection of cancer, 2003. *CA Cancer J Clin.* 2003; 53:27–43.

4 Tabar L, Duffy SW, Vitak B, et al. The natural history of breast carcinoma: what have we learned from screening? *Cancer.* 1999;86: 449–462.

5 Smith RA, Saslow D, Sawyer KA, et al. American Cancer Society guidelines for breast cancer screening: update 2003. *CA Cancer J Clin.* 2003;53:141–169.

6 USPSTF. Screening for breast cancer: recommendations and rationale. *Ann Intern Med.* 2002;137:344–346.

7 American College of Obstetricians and Gynecologists (ACOG). *ACOG Practice Bulletin.* Breast cancer screening. Number 42, April 2003.

8 Humphrey L, Helfand M, Chan B, et al. Breast cancer screening: a summary of the evidence for the U.S. Preventive Services Task Force. *Ann Intern Med.* 2002;137:347–360.

9 Chang H, Cole B, Bland K. Nonpalpable breast cancer in women aged 40–49 years: a surgeon's view of benefits from screening mammography. *J Natl Cancer Inst Monogr.* 1997;22:145–149.

10 Ernster V, Barclay J. Increases in ductal carcinoma in situ (DCIS) of the breast in relation to mammography: a dilemma. *J Natl Cancer Inst Monogr.* 1997;22:151–156.

11 Elmore JG, Barton MB, Moceri VM, et al. Ten-year risk of false positive screening mammograms and clinical breast examinations. *N Engl J Med.* 1998;338:1089–1096.

12 Feig SA, Hendrick RE. Radiation risk from screening mammography of women aged 40–49 years. *J Natl Cancer Inst Monogr.* 1997;22:119–124.

13 Oestreicher N, White E, Lehman CD, et al. Predictors of sensitivity of clinical breast examination. *Breast Cancer Res Treat.* 2002;76: 73–81.

14 Thomas DB, Gao DL, Ray RM, et al. Randomized trial of breast self examination in Shanghai: final results. *J Natl Cancer Inst.* 2002;94: 1445–1457.

15 Lewin J, Hendrick RE, D'Orsi CJ, et al. Comparison of full-field digital mammography with screen-film mammography for cancer detection: results of 4,945 paired examinations. *Radiology.* 2001;218: 873–880.

16 Leung JWT. New modalities in breast imaging: digital mammography, positron emission tomography, and sestamibi scintimammography. *Radiol Clin N Am.* 2002;40:467–482.

17 Freer TW, Ulissey MJ. Screening mammography with computer-aided detection: prospective study of 12,860 patients in a community breast center. *Radiology.* 2001;220:781–786.

18 Warren Burhenne LJ, Wood SA, D'Orsi CJ, et al. Potential contribution of computer-aided detection to the sensitivity of screening mammography. *Radiology.* 2000;215:554–562.

19 Gordon PB. Ultrasound for breast cancer screening and staging. *Radiol Clin N Am.* 2002;40:431–441.

20 Kolb TM, Lichy J, Newhouse JH. Comparison of the performance of screening mammography, physical examination, and breast ultrasound and evaluation of factors that influence them: an analysis of 27,825 patient evaluations. *Radiology.* 2002;225:165–175.

21 Gordon PB, Goldenberg SL, Chan NH. Solid breast lesions: diagnosis with ultrasound-guided fine-needle aspiration biopsy. *Radiology.* 1993;189:573–580.

22 Warner E, Plewes DB, Shumank RS, et al. Comparison of breast magnetic resonance imaging, mammography, and ultrasound for surveillance of women at high risk for hereditary breast cancer. *J Clin Oncol.* 2001;19:3524–3531.

23 Burke W, Daly M, Garber J, et al. Recommendations for follow-up care of individuals with an inherited predisposition to cancer. *JAMA.* 1997;277:997–1003.

24 Orel SG. MR imaging of the breast. *Radiol Clin N Am.* 2000;38: 899–913.

25 Dooley WC, Ljung BM, Veronesi U, et al. Ductal lavage for detection of cellular atypia in women at high risk for breast cancer. *J Natl Cancer Inst.* 2001;93:1624–1632.

26 Miki Y, Swensen J, Schattuck-Eidens D, et al. Isolation of BRCA1, the 17q-linked breast and ovarian cancer susceptibility gene. *Science.* 1994;266:66–71.

27 Wooster R, Bignell G, Lancaster J, et al. Identification of the breast cancer susceptibility gene BRCA2. *Nature.* 1995;378:789–792.

28 Ford D, Easton DF, Stratton M, et al. Genetic heterogeneity and penetrance analysis of the BRCA1 and BRCA2 genes in breast cancer families. *Am J Hum Genet.* 1998;62:676–689.

29 Malone KE, Daling JR, Neal C, et al. Frequency of BRCA1/BRCA2 mutations in a population-based sample of young breast carcinoma cases. *Cancer.* 2000;88:1393–1402.

30 Barnes-Kedar IM, Plon SE. Counseling the at risk patient in the BRCA1 and BRCA2 era. *Obstet Gynecol Clin N Am.* 2002;29:341–366.

31 Smith RA, Saslow D, Sawyer KA, et al. American Cancer Society guidelines for breast cancer screening: update 2003. *CA Cancer J Clin.* 2003;53:141–169.

32 Gail MH, Brinton LA, Byar DP, et al. Projecting individualized probabilities of developing breast cancer for white females who are being examined annually. *J Natl Cancer Inst.* 1989;81:1879–1886.

33 Claus E, Risch N, Thompson WD. Autosomal dominant inheritance of early-onset breast cancer. *Cancer.* 1994;73:643–651.

34 Euhus DM, Smith KC, Robinson L, et al. Pretest prediction of BRCA1 or BRCA2 mutation by risk counselors and the computer model BRCAPRO. *J Natl Cancer Inst.* 2002;94:844–851.

35 Statement of the American Society of Clinical Oncology. Genetic Testing for Cancer Susceptibility, adopted on February 20, 1996. *J Clin Oncol.* 1996;14:1730–1736.

36 Winawer SJ, Fletcher RH, Miller R, et al. Colorectal cancer screening: clinical guidelines and rationale. *Gastroenterology.* 1997;112: 594–642.

37 Stryker SJ, Wolff BG, Culp CE, et al. Natural history of untreated colonic polyps. *Gastroenterology.* 1987;93:1009–1013.

38 Winawer SJ, Shike M. Prevention and control of colorectal cancer. In: Greenwald P, Kramer BS, Weed DL, eds. *Cancer Prevention and Control.* New York: Marcel-Dekker; 1995:537–560.

39 Winawer SJ, Zauber AG, O'Brien MJ, et al. Randomized comparison of surveillance intervals after colonoscopic removal of newly diagnosed adenomatous polyps. *N Engl J Med.* 1993;328: 901–906.

40 Winawer SJ, Fletcher R, Rex D, et al. Colorectal cancer screening: clinical guidelines and rationale-update based on evidence. *Gastroenterology.* 2003;124:544–560.

41 USPSTF Recommendations 2003. *www.preventiveservices.ahrq.gov* accessed 11/3/2003.

42 Smith R, Cokkinides V, Eyre HJ. American Cancer Society for early detection of cancer, 2003. *CA Cancer J Clin.* 2003;53:27–43.

43 Levin B, Brooks D, Smith RA, et al. Emerging technologies in screening for colorectal cancer. *CA Cancer J Clin.* 2003;53:44–55.

44 Mandel JS, Bond JH, Church TR, et al. Reducing mortality from colorectal cancer by screening for fecal occult blood. *N Engl J Med.* 1993;328:1365–1371.

45 Hardcastle JD, O'Chamberlain J, Robinson MHE, et al. Randomised controlled trial of faecal-occult-blood screening for colorectal cancer. *Lancet.* 1996;348:1472–1477.

46 Kronborg O, Fenger C, Olsen J, et al. Randomised study of screening for colorectal cancer with faecal-occult-blood test. *Lancet.* 1996;348: 1467–1471.

47 Bini EJ, Rajapaksa RC, Weinshel EH. The findings and impact of nonrehydrated guaiac examination of the rectum (FINGER) study. *Arch Intern Med.* 1999;159:2022–2026.

48 !nSure, Summary of safety and effectiveness. Available at *http://www.insurefobt.com/scientific03.html.* Accessed November 2003.

49 Winawer SJ, Stewart ET, Zauber AG, et al. A comparison of colonoscopy and double-contrast barium enema for surveillance after polypectomy. National Polyp Study Work Group. *N Engl J Med.* 2000;342:1766–1772.

50 Dachman AH, Yoshida H. Virtual colonoscopy: past, present, and future. *Radiol Clin N Am.* 2003;41:377–393.

51 Lieberman DA, Weiss DG, Bond JH, et al. Use of colonoscopy to screen asymptomatic adults for colorectal cancer. Veteran Affairs Cooperative Study Group 380. *N Engl J Med.* 2000;343:162–168.

52 Imperiale TF, Wagner DR, Lin CY, et al. Risk of advanced proximal neoplasms in asymptomatic adults according to the distal colorectal findings. *N Engl J Med.* 2000;343:169–174.

53 Rex DK, Cutler CS, Lemmel GT, et al. Colonoscopic miss rates of adenomas determined by back-to-back colonoscopies. *Gastroenterology.* 1997;112:24–28.

54 Hara AK. The future of colorectal Imaging: computed tomographic colonography. *Gastroenterol Clin N Am.* 2002;31:1045–1060.

55 SEER cancer database. *www.seer.cancer.gov.* Accessed November 2003.

56 ACOG Practice Bulletin. Number 45, August 2003. Cervical Cytology Screening. *Obstet Gynecol.* 2003;102:417–427.

57 USPSTF Recommendations 2003. *www.preventiveservices.ahrq.gov.* accessed 11/3/2003.

58 Ho GYF, Bierman R, Beardsley L, et al. Natural history of cervicovaginal papillomavirus infection in young women. *N Engl J Med.* 1998; 338:423–428.

59 Pearce KF, Haefner HK, Sarwar SF, et al. Cytopathological findings on vaginal papanicolaou smears after hysterectomy for benign gynecological disease. *N Engl J Med.* 1996;335:1559–1562.

60 Nanda K, McCrory DC, Myers ER, et al. Accuracy of the Papanicolaou test in screening for and follow-up of cervical cytologic abnormalities: a systematic review. *Ann Intern Med.* 2000;132:810–819.

61 Sawaya GF, Brown AD, Washington AE, et al. Current approaches to cervical cancer screening. *N Engl J Med.* 2001;344:1603–1607.

62 Lee KAR, Ashfaq R, Birdsong GG, et al. Comparison of conventional Papanicolaou smears and a fluid-based, thin-layer system for cervical cancer screening. *Obstet Gynecol.* 1997;90:278–284.

63 Solomon D, Schiffman M, Tarone R. Comparison of three management strategies for patients with atypical squamous cells of undetermined significance: baseline results from a randomized trial. *J Natl Cancer Inst.* 2001;93:293–299.

64 Sherman ME, Lorincz AT, Scott DR, et al. Baseline cytology, human papillomavirus testing, and risk for cervical neoplasia: a 10-Year cohort analysis. *J Natl Cancer Inst.* 2003;95:46–52.

65 Bast RC, Siegal FP, Runowicz C, et al. Elevation of serum CA-125 prior to diagnosis of an epithelial ovarian carcinoma. *Gynecol Oncol.* 1985; 22:115–120.

66 Kramer BS, Gohagan J, Prorok PC, et al. A National Cancer Institute sponsored screening trial for prostatic, lung, colorectal, and ovarian cancers. *Cancer.* 1993;71:589–593.

67 Jacobs I, Davies AP, Bridges J, et al. Prevalence screening for ovarian cancer in postmenopausal women by CA-125 measurement and ultrasonography. *BMJ.* 1993;306:1030–1034.

68 van Nagell JR, DePriest PD, Reedy MB, et al. The efficacy of transvaginal sonographic screening in asymptomatic women at risk for ovarian cancer. *Gynecol Oncol.* 2000;77:350–356.

69 Jacobs I. Discussion: ovarian cancer screening. *Gynecol Oncol.* 2003; 88:S80–S83.

70 Schildkraut JM, Thompson WD. Familial ovarian cancer: a population-based case-control study. *Am J Epidemiol.* 1988;128:456–466.

71 Risch HA, McLaughlin JR, Cole DEC, et al. Prevalence and penetrance of germline BRCA1 and BRCA2 mutations in a population series of 649 women with ovarian cancer. *Am J Hum Genet.* 2001; 68:700–710.

72 ACOG Committee Opinion. *Routine Cancer Screening.* Number 247, December, 2000.

73 Rose PG. Endometrial carcinoma. *New Engl J Med.* 1997;336:640–649.

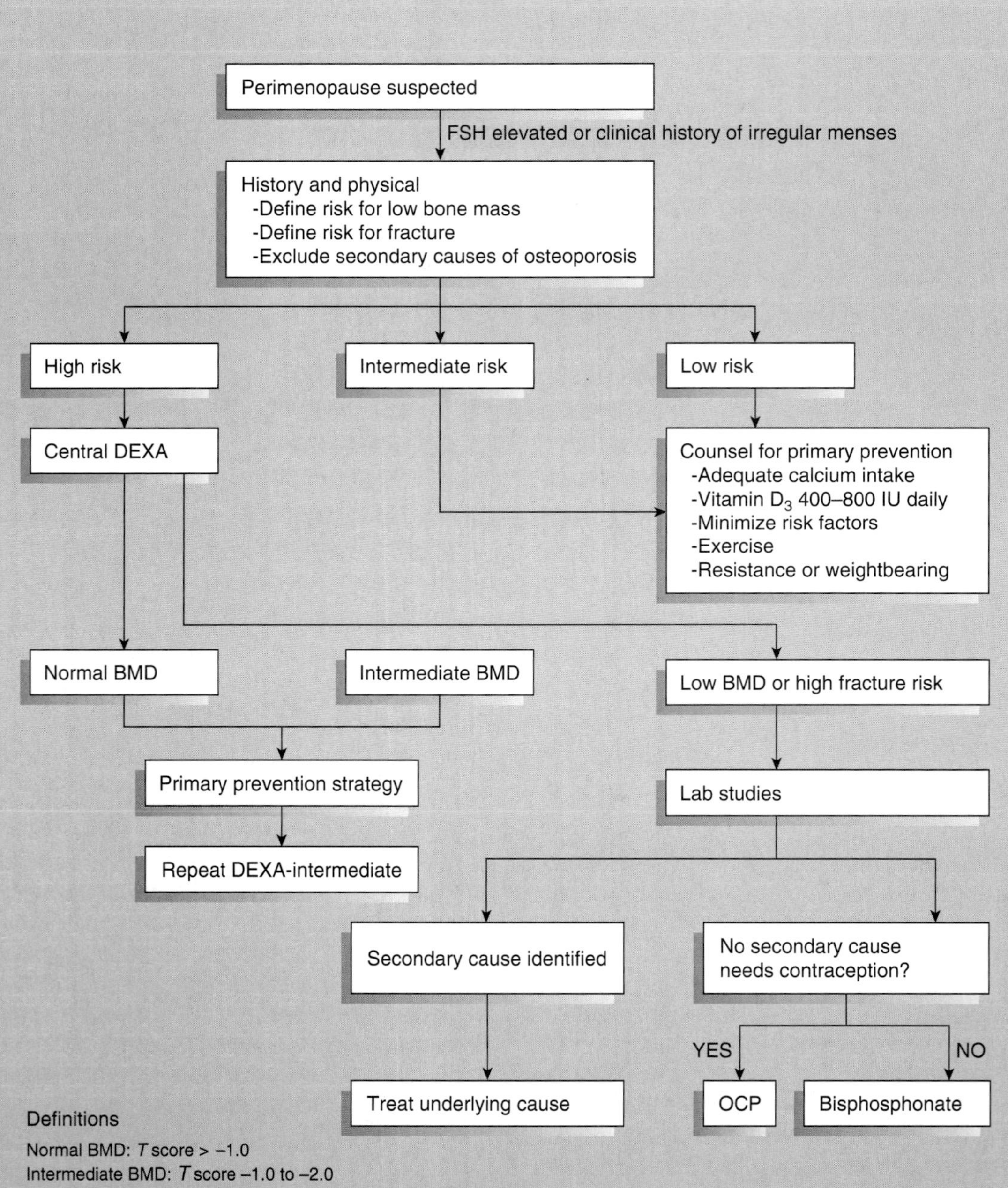

Perimenopause suspected
FSH elevated or clinical history of irregular menses
History and physical
-Define risk for low bone mass
-Define risk for fracture
-Exclude secondary causes of osteoporosis
High risk
Intermediate risk
Low risk
Central DEXA
Counsel for primary prevention
-Adequate calcium intake
-Vitamin D_3 400–800 IU daily
-Minimize risk factors
-Exercise
-Resistance or weightbearing
Normal BMD
Intermediate BMD
Low BMD or high fracture risk
Primary prevention strategy
Lab studies
Repeat DEXA-intermediate
Secondary cause identified
No secondary cause needs contraception?
YES
NO
Treat underlying cause
OCP
Bisphosphonate
Definitions
Normal BMD: *T* score > –1.0
Intermediate BMD: *T* score –1.0 to –2.0
Low BMD: *T* score < –2.0
High risk: Presence of two or more risk factors for low bone mass or fracture or identified secondary cause.
Intermediate risk: Presence of one risk factor for low bone mass or fracture.
Low risk: No independent risk factors for low bone mass or fracture.

23 Bone Health in the Perimenopause

Rebecca D. Jackson
W. Jerry Mysiw
Shubhangi Shidham

Introduction

Osteoporosis is a major public health issue facing postmenopausal women. The primary clinical consequence of osteoporosis is the fragility fracture. Low bone mass or osteoporosis contributes to an estimated 1.5 million fractures annually, including almost 300,000 hip fractures. Not only does osteoporosis result in pain, disability, and a reduction in the quality of life, but recent data suggest that both hip and vertebral fractures contribute to an excess mortality.

Although osteoporosis is a multifactorial disease reflecting a balance of environmental, genetic, lifestyle, and metabolic influences, the sex hormone milieu is a major factor influencing rates of bone turnover and bone loss. Thus, factors that influence estrogen exposure might have a dramatic and clinically important effect on subsequent development of osteoporosis and increased risk for fracture. Until recently, attention has been primarily focused on diagnostic strategies and interventions that prevent the bone loss after menopause, a time of dramatic declines in estrogen exposure. There is now an emerging body of data, however, to support a potential role of the perimenopause in the regulation of bone metabolism where perturbations in bone remodeling and bone loss can occur years before the development of significant estrogen deficiency. Careful evaluation and initiation of prevention and treatment strategies in high-risk individuals during this period of menopause transition might result in a substantial reduction of the burden of this common disease in the later postmenopausal years.

Epidemiology of Postmenopausal Osteoporosis

Osteoporosis is defined as a systemic skeletal disease characterized by compromised bone strength predisposing a person to an increased risk for fracture.[1] This current definition embraces the effects of bone mass, bone turnover, microarchitecture, and bone geometry as important determinants of bone strength that should be considered when assessing risk for fracture. In the United States, more than one in two postmenopausal White women will suffer at least one fracture due to osteoporosis during their lifetime.[2] In African American women, the fracture rate is approximately half as high.

The risk for bone loss and fractures after the menopause is increased in the presence of specific risk factors, some of which may be modifiable and a target for prevention strategies. The timing of the onset of the estrogen-deficient state of menopause has also been shown to have a significant impact on fracture risk years later. This concept might support early detection and intervention of women at risk for low bone mass or rapid bone loss at the perimenopause as early accentuated losses may have only a modest adverse effect on fractures in the immediate period but may lead to substantial burden of disease in later years.[3]

Pathophysiology of Estrogens on Bone Health

The quantity of bone mass at any time in adult life reflects the impact of the amount of bone attained during adolescence and the young adult years (peak bone mass) minus that bone which is lost through age, estrogen deficiency, or secondary factors. Estrogen plays a decisive role in both the initiation of bone growth and bone mass acquisition in adolescence and the rates of bone loss at the menopause transition. Lifestyle factors including physical activity and nutrition are also important components to achieving the peak bone mass and reducing rates of bone loss in later years.

The maximal attainable bone size and mass is genetically determined. During the acquisition of peak bone mass, the skeleton has its first vulnerable window when inadequate dietary calcium, immobilization, or decreased exposure to reproductive hormones could diminish the peak bone mass. This could clinically manifest itself years later as lesser skeletal reserve to accommodate menopause and age-related losses.

The bone mass remains relatively stable until the third to fourth decade of life when bone loss first slowly begins. Cross-sectional data, based on either clinical characteristics of perimenopause (as defined by irregular bleeding patterns) or transient increases in gonadotropin secretion suggest that bone mineral density (BMD) in perimenopausal women is reduced relative to that in premenopausal women.[4,5] Longitudinal data reveal that this lower BMD is a reflection of bone loss that occurs prior to the menopause.[6–13] Examination of the patterns of bone loss in the perimenopause suggest that although the magnitude of loss is greatest at sites rich in cancellous bone, significant rates of bone loss can be demonstrated at both the spine (1.8% per year) and hip (1.3% per year).[14] Since this is a time preceding the amenorrhea of estrogen deficiency, it has been postulated that anovulatory cycles and variations in menstrual patterns contribute to a hormonal pattern that is permissive to bone loss.[15]

As a woman enters menopause, her bone loss accelerates with the greatest decrement in bone mass occurring within the first 3–6 years of menopause. Rates of bone loss then slow in later menopause but continue through old age.

The advent of bone loss in the perimenopause with the accentuation of rates of loss in the early menopause reflects the effects of diminished estrogen and/or the accentuated gonadotropins on the process of bone remodeling. Bone remodeling is a dynamic process of self-repair and renewal that occurs at discrete bone multicellular units on the bone surface. The remodeling process has four basic steps: activation, resorption, reversal, and formation. Osteoclasts are recruited to the bone surface and in response to circulating cytokines, release proteolytic enzymes and acid onto the bone surface to digest organic matrix and dissolve bone mineral. Clinically, this resorptive phase of bone remodeling can be examined by measurement of breakdown products of Type I collagen (N-telopeptide [N-Tx], C-telopeptide [C-Tx], or deoxypyridinoline [DPD]). During bone resorption, there is also the release of a chemical mediator(s) that recruits osteoblasts to the bone surface through a coupled, coordinated process. During the slower process of bone formation, the osteoblast synthesizes collagen matrix (osteoid), which is then mineralized. Clinical assessment of bone formation can be performed by measurement of two serum markers of osteoblast function (bone-specific alkaline phosphatase [BSAP] and osteocalcin [OC]). For complete mineralization of the skeleton, an adequate supply of extracellular calcium and phosphate and sufficient 1,25 $(OH)_2$ vitamin D must be present.

At skeletal maturity in the young adult, the amount of bone formed is equal to the amount resorbed and bone mass is stable. However, any disruption of the remodeling cycle (increased or decreased activation of bone modeling, enhanced resorption, or diminished formation) can result in a net deficit in bone on completion of each cycle.

This imbalance in remodeling underlies the bone loss noted in response to estrogen deficiency at the menopause. As estrogen levels fall, there is an increase in release of interleukin-1 and tumor necrosis factor from peripheral blood mononuclear cells and interleukin-6 and granulocyte and macrophage colony-stimulating factors from osteoblast and stromal cells. The increased exposure of the bone microenvironment to these cytokines and growth factors results in activation of the osteoclasts with an increase in resorption. There is concurrent uncoupling of bone remodeling, with formation falling behind resorption that further accentuates the net loss of bone mass. Although there are less dramatic changes in estradiol during perimenopause, there are limited data to support that changes in bone remodeling, similar in nature although to a lesser magnitude, can occur during this early transitional period.

What is the Evidence to Link Changes in the Hormonal Milieu to Bone Loss?

KEY POINT

Markers of bone resorption are increased during the early perimenopause and remain elevated into the menopause.

The most consistent characteristic of the perimenopause is the presence of significant hormonal variability that can have a profound effect on bone remodeling and subsequent bone loss. In the early perimenopause, there is a transient rise in follicle-stimulating hormone (FSH) and inhibin during the follicular phase of the cycle associated with the higher percentage of anovulatory cycles. This higher FSH can drive the production of normal to higher than normal levels of estradiol in the luteal phase of the cycle.[16] As perimenopause progresses and a woman nears the time of menopause, the estradiol levels progressively fall. Thus, an evaluation of women in the perimenopause must consider the unique impact that these changing hormone patterns from the early to late perimenopause may have on diagnostic markers and choices of prevention and treatment interventions.

In response to perimenopause, there are significant increases in markers of bone resorption (DPD and N-Tx) and formation (OC and total alkaline phosphatase) that reflect increased bone remodeling.[14,17–19] With the transition to menopause, there are further increases in the magnitude of N-Tx suggesting that N-Tx might be a better reflection of the degree of bone remodeling and subsequent bone loss that is seen with the estrogen deficiency of menopause. In contrast, bone formation markers and estradiol are not significantly altered from premenopausal levels until menopause occurs.[19] Significant inverse correlations have been reported for markers reflecting increased bone turnover (BSAP, C-Tx, OC, and DPD) with 2-year change in BMD.[20]

KEY POINT

Bone loss in the early perimenopause correlates with increases in FSH.

The relationship between perimenopause and increased bone resorption is also supported by studies examining the effects of the perimenopause on the osteoprotegerin (OPG)- receptor activator of NF-kappa ligand (RANK-L) system. OPG is the decoy receptor for RANK-L and a potent inhibitor of osteoclastogenesis. Postmenopausal women have been shown to have higher circulating OPG levels than premenopausal women[21] and OPG levels directly correlate with age, urinary DPD, and FSH. There are also higher OPG and lower RANK-L levels seen in the perimenopause. Concordant with the association of OPG with higher rates of bone resorption in perimenopausal women, OPG directly correlated with N-Tx whereas the serum RANK-L is inversely correlated with OC.[22]

Examination of the effect of hormonal patterns on change in bone mass suggests that bone mass is lost prior to a substantial decrease in estradiol levels.[18,23] Rannevik and associates suggested that there was no significant association of hormone levels (as defined by estradiol) and BMD at the distal forearm.[24] Longitudinal studies have shown that perimenopausal women can lose up to 10.6% of their trabecular bone over 2 years, despite estradiol levels at 1 and 12 months that exceeded the mean values reported for premenopausal women.[19]

Bone mass in the perimenopause, however, is affected by the gonadotropin milieu.[5,18,23] For each tertile increase in FSH, there is a corresponding reduction in BMD[25] translating to a 0.5% decrement in BMD for each 5 mIU/mL increase in FSH. The reported relationship between BMD and FSH appears to be linear and is similar in women from all ethnic backgrounds. In contrast, there was no association of BMD with serum estradiol, total testosterone, or either free androgen or free estradiol index after adjusting for covariates.[5] These data support a role for changes in hormonal status as defined by FSH on enhancing bone resorption and contributing to a reduction in bone mass before the final menstrual period has occurred.

In summary, with the onset of perimenopause, there is an increase in some but not all markers of bone resorption relative to formation and attendant declines in BMD at both the spine and femoral neck.[19] The pathophysiology of this bone loss remains uncertain since it occurs before estrogen levels fall but the association with a rise in gonadotropins[5,18,23] suggests that a decline in follicle number or other subtle changes in menstrual function may underlie this effect. In the late perimenopause, data support that bone loss is directly related to estradiol concentrations and consistent with this relationship, OC has been shown to be a better predictor of bone loss than resorption markers in menopause.[12]

An important unresolved question is to determine if this early bone loss predisposes a woman to a greater fracture risk. There are no prospective data to support a direct effect of perimenopausal bone loss on increased fracture risk during the immediate perimenopausal period. There are however, some data to suggest that early, more significant bone loss, such as is seen with early menopause or premature ovarian failure results in a greater risk for fractures many years down the road.[3] Thus although data are limited at this time, it seems reasonable to consider that prevention of accentuated losses of bone mass at the perimenopause in vulnerable populations where peak BMD is low, might reduce the rate of fractures in later life when risk for fracture is clinically significant.

Evaluation of the Perimenopausal Woman for Bone Health

The guiding clinical questions used to assess risk for osteoporosis in a perimenopausal woman focuses on three specific issues. *What risk factors does a woman have that might predispose her to have a lower bone mass at she enters into the perimenopause? Are there any factors independent of bone density that might predispose her to a greater risk for fractures? Are there any secondary causes of osteoporosis that might predispose her to more rapid rates of bone loss?* The primary goal of the history and physical examination is to assess these risks to help determine the need for additional testing (Table 23-1).

FACTORS THAT CONTRIBUTE TO LOW BONE MASS

Low bone mass is an independent risk factor for fracture and BMD is utilized as a surrogate definition for osteoporosis. In any individual, the cause of low bone mass is likely to be multifactorial.

Table 23-1. **IMPORTANT RISK FACTORS ON HISTORY OR EXAMINATION**

LOW BONE MASS	*FRACTURE RISK*	*SECONDARY CAUSE*
Nonmodifiable	Skeletal factors	Endocrinopathies
Age	BMD and quality	Hypogonadism
Family history	Geometry	Hypercalciuria
Modifiable	Prior fracture	Hyperparathyroidism
Diminished estrogen exposure	Bone metabolism	Hyperthyroidism
	Increased resorption	Steroid excess (Cushing's)
Inadequate calcium intake	Low 25(OH) Vitamin D	Malabsorption
Excessive alcohol	Falls	Gastrectomy
Reduced physical activity	Frailty	Inflammatory bowel disease
Smoking	Fall mechanics	Celiac sprue
Medications	Cognitive impairment	Primary biliary cirrhosis
Glucocorticoids	Visual-proprioceptive disorders	Pancreatic insufficiency
Excess thyroid supplement		Neoplastic Disorders
Heparin	Medications	Multiple myeloma
GnRH agonist/antagonist	Obstacles	Hemoglobinopathies
Phenytoin	Other	Myeloproliferative disorders
Cyclosporine	Age	Gaucher's
Depo-Provera	Family history of fracture	Mastocytosis
	Low body weight	Inherited
	Cigarette smoking	Osteogenesis Imperfecta
		Ehler's Danlos
		Homocystinuria
		Osteomalacia
		Medications
		Other
		Immobilization
		Depression

Heritability or genetics accounts for 46–62% of the variance in BMD after adjustments for age, weight, height, and lifestyle. The impact of genetic factors is seen most dramatically during the acquisition of peak bone mass as bone formation rather than bone resorption appears to be strongly dependent on genetically-determined factors.

The second most important determinant of low bone mass is body weight and this accounts for 15–20% of the variance in BMD. Low body weight has also been shown to be a predictor of bone mass in the perimenopause. Although it had previously been hypothesized that the protective effect of high body weight is due to the higher body fat which can contribute to substantially higher estrogen levels and thus slower rates of bone loss in overweight and obese women, in the perimenopause, it is lean body mass that accounts for 38% of the variance of femoral neck BMD with no independent effect from the percentage of body fat.[26]

A reduction in estrogen levels occuring at menopause can result in increased rates of bone loss and diminished lifetime; estrogen exposure is an independent factor for low bone mass. Accentuated bone loss in the perimenopause, associated with higher FSH values[5] or a longer than average duration of perimenopause, might increase the risk for early development of osteoporosis.

Cigarette smoking has an adverse effect on bone mass through enhancement of estrogen metabolism and women who smoke transition into menopause at a younger age. Smoking has also been shown to be an independent risk factor for low bone mass at the perimenopause.[7] Alcohol has direct adverse effects upon osteoblast function and increases urinary calcium loses. Recent studies have suggested that heavy alcohol intake is deleterious to bone whereas moderate alcohol (<7 alcoholic beverages per week) is not.

Reduced physical activity can dramatically decrease bone mass as mechanical strain modulates bone formation. Physical activity may exert its greatest impact on osteoporosis through its regulation of the acquisition of genetically-determined maximal bone mass and size in childhood and adolescence.

Nutrition may also play a role in the pathogenesis of osteoporosis but there are limited studies examining the interaction of specific nutrients or patterns of eating with bone mass in the perimenopause. Epidemiological studies have shown that lifelong calcium intake is correlated with BMD at all ages. Factors that adversely affect calcium balance may also increase the risk for low bone mass including excessive caffeine intake, high protein intake, or excessive sodium intake.

There are also a host of other medical conditions that may contribute to excessive rates of bone loss and prematurely low bone mass and these should be considered during any risk assessment for osteoporosis. Most of these secondary causes of osteoporosis result in increased rates of bone resorption and bone loss and may be present at perimenopause. Autoimmune disorders such as subclinical hyperthyroidism present more frequently during the perimenopause or early menopause and can have adverse skeletal consequences. Depression has also been shown to be associated with a 7.8% lower bone mass in perimenopausal women.[27]

Factors that Directly Contribute to Risk for Fracture

Recent epidemiological studies specifically addressing the older postmenopausal woman have identified specific factors that may enhance the risk for a fragility fracture independent of their effect on bone density. These can be divided into factors that directly affect the amount and quality of the skeleton, bone metabolism, or increase the frequency and effect of falls. To date there are no data defining unique risk factors or confirming the role of these risk factors in perimenopausal women. Until such a time as an evidence-based recommendation can be made, it would be prudent to assess the four major risk factors for fracture identified in older women that might potentially define a higher risk subgroup of perimenopausal women: women with a prior history of nontraumatic fracture, a positive family history of fracture in a first-degree relative after age 50, current cigarette smoking, or body weight in the lowest quartile for age.

Data also suggest that rates of bone resorption may independently predict risk for fracture and in the perimenopause, increased rates of bone resorption are one of the first clinically apparent consequences of the changes in sex hormone environment. Due to inadequate dietary and supplement intake and use of sunscreens, the risk for low vitamin D stores may also be present and when significantly diminished, may be associated with more rapid rates of bone loss.

It is reasonable to conclude that factors that have been shown to affect peak bone mass or microarchitectural integrity will impact the subsequent risk for fracture throughout the life span but data defining the factors that might alter rates of bone loss in the perimenopause are lacking. Ongoing longitudinal studies such as the multiethnic Study of Women's Health Across the Nation (SWAN) that are examining risk factors and their affect on metabolic parameters through the perimenopause will help to better elucidate the clinical characteristics of women who may be at highest risk and deserving of more aggressive evaluation and follow up. Until then, use of those risk factors identified to be associated with osteoporosis in postmenopausal women will have to be judiciously applied in the clinical setting for the care of the perimenopausal woman.

Radiologic Studies to Define Bone Mass

BMD predicts fracture risk and estimates of the relative risk for fracture are typically based on the number of standard deviations that the bone density falls below the mean for a normal young adult population. In able-bodied postmenopausal women, there is an exponential rise in fracture incidence starting one standard deviation below the reference population. In general, for every 1 SD decrease in BMD, there is an approximate 1.8–2.2-fold increase in the relative risk for fracture at any skeletal site. Since low bone density is an excellent predictor of fracture risk, assessment of the BMD is the primary diagnostic method for osteoporosis.

Central dual energy x-ray absorptiometry (DXA) is considered the gold standard for determining BMD. Advantages of DXA include high precision, short scanning time, minimum radiation dose, low cost, and efficacy for follow up. Sites often assessed include the lumbar spine, hip, and distal radius, although the BMD at any skeletal site can be determined.

DXA scan results are expressed as areal BMD in grams of bone mineral content per cm^2 and are compared to two referent populations to generate the *T* and *Z* score. The *T* score, a comparison of an individual's BMD with mean values of 20–30-year-old White women, is expressed in standard deviations above or below this mean, whereas the *Z score* compares the BMD to a population of similar age, gender, ethnicity, and body weight.

Utilizing the well-defined relationship between the risk for fracture and bone mass, the World Health Organization developed three diagnostic categories based upon the *T* score: normal (BMD that is no more than 1 SD below the young normal reference population), osteopenia (BMD between 1 and 2.5 SD below the reference population), and osteoporosis (<2.5 SD below the reference population). However, it is important to realize that these criteria may have limitations for assessment of perimenopausal multiethnic populations of women as they have only been validated against databases containing primarily healthy postmenopausal White women. They therefore cannot be inferred to have the same degree of accuracy in reflecting fracture risk for perimenopausal women.

Lateral spine DXA scans are less influenced by degenerative changes and are sensitive measures of vertebral trabecular bone. Although there are data suggesting that the rapid cancellous bone loss in the perimenopause may be more easily evident on lateral DXA, there are no longitudinal studies to define the cut points necessary for consideration of intervention.

Peripheral x-ray absorptiometry techniques measure BMD at appendicular sites in distal radius or calcaneus. As peripheral bones are less sensitive to changes in BMD, peripheral DXA cannot be used for evaluation of treatment efficacy.

Quantitative computed tomography (QCT) is the only diagnostic method that can determine true volumetric density and may play a role in assessing bone mass in women with very small (or conversely, very large) bone volume. It can also isolate trabecular and cortical bone content and its greater sensitivity for detecting trabecular bone loss might enhance its utility as a tool for assessing bone mass in the perimenopause. However, because of the higher in vivo precision and accuracy errors and greater radiation exposure, it has had only limited clinical utility.

KEY POINT

There is insufficient scientific evidence to support universal bone mass screening at the perimenopause.

Quantitative ultrasound (QUS) has been developed as a measure of bone quality. As osteoporosis is a disease characterized by both reduction in bone mass and changes in microarchitecture, the measurements of ultrasound transmission velocity that are affected by trabecular separation, connectivity, and elasticity could discriminate structural changes in osteoporosis. It has shown some early promise in discriminating perimenopausal women at risk for osteoporosis but additional studies examining its long-term predictive value are needed.

Although there is consensus that densitometry techniques are reasonably precise and accurate, the primary clinical question facing the clinician is to determine which perimenopausal women are most likely to benefit from these diagnostic techniques. At present, there is no support for universal screening of perimenopausal women with DXA. Neither the American College of Obstetricians and Gynecologists (ACOG), the North American Menopause Society (NAMS), nor the National Osteoporosis Foundation (NOF) recommends routine BMD screening of perimenopausal women. A review of international guidelines on osteoporosis revealed that five of nine guidelines were opposed to uniform screening of perimenopausal women (INAHTA, European Commission, Canadian Task Force, British Columbia Office of Health Technology Assessment and United Kingdom Department of Health) with the other four agencies offered no recommendation citing insufficient scientific evidence (US Preventive Services Task Force, National Institutes of Health, Swedish Council of Technology Assessment in Health Care and Catalan Agency).[28] Based upon current evidence, DXA should be reserved for diagnostic or confirmatory purposes in individuals at high risk for low bone mass or fracture or those with evidence of an underlying health condition that would accentuate risk for bone loss and fracture. This information should be combined with other clinical and laboratory data where appropriate to propose a management plan.

Laboratory Evaluation

There are no evidence-based data to help determine the appropriate laboratory evaluation to assess risk for fracture in the perimenopause. Data support that FSH has an inverse relationship with BMD and explained the variability in BMD better than the clinical classification of irregular menstrual bleeding patterns. As a laboratory criterion suggestive of the perimenopause and a biomarker of risk for low bone mass, a follicular phase FSH might be helpful in stratifying risk, but it has not been demonstrated to correlate with fracture risk. It may have limited clinical utility in women with several risk clinical risk factors for osteoporotic fracture.

Estradiol levels less than 5 pg/mL are associated with lower BMD and increased risk for fractures, and thus assessment of total or free estradiol in specific late perimenopausal women may further define fracture risk. Its use in early perimenopause is limited by the wide fluctuations of sex hormones at that time. Both total and free estradiols are also limited in their utility as a biomarker of risk for bone loss as there is no defined threshold for estradiol where bone loss becomes evident.

Recent studies have shown that vitamin D deficiency is common and easily amenable to therapy. Measurement of 25(OH) vitamin D by methodology that allows for assessment of both D_2 and D_3 levels is an important factor in the clinical management of osteoporosis.

It might be predicted that markers of bone resorption (e.g., N-Tx, C-Tx, or DPD) and bone formation (OC, BSAP) would be helpful for assessing osteoporosis and guiding therapy choices but to date, their role in management of clinical osteoporosis is limited. However, the finding of an accentuated level of a bone resorption marker in an individual with low bone mass in the perimenopause might support consideration of medication for the prevention of bone loss.

Finally if treatment is planned, biochemical testing for renal and hepatic function, a complete blood count, serum calcium, phosphorus, and total alkaline phosphatase should be measured to screen for secondary causes of bone loss or factors that might influence treatment choices. In uncomplicated menopause or involutional osteoporosis, these lab studies will be normal. Additional testing as suggested by the history and physical examination should be performed to exclude secondary causes of osteoporosis when appropriate.

Option for the Prevention and Treatment of Perimenopausal Osteoporosis

Primary Prevention Strategies

The goal of primary prevention of osteoporosis is to minimize rates of bone loss during the perimenopause transition. These strategies should be discussed with all perimenopausal women. Prevention strategies should include avoidance of cigarettes, moderation in alcohol consumption, minimizing the use of medications that contribute to a negative calcium balance or bone loss, and assurance of regular physical activity and adequate calcium and vitamin D intake.

KEY POINT

Education regarding primary prevention strategies of adequate calcium, vitamin D_3, exercise, and smoking cessation should be given to all perimenopausal women irrespective of risk for low bone mass.

Recommendations for adequate calcium and vitamin D intake suggest a total daily intake of calcium from the combination of diet and supplements should meet 1000–1500 mg elemental calcium with vitamin D intake of 400–600 IU daily. Recent data suggesting the need to target 25(OH) vitamin D to 30 ng/mL or higher would necessitate vitamin D intakes of 700–800 IU daily. A recent prospective randomized trial has shown that the BMD in perimenopausal women supplemented with 500 mg calcium and 200 IU vitamin D daily was significantly higher than the BMD in women receiving placebo.[29]

Exercise stimulates bone formation directly and weight-bearing exercise contributes to the development and maintenance of bone mass. A systematic review of the efficacy of exercise for the prevention and treatment of osteoporosis among a diverse population of both pre- and postmenopausal women demonstrated trends suggesting that exercise increases or maintains bone density. Recent longitudinal data in women who remained physically active (jogging or volleyball) through the perimenopause showed no reduction in the rate of bone loss at the spine (–2.6% per year) or hip (–1.07% per year).[30]

PHARMACOLOGIC INTERVENTIONS

KEY POINT

Oral contraceptive use in the perimenopause will reduce markers of bone resorption and may slow bone loss, but have not been demonstrated to reduce fractures.

There are a number of medications that might be effective for preventing bone loss in perimenopausal women with low bone mass (defined as a *T* score <–2.0) or at marked increase for the risk of fracture (two or more risk factors for fracture or low bone mass or a secondary cause of osteoporosis). The best studied and probably most effective agent for the prevention of perimenopausal bone loss is hormone therapy (HT) formulated as an oral contraceptive. In contrast, there are no clinical trial data supporting the use of bisphosphonates or teriparatide in perimenopause although some insight into bisphosphonate use can be derived from prevention studies in the early menopause.

In oligomenorrheic perimenopausal women, low-dose oral contraceptive use has been shown to decrease urinary excretion of hydroxyproline (a marker of collagen degradation and bone resorption) and plasma OC with a reduction in bone QUS changes.[31] In addition, oral contraceptive use in the fourth decade of life has been suggested to reduce the risk of hip fractures in women decades later. Data from the Danish Osteoporosis Prevention Study in late perimenopausal and early postmenopausal women support greater BMD in HT users at both the proximal femur and spine.[32] They estimated that only 8.4% and 5.6% of women were nonresponders to HT at the femoral neck and spine, respectively, compared to 25% and 75% who were good responders to HT. Nonresponders were more likely to be smokers with low spine BMD and good responders were older, higher body weight and higher alcohol intake. Data from the 93,725 postmenopausal women in the observational arm of the Women's Health Initiative provided no support for a fracture benefit later in life for those women who had used oral contraceptives.[33]

Although the Women's Health Initiative has demonstrated that postmenopausal estrogen plus progestin is effective in decreasing the risk of clinical vertebral, wrist, hip, and total fractures, the increased risk of coronary heart disease, stroke, venous thromboembolism, and breast cancer has resulted in recommendation that other agents with a more favorable risk-benefit balance should be considered for the prevention and treatment of postmenopausal osteoporosis.[34] There are no comparable data available to assess the balance of benefits and risks of either oral contraceptives or HT for perimenopausal women. Additional studies carefully elucidating the effects of low-dose oral contraceptives in the perimenopause would allow women and their health-care providers to make informed decisions regarding their use. In an attempt to minimize these risks associated with oral HT, women have also explored the use of phytoestrogens as an estrogen alternative. In perimenopausal women, higher intake of genistein, a soy isoflavone, was not associated with higher BMD.[35]

Bisphosphonates, analogues of pyrophosphate, have consistently been shown to be effective agents for the prevention and treatment of postmenopausal osteoporosis. Alendronate, risedronate, ibandronate and cyclic etidronate have been shown to increase BMD at both the spine and hip in a dose-dependent fashion. They have also consistently resulted in a reduction in vertebral fracture incidence by 30–50% with efficacy that starts as early as 6–12 months after initiating treatment. Both alendronate and risedronate also decrease the rates of nonvertebral fracture. However, because fertility potential is still present in the perimenopause and bisphosphonate use might have a deleterious effect on fetal skeletal development, bisphosphonates should only be considered for use in perimenopausal women with assured birth control and no risk for pregnancy.

Calcitonin is a weak antiresorptive agent approved for treatment of established osteoporosis in postmenopausal women. At doses of 100 units subcutaneously daily, it has been shown to be ineffective at reducing bone turnover or BMD loss in the perimenopause.[36]

In summary, perimenopause is a time when patterns of sex hormones transition from fluctuating gonadotropins to decreasing estradiol culminating in loss of menses and menopause. During this time, bone resorption rapidly increases, at times to levels as great or greater than seen at menopause. Bone mass, primarily at cancellous or trabecular regions is lost at rates of 1–2% per year. Identifying perimenopausal women at high risk for osteopenia or rapid bone loss in the perimenopause through judicious use of DXA and laboratory studies offers the opportunity to initiate interventions to slow bone loss before the accelerated bone loss at early menopause puts them at greater risk for fracture for years to come. Although there are few evidenced-based analyses available to lay the foundation for recommendations, it is reasonable to apply the National Osteoporosis Foundation recommendations of initiating intervention in women at perimenopause who have significant reduction in bone density ($T < -2.0$) or in individuals with somewhat higher bone density but additional risk factors or an identified secondary cause of osteoporosis. HT has been shown to be effective at preventing bone loss. Although there are no clinical trials of bisphosphonates in perimenopause, their efficacy in preventing bone loss at menopause justifies consideration of their use in women with significantly diminished bone mass who are at no risk for pregnancy. These interventions provide benefit beyond that seen with ensuring adequate calcium, vitamin D, and regular exercise. There is evidence to suggest that the benefits of preventing further bone loss is these high-risk women might reduce the risk of fractures decades in the future and thus the morbidity and associated mortality of osteoporosis.

Guiding Questions

- Are there specific risk factors that can be identified that might contribute to risk for low bone mass or fractures?
  - Does the woman have a low body weight relative to age-matched peers?
  - Does she currently smoke?
  - Does she have a history of anovulation or menstrual disturbances that might contribute to early losses in bone mass?
  - Did she use hormonal contraceptives and if so, what types?
  - Is there a strong family history of low bone mass or fragility fractures?
  - Does she have a past history of depression or are there signs and symptoms of dysthymia present that might have an adverse skeletal risk?
- Are there biochemical features that put her at specific risk for rapid loss of bone mass?
  - If ordered, is the FSH sufficiently elevated to suggest a significant adverse risk?
  - Is she vitamin D deficient or insufficient?

- Are her estradiol levels markedly diminished? An estradiol <5 pg/mL places a woman at the greatest relative risk for bone loss and fracture.
- Is there any evidence of subclinical hyperthyroidism?
- Assessing primary prevention strategies
  - Is the total daily calcium intake (dietary and supplement) equal to or greater than 1000 mg elemental calcium?
  - Does the woman take a multivitamin or vitamin D supplement, drink milk or have sufficient sunlight exposure to ensure the equivalent of 600–800 IU vitamin D daily?
  - What is her current exercise regimen? Is there any impediment to an exercise regimen that would intermittently load the skeleton?
- Assessing the need for pharmacologic intervention to prevent bone loss
  - Is the bone mass sufficiently low (T score <–2.0) to place the woman at risk for significant bone loss or is her fracture risk for the next 5–10 years sufficiently high to warrant pharmacologic treatment?
  - Are there any secondary causes of osteoporosis that might accentuate her risk for low bone mass, bone loss, or fracture?
  - Is there any contraindication to consideration of oral contraceptive (or HT) use such as a history of breast cancer, coronary heart disease, or venous thromboembolism?
  - Does the patient have a reliable form of birth control that might allow for consideration of bisphosphonate use?

Discussion of Cases

Case 1

A 46-year-old White woman presents to your office to discuss her concerns regarding her risk for osteoporosis. She has begun to note irregular menses with cycle length varying from 25 to 40 days over the past year and some minor flushes occurring primarily at night. Her 68-year-old mother was recently diagnosed with osteoporosis after having a vertebral compression fracture. She wants to know whether she needs further evaluation to determine her risk for osteoporosis.

What diagnostic approach should you use first?

It would be important to know the potential risk factors that this women might have that would suggest that she is at risk for low bone density or increased risk for fracture. A careful history and physical examination focusing on risk factors for low bone mass, risk for fractures, and secondary causes of osteoporosis would be warranted. This is also an important opportunity to stress prevention strategies including modification of lifestyle factors, such as exercise patterns, nutrition, smoking, and alcohol intake and to teach her proper body mechanics to reduce risk for compression fractures. Measurement of baseline height with a wall-mounted stadiometer will come in handy in later adult years, as a loss of height of 1 in. or greater is the most sensitive finding of a new compression fracture.

During her history, you determine that she had a wrist fracture last year while walking the dog, used to smoke 1 ppd until 5 years ago and believes she is lactose intolerant. She tries to remember to take a calcium supplement at least once a day but rarely remembers to take a multivitamin.

Based upon these factors, is further diagnostic testing warranted?

ACOG, NAMS, NOF, and multiple other published guidelines do not recommend routine bone density screening of perimenopausal women. However, this woman has several risk factors that might predispose her to low bone mass and fracture. If information resulting from performance of this diagnostic test would affect the choice of treatment strategies employed, then it would be appropriate to order a central DXA of spine and femur.

She underwent DXA and was found to have a lumbar spine *T* score—1.5 and total hip *T* score—0.9.

What is the most appropriate treatment option based upon her clinical presentation?

Although she has had a personal history of fracture, given the modest reduction in bone mass, counseling regarding primary prevention strategies now would be appropriate. Given her age, clinical characteristics and bone mass, her current risk for fractures is low. Oral contraceptive should only be considered if initiated for contraception or symptom management rather than as primary intervention to prevent bone loss but if initiated should diminish bone loss during the transition. Checking the 25(OH) vitamin D_3 level might be warranted to ensure that she has adequate vitamin D stores. A plan for follow-up testing should be developed.

References

1 Osteoporosis Prevention, Diagnosis and Therapy. NIH Consensus Development Conference. Bethesda, MD; 2000:17:1–45.

2 US Department of Health and Human Services. *Bone Health and Osteoporosis: A Report of the Surgeon General.* Rockville, MD: US Department of Health and Human Services. Office of Surgeon General; 2004.

3 van Der Voort DJM, van Der Weijer PHM, Barentsen R. Early menopause: increased fracture risk at older age. *Osteoporos. Int.* 2003; 14:523–531.

4 Perrone G, Galoppi P, Capro O, et al. Lumbar and femoral bone density in perimenopausal women with irregular cycles. *Int J Fertil Menopausal Stud.* 1995;40:120–125.

5 Sowers MR, Finkelstein JS, Bondarenko I, et al. The association of endogenous estrogen hormone concentrations and bone mineral density measures in pre- and perimenopausal woman of four ethnic groups: SWAN. *Osteoporos. Int.* 2003;14:44–52.

6 Recker RR, Lappe JM, Davies M, et al. Change in bone mass immediately before menopause. *J Bone Miner Res.* 1992;7:857–862.

7 Sowers MFR, Clark M, Hollis B, et al. Radial bone mineral density in pre- and post-menopausal women: a prospective study of rates and risk factors for loss. *J Bone Miner Res.* 1992;7:647–657.

8 Fujiwara S, Funkunaga M, Nakamaura T, et al. Rates of change in spinal bone density among Japanese women. *Calcif Tissue Int.* 1998;63:202–2079.

9 Riggs BL Wahner HW, Meltin III LJ, et al. Rates of bone loss in the appendicular and axial skeletons of women. *J Clin Invest.* 1986;77: 1487–1491.

10 Recker R, Lappe J, Davies K, et al. Characterization of perimenopausal bone loss: a prospective study. *J Bone Miner Res.* 2000;15:1965–1973.

11 Citron JT, Ettinger B, Genant HK. Spinal bone loss in estrogen-replete calcium-replete premenopausal women. *Osteoporos Int.* 1995;5: 228–233.

12 Slemenda C, Hui SL, Longcope C, et al. Sex steroids and bone mass. A study of changes about the time of menopause. *J Clin Invest.* 1987; 80:1261–1269.

13 Pouilles JM, Tremollieres F, Ribot C. The effects of menopause on longitudinal bone loss from the spine. *Calcif Tissue Int.* 1993;52: 340–343.

14 Seifert-Klauss V, Mueller JE, Luppa P, et al. Bone metabolism during the perimenopause transition: a prospective study. *Maturitas.* 2002; 41:23–33.

15 Sowers MFR, Galuska D. Epidemiology of bone mass in premenopausal women. *Epidemiol Rev.* 1993;15: 374–398.

16 Prior J. Perimenopause: the complex endocrinology of the menopausal transition. *Endocr Rev.* 1998;19:397–428.

17 Hoshino H, Kushida K, Takahashi M, et al. Changes in levels of biochemical markers and ultrasound indices of os calcis across the menopause transition. *Osteoporos Int.* 2000;11:128–133.

18 Ebeling P, Atley LM, Guthrie JR, et al. Bone turnover markers and bone density across the menopause transition. *J Clin Endocrinol Metab.* 1996;81:3366–3371.

19 Seifert-Klauss V, Laakmann J, Rattenhuber J, et al. Bone metabolism, bone density and estrogen levels in perimenopause: a prospective, 2-year study. *Zentrabl Gynakol.* 2005;127:132–139.

20 Rosenbrock H, Seifert-Klauss V, Kaspar S, et al. Changes of biochemical bone markers during the menopause transition. *Clin Chem Lab Med.* 2002;40:143–151.

21 Oh KW, Rhee EJ, Lee WY, et al. The relationship between circulating osteoprotegerin levels and bone mineral metabolism in healthy women. *Clin Endocrinol.* 2004;61:244–249.

22 Jacka FN, Zhao HY, Ning G, et al. Relationships between the changes of serum levels of OPG and RANK-L with age, menopause, bone biochemical markers and bone mineral density in Chinese women aged 20–75. *Calcif Tissue Int.* 2005;76:1–6.

23 Nilas L, Christiansen C. The pathophysiology of peri- and postmenopausal bone loss. *Br J Obstet Gynaecol.* 1989;96:580–587.

24 Ravennik G, Jeppson S, Johnell O, et al. A longitudinal study of the perimenopause transition: altered profiles of steroid and pituitary hormones, SHBG and bone mineral density. *Maturitas.* 1995;21: 103–113.

25 Garton M, Martin J, New S, et al. Bone mass and metabolism in women aged 45–55. *Am J Clin Nutr.* 1996;44:563–570.

26 Li S, Wagner R, Holm K, et al. et al. Relationship between soft tissue body composition and bone mass in perimenopausal women. *Maturitas.* 2004;47:99–105.

27 Jacka FN, Pasco JA, Henry MJ, et al. Depression and bone mineral density in a community sample of perimenopausal women: Geelong Osteoporosis Study. *Menopause.* 2005;12:88–91.

28 Rossignol M, Moride Y, Perreault S, et al. Recommendations for the prevention of osteoporosis and frailty fractures: international comparison and synthesis. *Int J Technol Assess Health Care.* 2002;18: 597–610.

29 DiDaniele N, Carbonelli MG, Candelero N, et al. Effect of supplementation of calcium and vitamin D on bone mineral density and bone mineral content in peri- and pos-menopause women; a double-blind, randomized controlled trial. *Pharmacol Res.* 2004;50:637–641.

30 Goto S, Shigeta H, Hyakutake S, et al. Comparison of menopause-related changes in bone mineral density of the lumbar spine and the proximal femur in Japanese female athletes: a long-term longitudinal study using dual-energy X-ray absorptiometry. *Calcif Tissue Int.* 1996;59:461–465.

31 Gambacciani M, Cappagli B, Ciaponi M, et al. Hormone replacement therapy in the perimenopause: effect of a low dose oral contraceptive preparation on bone quantitative ultrasound characteristics. *Menopause.* 1999;6:43–48.

32 Rejnmark L, Vestergaard P, Tofteng CL, et al. Response rates to oestrogen treatment in perimenopausal women: 5-year data from the Danish Osteoporosis Prevention Study (DOPS). *Maturitas.* 2004;48:307–320.

33 Barad D, Kooperberg C, Wactawski-Wende J, et al. Prior oral contraception and postmenopausal fracture: a Women's Health Initiative observational cohort study. *Fertil Steril.* 2005;84:374–383.

34 Writing group for the Women's Health Initiative Investigators. Risks and benefits of estrogen plus progestin in healthy postmenopausal women: principal results from the Women's Health Initiative randomized controlled trial. *JAMA.* 2002;288:321–333.

35 Greendale GA, FitzGerald G, Huang MH, et al. Dietary soy isoflavones and bone mineral density: results from the Study of Women's Health Across the Nation. *Am J Epidemiol.* 2002;155:746–754.

36 Arnala I, Saastamoinen J, Alhava EM. Salmon calcitonin in the prevention of bone loss at perimenopause. *Bone.* 1996;18:629–632.

24 Alternative Medicine Use

Maida Taylor

Introduction

In the wake of the Women's Health Initiative, women bothered by the symptoms of the climacteric are now also bewildered by abrupt shifts in the view of hormone therapy. Many have turned to nonprescription therapy. The abuse and misuse of the term *natural* hormone has escalated dramatically and the promotion of alternatives to hormone therapy has also accelerated. As women become increasingly distrustful of doctors, drugs, drug companies, and the whole medical establishment, they unjustifiably assume that over-the-counter supplements and botanicals are safe and effective, just because they are on store shelves. They often buy expensive products with little or no evidence of efficacy and no documentation of safety.

KEY POINT

Alternative medicine encompasses several systematic medical practices based on physical assessments that differ from the physiology used in Western medicine.

This confluence of events makes it ever more important for practicing physicians and other providers of health services to be knowledgeable about complementary and alternative practices, or at the least, be able to secure adequate information from reliable sources in a timely and efficient manner.

Defining Complementary and Alternative Medicine

Alternative medicine encompasses several systematic medical practices based on physical assessments that differ from those used in Western medicine. Examples include traditional Chinese medicine (TCM), a system defining health in terms of the balance of an essential life force called Qi (pronounced Chee). Acupuncture is said to support wellness and to treat disease by regulating the flow of Qi along meridians that course through the body. Mind-body systems of medicine support health by using conscious and unconscious influences of mind over bodily processes. Manipulative and body-based practices include chiropractic, osteopathy, and massage. Meditation, hypnosis, music, and prayer fall into the area of mind-body practice. Somewhat related to mind-body medicine are so-called energy modulating modalities, which supposedly reorder bioelectric fields of the body. Examples include therapeutic touch, Qi Gong treatment, and magnets. The most recognizable and widely employed practices are biologic-based therapies like botanical medicines, dietary supplements, vitamins, minerals, and orthomolecular medicine.

Extent of Usage of CAM

CAM practice can be narrowly defined, restricting the rubric to the use of unconventional therapies. CAM can also be sweepingly broad in scope, when the term is used to include diet, nutrition, prayer, and the use of vitamins and mineral supplements. Depending on the definition, estimates of CAM usage range from less than 10% to over 60%.

The Federal Food and Drug Administration (FDA) in the United States restricts the advertising claims that vitamin and supplement manufacturers can make; nonetheless, overtly and covertly, the purveyors promise benefits far beyond those allowed by the FDA. *Mood* suggests treatment of depression, *prostate health* means therapy for benign prostatic hypertrophy, two therapeutic claims that may, in fact, be true for some botanical offerings. The line between fact and fiction begins to blur as claims for *appetite control* appear to promise weight loss without diet or exercise; *wellness* means suspending the aging process, and *high fiber* means cancer prevention.

Appeal of CAM

Users of alternatives are not dissatisfied with conventional allopathic medicine. Astin[1] (1998) questioned over 1000 individuals about the use of alternative medicine. The highest rates of use occurred in persons age 35–49 and 50–64, 42% and 44%, respectively. Reasons for using CAM include (1) dissatisfaction with conventional medicine as ineffective, impersonal, overly technological or costly, or yielding adverse outcomes; (2) A need for personal control, viewing alternatives as less authoritarian, more empowering, and affording greater personal autonomy; (3) philosophical congruence, a perception that alternatives are more compatible with personal values and personal ethical and religious beliefs. Users of alternatives have higher levels of education, but somewhat poorer health status. They claimed to be more holistic in their orientation to health, and are also more likely to have had a transformational experience impacting their view of the world and their values. Many had chronic health conditions like anxiety, back problems, chronic pain, and urinary tract that are often poorly managed by conventional medical care. Individuals who hold beliefs and values consistent with environmentalism, feminism, spirituality, and personal growth psychology are also more likely to use CAM.

Common CAM Treatments

While every system within the CAM world offers interventions to address symptoms of the climacteric, the most commonly employed systems are botanical medicine, so-called natural plant-based hormones, and mind-body therapies, which include meditation, movement, or a combination of both.

While the term *herbal* defines medicines made from the herbaceous portions of plants, namely the leaves and stems, *botanical* denotes foods and supplements made from any plant part—leaves, stems, seeds, fruits, flowers, and roots. Estimates are that 30% of our current pharmacopoeia is derived from old plant medicines, still grown in open fields, or a phytochemical that is now synthesized in the laboratory setting. Different plants are used for different therapeutic purposes, and different parts of the same plant may be used for different complaints. In discussing the role of CAM in treating the perimenopausal woman, most of the information will center on botanical medicines as interventions.

Estimates are that between 30% and 60% of women are using alternative interventions for menopause, including so-called *natural* estrogens; plant estrogens (which should be termed *phyto-SERMs*, since they function as selective estrogen receptor modulators); herbal medicines and acupuncture. Botanicals, herbals, and many steroid products are sold over the counter and

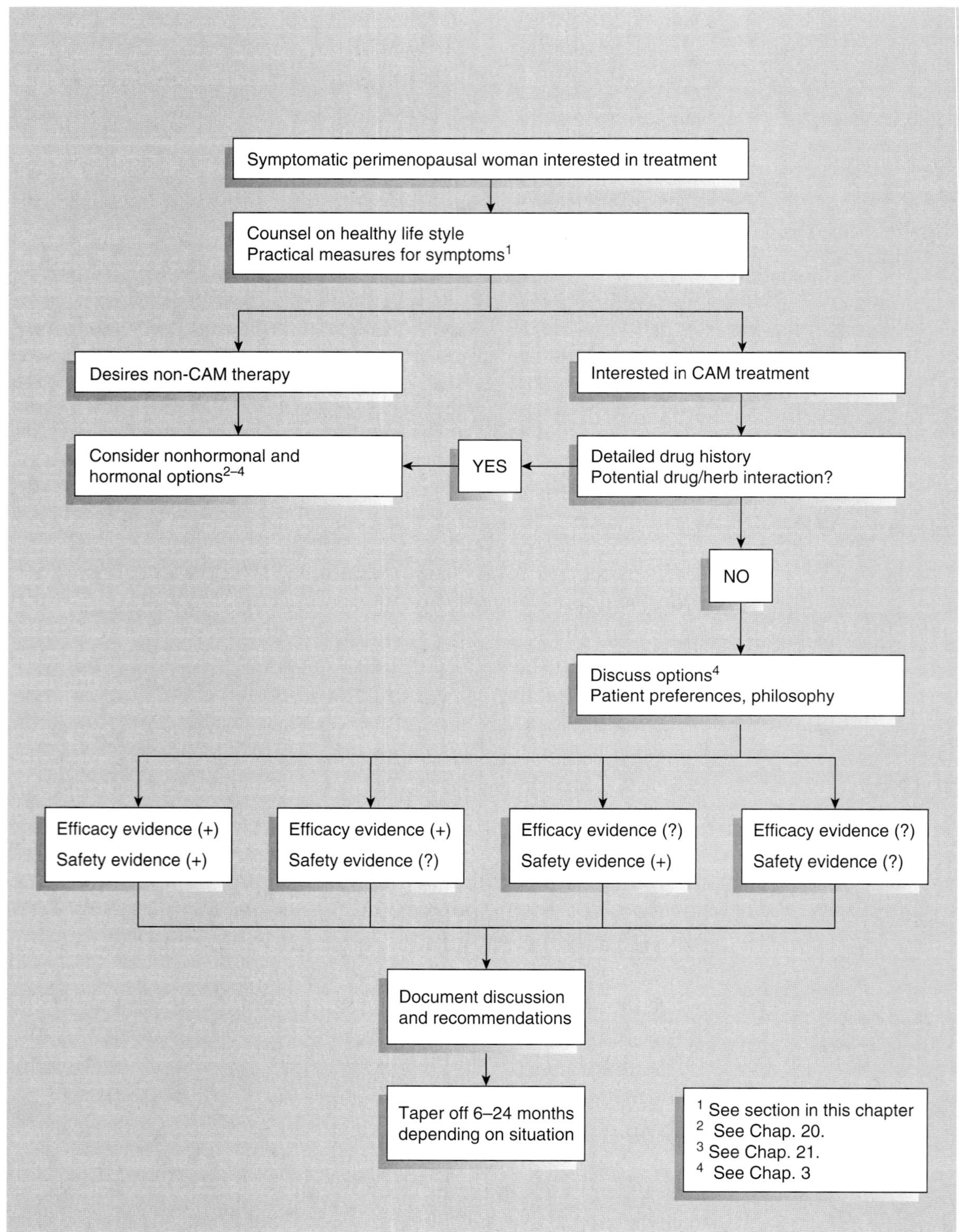
Symptomatic perimenopausal woman interested in treatment
Counsel on healthy life style
Practical measures for symptoms[1]
Desires non-CAM therapy
Interested in CAM treatment
Consider nonhormonal and hormonal options[2–4]
YES
Detailed drug history
Potential drug/herb interaction?
NO
Discuss options[4]
Patient preferences, philosophy
Efficacy evidence (+)
Safety evidence (+)
Efficacy evidence (+)
Safety evidence (?)
Efficacy evidence (?)
Safety evidence (+)
Efficacy evidence (?)
Safety evidence (?)
Document discussion and recommendations
Taper off 6–24 months depending on situation
1 See section in this chapter
2 See Chap. 20.
3 See Chap. 21.
4 See Chap. 3

some do in fact provide clinically significant impact on hormonal functions. Despite scant clinical study, many people believe botanical medicines are safe and effective because of their long history of use. In other words, persistence of a practice is assumed to be adequate proof.

Research and Regulatory Issues Relating to Botanical Medicines

Consumer demand, coupled with the support of the U.S. Congress, led to legislation that has helped to cement the seeming legitimacy of complementary and alternative medicine (CAM) in the United States. In 1992, the office of Alternative Medicine was started as a branch of the National Institutes of Health, with minimal funding, $2 million, and even that small amount was thought by many to be a waste of tax money. Now, the National Center for CAM, with a budget of $89 million, has become a major provider of funding for research on CAM practices. The Dietary Supplement Health and Education Act (DSHEA) exempts botanical medicines from drug regulatory processes by classifying them as dietary supplements. Supplements can be sold without oversight and testing by the FDA. Unfortunately, in contradistinction to pharmaceutical products, which are required to document efficacy and safety as part of the drug approval process, botanical medicines are exempt. And in fact, the burden of proof lies with the agency to demonstrate lack of efficacy and lack of safety. This mandate is unfunded. In January 2005, the Institute of Medicine issued a report that called upon Congress to work toward amending DSHEA in order to achieve quality-control standards and more accurate labeling in this field (*http://national-academies.org*).

Toxicity, Contamination, and Adulteration

Adulteration and contamination are not uncommon. Study of Chinese patent medicines in California found 30% adulterated with pharmaceuticals; herbal cold remedies contained pseudoephedrine, aphrodisiacs were topped off with methyl testosterone, arthritis remedies tested positive for ibuprofen.[2] Moreover, botanical medicines may vary in potency with climatic and seasonal growing conditions and variable processing. Different lots from the same manufacturer may vary widely, and products from different manufacturers also vary greatly. Contamination may occur during growing, picking, processing, and packaging.

Estimates are that only 10% of adverse reactions to prescription drugs are reported, and it is estimated that less than 1% of

KEY POINT

Incidence of an adverse reaction in 1 in 1000 users means one has to treat 4800 patients to see two events

such events are reported for alternative treatments. Traditionalists claim experiential evidence of safety for alternative remedies is sufficient. Recently, DeSmet defined just how little an individual practitioner would really know from personal clinical experience. Data collection and study are essential if we are to protect patients from unsafe practices. "If a herb caused an adverse reaction in 1 in 1000 users, a traditional healer would have to treat 4800 patients with that herb (i.e., one new patient every single working day for more than 18 years) to have a 95 percent chance of observing the reaction in more than one user."[3]

Problems inherent in botanical medicines include the following:[4,5]

- Quality
- Efficacy
- Safety
- Lack of standardization
- Adulteration
- Potential drug-herb interactions
- Lack of reporting of adverse events
- Variation in active constituents batch to batch, season to season, and so forth.

Chaparral has been associated with nonviral hepatitis, and fulminant liver failure requiring transplant. Comfrey, commonly brewed as a tea, is known to cause lung, kidney, gastrointestinal (GI), and hepatic toxicity. Recently regulators and health workers have called for a ban on ephedra (Ma Huang), an herbal with adrenergic activity used as a stimulant (herbal ecstasy), and weight loss aid, after numerous deaths across the United States. Ephedra has been associated with palpitations, arrhythmias, stroke, psychosis, and hypertension. *Lobelia* (Indian tobacco) can cause autonomic dysfunction with resultant respiratory depression, hypotension, coma, and death. Other serious or potentially lethal botanical medicines are listed in De Smet's excellent summary.[4] Other problems recently reported in the literature include the following:

- Contamination of PC Spes, an herbal to treat prostate problems. In one report, the product was contaminated with warfarin, since both pills were packed on the same production line.

In another instance, the drug was contaminated with alprazolam (Xanax). And finally some lots have been found to contain indomethacin and diethylstilbestrol.[6] The FDA ordered a nationwide recall of PC Spes because of the possible contamination.

- Examination of *Echinacea* products by an independent testing laboratory in 2001 found highly variable amounts of the phenolic compounds between brands and between lots of a single brand. *Echinacea* and other herbals have been found to contain wide ranges of organochlorine pesticides, lead, arsenic, and other heavy metals, particularly in products grown in India and China. Researchers at the National Institutes of Health recently looked for sourcing of product for a clinical trial of glucosamine and chondroitin for treatment of arthritis. They could not find a producer capable of producing consistent batches. The NIH manufactured the product used in the trial.

These are just a few representative cases of the problems inherent in using botanical medicines. This emphasizes the need to identify high quality products from reliable manufacturers.

On February 28th, 2004, the FDA and the Department of Health and Human Services jointly announced a ban on ephedra.[7] The action was prompted by review of some 16,000 adverse event reports. A RAND review of cases enumerated two deaths, four heart attacks, nine strokes, one seizure, and five psychiatric cases involving ephedra with no other contributing factors. The FDA press release cited a study that noted while "ephedra-products make up less than one percent of all dietary supplement sales, these products account for 64 percent of adverse events associated with dietary supplements." The director of FDA issued a special warning about use of ephedra during intense athletic activity, use with caffeine and other stimulants, use by persons on diets that stress the cardiovascular system, and use in those under age 18. A special word of caution also needs to be added about persons with eating disorders, body-image disorders, and mood disorders. These are the patients who are likely to abuse ephedra and who are also likely to manifest a high rate of severe adverse events. This move by the FDA is a bold step toward protecting the public health from commercialism. Sincere but misguided overpromotion of products and bold-faced fraud short circuit our ability to validate the scientific utility of CAM modalities.

Use of CAM for Hot Flushes

Soy Foods and Isoflavone Isolates

KEY POINT

Study designs vary greatly with different entry criteria, different treatments, different patient populations.

The use of soy in perimenopausal women has not been specifically addressed. Studies of soy have included only postmenopausal women. The results are mixed. The outcomes are difficult to compare since there are different amounts of soy protein in differing food stuffs with different amounts of the active component, the isoflavones. Moreover, studies have been of very short duration, often less than 3 months. Representative studies include Washburn,[8] where women were given 20 g soy protein with 34 mg isoflavones or a 20 g carbohydrate complex for 1.5 months. Hot flushes decreased in severity but not frequency in the treatment group. Albertazzi[9] studied more than 100 women with seven or more hot flushes per day, and randomized them to a 60 g soy protein supplement with 76 mg isoflavones or to a casein control. Hot flushes decreased by 45% in the treatment arm, compared to only a 30% decrease in the control group. Murkies[10] gave women a soy flour supplement. After 3 months, the soy group evidenced a 40% reduction while the controls-fed wheat flour experienced about a 25% decline. The difference was not statistically significant.

In 2001, Knight et al.[11] conducted a randomized, double-blind, placebo-controlled, parallel-group trial with 24 postmenopausal women. After 3 months of treatment, women on a dietary beverage with 60 g of soy protein, and a total isoflavone concentration of 134.4 mg were compared to a control group ingesting the same shake but an isoflavone-poor version. There were no observed differences in hot flushes, Greene Menopause Symptom Scores, vaginal maturation values, levels of follicle-stimulating hormone (FSH) or sex hormone-binding globulin (SHBG), or bone turnover markers. The soy group had a 25% dropout rate from the study, because of bad taste. Other studies have also had very high discontinuation rates in the soy arms due to GI distress, gas, cramps, and stomach pains.

Contradiction and ambiguity continue regarding soy foods and hot flushes. Recently Burke et al.[12] did a study which included 241 moderately symptomatic women with 2.6–4.2 flushes per day, randomized into one of three groups. All women received 25 g of protein, but the amount of isoflavone was stratified in the soy: (1) isoflavone free soy protein, (2) soy with 42 mg isoflavones, and (3) soy with 58 mg isoflavones. During the 2-year study period, a reduction in the number and severity of vasomotor symptoms was observed in all three treatment groups but no significant differences were seen. The protein-only group decreased from 3.5 to 0.8 vasomotor symptoms per day, while the high and low isoflavone groups decreased from 3.2 to 1.3 and 2.6 to 1.5, respectively. Women in the soy with isoflavones group had a more rapid decline but ultimately all subjects reached the same place. There was no true placebo group in this study, so it is unclear if the decline just represents the natural "decline" of symptoms over time. Soy proponents have suggested that when study subjects experience more symptoms, soy appears to offer some benefits. Effects are difficult to measure when the rate of flushing is low.

A large study was published which examined the role of isoflavones in cognitive function, bone mineral density, and plasma lipids in postmenopausal women. A total of 202 healthy postmenopausal women aged 60–75 years in the Netherlands were assigned randomly to 25.6 g of soy protein containing 99 mg of isoflavones (52 mg genistein, 41 mg daidzein, and 6 mg glycetein) or a total milk protein powder on a daily basis for 12 months. Many tests of cognition and dementia were included in the protocol: Mini-Mental State Examination; Rey Auditory Verbal Learning Test, Digit Span forward and reversed, Doors test; Digit Symbol Substitution and Trailmaking, A1, A2, and B; Verbal Fluency A and N, and the Boston Naming Task. Bone mineral density tests of the hip and lumbar spine were performed with dual-energy x-ray absorptiometry. Lipid profiles were obtained. Useful data were collected for 175 subjects. At the end of 1 year with relatively good compliance on the part of study subjects, no significant differences in cognitive function, bone mineral density, or plasma lipids were detected.[13]

Soy- and Red Clover-Based Isoflavone Supplements

Soy and red clover, *Trifolium pratense*, are legumes, and rich sources of a large number of phytochemicals and sterols. While soy is the most common source of isoflavones in the human diet, red clover is the richest source of isoflavones of any plant. Red clover is also a rich source of coumestans, phytochemicals with steroid-like activity. Proponents claim Isoflavone isolates provide the same benefits as whole soy foods, but evidence is lacking to support such claims.

Trials of various isoflavones isolates for hot flushes have been equivocal. A red-clover derived commercial preparation containing 40 mg total isoflavones was given to 51 women while 43 women received placebo. Baber[14] found after the 6-month crossover trial that the product was not more effective than placebo. Hot flush frequency decreased 18% and 20% in treatment and placebo, respectively. No differences were seen in other symptoms (Greene Scale) or endometrial thickness (ultrasound). Knight studied the same product[15] using isoflavone 40 mg, 160 mg, or placebo for 12 weeks. Hot flush frequency decreased 35, 29, and 34%, respectively. There were no differences from baseline in FSH or SHBG.

In another trial thirty women with more than 12 months' amenorrhea experiencing more than five flushes per day were enrolled in a randomized trial, which included a 4-week placebo run in, followed by 12 weeks of treatment or placebo.[16] The active treatment arm received an 80-mg isoflavone tablet (Promensil). End points included hot flushes per day and changes in Greene Climacteric Scale Score. Hot flushes decreased 16% during the run-in phase. During the subsequent double-blind phase, a further, statistically significant decrease of 44% was seen in the isoflavone group ($P < 0.01$), whereas no further reduction occurred within the placebo group. Greene score was lower by 13% in the treatment arm only and remained unchanged in the placebo group.

In counterpoint, a much larger study done by Tice et al. included 252 menopausal women, aged 45–60 years, with a higher degree of symptomatology.[17] Like FDA registration trials, the participants had to have at least 35 hot flushes per week (7 or more per day). After a 2-week placebo run-in, women were then randomly assigned to Promensil (82 mg of total isoflavones per day), Rimostil (57 mg of total isoflavones per day), or an identical placebo, and followed for 12 weeks. Two hundred and forty-six (98%) completed the 12-week protocol, and 97% of study drug tablets were consumed, very high retention and compliance rates. The reductions in mean daily hot flush count at 12 weeks were similar for the Promensil (5.1), Rimostil (5.4), and placebo (5.0) groups, approximately 30–40% over the time period of the study.

Quality-of-life measures and Green Climacteric Scale scores were similar in all groups.

In a report by Faure, a standardized soy extract was studied in 75 women with at least 7 hot flushes per day who were within 6 months of menopause.[18] Women were given Phytosoya (with 70 mg of genistin and daidzin) or placebo. After 16 weeks, treatment group evidenced a 61.2% reduction in symptoms compared to only a 20.8% reduction in the placebo group. When responders were defined as those with at least a 50% reduction, 65.8% of women in the treatment group were classed as responders, with only 34.2% in the placebo group. Fifteen and thirty-nine percent of women withdrew during the course of the study.

In summary, soy foods may be of some limited value in the treatment of vasomotor symptoms. The degree of benefit is highly unpredictable. Many people, particularly, Northern Europeans and Caucasian Americans, cannot convert genistin and daizdin to genistein and daizdein, the active aglyconic metabolites, and may not benefit from a soy rich diet. Since soy foods eaten in traditional dietary quantities are harmless, and may offer some theoretical health benefits, like improvements in cholesterol (again the evidence is somewhat confusing and contradictory), and decreases in the rate of bone mineral density decline, they are a relatively foolproof recommendation. But one should not overstate the benefits.

Be sure to advise women to buy soy foods that actually have isoflavones. Tofu packed in white plastic tubs often is alcohol washed which removes the isoflavones. Many brands of tofu, soy milk, and soy snack, conscious of consumer demands, list the isoflavone content on the packaging, next to the United States Department of Agriculture (USDA) nutritional label. The use of soy foods may also appeal to the ethical and philosophical tenets and beliefs of many women. We all need to be aware that 50% of the calories in soy come from fat, albeit, a good fat, but fat nonetheless. Recommend low-fat tofu and soy milk, fat-reduced soy nuts, and so forth. Again the USDA food labels are helpful in identifying soy foods that have better nutritional balance with 20–30% of the calories from fat. There is insufficient proof of the safety and efficacy of clover or soy-based isoflavone isolates in tablet form to support their use. Isoflavones isolates cost around $22 to $50 per month. Evidence does not support this expenditure.

Black Cohosh (*Cimicifuga racemosa* L. Nutt, Family, Ranunculaceae)

Black cohosh goes by many folk names including black snakeroot and bugbane. Lydia Pinkham's Vegetable Compound was based on black cohosh plus 18% ethanol and the amount of black cohosh is said to be similar to the amount in current commercial preparations. In Europe and the United States, an ethanolic extract is sold over the counter as Remifemin and is on the list of botanicals approved by the Germany Commission E for the treatment of the climacteric and for premenstrual syndrome (PMS), and dysmenorrhea. Prior to the recognition of a potential link between estrogen and breast cancer, the basic science research of the manufacturer sought to prove that black cohosh had estrogenic activity. The company however took a different tack after 1990, trying to characterize black cohosh as something other than estrogen.

Seven of eight published trials did not use placebo controls and seven of eight are only available in German. Duker (1991) compared black cohosh to placebo using 40-mg twice daily (twice the "standard" dose) and found Remifemin suppressed hot flushes about 25% better than placebo in the 2-month trial. Stoll (1987) gave 40-mg twice daily versus conjugated equine estrogen (CEE) 0.625 mg and with placebo. The herbal remedy provided good relief, while estrogen performed no better than placebo, a finding difficult to explain. The study included premenopausal, perimenopausal, and postmenopausal women. Another study by Lehmann-Willenbrock of postmenopausal women included 60 subjects under the age of 40. A careful reading of the abstract and text reveals that though these women had all had a hysterectomy, they had one or both ovaries retained.

The most recent publication on black cohosh was done in 85 breast cancer survivors. Subjects received placebo or black cohosh 20-mg twice daily. Both treatment and placebo groups evidenced significant declines in the number and intensity of hot flushes over time, but the differences between the groups were not statistically significant. This study may not be applicable to all breast cancer patients because 59 of the 85 women were on tamoxifen. The lack of efficacy in tamoxifen-treated women may not apply to breast cancer patients not on tamoxifen or to other menopausal subjects. Of the women assigned to black cohosh, only 9 were not taking tamoxifen. These findings do not completely squash all hopes regarding black cohosh.[19] Further trials with meticulous study design are needed.

While both the manufacturer and the German Commission E, a regulatory body in Germany, which oversees the manufacture and use of botanical medicines, assure us that black cohosh is safe, there are some unanswered questions. Recent studies looking at endometrial thickness, maturation index of the vaginal epithelium, serum luteinizing hormone (LH), FSH, estradiol, and prolactin[20] confirm that black cohosh does not exhibit peripheral estrogenic effects. Black cohosh does not cause changes in renal, hepatic, or coagulation functions, and has no major side effects save for some minor GI complaints. Recently an animal study raised concerns about the safety of black cohosh. Reported on the health wire services in summer 2003 was an abstract from a Duquesne University study presented July 12 at the American Association for Cancer Research annual meeting in Washington, DC. Mice received amounts of black cohosh comparable 40 mg a day, the amount normally recommended to treat menopausal symptoms, for 12 months. While black cohosh did not seem to increase the risk of mice developing breast cancers, it did find that in mice with mammary tumors, black cohosh increased the number of tumors that metastasized to the lung. Many conventional and alternative practitioners have been recommending black cohosh to breast cancer survivors. While this animal model is not definitive proof, it does cast a shadow over the use of the product. There is no official registry of adverse outcomes in women taking the herbal supplement.

At this point, it might be advisable to consider the use of black cohosh in women with symptoms for limited periods of time. Women at high risk for breast cancer should be given appropriate informed consent, just as one might for using estrogen in such women.

Dong Quai, *Angelica sinensis* also Called Dang Gui, Tang Kuei

Dong Quai (*Angelica polymorpha* Maxim. var sinesis Oliv., aka *A. sinensis* [Oliv.] Diels) is a type of angelica. The root is used as the female balancing agent in TCM, and is a panacea for almost every gynecologic ailment, including hot flushes, dysmenorrhea, oligomenorrhea, PMS, amenorrhea, and menopausal syndrome. It is also recommended as a laxative and antispasmodic, and as a treatment for insomnia, anemia, and hypertension. Dong quai is said to be "a warm herb that both circulates and nourishes blood, is also good for strengthening someone who is underweight, frail, anemic and chilly." Dong quai is supposedly estrogenic, since it has been associated with episodes of uterine bleeding and has uterotropic effects in ovariectomized rats. There are no studies of dong quai specifically directed toward the perimenopause. Hirata et al.[21] studied 71 women with FSH over 30 mIU/mL and randomized them to either 4.5 g dong quai per day or placebo. The outcomes, based on patient diaries and Kupperman index found no differences in FSH, LH, estradiol, vaginal maturation index, and endometrial thickness. Critics suggested that the study design was inadequate since dong quai is never given alone, but rather, always used in concert with other herbs, and that interaction of the botanicals provides a synergy needed for clinical effects. Nonetheless, in the real world, dong quai is promoted and sold as a single botanical, often in very low doses, far lower than the 7–12 g used by some TCM practitioners. Considering the lack of efficacy and its potential for anticoagulation and herb-drug interactions, practitioners should advise women to avoid dong quai.

Evening Primrose (Evening Primrose, Evening Star, *Oenothera biennis* L. Family Onagraceae)

The evening primrose is a lovely flowering plant, often a volunteer in many gardens, and is a rich source of the linolenic acid, a type of omega-3 essential fatty acid. Other sources include cold-water fish, canola oil, soybean oil, and a few vegetable oils. Gamma linolenic acid (GLA) comes from seed oils of current, borage, and evening primrose. These fatty acids are eicosanoid precursors and are part of cell membranes. The pathway for dietary GLA leads to dihomo-gamma-linolenic acid (DGLA), which in turn is converted by inflammatory cells to 15-(*S*)-hydroxy-8,11,13-eicosatrienoic acid and prostaglandin E1, with potent anti-inflammatory activity. GLA and DGLA appear to affect inflammatory processes by regulating T-lymphocytes and GLA inhibits angiogenesis, and thus, evening primrose is recommended for a number of inflammatory and autoimmune processes. In reproductive medicine, evening primrose oil (EPO) is used to treat mastalgia and mastadynia. Blommers et al. recently reported a trial of evening primrose and fish oil for severe chronic mastalgia. There was no difference seen in women in any of the groups, where corn oil and corn oil plus wheat germ oil used as controls.[22] The most publicized uses have been for PMS and menopausal symptoms. There are seven studies of EPO for PMS, with five of the seven using blinding and randomization. The responses to EPO were no better than placebo.[23,24] Null results were also found in the one well-constructed clinical trial using EPO for menopause.[25]

GINSENG (*PANAX GINSENG*)

The genus name for many types of ginseng, panax, derives from the word panacea, meaning cure all. (There has also been one case of uterine bleeding occurring after a woman used a ginseng containing face cream.) Ginseng is widely promoted as a performance-enhancing supplement, promising stamina, speed, and endurance. For women, ginseng sings the most provocative of siren songs: the promise of weight loss without dieting or exercise. Different ginsengs are reputed to have different effects. Korean or Chinese ginseng claims more stimulant, aphrodisiac, digestive, and anabolic effects and is promoted as a health tonic for the elderly. American ginseng is offer as the best "adaptogen." Siberian ginseng is supposed to be the best for athletic performance and endurance. Unfortunately, most of the literature on *Eleutherococcus* is in Russian and not accessible in English for studies done by the Soviet military and Olympic trainers.

Regarding menopause, specifically, Wiklund recently reported a relatively large and long-term study of a branded product, Ginsana 115, the active ingredient in a commercial product sold in the United States and Europe, Ginsana. A randomized, multicenter, double-blind, parallel-group study was done in 384 postmenopausal women over 16 weeks. Physiological measures included FSH, estradiol levels, endometrial thickness, maturity index, and vaginal pH. The primary end point (total score of the PGWB index) showed a tendency for a slightly better overall symptomatic relief ($P < 0.1$). Scales for depression, well-being, and health subscales also improved favoring ginseng compared with placebo, but the study was not powered to "prove" these secondary outcomes. Ginseng had no effect on FSH and estradiol levels, endometrial thickness, maturity index, and vaginal pH and hot flushes were no better in the treatment versus placebo arms.[26]

TOPICAL PROGESTERONE, WILD YAM AND *DIOSCOREA*

Progesterone creams are sold over the counter in health food stores in menopause and perimenopausal supplements. Progesterone is absorbed through the skin. Claims for topical progesterone were promulgated by Dr. John Lee who claimed to have a large group of women who evidenced large increases in bone mass with this remedy, as well as alleviation of many symptoms of the climacteric. Leonetti and Anasti tried to replicate Lee's effort.[27] They assigned 102 healthy women within 5 years of menopause to transdermal progesterone cream or placebo. Women used a quarter teaspoon of cream (containing 20-mg progesterone or placebo) to the skin daily plus multivitamins and calcium 1200 mg. Bone density and serum chemistries were repeated after 1 year. Thirty of the 43 (69%) women in the treatment group and 26 of the 47 (55%) women in the placebo group complained initially of vasomotor symptoms. Improvement or resolution was noted from diaries in 25 of 30 (83%) treatment subjects and 5 of 26 (19%) placebo subjects ($P < 0.001$). No differences were found in bone mineral densities between the groups.

Recently, progesterone creams have been promoted by word of mouth and in consumer seminars as substitutes for oral progestational therapy in women taking exogenous estrogens. Short term, this approach may limit hyperplasia. Long-term studies need to be done. Serum levels of progesterone via the transdermal route are highly variable. Women who choose to use progesterone cream in lieu of oral progestin while using supplemental estrogens should be evaluated with annual endometrial biopsy, just as though they were taking unopposed estrogen.

Wild yam creams contain yam extract from *Dioscorea villosa*, the Mexican yam and are supposed to increase endogenous production of natural progesterone and other adrenal sex steroids like dehydroepiandrosterone (DHEA). There is no pathway for conversion of *Dioscorea* to progesterone in vivo. Moreover, Mexican yam extract more correctly should be thought of as estrogenic, since the yams contain diosgenin, a plant phytoestrogen. Most creams on the market do not contain any yam extract. Many contain progesterone or progestins like medroxyprogesterone acetate and some have even been found to be adulterated with estrogens. Natural medicine advocates admit that a "wild yam scam" has been perpetrated. A 1-month supply costs more than a month supply of CEE or estradiol cream. Any woman who presents with vaginal bleeding after using such creams needs to have her endometrium evaluated with appropriate biopsy and ultrasound studies.

Use of CAM for Cognition and Memory

GINKGO (*GINKGO BILOBA*)

Ginkgo, also known as maidenhair tree, Asiatic ginseng, Chinese ginseng, and wonder of the world, is a very old tree whose leaf extract contains a variety of active flavonoids and terpenes. The plant has been used for medicinal purposes in TCM for hundreds of years. It is purported to slow aging, to enhance cerebral blood flow, and to prevent or treat multi-infarct dementia (MID), Alzheimer's (AD), and memory loss. It is also used to treat circulatory disorders, tinnitus, PMS, impotence, stroke, shock, headaches, hyperlipemia, hepatitis, asthma, colitis, and cochlear deafness. Ginkgo does increase blood flow and tissue perfusion, and stimulates the production of prostaglandins. It also has some catecholamine activity.

Clinical trials have found improvements in cognitive symptoms in AD and MID. It has been suggested that the improvements result from increased blood flow, and decreased red blood cell aggregation and blood viscosity. There are a few well-designed studies of cognitive function in patients with dementias with small improvements in function. But clinical studies on cognition and memory in otherwise healthy individuals have been less encouraging. There are no studies of midlife perimenopausal women. Ginkgo has been found to be an effective therapy in antidepressant-induced sexual dysfunction.[28] The dose advocated for this indication is 60–240 mg per day.

Since ginkgo causes decreased platelet and red cell aggregation, care should be exercised in recommending it to patients on anticoagulants, aspirin, and nonsteroidal anti-inflammatories. Spontaneous subdural, subarachnoid, retinal, and other bleeds have been reported.

Use of CAM for Depression and Mood

Kava (*Piper methysticum*)

The kava shrub is grown in the south Pacific and the roots contain pharmacologically-active compounds known as kavapyrones. Kava drinks are used in many ritual settings in the Pacific islands for spiritual and amusement purposes. The most commonly studied product is an extract called WS 1490, which contains 70% kavapyrones. Kava acts very much like the benzodiazepines. Suggested sites of action include the limbic center and gamma-aminobutyric acid (GABA) receptors. Kava does not bind directly to benzodiazepine receptors, however. Kava also inhibits norepinephrine uptake, antagonizes dopamine, inhibits monoamine oxidase (MAO)-B, and decreases glutamate release but does not interact with opioid receptors. Seven randomized trials have been done, most often comparing kava to benzodiazepines. Overall impressions are that kava provides significant reductions in anxiety scores, but the sample sizes are small, and the criteria for admission to the trials have been quite variable. While not studied specifically in perimenopause or menopause, kava offers some interesting possibilities in treating anxiety and insomnia. Side effects include disorientation and intoxication. Alcohol and the use of other sedative hypnotics may potentiate kava's effects.

Since 1999, health-care professionals in Germany, Switzerland, and the United States have seen cases of severe hepatic toxicity possibly associated with the consumption of kava. Eleven patients who used kava products had liver failure and underwent liver transplantation. On March 25, 2002, in response to five such case reports (four in Europe and one in the United States), the FDA issued a consumer advisory. At least two cases have occurred in the United States. Sales of kava have been halted in several European countries.[29]

ST. JOHN'S WORT (*HYPERICUM PERFORATUM*)

Extracts of this flower have been used for hundreds of years to treat mild-to-moderate depression. The constituents include hypericin, pseudohypericin and flavonoids. Several mechanisms of action for the psychotropic effects of St. John's wort (SJW) have been proposed but not confirmed. These include (1) inhibition of monoamine oxidase (MAO) and catechol methyl-transferase (COMT), (2) decreased corticotropin releasing hormone lowering levels of cortisol or affecting GABA receptors in the brain, and (3) serotonin receptor blockade. SJW inhibits norepinephrine, serotonin, and dopamine reuptake. Hypericin, once thought to be the primary active ingredient, serves as a standardization marker for commercial alcohol extract products. Hypericin does not appear to be an MAO inhibitor. Products were often standardized to contain 0.3% hypericin, but now preparations are commonly standardized to the hyperforin content, thought to be the active ingredient. SJW extracts are popular remedies for dysphoria, depression, seasonal affective disorder, and other affective problems.

Most studies of SJW have compared the herb to tricyclic antidepressants often at subtherapeutic doses. Trials comparing SJW to selective serotonin reuptake inhibitors (SSRIs) are limited by small size, no placebo arm, short duration, and differing preparations. Fifteen controlled trials have been assessed in a meta-analysis by Linde. Combined analysis of 1757 cases found that hypericin in doses less than 1.2 mg per day led to a 61% improvement in mild-to-moderate depression, while higher doses up to 2.7 mg per day produced a 75% improvement. The herb appears to be ineffective for severe depression. In a large National Institutes of Mental Health-sponsored study,[30] SJW was ineffective in treating major depression; the SSRI used in the trial was also relatively ineffective as well and had a higher incidence of side effects.

Side effects with SJW include dry mouth, dizziness, constipation, GI upset, sedation, fatigue, and confusion. SJW is potentially photosensitizing, and concern has been stated regarding increased risk of cataracts. A body of literature is emerging documenting numerous drug-herb interactions with SJW. SJW lowered levels of the protease inhibitor, indinavar, lowering serum levels so profoundly as to render the drug ineffective.[31] SJW (*Hypericum perforatum*) drug-herb interactions[32] include potential interactions with serotonin reuptake inhibitors, and decreased bioavailability of digoxin, theophylline, cyclosporin, and phenprocoumon and lower the levels of oral contraceptives, calcium antagonists, metoprolol, propranolol, phenytoin, rifampin, midazolam, and other anesthetics, with SJW acting as potent upregulator of the cytochrome P450 system, particularly CYP3A. SJW induces changes in the drug efflux transport *P*-glycoprotein and subsequently may affect levels of drugs which are metabolized through this pathway.[33] Anesthesiologists ask that patients discontinue of all botanicals at least 2 weeks prior to elective surgery.

Use of CAM for Sleep Dysfunction

VALERIAN (*VALERIANA OFFICINALIS* L. VALERIANACEAE) Common valerian or garden heliotrope, has been used for ages as a tranquilizer and soporific. The active component has not been identified, but is thought to be a GABA derivative. Note that a similar GABA-like compound has been found in chamomile, which also is suggested as an herbal sleep remedy and sedative. Before the advent of benzodiazepines and barbiturates, many psychiatric illnesses were treated with valerian. There is no demonstable toxicity, and the herbal toxicity degrades rapidly. There have been a few reports of dystonic reactions and visual disturbances, perhaps due to interactions with other drugs. Tea or alcohol tincture produce mild, sedating and calming effects without the lingering metabolites seen after taking benzodiazepams. After L-tryptophan was taken off the market, valerian enjoyed an upsurge in use. Studies on sleep architecture have found that valerian reduces sleep latency, prolongs stage 2 nonrapid eye movement (NREM) sleep, and decreases rapid eye movement (REM) and slow-wave sleep (SWS) duration.[34] Other EEG studies have failed to confirm these findings. While adverse events are rare, a recent case report attributed high output congestive heart failure, tachycardia, and delirium to acute withdrawal after prolonged use of large amounts of valerian.[35] Alcohol and sedative-hypnotics should not be used with valerian.

What's the Evidence?

In general, botanical products, other supplements, and alternative practices have been less rigorously studied than prescription drugs. There is no consistent methodology or standard for testing botanicals and supplements, and each product needs to be assessed individually. As with conventional pharmaceuticals, every study needs careful review and scrutiny. In addition to the references cited in this chapter, the National Center for CAM Web site (*http://nccam.nih.gov/health/*) provides information that may be helpful to the clinician.

Conclusions

CAMs are increasingly popular for management of symptoms during the perimenopause and beyond. Given the current uncertainties and bad press about hormonal regimens, women are seeking kinder gentler alternatives to conventional pharmaceutical interventions for symptom relief.

KEY POINT

Provide accurate information on safety and efficacy of alternative treatments.

When counseling women on the use of botanicals in place of conventional hormone treatment, wise counsel would include a careful assessment of all options. Such counseling should include (1) documentation of the severity of symptoms; (2) evaluation of the supporting evidence for efficacy and safety of alternatives; (3) adequate informed consent; (4) follow-up care at a reasonable interval of time to assess efficacy and safety; and (5) when appropriate referral to a qualified provider of specialty care for acupuncture, cognitive behavioral therapy, and meditation and other CAM modalities. CAM practices fall into four major classes[36]:

- Those with both confirmed safety and efficacy
- Those with evidence supporting safety, but evidence regarding efficacy is inconclusive

- Those with evidence supporting efficacy, but evidence regarding safety is inconclusive
- Those that are documented to carry serious risk or inefficacy

The decision to use over-the-counter botanicals ultimately lies with the patient, since access cannot be denied. Care should not be denied if a woman selects an unproven remedy. As long as the plant medicine has no known major toxicities, guidance not dismissal seems to be the most compassionate course. Many women find that their alternative medications prove to be less helpful and will, if lines of communication are kept open, return for further counseling and treatment. As the perimenopause progresses, complaints and symptoms may change. Support, kindness, and time may be the best medicine of all during the uncertainties and instabilities of the menopausal transition.

Discussion of Cases

CASE 1

A 51-year-old perimenopausal woman presents with symptoms of night sweats, disordered sleep, vaginal dryness, and irritability. Her last menstrual period was 6 weeks ago. She finds the symptoms distressing, mostly the fatigue from sleep loss. She does not want to take hormones under any circumstance since her older sister developed breast cancer after 6 years on hormones. She had been struggling with her symptoms for several months when she wandered into a local health food store and was intrigued by the array of choices. She asks if the two products she bought are safe, and she wants to know what other supplements might be useful in treating her symptoms.

- Assess sleep disorder—increased sleep latency, early waking, night sweats
- What has she tried in the past?
- What has she brought in with her?
- Discuss valerian and chamomile and other botanicals which have limited proven efficacy but are also generally safe and might have some value
- While valerian is thought to bind to receptors for the neurotransmitter GABA, appears to shorten sleep latency, and seems to improve sleep quality, it is not appropriate for the acute treatment of insomnia. Rather it promotes a natural sleep state with several weeks of use, and it appears to do so without dependency or other adverse events associated with pharmaceutical sleep medications.[37]
- Chamomile is used for insomnia as a tea or as aromatherapy and is generally regarded as safe. It can also be taken as a capsule or a tincture. Alternatively, dried chamomile flowers in cheesecloth are placed under the tap in a bath to produce a relaxing feeling. Remember to avoid this herb in persons with known allergy to ragweed as both plants belong to the daisy family.

- Lavender, lemon balm, passion flower, and hops and all cited for insomnia, restlessness, and anxiety, and are all generally safe as teas or as aromatherapies.[38]
- Discuss sleep hygiene. Behavioral interventions include the following:
  - No exercise after 6 PM
  - No caffeine after 3 pm
  - Avoid naps
  - Avoiding large meals and excessive fluid intake before sleeping lessen the likelihood of indigestion, gastroesophageal reflux and nocturia
  - Warm baths and head wraps may help
  - Light, sound, music, and aromatherapy machines may also help some people.
- Arrange follow up visit
- Consider pharmaceutical sleep aids if botanicals fail.

Case 2

A 45-year-old presents with 6 months of amenorrhea. She has minimal symptoms but wants to know what sort of supplements and nutritional products she can take to maximize her health in the long term. She wants to know what she can do to lower her risk of heart disease, stroke, breast cancer, and osteoporosis. She has heard that soy provides all the benefits of estrogen without the risks. She is interested in a soy-based diet. She also heard that yams contain chemicals that provide estrogen-like benefits. She wants to know if soy tablets will provide the same benefits as soy diets in the long term.

- Assess personal risk factors for cardiovascular disease such as smoking, obesity, diabetes, lipids, inactivity
- Assess familial health risks such as osteoporosis, and cancer history
- Review dietary history, weight history, reproductive history
- Perform appropriate midlife health screening such as mammography, stool guaiac, lipid screen, bone mineral density if indicated
- Encourage exercise
- Counsel on nutrition with the following information:
  - Vitamin and mineral supplements of known value—multivitamin with folate, calcium 1500 mg per day (in a woman not on hormone therapy, vitamin D or vitamin D analogues are useful supplements in menopausal women. Current recommendations range from 400 to 800 IU a day. Vitamin D analogues include calcitriol 0.25 mg, ergocalciferol 800 IU, or cholecalciferol 800 IU (20 μg) orally each day.
  - Soy foods and their role in nutrition and long-term health. Epidemiological data show that high soy intake correlates with lower cancer risk. There are no trials as yet that show lower rates of cancer in women placed on a high soy diet nor are there trials that show that women with breast cancer given a soy diet experience lower rates of recurrence. Some studies are underway looking at these end points.
  - Soy protein 20–50 g per day lowered cholesterol 10–15% in some studies. Other studies found no effect. Nonetheless the FDA has designated soy as a heart healthy food and recommends 25 g per day. The lipid effects are thought to be a direct effect of protein, independent of lower fat intake associated with soy diets (see lack of efficacy of soy tablets further).

Antioxidant properties of soy and many other vegetables may help to prevent lipid oxidative damage, and oxidative damage associated with malignancy. Genistein may inhibit coagulation and thrombus formation thereby protecting against coronary disease.

- Osteoporosis effects are uncertain and appear to be small. Soy appears to slow bone resorption. This may be due to a decrease in intake of nitrogen in a meat-based diet. Nitrogen is thought to promote bone resorption.
- Soy may help mild-to-moderate hot flushes in amounts over 80 mg per day (a high Asian intake), but the trial outcomes have been inconsistent

- Vitamins, minerals, and other supplements of unproven value:
    - Soy and clover-based isoflavone tablets have not shown consistent impact on hot flushes or on lipids. Their long-term safety cannot be assumed
  - Yams—The yams that have steroid-like compounds are not the yams or sweet potatoes in the supermarket. The yams with high content of steroid-like molecules are not grown as food crops (*Dioscorea villosa* or mexicana) One would have to eat large amounts and eat them raw to get any steroid-like effects. Most yam creams contain very little or no yam and even if they did, it would not work as a real hormone. The same is true for yam tablets. Many yam creams are adulterated with progesterone, progestins like medroxyprogesterone acetate, and even estrogens. They should not be regarded as safe or *inactive placebos*.
  - Magnesium—Low magnesium has been implicated as having a role in coronary disease and diabetes. New research suggests that those with higher magnesium have greater ability to utilize insulin. A diet rich in whole grains, beans, seeds, nuts, fish, and leafy greens should provide adequate magnesium intake. "One ounce of sunflower seeds contains 100 milligrams; almonds, 85; cashews, 75; wheat germ, 70; brazil nuts, 65; dark chocolate, 35. A half cup of cooked spinach, Swiss chard, or cooked beans contains 60 to 80 milligrams. Three ounces of many kinds of fish has 50 to 90 milligrams."[39] Hard water provides magnesium. Supplements also help with GI motility, help mitigate the constipation associated with calcium supplements and aid in calcium absorption. While magnesium deficiency is not common, supplements are not generally harmful.
  - Other trace minerals like boron and selenium have not been shown to provide any consistent benefits in persons with normal nutrition.
- Discuss course of perimenopause and possibility of symptoms later on and need for ongoing relationship and care.

References

1 Astin J. Why patients use alternative medicine: results of a national study. *JAMA*. 1998;279(19):1548–1553.

2 Ko RJ. Adulterants in Asian patent medicines. *N Engl JMed*. 1998; 17;339(12):847.

3 De Smet PAGM. Health risks of herbal remedies. *Drug Saf.* 1995;13: 81–93.

4 De Smet PAGM. Drug Therapy: Herbal Remedies. *New Engl J Med.* 2003;347:2046–2056.

5 Marcus D, Grollman AP. Botanical medicines—the need for new regulations. *N Engl J Med.* 2003;347:2073–2076.

6 Sovak M, Seligson AL, Konas M, et al. Herbal composition PC-SPES for management of prostate cancer: identification of active principles. *J Natl Cancer Inst.* 2002;94(17):1275–1281.

7 *http://www.fda.gov/bbs/topics/NEWS/2003/NEW00875.html*

8 Washburn S, Burke GL, Morgan T, et al. Effect of soy protein supplementation on serum lipoproteins, blood pressure, and menopausal symptoms in perimenopausal women. *Menopause.* 1999;6:7–13.

9 Albertazzi P, Pansini F, Bottazzi M, et al. Dietary soy supplementation and phytoestrogen levels. *Obstet Gynecol.* 1999;94(2):229–231.

10 Murkies AL, Lombard C, Strauss BJ, et al. Dietary flour supplementation decreases post-menopausal hot flushes: effect of soy and wheat. *Maturitas.* 1995;21(3):189–195.

11 Knight DC, Howes JB, Eden JA, et al. Effects on menopausal symptoms and acceptability of isoflavone-containing soy powder dietary supplementation. *Climacteric.* 2001;4(1):13–18.

12 Burke GL, Legault C, Anthony M, et al: Soy protein and isoflavone effects on vasomotor symptoms in peri- and postmenopausal women: the Soy Estrogen Alternative Study. *Menopause.* 2003;10(2):147–153.

13 Kreijkamp-Kaspers S, Kok L, Grobbee DE, et al. Effect of soy protein containing isoflavones on cognitive function, bone mineral density, and plasma lipids in postmenopausal women: a randomized controlled trial. *JAMA.* 2004;292(1):65–74.

14 Baber RJ, Templeman C, Morton T, et al. Randomized placebo-controlled trial of an isoflavone supplement and menopausal symptoms in women. *Climacteric.* 1999;2:85–92.

15 Knight DC, Howes JB, Eden JA. The effect of Promensil™, an isoflavone extract, on menopausal symptoms. *Climacteric.* 1999;2:79–84.

16 van de Weijer PH, Barentsen R. Isoflavones from red clover (Promensil) significantly reduce menopausal hot flush symptoms compared with placebo. *Maturitas.* 2002;42(3):187–193.

17 Tice JA, Ettinger B, Ensrud K, et al. Phytoestrogen supplements for the treatment of hot flashes: the Isoflavone Clover Extract (ICE) Study: a randomized controlled trial. *JAMA.* 2003;290(2):207–214.

18 Faure ED, Chantre P, Mares P, et al. Effects of a standardized soy extract on hot flushes: a multicenter, double-blind, randomized, placebo-controlled study. *Menopause.* 2002;9(5):329–334.

19 Jacobson JS, Troxel AB, Evans J, et al. Randomized trial of black cohosh for the treatment of hot flashes among women with a history of breast cancer. *J Clin Oncol.* 2001;19(10):2739–2745.

20 Schaper & Brummer GmbH & Co KG. Remifemin®: The Herbal Preparation for Gynecology: Scientific Brochure. Salzgitter, Germany: Schaper & Brummer, 1997 *http://www.schaper-bruemmer.de*

21 Hirata JD, Swiersz LM, Zell B, et al. Does dong quai have estrogenic effects in postmenopausal women? A double-blind, placebo-controlled trial. *Fertil Steril.* 1997;68(6):981–986.

22 Blommers J, de Lange-De Klerk ES, Kuik DJ, et al. Evening primrose oil and fish oil for severe chronic astalgia: a randomized, double-blind, controlled trial. *Am J Obstet Gynecol.* 2002;187(5):1389–1394.

23 Budeiri D, Li Wan Po A, Dornan JC. Is evening primrose oil of value in the treatment of premenstrual syndrome? *Control Clin Trials.* 1996;17(1):60–68.

24 Collins A, Coleman G, Landgren BM. Essential fatty acids in the treatment of premenstrual syndrome. *Obstet Gynecol.* 1993;81:93–98.

25 Chenoy R, Hussain S, Tayob Y, et al. Effect of oral gamolenic acid from evening primrose oil on menopausal flushing. *BMJ.* 1994;308:501–503.

26 Wiklund IK, Mattsson LA, Lindgren R, et al. Effects of a standardized ginseng extract on quality of life and physiological parameters in symptomatic postmenopausal women: a double-blind, placebo-controlled trial. Swedish Alternative Medicine Group. *Int J Clin Pharmacol Res.* 1999;19(3):89–99.

27 Leonetti HB, Longo S, Anasti JN. Transdermal progesterone cream for vasomotor symptoms and postmenopausal bone loss. *Obstet Gynecol.* 1999;94(2):225–228.

28 Cohen AJ, Bartlik B. Ginkgo biloba for antidepressant-induced sexual dysfunction. *J Sex Marital Ther.* 1998;24(2):139–143.

29 Hepatic toxicity possibly associated with kava-containing products—United States, Germany, and Switzerland, 1999–2002. *MMWR Morb Mortal Wkly Rep.* 2002;51(47):1065–1067.

30 Hypericum Depression Trial Study Group. Effect of *Hypericum perforatum* (St John's wort) in major depressive disorder: a randomized controlled trial. Hypericum Depression Trial Study Group. *JAMA.* 2002;287(14):1807–1814.

31 Piscitelli SC, Burstein AH, Chaitt D, et al. Indinavir concentrations and St John's wort. *Lancet.* 2000;355:547.

32 Fugh-Berman A. Herb-drug interactions. *Lancet.* 2000;355(9198):134–138.

33 The Medical Letter, Drug Interactions with St. John's Wort, Jun 26, 2000 42:

34 Leathwood PD, Chauffard F, Heck E, et al. Aqueous extract of valerian root improve sleep quality in man. *Pharmacol Biochem Behav.* 1982;17: 65–71.

35 Garges HP, Varia I, Doraiswamy PM. Cardiac complications and delirium associated with valerian root withdrawal. *JAMA.* 1998;280: 1566–1567.

36 Cohen MH, Eisenberg DM. Potential physician malpractice liability associated with complementary and integrative medical therapies. *Ann Intern Med.* 2002;136(8):596–603.

37 Schulz V, Hansel R, Tyloer VE. *Rational Phytotherapy: A Physicians' Guide to Herbal Medicine.* Berlin: Springer-Verlag; 1998:81.

38 The Complete German Commission E Monographs. *Therapeutic Guide to Herbal Medicines.* Klein J, eds. Austin, TX: American Botanical Council; 1998.

39 *http://www.berkeleywellness.com/html/ds/dsMagnesium.php* UC Berkeley Wellness Letter, January 2002.

Index

Page numbers followed by *f* refer to figures; page numbers followed by *t* refer to tables.

E

Q

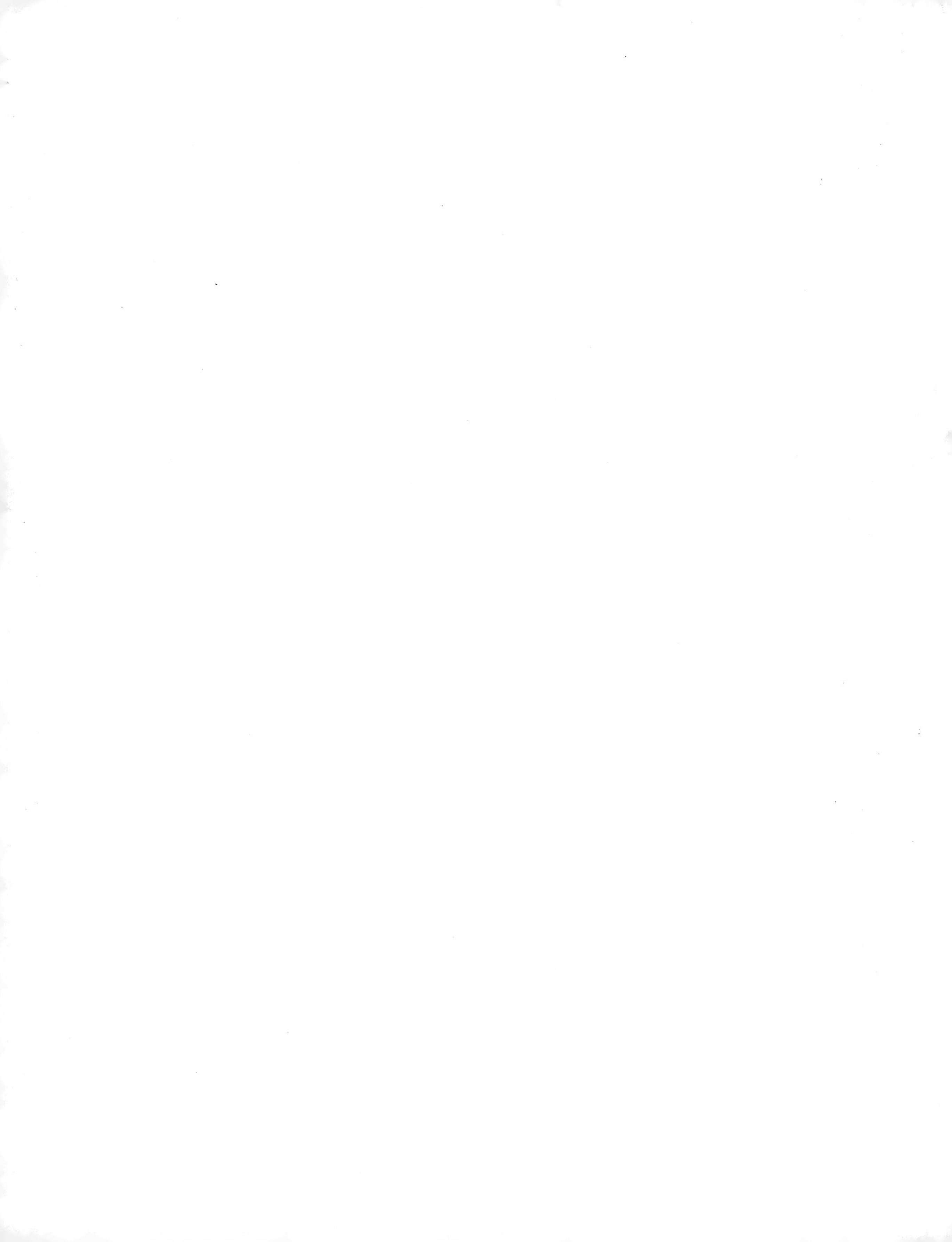